China's Commercial Health Insurance

This book examines the financing of China's health system, argues that present arrangements are not adequate, and proposes an increased role for commercial health insurance as a way of overcoming the difficulties. Highlighting that China's present social medical insurance system can only cover basic medical services, with the result that many Chinese people with higher incomes are going abroad for high-quality medical services and that doctors are not bringing in the salaries and obtaining the social status they expect, the book suggests that commercial health insurance offers a possible solution, in that it can help meet the demand of higher-income groups for better healthcare services while at the same time increasing the income of more competent medical professionals. The book goes on to consider the current state of China's commercial health insurance industry, outlining the various challenges that the industry needs to overcome if it is to fulfil an increased role, challenges such as greater specialization, increased capacity, structural reform, improved regulation, and closer integration with China's medical reform program.

China Development Research Foundation is one of the leading economic thinktanks in China, where many of the details of China's economic reform have been formulated. Its work and publications therefore provide great insights into what the Chinese themselves think about economic reform and how it should develop.

Routledge Studies on the Chinese Economy

Series Editor: Peter Nolan
Director, Centre of Development Studies; Chong Hua Professor in Chinese Development; and Director of the Chinese Executive Leadership Programme (CELP), University of Cambridge

Founding Series Editors
Peter Nolan
University of Cambridge
and
Dong Fureng
Beijing University

The aim of this series is to publish original, high-quality, research-level work by both new and established scholars in the West and the East, on all aspects of the Chinese economy, including studies of business and economic history.

68 **The Silk Road and the Political Economy of the Mongol Empire**
   Prajakti Kalra

69 **The Evolution of China's Banking System, 1993–2017**
   Guy Williams

70 **China and the West**
   Crossroads of Civilisation
   Peter Nolan

71 **Wind Power in China**
   Ambiguous Winds of Change in China's Energy Market
   Julia Kirch Kirkegaard

72 **Multinationals, Global Value Chains and Governance**
   The Mechanics of Power in Inter-firm Relations
   Peter Hertenstein

73 **China in the Asian Financial Crisis**
   Peter Nolan

74 **China's Commercial Health Insurance**
   China Development Research Foundation

75 **Finance and the Real Economy**
   China and the West since the Asian Financial Crisis
   Peter Nolan

China's Commercial Health Insurance

China Development Research Foundation

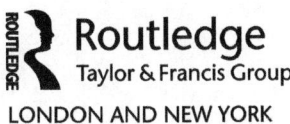

Routledge
Taylor & Francis Group

LONDON AND NEW YORK

First published 2021 by Routledge

2 Park Square, Milton Park, Abingdon, Oxon OX14 4RN
605 Third Avenue, New York, NY 10017

Routledge is an imprint of the Taylor & Francis Group, an informa business

First issued in paperback 2022

Publisher's Note

The publisher has gone to great lengths to ensure the quality of this reprint
but points out that some imperfections in the original copies may be apparent.

British Library Cataloguing-in-Publication Data
A catalogue record for this book is available from the British Library

Library of Congress Cataloging-in-Publication Data
A catalog record has been requested for this book

ISBN: 978-0-367-31323-4 (hbk)
ISBN: 978-1-03-233597-1 (pbk)
DOI: 10.4324/9780429340406

Typeset in Times New Roman
by Wearset Ltd, Boldon, Tyne and Wear

Contents

Research team members   vii

Preface   ix

LU MAI

Foreword   xi

FANG JIN

Acknowledgments   xiv

1 **Main Report: Research project on China's commercial health insurance**   1

CDRF RESEARCH GROUP

2 **Research Topic 1: Research on the supply of commercial health insurance in China**   43

YU GUIFANG AND WANG QIGUO

3 **Research Topic 2: Research on the demand for commercial health insurance in China**   110

TAO CUNWEN, ZHOU HUA, AND BAI WENJUAN

4 **Research Topic 3: Role of and development model for commercial health insurance in China**   198

SHI XIAOJUN, WANG AORAN, AND FENG PENGCHENG

5 **Research Topic 4: Policies and regulations relating to commercial health insurance**   303

ZHU MINGLAI

6 **Research Topic 5: Impact of comprehensive medical reform on commercial health insurance**   366

ZHU HENGPENG, ZAN XIN, AND SUN MENGTING

7 **Survey report on demand for commercial health insurance in China** 416

QIU YUE AND GUO PEI

Index 476

Research team members

Team advisor

Lu Mai, Vice Chairman, Secretary General, Research Fellow, China Development Research Foundation

Team leader

Fang Jin, Deputy Secretary General, Research Fellow, China Development Research Foundation

Team coordinator

Qiu Yue, Deputy Director of Research Department II, Associate Research Fellow, China Development Research Foundation

Authors of topic reports

Research on the supply of commercial health insurance

Yu Guifang, Deputy Director, Policy Research Department, China Insurance Regulatory Commission (CIRC)
Wang Qiguo, Postdoctoral Researcher, Policy Research Department, China Insurance Regulatory Commission (CIRC)

Research on the demand for commercial health insurance

Tao Cunwen, Professor, Central University of Finance and Economics
Zhou Hua, Associate Professor, Central University of Finance and Economics
Bai Wenjuan, Qinghai branch of the National Development Bank

Role of and development model for China's commercial health insurance

Shi Xiaojun, Professor, Renmin University of China
Wang Aoran, Doctoral Candidate, Renmin University of China
Feng Pengcheng, Manager and Senior Economist, China Life

Policies and regulations relating to commercial health insurance

Zhu Minglai, Professor, Nankai University

Impact of comprehensive medical reform on commercial health insurance

Zhu Hengpeng, Deputy Director of Institute of Economics, Research Fellow, Chinese Academy of Social Sciences
Zan Xin, Assistant Director of Public Policy Research Center, Chinese Academy of Social Sciences
Sun Mengting, Research Assistant, Public Policy Research Center, Chinese Academy of Social Sciences

Survey report on demand for commercial health insurance in China

Qiu Yue, Deputy Director of Research Department II, Associate Research Fellow, China Development Research Foundation
Guo Pei, Project Director of Research Department II, Assistant Research Fellow, China Development Research Foundation

Project officer

Guo Pei, Project Director of Research Department II, Assistant Research Fellow, China Development Research Foundation

Preface

China's economy has sustained rapid growth since the start of Reform and Opening Up, to the extent that per capita GDP surpassed USD 8,000 in 2016. With the ongoing rise in people's income and the rapid expansion of a middle class, people are now demanding better and more diversified healthcare.

Everybody wants a long and healthy life, and people are also willing to put out the effort to pay for health. At present, however, China's social medical insurance system can only cover basic medical services. It cannot satisfy the diverse medical demands of people with different levels of income. Two phenomena are emerging as a result. First, people with higher income are going abroad for high-quality medical services. Second, China's medical services system is showing a deficit. Meanwhile, doctors are not bringing in the salaries and obtaining the social status they deserve. Commercial health insurance offers a possible solution: it can help meet the demand of higher-income groups for better healthcare services while at the same time increasing the income of more competent medical professionals. It can lead to better ways of handling healthcare needs in the country while improving medical conditions in general.

Because of this, commercial health insurance should be regarded as an important component of China's medical security system. It is a key path toward meeting people's multi-tiered, diversified healthcare needs, and it can play a vital role in deepening China's medical reform. It can be a major force in pushing forward the Healthy China Initiative. The country's commercial insurance industry still faces many challenges if it is to achieve these things, however. At present, the effective supply of such insurance is insufficient and the level of specialization is low, making it hard to shift demand in its direction. Commercial insurance has not yet begun to assume the role it should play in deepening China's medical reform, nor has the regulatory system governing insurance been updated to meet changing times.

Our research has explored a number of topics relating to China's commercial health insurance, including supply and demand, positioning of the industry, and regulatory aspects. We have looked at the relationship between commercial health insurance and the comprehensive plan for medical reform and have evaluated how to push forward the development of commercial health insurance through a number of measures: supply-side structural reform, transformation of demand, regulatory aspects, and improvement of the mechanisms that go along with China's medical reform program. Our work should be considered explorative in nature. We hope it will encourage others to carry on further discussion and research, including experts, government authorities, companies in the industry, and also people in society at large.

Lu Mai
Vice Chairman, Secretary General
China Development Research Foundation
September 2017

Foreword

Good health is the foundation for the all-round development of human beings and is something that all people strive to achieve. Right now, however, China is facing a complex situation in which a number of factors are impacting health in a negative way. Health problems are being compounded by such challenges as industrialization, urbanization, an aging population, and constantly changing lifestyles. Chronic disease is rapidly increasing as the population ages. Not only is this driving up the demand for healthcare but it is intensifying the rise in medical costs. In addition, a middle class is quickly expanding as standards of living improve, leading to greater demand for such health-related services as better access to doctors, fitness, and caring for the elderly.

To a certain degree, the development of commercial health insurance can fill in for the inadequacies of China's basic medical insurance system. It can increase sources of income for medical security and it can contribute somewhat toward meeting the demand for diversified, multi-tiered health insurance products and services. In fact, China's government and the various departments involved have been very aware of this since 2009, when the New Medical Reform program was launched. A number of key documents have been published that aim to promote the development of commercial health insurance in the country.

This is the context in which the China Development Research Foundation (CDRF) created a task force in 2016 to study commercial health insurance in China. Over the past year and a half, the task force has conducted in-depth research on the subject, including such aspects as supply and demand, positioning and sector development, regulation, and the relationship between commercial health insurance and the overall medical reform program. During this process, the task force not only drew on the extensive experience of Chinese and international experts but it conducted a fairly large questionnaire-type survey on the demand for commercial health insurance products among urban and rural residents. This was able to collect large amounts of first-hand data.

In the course of researching and assembling this Report, the research group held a number of forums and three international conferences, and it carried out field surveys in the United States, Shanghai, and Jiangyin and Taicang in Jiangsu province. After a year and a half of hard work, the team completed five reports on specific topics: 'Research on the supply of commercial health insurance in China' (by Yu Guifang and Wang Qiguo), 'Research on the demand for commercial health insurance in China' (by Tao Cunwen, Zhou Hua, and Bai Wenjuan), 'Role of and development model for commercial health insurance in China' (by Shi Xiaojun, Wang Aoran, and Feng Pengcheng), 'Policies and regulations relating to commercial health insurance' (by Zhu Minglai), and 'Impact of comprehensive medical reform on commercial health insurance' (by Zhu Hengpeng, Zan Xin, and Sun Mengting). It also completed a report on the survey: 'Survey report on demand for commercial health insurance in China.'

The 'Main report,' included here, consolidates the work of all of the research, survey, and specific reports. It reviews the achievements made by China's commercial health insurance so far, analyzes challenges to further development, and points the way to future directions and areas for growth. This research report, *China's Commercial Health Insurance*, summarizes the final results.

The smooth completion of this task would not have been possible without the hard work of all our researchers and the generous support of many other experts and units. The Pharmaceutical Research and Manufacturers of America (PhRMA) not only provided generous financial support, but also helped with connections to well-known international authorities in the field. It also arranged for our field survey in the United States. Our special thanks go to Ms. Jennifer Osika, Deputy Vice President for International Affairs, consultant Mr. Olin L. Wethington, assistant consultant Ms. Judith Logan, and Director of International Affairs Ms. Amey Sutkowski for their hard work. During our field trip to Boston, Professor Michael Chernew of the Harvard University organized a forum, and invited various medical and health insurance experts to introduce the U.S. medical system and health insurance system to us. Within China, the city governments of Jiangyin and Taicang provided excellent arrangements for us, while the Taikang Insurance Company and United Family Hospital provided us with excellent opportunities for exchange of ideas and learning. We also received strong support from the Public Opinion Survey Center of the National Bureau of Statistics in terms of questionnaire design, actual execution in the field, and collection of data.

Inside CDRF, Lu Mai, Vice Chairman and Secretary General, provided us with invaluable suggestions about the design of the research; Deputy Director Qiu Yue of Research Department II was specifically responsible for advancing the subject and overseeing research on the questionnaire. She and Project Director Guo Pei organized the research teams on specific topics as well as overseeing the preparatory work and the writing of reports. Assistant President of the China Development Press, Zhang Shiyu, and Editor Fan Pengyu, provided enormous support and enabled the smooth publication of this volume.

We hope that our research findings will provide scientific backing for evidence-based policies as the government pushes forward the development of commercial health insurance and as it improves upon China's system of medical safeguards. We hope it can serve as a valuable reference in the country's Healthy China initiative. At the same time, we look forward to having more experts, government authorities, people in the industry, and people from society at large become involved in researching, discussing, and focusing on the whole field of healthcare in China in order to push forward the growth of commercial health insurance and meet the goals of 'Healthy China 2030.'

Finally, as head of the research group and on behalf of the China Development Research Foundation, I want to express my sincere appreciation to all members of the team for bringing this project to a smooth completion. Thank you to everyone in the research group, to the units that were involved, and to each and every individual for your help and support.

Fang Jin
Deputy Secretary General
China Development Research Foundation
September 2017

Acknowledgments

Foreign experts

Michael Chernew	Leonard D. Schaeffer Professor of Health Care Policy, Harvard Medical School
Roberta Lipson	CEO, Chindex International
Christian Wards	Director of Group Healthcare, AIA Group
Liz Fowler	Vice President, Global Health Policy, Johnson & Johnson
Davout Yean	Chief Strategy Officer, American International Group (AIG) Business Consulting
Jeff Wu	CEO, EnsurLink
Jennifer Osika	Deputy Vice President, PhRMA
Linda Distlerath	Deputy Vice President, PhRMA
Kevin Haninger	Deputy Vice President, PhRMA

Chinese experts

Yu Guifang	Deputy Director, Policy Research Department, China Insurance Regulatory Commission (CIRC)
Tao Cunwen	Professor, Central University of Finance and Economics
Shi Xiaojun	Professor, Renmin University of China
Zhu Minglai	Professor, Nankai University
Zhu Hengpeng	Deputy Director of Institute of Economics, Research Fellow, Chinese Academy of Social Sciences
Wang Qiguo	Postdoctoral researcher, Policy Research Department, China Insurance Regulatory Commission (CIRC)
Zan Xin	Assistant Director of Public Policy Research Center, Chinese Academy of Social Sciences

1 Main Report

Research project on China's commercial health insurance[1]

CDRF Research Group

1.1 RESEARCH BACKGROUND AND SIGNIFICANCE

Health is central to the pursuit of the overall development of human beings. It forms the foundation for economic and social development and therefore is an important indicator of a country's strength and prosperity. Health is also an aspiration common to all mankind. Since the reform and opening up, China has seen rapid development of its health sector, continuous improvement of its healthcare and health security system, and significant improvement in the level of health of its people in general. Among all these, the healthcare security system has consistently received close attention from the government and people, since it lays the financial and material foundation for people to receive adequate healthcare.

The concept of promoting a 'Healthy China' in terms of policy support was first set forth at the fifth plenary session of the 18th CPC National Congress in October 2015. At the 2016 National Health Conference, Chinese President Xi Jinping stressed that the policy goal of moderate prosperity for all people in China is impossible without making health a priority and a strategic part of development goals. In his report to the 19th CPC National Congress, President Xi went further in saying that 'a healthy population is an important symbol of national strength and prosperity,' that 'it is imperative that we implement the Healthy China strategy' and 'that we improve upon national healthcare policies and provide comprehensive lifelong healthcare services to the general public.'

The 19th CPC National Congress report also pointed out that the principal social contradiction facing China now is the contradiction between unbalanced and insufficient development and the ever increasing demands of people for a better life. With the improvement in socio-economic conditions in recent years, there has been a commensurate increase in the demand for better healthcare services and health security system. There is ever-mounting pressure in China to provide better safeguards for people's health.

On the one hand, demand for healthcare services and health security is increasing in China. This is due to a shift in the spectrum of diseases, the aging of the population, the improvement in incomes, change in the structure of consumption, and the increase of people's awareness of health.

Chronic non-communicable diseases are spreading at an alarming rate. Within two decades, the prevalence of chronic disease is expected to double or even triple among Chinese above the age of 40. The prevalence of diabetes will be the highest; the prevalence of lung cancer will be five times what it is now.[2] In 2012, the mortality rate due to chronic disease among the Chinese population in general was 533 per 100,000, accounting for 86.6% of total deaths. Cardiovascular diseases, cancer, and chronic respiratory diseases were the main causes, accounting for 79.4% of total deaths.[3] The problems of an aging population and the increase in the number of patients with chronic diseases have led to a significant increment in demand for health services and health security.

Meanwhile, China's middle class is growing rapidly and the demand for better and more diverse healthcare is increasing. According to the *Blue Book of China's Society*, published by the Chinese Academy of Social Sciences (CASS), the middle-income class currently accounts for 37.4% of China's total population. In the next few years, assuming that household income continues to grow at a rate of 6.5% and that the distribution of income remains the same, China's middle-income class will be 43% of the population by 2020 and will surpass 50% by 2025.[4] This growing group of people will increasingly be demanding more differentiated and customized healthcare choices in addition to greater accessibility to healthcare. Outbound medical tourism has been growing in recent years. According to the *2016 Online Medical Tourism Report* by Ctrip Tourism, the number of customers signing up for outbound medical tourism through this platform in 2016 was five times what it was in 2015. It is estimated that more than 500,000 people are leaving China for medical tourism every year. On this particular platform, the per capita cost of outbound medical tourism exceeds RMB 50,000, which is about ten times the cost of ordinary outbound tourism. Reinforcing this data is the *Research Report on the Outbound Medical Tourism Marketin China 2016*,[5] which notes that China is expected to become a major source of medical tourists in the future as its people become more aware of health issues and more accustomed to going abroad for healthcare. Outbound medical tourism is gaining momentum as the growing middle-income class seeks to upgrade consumption of all kinds, which includes demanding higher-quality medical and healthcare services.

On the other hand, financial pressures on the country's health security system are enormous, as is the burden of healthcare on individuals. Economic development has entered a new period of what is regarded as normal, with the government's fiscal revenues increasing at a slower rate while medical and healthcare costs are rapidly rising.

For a long time now, China has been maintaining a fairly fast increase in total health expenditures and in government investment in the health sector. According to data from the National Health and Family Planning Commission (NHFPC), China's total health expenditures increased by 14 times over the past 20 years. From RMB 220 billion, they reached RMB 3.17 trillion in 2013. This rate of growth exceeds that of both OECD (Organisation for Economic Co-operation and Development) countries and other BRIC (Brazil, Russia, India, and China) countries. It is related to the rapid economic growth of China's economy and can be attributed largely to the substantial increase in government healthcare expenditures. This includes the very large government subsidies for social medical insurance (see Figures 1.1 and 1.2). According to the white paper entitled *Development as a Right: China's Philosophy, Practice, and Contribution*, published by the State Council Information Office at the end of 2016, China's total government spending on healthcare came to RMB 1.3154 trillion in 2016, which was 4.1 times higher than it had been in 2008, prior to when China's New Medical Reform was initiated (RMB 318.2 billion). The 2016 figure was also 10% more than the figure in 2015.

Over the long run, China's figures hold the prospect of a severe crisis in spending ability. Since 2009, when the New Medical Reform began, payments out of China's medical insurance fund have constantly increased. Some research indicates that the majority of employees' medical insurance funds across the country will face a gap in funding their payment obligations around 2020. By 2024, the total gap[6] will reach RMB 735.3 billion, putting the system severely in the red.[7] Meanwhile, the increase in medical costs also places Chinese residents under heavy pressure. According to a nationwide survey of people caring for elderly at home, medical expenses constitute one-quarter of total household expenditures. The average figure of RMB 1,039.8 per month was second only to basic living expenses. The survey covered respondents and their spouses in ten major cities across the country.[8]

Generally speaking, the problem of limited financial resources and inadequate social security systems will only become more pronounced as time goes on, given China's economic and social development, its shifting pattern of diseases, and the increasing pace at which its population ages. The government will

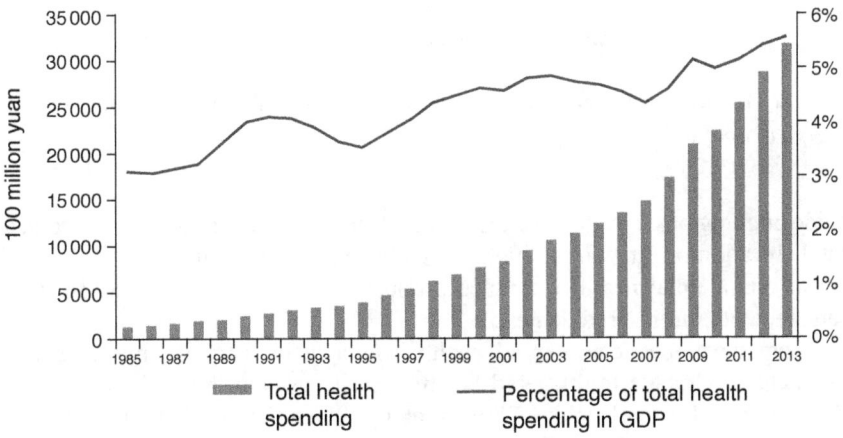

Figure 1.1 Total healthcare expenditures in China.

Source: Health Development Research Center, National Health and Family Planning Commission, 2014.

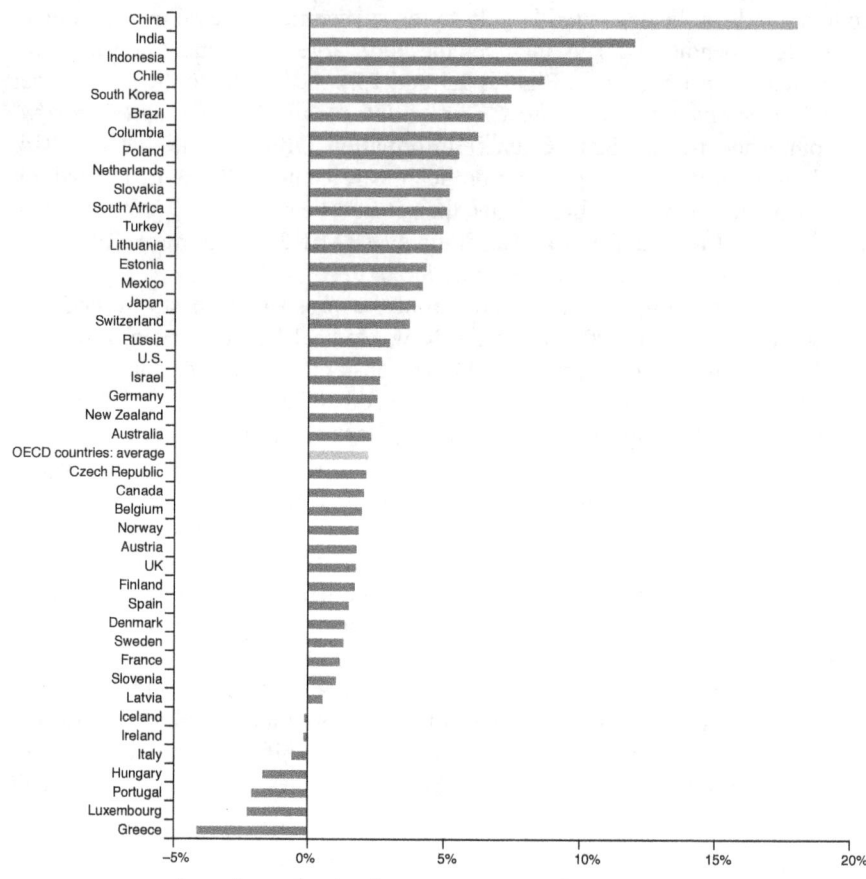

Figure 1.2 Annual growth rate of government spending on healthcare by country.
Source: OECD, 2015.

provide ongoing basic healthcare security that 'insures the basics'—this is fundamental. In addition, it will be highly significant, however, to have a plentiful
array of commercial health insurance products and services as a way to meet
diversified and multi-tiered demand.

A more developed commercial health insurance industry is important as a
component of China's multi-tiered health security system, but it is also inherently necessary for the Healthy China strategy. Since the New Medical Reform
was initiated in 2009, the Chinese government has attached great importance to
developing commercial health insurance and has issued a number of important
policy documents in that regard (see Table 1.1). In 2004, the *Opinions of the
General Office of the State Council on accelerating the development of commercial*

Table 1.1 Summary of commercial health insurance policies introduced in recent years

Year	Title of document	Issuing authority	Policies related to commercial health insurance
September 2006	Health insurance administration measures	CIRC	**First health insurance administration policy**
March 2009	Opinions for deepening the healthcare reform	State Council	We should 'encourage commercial insurance companies to develop diverse health insurance products to meet different needs … and actively promote the health insurance management model under which the government **procures health insurance services from qualified commercial insurance companies.**'
May 2009	Opinions on the further participation of the insurance industry in the healthcare reform and the construction of the multi-tiered health security system	CIRC	We should 'vigorously promote the development of commercial health insurance to meet the diverse needs … **encourage commercial insurers to actively participate in basic medical insurance management** … and to **actively explore different ways to participate in the construction of the healthcare system**.'
March 2012	The Notice of the State Council on issuing the plan and implementation program for deepening healthcare reform during the 12th Five-Year Plan period	State Council	We should 'encourage commercial insurance companies to develop health insurance products other than basic medical insurance products, including long-term care insurance and special illness insurance, to meet diverse healthcare needs' and 'encourage enterprises and individuals to participate in commercial health insurance and various supplementary insurance schemes and implement preferential tax treatment and other related preferential policies.'

continued

Table 1.1 Continued

Year	Title of document	Issuing authority	Policies related to commercial health insurance
August 2012	Advice for promoting urban and rural critical illness insurance	National Development and Reform Commission (NDRC), Ministry of Finance, Ministry of Health, Ministry of Civil Affairs, Ministry of Civil Affairs and CIRC	The document provides that urban and rural critical illness insurance services should be 'purchased from commercial insurance companies,' points out that insurance procurement and contract management should be standardized, and sets out the basic participation criteria for commercial insurance companies
September 2013	Several Opinions of the State Council on promoting the development of the healthcare sector	State Council	We should 'encourage commercial insurance companies to invest in the healthcare sector by investing new projects and participating in restructuring, trusteeship, operation of companies established by the government, etc.' and 'support the development of commercial health insurance products that are supplemental to basic medical insurance, encourage commercial health insurance companies to offer urban and rural critical illness insurance products, and expand the coverage of commercial health insurance.'
August 2014	Opinions of the State Council on accelerating the development of the modern insurance industry	State Council	We should 'encourage insurers to develop commercial health insurance products such as medical insurance, illness insurance and loss of income insurance to supplement basic medical insurance' and 'the government can entrust insurance companies to manage insurance funds or purchase insurance products and services directly from insurance companies.'

Date	Document title	Issuing body	Content
October 2014	*Opinions of the General Office of the State Council on accelerating the development of commercial health insurance*	State Council	We should strive to '**increase the supply of commercial health insurance ... so that commercial health insurance can play its role in deepening the healthcare reform, driving the development of health services and promoting economic upgrading**' and 'encourage commercial insurance companies to manage urban and rural critical illness insurance funds and standardize relevant market activities ... and encourage commercial insurance companies to participate in the management of various health insurance funds.'
December 2015	*Notice on the trial implementation of the policy of preferential individual income tax treatment for premiums paid for commercial health insurance products*	Ministry of Finance, State Administration of Taxation, and CIRC	The notice listed the pilot areas and set out regulations for commercial health insurance products and preferential individual income tax treatment and announced that the policy would come into force on January 1, 2016 in the pilot areas
August 2016	*Outline of the Healthy China 2030 Plan*	State Council	The document outlined the goal of 'achieving further development of the modern commercial health insurance sector and significantly raising the percentage of payouts of commercial health insurance schemes in total health spending by 2020.'
December 2016	*Notice of the State Council on issuing the plan for deepening healthcare reform during the 13th Five-Year Plan period*	State Council	'We should allow commercial health insurance providers to play to their strengths in actuarial science, specialty services, risk management, and other fields, encourage them to participate in the health insurance sector to diversify the competitive landscape ... diversify health insurance products, vigorously develop consumer-driven health insurance ....'

continued

Table 1.1 Continued

Year	Title of document	Issuing authority	Policies related to commercial health insurance
May 2017	*Opinions of the General Office of the State Council on encouraging the private sector to provide multi-tiered and diversified healthcare services*	State Council	We should 'encourage commercial insurance companies to work together with health management facilities to develop health management insurance product and encourage commercial insurance companies and healthcare facilities to develop insurance products for special care, innovative therapies, advanced examination services, the use of high-value medical devices, etc.'
June 2017	*Notice on the nationwide trial implementation of the policy of preferential individual income tax treatment for premiums paid for commercial health insurance products*	Ministry of Finance, State Administration of Taxation, and CIRC	The Notice provided that, from July 1, 2017 onwards, the policy of preferential individual income tax treatment for premiums paid for commercial health insurance products would be implemented on a nationwide scale

health insurance explicitly declared the intent to 'increase the supply of commercial health insurance so that commercial health insurance can play a vital role in deepening healthcare reform, driving the growth of the healthcare services industry, and enhancing effective economic upgrading.' In 2015, the China Insurance Regulatory Commission (CIRC), the Ministry of Finance, and other departments jointly issued the *Notice on the trial implementation of the policy of preferential individual income tax treatment for premiums paid for commercial health insurance products*. This was aimed at promoting the development of commercial health insurance via tax incentives. In the same year, the State Council issued *Opinions on promoting the development of critical illness insurance products targeting urban and rural residents*, which was aimed at encouraging commercial health insurance companies to offer critical illness insurance products to urban and rural residents. The *Outline of the Healthy China 2030 Plan*, issued in 2016, set forth the goal of creating a multi-tiered health security system with basic medical insurance as the main component and other forms of supplementary health insurance and commercial health insurance as supporting components. This was to encourage companies and individuals to participate in health insurance plans and various supplementary plans. The *Outline of the Healthy China 2030 Plan* also set forth the goal of 'achieving further development of the modern commercial health insurance sector and significantly raising the percentage of compensation by commercial health insurance plans in total healthcare spending by 2020.' In 2017, the *Notice on the nationwide trial implementation of the policy of preferential individual income tax treatment for premiums paid for commercial health insurance products* provided that, from July 1, 2017 onwards, the policy of preferential individual income tax treatment for premiums paid for commercial health insurance products would be implemented on a nationwide basis.

The situation described above was the context in which the CDRF created a task force in 2016 to study commercial health insurance in China. Over the past year and a half, the task force has conducted in-depth research on the subject, including such aspects as supply and demand, positioning and [sector] development, regulation, and the relationship between commercial health insurance and the overall medical reform program. During this process, the task force not only drew on the extensive experience of Chinese and international experts but it conducted a fairly large questionnaire-type survey on the demand for commercial health insurance products among urban and rural residents. This survey collected large amounts of first-hand data from roughly 20,000 sample respondents in 43 cities and districts, including the 3 municipalities directly administered by the Central Government.[9]

This 'Main report' reviews achievements made in commercial health insurance so far, identifies key challenges, and points to future directions and areas for further development. It is based on information in the five research reports as well as data from the field survey. We hope that this study will provide scientific backing and reference material to assist policymakers in making evidence-based decisions that promote the development of commercial health insurance in

China. We hope it will contribute to improving China's medical safeguards system, and achieving the goal of a Healthy China.

1.2 ACHIEVEMENTS MADE TO DATE IN PROMOTING THE DEVELOPMENT OF COMMERCIAL HEALTH INSURANCE IN CHINA

Under the impetus of government policies and a growing diversification of healthcare needs in the country, China's commercial health insurance industry has achieved tremendous growth. The comprehensive strength of the industry has increased significantly since the country entered into its 12th Five-Year Plan period. Health insurance is the fastest growing industry within the insurance sector as a whole.

We first look at the situation from the perspective of the supply side and the levels of health security. The latest statistics show that premiums taken in by commercial health insurance companies in China grew from RMB 57.4 billion in 2009 to RMB 403.4 billion in 2016. This reflects an average annual growth rate of 27.6%, a much higher figure than the average annual growth of life insurance in the same period. Health insurance premiums went from 6.95% of total personal insurance premiums to 18.2%; health insurance compensation increased by 3.6 times, from RMB 21.7 billion to RMB 100.075 billion. Meanwhile, the insurance density[10] of health insurance increased from RMB 43 in 2009 to RMB 292 in 2016, while the health insurance penetration[11] (that is, health insurance premiums as a percentage of GDP) increased from 0.16% in 2009 to 0.54% in 2016 (see Figures 1.3, 1.4, and 1.5).

Second, commercial health insurance companies have been active in insuring critical illness in both urban and rural areas. By the end of September 2016, 16 insurance companies had taken on the handling of critical illness insurance in 31 provinces, autonomous regions, and directly administered cities. In so doing, they were providing critical illness insurance to 1.05 billion urban and rural residents. In 2016, actual reimbursements of medical expenses related to critical illness increased by 13.16 percentage points on average. Expenses related to critical illness have gone down considerably for residents in certain cities and rural areas. The largest reimbursement in 2016 came to RMB 1,116,000.

Third, commercial health insurance companies have been proactive in providing all kinds of health insurance services and participating in the building of the healthcare safeguards system. From 2010 to the end of September 2015, the insurance sector has been authorized to manage a cumulative total of RMB 86 billion worth of health insurance funds. It has paid out RMB 55 billion in compensation. Premium income of commercial health insurance reached RMB 71.1 billion; commercial health insurers paid out RMB 57.5 billion in reimbursements and served a cumulative total of more than 300 million person-visits. At the same time, in the course of handling all kinds of management services relating to health insurance, commercial health insurance companies have experimented

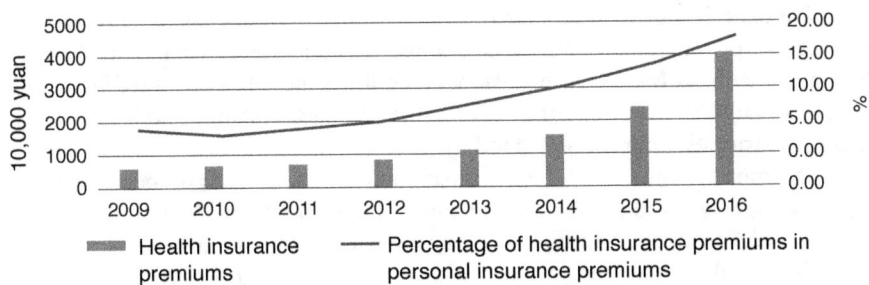

Figure 1.3 Health insurance premiums and percentage of health insurance premiums in life insurance premiums.

Source: Topic report of the task force, entitled 'A Study of the Supply of Commercial Health Insurance Products.'

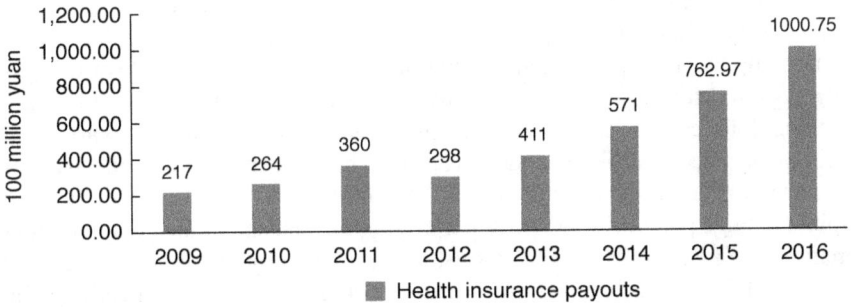

Figure 1.4 Health insurance payouts.

Source: Research Topic 1: Research on the supply of commercial health insurance in China, in this volume.

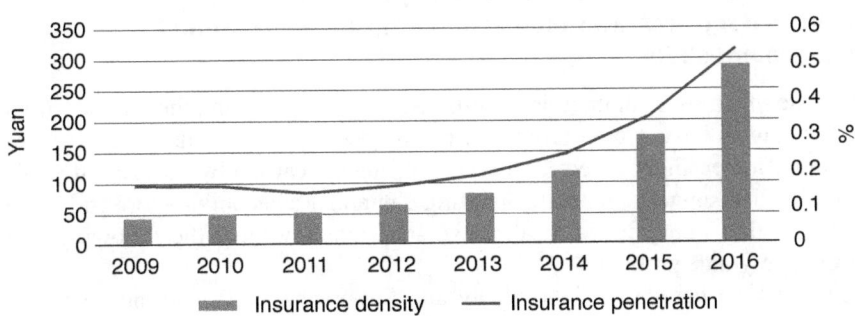

Figure 1.5 Density and penetration of health insurance.

Source: Research Topic 1: Research on the supply of commercial health insurance in China, in this volume.

with new methods and developed a number of unique models while building up extensive experience. Such models include the 'entrusted management model' as adopted in Luoyang, Henan Province (Luoyang Model) and in Jiangyin, Jiangsu Province (Jiangyin Model), the 'insurance contract model' as adopted in Jiande City, Zhejiang Province, and the 'public–private partnership model' adopted in Pinggu District, Beijing (Pinggu Model).

Furthermore, commercial health insurance companies have been actively exploring new ways to participate in China's medical reform, including ways to invest in public medical institutions. They have achieved a measure of success in strengthening the regulation of the healthcare sector and in lowering unreasonable medical expenses.

1.3 MAJOR CHALLENGES FACED BY CHINA'S COMMERCIAL HEALTH INSURANCE SECTOR

Despite fairly rapid growth, China's commercial health insurance industry remains in its infancy. Major problems faced by the industry include the lack of effective supply, insufficient transformation of demand, and a backward regulatory system. More specifically, the industry's problems can be divided into the following four categories: (1) insufficient effective supply, limited variety of product offerings, insufficient guarantees and health services, and the lack of specialized professional management; (2) inability to shift or transform demand despite the huge potential, and weak policy support that should be guided by that demand; (3) failure to date of the industry to play its proper role in the medical reform; and (4) a regulatory system that is not in tune with the needs of the times, that lacks a targeted approach, and that lacks the necessary set of accompanying policies.

1.3.1 Insufficient effective supply, limited variety of product offerings, insufficient health security provisions, lack of healthcare services, and the need to upgrade professional management skills

The scale of China's commercial health insurance industry and the number of its market players have grown rapidly in recent years. Services and products[12] are becoming increasingly diverse. However, problems caused by the lack of sufficient effective supply to meet the growing demand are becoming more and more serious. China's commercial health insurance industry faces the following five major supply-side problems.

First, China has insufficient supply and low insurance density and penetration. Insurance density and insurance penetration are indicators used to measure the level of development of an insurance market. They reflect the status of the insurance industry in an economy and how much each of the residents in a geographic area spends on insurance in terms of premiums. During 2009–2016, both the density and penetration of commercial health insurance rose slowly. In 2016, per capita commercial health insurance premiums came to about RMB 292. In the aggregate, health insurance premiums accounted for 0.54% of GDP in that year. By way of contrast, in the United States and Germany, per capita commercial health insurance premiums in 2013 came to about the equivalent of RMB 16,800 and RMB 3,071, respectively.[13] Health insurance enjoys a very small market compared to property insurance, personal insurance, life insurance, casualty insurance, and other insurance products. While health insurance premiums went from 6.95% to 18.2% of total personal premiums between 2009 and 2016, this was still much lower than in mature insurance markets, where the figure is around 30%.[14]

Second, commercial health insurance products in the Chinese market are overly uniform, with little diversity in what is offered. Products covering critical illness and medical costs occupy a dominant position in the market, while insurance to cover the costs of nursing care and loss of income due to disability is seriously inadequate. Statistics show that premiums for insurance for specified diseases came to RMB 114,121 billion in 2015, a sum that accounted for 47.34% of all commercial health insurance premiums. Medical insurance (for hospitalization) accounted for 36.11%. Nursing care insurance accounted for 16.42%, while disability insurance accounted for only 0.13%.[15] Meanwhile, although insurance for hospitalization enjoys a large market share (36.11% of commercial health insurance), in fact many of its functions are redundant in that they duplicate the existing basic medical insurance plans. There are few products that are truly supplemental to basic medical insurance. The results of the CDRF survey show that respondents purchased commercial health insurance products that exhibited a similar pattern, in that insurance for critical illness was dominant while insurance for loss of income due to disability or for nursing care was modest (see Figure 1.6).

In addition, China's commercial health insurance products are structured to look like life insurance products. To be more specific, most commercial health insurance products resemble money management products and are savings-based. Their design usually focuses on dividends and a return on premiums. In this respect, they are notably like life insurance and casualty insurance. With regard to sales channels, health insurance is often sold in the form of 'add-ons,' or is bundled together with other insurance products. The development of health insurance therefore becomes secondary to the design of primary insurance products and the security health insurance provides is actually very limited.

Third, the level of protection offered by commercial health insurance products is limited. Statistics show that actual reimbursements paid out by health insurance in China accounted for only 1.93% of national healthcare spending in 2015. In Germany, Canada, France, and other developed countries, the figure is more than 10%. In the United States, it is 37%. In 2015, reimbursement spending by commercial health insurance accounted for only 6.27% of personal healthcare spending in China. Clearly, the degree of protection provided by commercial health insurance is highly limited (see Figure 1.7).

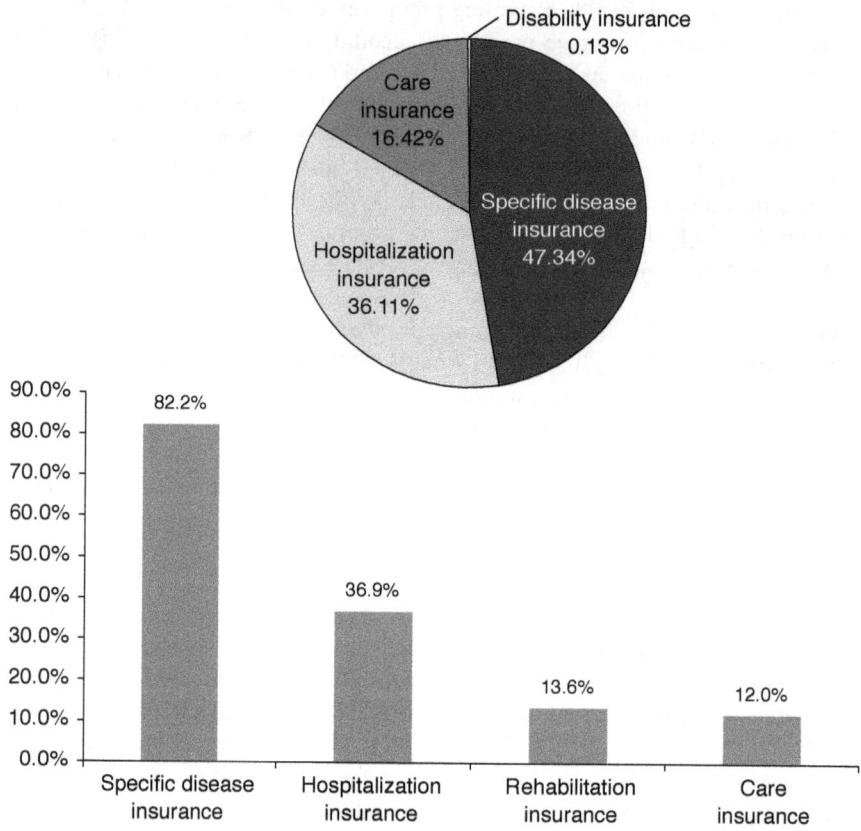

Figure 1.6 Types and percentages of health insurance purchased by respondents.

Source: Research Topic 2: Research on the demand for commercial health insurance in China, in this volume.

Fourth, a whole-process service model has not yet been established in China, and insurance products are insufficiently aligned with healthcare services. At present, commercial health insurance products in China remain stalled at a level of 'plain old health insurance.' Health insurance products covering health management services are rare, and the industry still cannot meet the diverse needs of Chinese residents for differentiated health insurance products. The results of the CDRF survey show that 23.9% of the respondents thought that 'the lack of appropriate health management and healthcare services' was one of the top three problems faced by the commercial health insurance industry at present. In the meantime, health management services have a significant impact on purchasing decisions related to commercial health insurance products. The results of the CDRF survey show that the top three items of value-added services that affect

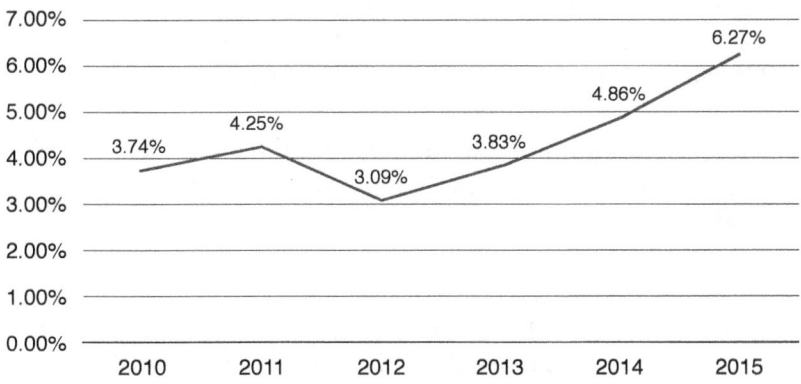

Figure 1.7 Payouts of health insurance schemes during 2010–2015 (expressed as percentage of personal health spending).

Source: Based on data from *Yearbook of China's Insurance 2001–2016*.

respondents' decision to purchase health insurance products are the following:
physical examinations (41.6%), appointment-booking services in public hospitals (35.3%), and healthcare management services (31.8%). Analysis of
China's different regions shows that the demand for healthcare management services in developed areas is relatively higher than it is in less developed areas.
The demand of urban residents for value-added services of health insurance is
higher than that of rural residents. In addition, as incomes rise, the demand of
the respondents for advance booking of appointments in public hospitals and for
direct overseas medical services increases.

Fifth, not enough companies specialize in providing health insurance products. The market for supplying health insurance is dominated by life insurance
companies and property insurance companies. Health insurance companies that
specialize in providing health insurance products have only a small market share.
More than 100 insurance companies are qualified to offer commercial health
insurance products in China, but only eight are companies that actually specialize
in health insurance. These eight, meanwhile, are still in the exploratory stage of
operations and face many operational challenges. In addition, because most
health insurance products are offered as add-ons to life insurance plans, health
insurance companies often integrate features of life insurance products into the
design of their own products—they copy the business philosophy and operating
models of life insurance companies. In fact, there should be a significant difference between health insurance and life insurance in terms of product design,
actuarial pricing, protection functions, risk prevention, review of claims,
payment of benefits, and so on. The business of a health insurance company is
affected by many stakeholders, including the insured, healthcare facilities, and
health insurance authorities. Health insurance companies face a variety of risks

such as information asymmetry, adverse selection, moral hazard, and changes in healthcare policies. The difficulties of such specialized operations are substantial. At present, Chinese insurance companies lack a clear understanding of specialized health insurance operations and specialized business models.

1.3.2 The massive amount of potential demand in China has not yet been realized, and policies that are guided by demand are not yet strong enough

As China moves further in implementing comprehensive medical reform, its residents are becoming more aware of the risks of not having health insurance. The role played by commercial health insurance in meeting their diverse needs is increasingly important, yet the actual demand of the market remains far smaller than the potential demand. The results of the CDRF survey show that only 26.2% of the respondents had purchased health insurance, while 41.3% of the respondents intended to purchase commercial health insurance products in the coming year. The disparity between effective demand and potential demand is enormous. Four primary factors are behind the failure of China's commercial health insurance industry to transform the potential demand of Chinese residents into effective demand.

First, basic medical insurance programs are gradually improving coverage and increasing benefits. This has led to a debate among scholars about the relationship between such government-funded insurance and commercial insurance. Some feel that publicly funded insurance squeezes out some commercial health insurance products. Given a limited amount of financial resources in the society, an increasing supply of basic medical insurance will reduce the demand for commercial health insurance. Others argue that the two should be able to supplement and reinforce each other. Since the 18th CPC National Congress, the Chinese government has been striving to build a social security system that 'covers all people, meets people's basic demands, and is multi-tiered and sustainable.' Social medical insurance emphasizes coverage for all and very basic benefits, while commercial health insurance highlights tiered and flexible services that can make up for the inadequacies of social insurance. Meanwhile, ongoing development of China's social medical insurance should also serve the purpose of improving people's understanding of insuring risk, and thus increase the demand for commercial health insurance.

Second, commercial health insurance products on the market tend to resemble one another and also overlap in function with the protections offered by China's basic medical insurance. The market therefore lacks differentiated products tailored to meet the diverse needs of residents. The results of the CDRF survey show that 13.1% of the respondents who had bought health insurance products believed that the protections offered by commercial health insurance products 'overlapped with basic medical insurance programs.' Basic medical insurance programs offer protection for only the most basic medical services. Instead, commercial health insurance products should design products that meet different needs of different groups. As it currently exists, however, the commercial health insurance industry is unable to meet the demand for personalized, diversified health insurance products. Products such as disability insurance due to loss of income and long-term care insurance remain in their infancy. Long-term care insurance products on the market are similar to annuities and fail to provide any real safeguards with respect to health problems.

Other factors affecting the inability of the industry to transform potential demand into effective demand are the lack of sufficient awareness in China about health risks and also insufficient purchasing power with which to buy insurance. The CDRF survey shows that the percentage of people who actually purchase health insurance products varies significantly across groups of different education levels. Purchase of health insurance products and level of education are positively correlated. 'Higher education' equates to 'higher purchase rate.' People with a master's degree or higher purchased insurance at a maximum rate of 39%, while those with only a primary education or lower bought insurance at a maximum rate of 10.4%. Another factor that affects the demand for commercial health insurance is disposable income.[16] In 2016, China's annual per capita disposable personal income was RMB 23,821, representing a real increase of 6.3% over 2015. In the same year, China's GDP grew by 6.7% and medical expenses by 12.3% over 2015. Per capita disposable income grew at a much lower rate than medical expenses and somewhat lower than GDP. Insufficient purchasing power of consumers is one of the primary reasons the industry has failed to transform potential demand into effective demand. The CDRF survey shows that the percentage of respondents who purchase health insurance products increases with level of income. Those with an annual income of RMB 250,000–500,000 and higher purchased health insurance at the highest rate (49.5% and 49.0%, respectively) while those with an annual income of less than RMB 10,000 purchased at the lowest rate (14.2%) (see Figure 1.8).

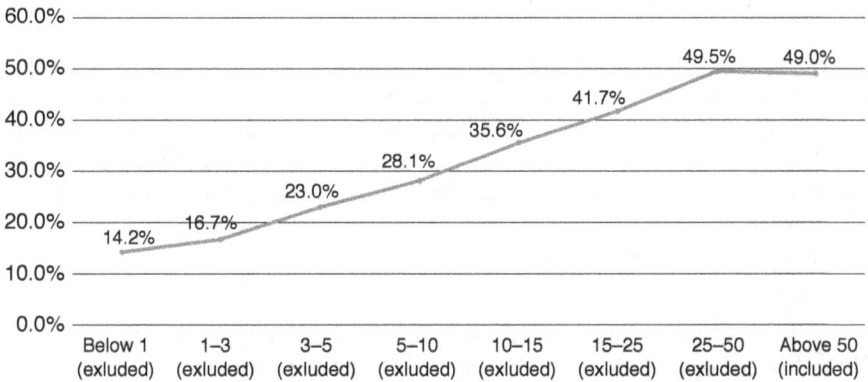

Figure 1.8 Percentage of respondents who purchased health insurance by level of family income (10,000 yuan).

Source: Research Topic 2: Research on the demand for commercial health insurance in China, in this volume.

Finally, policies that are focused on demand are not sufficiently strong to provide real support for the commercial health insurance industry. The most obvious problem is that preferential tax policies are too small to attract customers to products. In January 2016, the China Insurance Regulatory Commission formally issued the *Notice regarding the development of health insurance products that enjoy preferential individual income tax treatment*. By the end of 2016, 13 insurance companies were providing health insurance products that qualified for preferential individual income tax treatment in 31 provinces and cities of the country. They had signed up 54,370 qualified policies which brought in RMB 92 million in premium income. In terms of actual results, insurance companies received 506 claims in 2016 from 401 customers who had purchased health insurance products that were qualified for preferential individual income tax treatment. They paid out a total of RMB 2.02 million in benefits, which came to an average of RMB 5,054 per person.

The CDRF survey shows that only 16% of the respondents were even aware of this preferential tax incentive. In fact, since the start of its implementation, many people have felt it to be ineffective. It faces the following three main problems. First, the tax benefit is too small. In pilot areas where the policy has been applied, individuals that buy the relevant health insurance are allowed to deduct a maximum of RMB 2,400 per year from their income in figuring their income tax. This is equivalent to raising the threshold of income at which tax begins by RMB 200 per month. The specific amount of untaxed income is linked to the actual income of the person buying health insurance, with the amount of avoided tax coming out to a range of RMB 72 to 1,080 per year. In reality, however, China has just 28 million people who are obliged to pay individual income tax, a figure that represents less than 2% of the total population. On top of that, more than 80% of people who do pay individual income tax pay at a rate of 10% or lower, and the great majority of people can claim deductions of only RMB 72 per year or RMB 240 per year. The preferential tax benefit is therefore not strong enough to be effective.

Second, the products on the market are not attractive enough. Only people who pay individual income tax can buy health insurance products that are qualified for preferential tax treatment. A large number of such people have already enrolled in at least one supplementary health insurance plan, which duplicates protections offered by the preferential-tax product. This lowers the appeal of buying such products. Third, the enrollment process is cumbersome, which cuts the enthusiasm of potential purchasers.

1.3.3 The commercial health insurance industry has not yet played its proper role in furthering reform of China's medical, pharmaceutical, and healthcare system

As China's economy continues to grow, society continues to progress, and the medical reform proceeds, the government is more willing than ever to support the development of commercial health insurance. It has expressed its policy intent in this regard. The role of commercial health insurance in China's overall medical reform is consequently gradually changing. Commercial insurance is not only an important part of the country's health security system, but is also expected to help break into deeper realms of reforming the system. In this regard, it is hoped that China's commercial insurance companies will play a role in the following three respects.

First, they are expected to provide differentiated health insurance products that supplement basic medical insurance programs and meet multi-tiered, diversified, health security needs of customers. In the meantime, they should play a role in sharing the costs of medical expenses and should thereby reduce people's economic burden. The scope of health services covered by commercial health insurance may include services for special needs, innovative therapies, advanced diagnostic methods, services using high-value medical equipment and various other high-value medical services, as well as health management and nursing care. Second, as specialized, market-oriented entities, commercial health insurance companies are expected to offer expertise. They are expected to participate in the management of basic medical insurance and to supplement the tasks covered by supplemental health insurance, critical illness insurance, and other insurance funds. They should work together with basic medical insurance to achieve an organic synthesis of public and private resources. Commercial health insurance companies should play a role in reducing unreasonable medical expenses and curbing the rapid rise in those expenses by improving the efficiency of basic medical insurance management through appropriate product design, accurate forecasting, and control of risk. Third, commercial health insurance companies are encouraged to become deeply involved in the provision of healthcare. They may set up medical facilities or create a platform to facilitate their cooperation with medical, nursing, and other facilities, to better regulate medical services, control medical costs, and promote the optimal allocation of medical resources. Meanwhile, they can help expand the funding of hospitals and income sources for physicians. This should be helpful in motivating physicians to provide better, safer, more efficient, and more reliable services. In the UK, many physicians spend 70% of their working hours within the National Health Service (NHS) system, which generates half of their income. They spend the other 30% serving patients covered by commercial insurance, which constitutes the other half of their income.

However, constrained by the policy environment surrounding medical, pharmaceutical, and healthcare systems in China, and affected by its own insufficient development, the commercial health insurance industry has failed to play a vital role in furthering reform of the institutional structures that relate to medicine, pharmaceuticals, and healthcare. The industry is facing the following three major problems.

First, it does not yet function in a way that can meet the needs of multi-tiered healthcare demand, and it certainly has not made a contribution to helping physicians earn the income that they deserve. In 2015, commercial health insurance payouts accounted for only 2.6% of the revenue of medical facilities in the country. The payouts of China's basic medical insurance programs accounted for another 41.7%, which means that nearly half of medical expenses were paid for by patients themselves.[17] The reasons are as follows. On the one hand, most medical facilities in China are public institutions. It is therefore hard for commercial health insurance companies to optimize the allocation of medical resources through market mechanisms. As a result, commercial companies also fail to improve product quality and fail to cultivate a larger group of customers for commercial health insurance.

In addition, some local governments do not fully understand the different roles of basic medical insurance and commercial health insurance. They attempt to meet the health security needs of their constituencies by raising the protections offered by basic medical insurance programs to an improperly high level. This is not in accord with the principle that basic medical insurance should provide a 'basic level of safeguards' and it also squeezes out commercial health insurance products.

Second, as they take on the handling of China's basic medical insurance programs, commercial health insurance companies have not in fact raised the levels and quality of those programs as intended. They have not led to a synergy among medical insurance, medical treatment, and pharmaceuticals. The essential idea of having commercial insurance 'handle' basic medical insurance programs has been that the government purchases services and itself returns to the functions of policy formulation and regulation. This then allows for a separation between government oversight of the system and actual handling of the system. The idea has been that commercial insurance should be the authorized party handling basic medical insurance, using its specialized expertise to design products, control risk, and raise efficiencies. At the current time, however, commercial insurance companies have no ability whatsoever to influence such things as funding levels or insurance benefits—all of these things are decided unilaterally by local governments. Commercial insurance companies are simply the entities that execute administrative commands. They function merely as the cashiers of basic medical funds and not as suppliers of agreed-upon services.[18] For example, the terms of public procurement tenders for critical illness insurance are currently decided by the government without consulting commercial health insurance companies. Government proceeds according to the principle of balancing income and expenses, conserving principal while allowing for a modest profit, while critical illness insurance is in fact a quasi-public good. Commercial health insurance companies need to take advantage of their expertise and launch products after they have made accurate predictions based on incidence of disease, medical expenses, size of the population, and so on. Proceeding only according to a government-led tendering process may affect the stable and sound operations of insurance funds. Furthermore, commercial insurance companies have extremely limited ability to negotiate with local governments. The top-level design of the whole system has not allocated any authority to those handling insurance programs to provide regulatory oversight or punish offenses. When it comes to developing new products and managing health insurance processes, commercial health insurance companies have little power.

Third, commercial health insurance companies have not yet fulfilled their proper functions when it comes to participating in the provision of healthcare, evaluating and controlling risk, and optimizing the allocation of medical resources. China's healthcare system is dominated by public institutions. Insurance companies are in a weak bargaining position when negotiating with public hospitals. They are forced into the passive position of simply being the party that pays out the reimbursements. This makes it hard for them to establish any deep-seated cooperative mechanisms that can affect doctors' behavior and medical and drug costs. Currently, insurance benefits are paid on an item-by-item basis which can be easily manipulated to induce demand. Meanwhile, insurance companies mainly handle payments based on documents issued by hospitals that come from reimbursement claims from patients. It is hard for them to engage in monitoring and constraining behavior during the whole medical process. It is therefore hard to control medical costs and it is hard to form a link with hospitals that allows each to share both risks and benefits. In addition, the lack of data is still one of the major obstacles to the participation of commercial health insurance companies in provision of healthcare. On the one hand, there is no effective data-sharing mechanism between insurance and healthcare industries and social security, or even within an insurance company. Furthermore, digitization is at an early stage in the medical industry as a whole. Medical records are not standardized, so that insurance companies lack the ability to analyze medical statistics as well as the ability to make accurate forecasts. On the other hand, insurance companies themselves have inadequate amounts of data and inadequate experience in doing statistical analysis. The basis on which the industry can become 'information-ized' is quite weak.

1.3.4 Outdated regulatory system that does not meet the demands of changing times, insufficient focus, and a lack of supporting policies

Commercial health insurance has grown rapidly in recent years, but it is functioning within a regulatory system that cannot meet immediate demands, let alone long-term needs. China's commercial health insurance industry is facing the following three major regulatory problems.

First, the administrative level at which rules are established is low, while some administrative regulations are outdated and no longer relevant. So far, there is no law relating to commercial health insurance in China. The only regulation related to commercial health insurance is the *Health Insurance Administrative Measures* issued by the China Insurance Regulatory Commission. These measures belong to a category of rules and regulations called 'departmental bylaws,' which have less force of law than either 'laws' or 'administrative regulations.' In recent years, China's health insurance industry has developed rapidly and reform of its medical, pharmaceutical, and healthcare structures has moved into deeper territory. The commercial health insurance industry is faced by many new problems and challenges in its effort to participate in building the healthcare system. Yet it has already been ten years since the *Health Insurance Administrative Measures* was introduced in 2006. The regulations no longer meet the real-time needs of the health insurance industry. Only under an effective legal system can the commercial health insurance industry operate according to the law and be regulated according to the law and thus push health insurance in general on to further development.[19]

Second, the lack of supporting policies that are external to the industry is not conducive to having commercial insurance companies become willing to participate in the building of the health insurance system and the healthcare system. This is a problem when it comes to having commercial insurance participate in the basic medical insurance system—the various parts of China lack a unified tendering system, they lack management standards, performance evaluation standards, and standard operating procedures. With respect to authorizing insurance companies to handle critical illness insurance funds, various localities have been exploring ways to allow commercial insurance companies to play a role suited to each place, but they have not established a science-based regulatory oversight system. Specifically, there are no regulations or standards on how critical illness insurance plans should be funded—should they be financed by allocating a portion of the funds of the 'new rural cooperative medical insurance' and the 'urban and rural residents' basic medical insurance,' or should they set up their own funds just for critical illness insurance plans? There are also no unified standards on how commercial health insurance companies should participate in the management of critical illness insurance plans with respect to the bidding process for tenders, the scope of services, and performance evaluations. In order to participate in the building of China's healthcare system, some large commercial insurance companies have begun to invest in healthcare facilities and to set up supply chain networks for the health sector, but they lack guidance and specific policies and regulations at the national level. Meanwhile, selling health insurance through Internet channels is developing rapidly but the follow-up procedures are at an early stage, including how to sign contracts with customers, provide follow-up service, and handle claims. The industry is in urgent need of regulatory rules related to new sales and servicing models.

Third, there are no effective rules on how to differentiate between health insurance and other insurance products, so that it is difficult for customers to tell them apart. Due to its own unique nature, however, health insurance is a quasi-public good. It is different from life insurance in terms of actuarial principles, risk control, operating models, and so on. Although the *Health Insurance Administration Measures* issued in 2006 did set forth explicit rules on qualifications and business management, such rules are not followed in actual practice. In China, essentially all property and life insurance companies can provide health insurance products, and business models copy property or life insurance models. Specialization or differentiation is highly limited. There is an urgent need to improve upon the regulatory system and the business standards that govern commercial life insurance, including such things as accounting standards, actuarial procedures, and risk management.

1.4 FUTURE DIRECTIONS AND KEY AREAS OF DEVELOPMENT OF COMMERCIAL HEALTH INSURANCE

As mentioned above, the contradiction between the current health insurance situation and the current need for better health insurance is becoming acute. That is, the country has low levels of safeguards under the basic medical insurance program, and limited funding, but it is facing a rapidly aging population and changes in the spectrum of disease as its society and economy develop. Commercial health insurance can help meet the increasingly diverse and multi-tiered health insurance needs of customers. It can improve the multi-tiered health security system and is in line with the inherent requirements of the Healthy China strategy.

China's commercial health insurance still faces a number of challenges. Given what has been described above, we believe that we should adhere to the principle of innovative growth and should push forward with supply-side reform regarding China's commercial health insurance. We should increase awareness of insurance among the population by increasing policy support, and should promote the transformation of potential demand into effective demand. We should deepen the process of reforming our medical institutional structures through promoting the development of the commercial health insurance industry. We should create an effective commercial health insurance regulatory system. To be specific, developing China's commercial health insurance should focus on coordinated efforts to further progress in the following four key areas.

1.4.1 Promote innovation and push forward structural reform of the supply side

1.4.1.1 Strengthen innovation in products and service procedures to meet the demand for multi-tiered health insurance

Commercial health insurance companies should focus on market research and take guidance from the needs of the public as they set up products and servicing systems to meet multi-tiered demand for health insurance.

On the one hand, they should actively experiment with innovative products that target specific regions, types of illness, and groups of people. One of China's major problems in this regard is the lack of product diversity. According to the results of the CDRF survey, 12.3% of all respondents believed that this is one of the reasons for the inadequacies of health insurance.

First of all, one of the key principles of product innovation is to aim for the right target. China is vast and its economic and social development varies across the country. People's spending habits and health needs also vary greatly across regions.

The CDRF survey showed that there was tremendous variation across regions of China with respect to the purchase of at least one of the four major health insurance products and with respect to the intent to purchase in the coming year (see Table 1.2.) In the northeastern region, the percentage of respondents who

Table 1.2 Percentage of respondents who had purchased health insurance products and the percentage of respondents who expressed willingness to purchase in the next year by type of products (%)

Region	Critical illness insurance		Insurance for outpatient services and hospitalization		Rehab insurance		Care insurance		Other products	
	Had purchased	Intended to purchase	Had purchased	Intended to purchase	Had purchased	Intended to purchase	Had purchased	Intended to purchase	Had purchased	Intended to purchase
Municipalities directly under Central Government	78.9	84.7	40.4	49.8	11.5	25.5	9.5	21.8	9.4	2.4
Eastern Region	85	83.8	38	51.4	15.7	28	13.9	23.6	5.9	1.2
Central Region	82.1	80.4	32.4	44.8	12.1	22.2	10.8	17.9	9.1	2.2
Western Region	78.2	81.5	38.2	50.5	13.8	25.6	12	19.9	13.3	3.4
Northeast Region	89.1	87.7	31.1	50	12	30.9	12.9	27.3	7.8	3.6

Source: CDRF survey report, 'Survey report on demand for commercial health insurance in China.

had purchased critical illness insurance was highest, 89.1%. In the three cities that are administered directly by the Central Government, the percentage of respondents who had purchased insurance for outpatient services and hospitalization fees was highest, 40.4%. In China's eastern region, the percentage that had purchased rehabilitation and nursing care insurance was fairly high, 15.7% and 13.9% respectively. All of these choices were affected by the level of economic development and extent of an aging population in that specific area, among other factors. With respect to the types of health insurance that respondents intended to buy in the coming year, respondents in the northeastern region expressed greatest willingness to purchase critical illness insurance products—87.7% chose this type of insurance. In the eastern region, a majority of respondents (51.4%) expressed willingness to purchase outpatient services and hospitalization insurance. In the northeast, the percentage of people intending to buy rehabilitation and nursing care insurance was higher than in other regions. Internet-based big data platforms can be used as the basis for 'smart' statistical analysis of consumers, which then can help design health insurance products that are appropriate to local populations.

Second, insurance companies should develop personalized health insurance products that are based on the disease spectrum and the specific needs of different population groups, and they should expand the scope of protections. To reduce the costs of osteoporosis treatment in Germany, Barmer GEK and DAK-Gesundheit (two German health insurance funds) have analyzed patient data collected from multiple regions to find the most cost-effective treatment solution for this disease. Based on the results of their analysis, they incorporated an innovative drug into the scope of coverage. Some insurance companies in China are already developing insurance products that are specifically for diabetes. Collecting and analyzing patient data through certain methods in order to tailor products for specific critical illnesses can help meet the diverse needs of patients. For example, an insurance company launched a lifelong critical illness insurance plan that covers a number of illnesses. In addition to those covered by conventional illness insurance, it also covered more than 20 kinds of common diseases, to provide the insured with more comprehensive protection. Some insurance products are tailored to meet the health needs of the elderly population. Such products relax restrictions on the age of the insured and allow senior citizens to renew their policies and maintain coverage. China also encourages insurance companies to offer more long-term care insurance and disability insurance products to meet the diversified, multi-tiered, long-term protection needs of senior citizens.

In another regard, we should encourage insurance companies to use Internet technology, develop innovative models for handling claims, and improve the efficiency of their service. The CDRF survey shows that 30.2% of respondents held the view that the complex claims process and delay in reimbursement rank foremost among problems with health insurance in China. The speed of handling claims was the second most important factor considered by respondents when choosing health insurance products—21.5% of respondents chose this item. The importance of prompt servicing of claims is evident. At present, insurance companies have launched claims platforms that are connected with the platforms of healthcare facilities. Eligible customers can submit applications at the time of hospitalization and receive direct settlement after discharge, which greatly improves the efficiency of claims handling. Some insurance companies use such platforms as WeChat official accounts to provide information on insurance products, purchasing channels, follow-up services, and so on. Customers can use such platforms to pay premiums and submit claims by themselves, which allows them to enjoy a smooth, convenient, service experience. Another example is that of the Aviva Group in Singapore which, in 2015, launched a mobile application called Aviva Claim Connect. This allows users to submit claims electronically with scans of relevant documents and receive updates on the status of claims, which saves time for both the insurance company and the customer.

1.4.1.2 Vigorously develop 'consumption-type' health insurance products and promote supply-side structural reform

With respect to future trends and customer demands, commercial health insurance companies should gradually weaken the 'life insurance' and 'financial management' features of their health insurance products and focus on 'consumption insurance' that does not provide a financial return on premiums but instead focuses on healthcare safeguards. We should encourage commercial health insurance companies to offer products that can be integrated with China's basic medical insurance, in order to gradually push forward structural reforms that deal with the supply side.

Currently, China's commercial health insurance market is dominated by disease-specific insurance, particularly critical illness insurance products that offer a return benefit on the premium. The market share of consumption-type products is very small. The *Plan of the State Council for deepening reform of medical, pharmaceutical, and healthcare structures during the 13th Five-Year Plan period* first put forth the task of 'developing consumption-type health insurance' and called for putting major effort into this initiative. Consumption-type insurance is insurance that allows for reimbursement on presentation of claims. It provides compensation on an on-going basis for medical expenses related to health problems over the course of a lifetime. In contrast to insurance products that provide a return on investment, consumption-type health insurance does not provide investment benefits—instead it provides safeguards to cover the cost of medical problems.

According to a report put out by the Boston Consulting Group (BCG) and Munich Re,[20] as China's middle-class and wealthy populations grow, more and more people hope to receive better medical and healthcare services through this kind of reimbursement-type health insurance policy. They hope to provide their families with more solid safeguards. China's basic medical insurance system currently provides broad coverage in terms of the country's population but very low levels of safeguards. It cannot yet satisfy a high-level, multi-tiered demand for insurance protection. Some consumption-type insurance products are being launched by domestic insurance companies, and the key reason they are being well received is their design. These products break through the restrictions imposed by the official list of items covered on the catalogue that applies to social insurance. No longer are claims processed just according to secondary reimbursement by the basic medical insurance system. Instead, a portion of claims are reimbursed for out-of-pocket expenses. Meanwhile, insurance will not be denied due to the customer's health (pre-existing conditions). Such products provide better health protection and are widely welcomed by consumers. They have triggered a wave of support for reimbursement-type (consumption-type) health insurance. With respect to product design, the CRDF survey also shows that respondents (49.3%) were most concerned about scope of items covered by insurance and percentage of costs that it reimburses.

1.4.1.3 Actively develop insurance products for health management that are guided by the concept of 'greater health'

As people's living standards and health awareness improve, their demand for health management, preventive medicine, chronic disease management, rehabilitation, and other services will increase. In order to develop commercial health insurance, it will become necessary to integrate policies with an expanded scope of services. Services are transitioning from being 'just reimbursement of medical expenses' to 'integrating preventive measures with management of procedures and post-procedure reimbursement of medical expenses.' Guided by the concept of 'greater health,' we must vigorously develop health insurance products that are tied in to healthcare management services. Meanwhile, better assessment of health risks and better evaluation of the results of interventions will help us find suitable development models for managed care in China.

In recent years, commercial health insurance companies in developed countries have generally incorporated health management services into health insurance services. In addition to simply providing health insurance services, they provide customers with a full range of health security services to meet their multi-tiered health security needs. These include providing health consulting, a 'green channel' that expedites visits with doctors, and management of health-related funds. On the one hand, these efforts educate the person being insured, in order to prevent illness or the worsening of any given condition. On the other hand, they help medical service providers manage the health of the insured more effectively. They improve the results of treatment, which can reduce medical expenses and thus improve the ability to control risk.

The U.S. health insurance market can serve as an example. Products and services offered by commercial health insurance companies in the United States focus heavily on health management and disease prevention. In 1973, the U.S. enacted the Health Maintenance Organization Act to encourage the development of health maintenance organizations (HMOs). The idea was to change the traditional medical insurance model gradually into a model for managed care, and to integrate health management with health insurance. Specific management measures include a wide range of preventive healthcare services such as disease screening, comprehensive physical examinations, and dental care. The participant in a given insurance plan can choose to include these in the list of reimbursable items, with costs being either partially or fully reimbursed. Insurance companies also began to carry out a variety of health promotion activities to encourage participants to get healthier, such as quitting smoking, keeping fit, reducing stress, and so on. They offered material incentives toward reaching fitness goals. Some insurance companies sign contracts with professional health management agencies and health clubs to offer discounts and other benefits. Statistics indicate that 55% of total health insurance benefits in the U.S. are paid to 20% of patients with chronic diseases. Another 20% of total benefits are paid to the 15% of the population with a sub-optimal health status. Meanwhile, the main intervention method for people with chronic conditions is health management services.

British health insurance companies are also focusing on such things as health education, prevention of disease, and management of chronic disease as a way to prevent the worsening of conditions and to control medical costs. For example, the UK-based health insurance company Bupa provides a wide range of health management services, including a health hotline, occupational health education, and physical examinations and stress management, in order to 'prevent, mitigate, and treat disease.'

In China, the role of commercial health insurance companies should therefore expand from simply being health insurance providers to becoming health insurance-plus-health management service providers. They should attempt to reduce the incidence of disease among customers and their own loss rates by providing comprehensive health risk management services. Insurance companies should offer not only protection from medical expenses, but they should provide the insured with pre- and post-event health management services. They should aim to improve people's health and reduce costs through data collection and analysis, health interventions, health assessments, and feedback on evaluations. In the process of managing health, they can employ many current advanced health management technologies, including wearable equipment, various kinds of implants, big data analysis, and Internet tools.

1.4.1.4 Further improve the specialization of commercial health insurance

There are substantial differences between health insurance and life insurance or property insurance in terms of actuarial practices, risk management, and scope of operations. The areas impacted by health insurance are broad and require a high level of specialization. Health insurance companies should therefore focus on the gathering and analysis of data. They should build up teams of professionals and strengthen interactions with health-related industries. In all ways, they should further the specialization and professionalization of the health insurance industry.

First, health insurance should be run by specialized health insurance companies. The experience of developed countries indicates that fierce market competition will push general insurers to evolve into more specialized insurers. Health insurance becomes more and more specialized at the company level. Historically, in developed countries, comprehensive or general insurance companies initially could be divided into two major categories, life insurance companies and property insurance companies. As life insurance and personal financial services markets became saturated, the speed at which life insurance developed slowed down. In contrast, health insurance began to experience swift growth due to such things as an aging population and the development of medical technology. A number of companies shifted the core focus of their business toward health insurance. As a result, health insurance has gradually become differentiated from life insurance, annuities, and so on, and taken a path toward specialized operations. In 2000, the U.S. insurer Aetna sold its life insurance and financial services businesses and transformed itself—it went from being a comprehensive financial group to being a specialized health insurance company. In 2004, the U.S.-based insurance company Cigna also announced a reorganization that shifted its focus to healthcare. Meanwhile, in Germany, the health security system is dominated by social insurance and the law provides that only a specialized insurance company can offer health insurance products.

Second, we should develop underwriting and claims management systems that are specific to health insurance. We should gradually set up unified business standards for how to manage health insurance underwriting, including unified codes for diseases, surgeries, medical service providers, and medical service projects. In addition, insurance companies should establish an effective and strict claims management system and use advanced-technology means to improve the efficiency of claims handling. On top of that, they should clarify the authority and limits to authority of claims handling at all levels of government organizations, and they should set up a system for discussing major cases for which claims are difficult to determine.[21]

Third, we should set up a special information management system suitable for health insurance, and make a continual effort to strengthen our ability to analyze consumer data. Powerful data analysis is not only an important tool to identify different needs of customers, but also a useful tool in developing new products. In western countries, some insurance companies have begun to explore ways to use posts on social media as an important way to mine data on consumer preferences and risk data. At the same time, we should create an information system with functions that raise the level of specialization of the health insurance business. Such things would include process management, early warning of risk, automatic insurance underwriting, automatic claims handling, and ability to make inquiries of medical institutions and medical services.

Fourth, we should strengthen the training of personnel involved in professional health insurance management, including technical and marketing teams. We should establish and improve upon a science-based, specialized health insurance management system. We should develop a standard health insurance personnel qualifications system, including examinations and other qualification platforms, to improve the professional quality of health insurance management personnel. Insurance companies may also recruit health insurance professionals and introduce advanced management technology through various channels (for example, by cooperating with relevant colleges and universities).[22]

1.4.2 Raise awareness of health insurance among the population, strengthen supportive policies, and continue to push for transforming potential demand into effective demand

1.4.2.1 Raise awareness of health insurance among the population by distributing relevant information on various forms of media

First, we should make use of all possible forms of media in order to strengthen educational efforts and broaden knowledge about health insurance for a variety of groups of people. The aim is to turn potential demand for commercial health insurance into actual purchasing of insurance. The CDRF survey shows that most customers (45.1%) get information on health insurance from insurance company salespeople. Only 19.3% of customers get health insurance information via mobile phone or the Internet, and only 6.2% through traditional media. This indicates that the role of different types of media in the transmission of information related to commercial health insurance has not been fully exploited. We can draw on the experience of other countries in this regard.

In 1977, the South Korean Ministry of Finance announced that 1977 was to be regarded as the 'year of insurance,' and the government launched an insurance education program. The insurance industry actively participated in government activities. Through television, newspapers, advertising, and other public media, it vigorously promoted knowledge about insurance, with excellent results. Because of strong support from the government, over the next decade the Korean life insurance industry grew at an average annual growth rate of 51%. This was much higher than the average annual growth rate of Korea's GDP over the same period, which stood at 21%. The United States serves as another example. In the U.S., state governments or state insurance regulators educate consumers about health insurance by issuing informative consumer manuals, organizing seminars, distributing educational materials, and so on. There are many not-for-profit organizations in the United States that focus on insurance education. They target a range of people, from ordinary consumers to students.[23]

Second, in order to deal with a consumer psychology that distrusts health insurance products, we should tackle the problem from a number of different angles including consumer education, full information disclosure about the industry, proper handling of complaints, and so on. Commercial insurance companies should provide accurate, comprehensive, easy-to-understand product information. They should analyze the most outstanding problems that infringe upon consumer rights and interests, and protect consumers from being cheated by hidden terms, unilateral demands, and other forms of fraud. Next, commercial health insurance companies should establish an information disclosure platform that is unified and standard across the industry in order to disclose companies and products that defraud consumers. It should put the latter on an industry or product blacklist.

Third, commercial health insurance companies should improve the handling of health insurance complaints, and devise other supporting systems and platforms that make sure customers have no regrets about buying their products. Japan's insurance company, LifeNet, can serve as an example. It uses website interface design and navigation systems to guide customers to detailed information about their insurance products. These integrate animation and sound effects into product presentation in order to support informed consumer decision making. The company does not advocate a hard sell, persuasion, or other traditional means of selling product. Instead, it provides customers with a platform to learn about insurance. On this platform, customers can also learn general knowledge about insurance and how to develop insurance plans. If customers have other questions, they can call the toll-free number or email the address provided on the company's website. This approach improves consumers' understanding of insurance. It provides them with access to knowledge while also promoting insurance products.

1.4.2.2 Improve tax incentives, increase the strength of benefits, and improve the design of overall government policy with respect to insurance

Health insurance, as a quasi-public good, plays an indispensable role in the provision of multi-tiered health security for people. All countries generally provide policy support to commercial health insurance companies, and tax policies are the most important method by which they do this. The great majority of developed and developing countries provide tax incentives for those who invest in and those who operate commercial health insurance companies. They encourage and support the development of health insurance. The United States, France, Germany, Australia, and South Africa are among such countries.

The Australian government provides subsidies for premium payments to people of different income levels and ages, and this has achieved good results. In 1998, Australia launched the Commercial Health Insurance Incentive Act, which stipulated that eligible Australians were allowed a 30% private health insurance rebate from the government, starting in 1999. In 2005, the Australian government began to offer a 35% private health insurance rebate to customers between 65 and 69 years of age, and a 40% rebate to customers over 70 years of age. In addition, Australia also plans to reduce the subsidy to the affluent population. In 1999, less than 6 million Australians purchased health insurance. By 2017, more than 10 million people in Australia participated in commercial health insurance, accounting for more than 47% of the country's population.

The U.S. government mainly offers tax incentives for those participating in group health insurance, individual health insurance, and health insurance for self-employed individuals. In the case of group insurance, the government excludes employers' contributions to group health plans from taxation, and there is no upper limit. For individual coverage, the out-of-pocket expense or $2,700 ($5,400 for families), whichever is larger, is deductible. Since 2007, self-employed individuals may claim a deduction for 100% of commercial health insurance premiums they paid.[24]

In looking at the international experience and China's own current situation, it seems possible for China to improve upon its commercial health insurance tax incentives by adopting the following three methods.

First, China can increase the amount of the deduction. Each Chinese resident is currently allowed a maximum of RMB 2,400 in tax deductions for premiums paid out for commercial health insurance. In contrast, in the 1990s, each resident in Taiwan was allowed a total deduction of RMB 4,800 for premiums paid for commercial health insurance. Given the comparison with Taiwan, the maximum tax deduction in Mainland China needs to be further increased. At the same time, in order to encourage government units to buy commercial health insurance, China should allow non-corporate units to take a partial deduction on the supplementary health insurance premiums they pay on behalf of employees.

Second, China can increase protections and coverage. We recommend that Chinese health insurance companies engage in R&D to create products that are connected with the existing safeguards system. At the same time, on a pilot-project basis, we recommend that the government offer tax incentives for certain disease-specific products. Meanwhile, the groups that are eligible for tax incentives should be expanded. China may draw on the experience of Australia and offer differentiated tax incentives to different groups of people by income and age. Some cities may engage in trial implementation of a family-based health insurance tax incentive policy, allowing the insured to purchase insurance for their minor children, spouses, parents, and other immediate family members, in order to increase health insurance coverage.

Third, China can simplify procedures. China should develop an industry-wide standard catalogue for health insurance products that are eligible for tax incentives other than the social security catalogue. We should explore different ways, including an electronic information platform, to simplify the tax rebate process and thereby increase the willingness of customers to purchase commercial health insurance.

1.4.2.3 Expand the pilot program relating to personal account balances and encourage residents to purchase commercial health insurance products

The government should introduce a policy that stipulates that individual account balances in the urban employees' basic medical insurance fund can be used to purchase commercial health insurance or other healthcare products. This will help meet the multi-tiered health needs of the population. Employees in Shanghai are already allowed to use the balance in their basic medical insurance accounts to buy commercial medical insurance products. The pilot program of this policy has achieved remarkable results. The municipal government of Shanghai has worked with insurance companies to develop hospitalization insurance and critical illness insurance products that can be purchased using the balance in individuals' basic medical insurance accounts. This makes it more manageable for them to purchase commercial health insurance, and greatly improves the link between commercial health insurance and urban employees' basic medical insurance. In addition, more than ten cities, including Nanjing, Suzhou, Nantong, Shenzhen, Chengdu, and Tai'an, have encouraged residents to use their basic medical insurance card to pay for fitness products and services. Suzhou, Suqian, Liuzhou, Lanzhou, and other cities also allow employees to use the funds in their basic medical insurance account to pay for physical examinations and vaccines for such things as hepatitis B, influenza, and rabies.

1.4.3 Deepen China's Medical Reform and promote the development of commercial health insurance

The deepening of China's Medical Reform is a prerequisite for further development of commercial health insurance. The direct goal of Medical Reform is to increase access to medical services and reduce medical costs. At a deeper level, however, the purpose is to create a virtuous cycle that allows for well-functioning, high-quality, and efficient healthcare and health security systems to improve people's livelihood and welfare. With the deepening of the Reform, China's medical safeguards system should improve as the role and the scope of basic medical insurance protections are further clarified. The synergy between social security and commercial insurance should come into play. The status of commercial insurance companies as 'partners' with government in the basic medical insurance system will be further affirmed as companies supplement basic medical insurance programs more effectively. Instead of being 'squeezed' out of the market by basic medical insurance programs, commercial insurance products will gain a broader consumer base as the demand for commercial health insurance products increases. At the same time, an organic combination of the dual mechanisms of government and market will gradually build a multi-tiered health services supply system. Commercial health insurance companies will no longer be limited to doing business with public hospitals. As public hospitals lose the advantage of holding monopoly power in the future, commercial health insurance companies will find that their negotiating position is greatly improved. Their ability to amass a considerable amount of statistical data will also increase, as well as their ability to design products and control risk. They will become stronger and substantially more able to supply insurance products. In specific terms, we should focus on the following four tasks in order to deepen the Healthcare Reform and effectively promote the development of commercial health insurance.

1.4.3.1 Define the boundaries between commercial health insurance and basic medical insurance and clarify the responsibilities of the government and the market

In order to build a multi-tiered health security system in China, we need to enable the coordination of government and market. This requires that we adhere to the fundamental principle of having the government offer basic protection while the market achieves a multi-tiered diversification of insurance products. It means that we go further in clarifying that, given the limited resources available, 'basic medical insurance' gives priority to ensuring that basic needs are met. We maintain the principle of 'the basic level.' We therefore pull back the boundaries within which we finance basic medical insurance and grant commercial health insurance more room to grow. At the same time, we set up a social [public] health insurance system that operates at a basic level but that provides broad coverage on a unified basis for everyone in the country. We thereby change a situation in which less developed regions are disadvantaged relative to more developed regions, and we ensure more sustainable operation of insurance funds.[25] Meanwhile, using market-oriented means, commercial health insurance should be able to satisfy the more multi-tiered and diversified healthcare security needs of people.

Specifically, as necessary supplements to basic medical insurance, commercial health insurance products should focus on insuring the following health costs: (1) the self-pay percentage mandated by basic medical insurance, and the amount of expenses that exceed the cap on basic medical insurance programs; (2) drugs and services not included in the basic medical insurance list, including imported drugs and physical examinations; (3) expenses of drugs and services provided by non-designated health service facilities, such as rehabilitation centers, VIP beds, private clinics, etc.; (4) costs related to various forms of income subsidies and nursing allowances.

1.4.3.2 Separate management and operating functions in terms of how commercial health insurance companies participate in the management of basic medical insurance funds, and reaffirm the 'partner' status of commercial health insurance companies

Both international and domestic experience indicates that commercial health insurance companies should not serve merely as 'cashiers.' Instead, their innovative concepts and professional operating models should be assimilated into public healthcare departments in a form of public–private cooperation. The government departments in charge of health insurance should no longer involve themselves with micro-management of insurance funds. Instead, commercial insurance companies which sign contracts with the authorities should be responsible for assessment, planning, procurement, performance reviews, and design of special products other than basic insurance programs. This model will improve the efficiency and quality of medical services. The health insurance authorities will focus on industry regulation, keeping the industry in good order and functioning smoothly. In this respect, we can draw on the experience of the UK and the United States.

In 2007, the British government introduced a plan called the 'Framework for procuring External Support for Commissioners' (FESC), which encourages private insurers to participate in the management of the national healthcare system. The FESC issued by the UK Department of Health (DOH) allows qualified commercial insurers to provide the National Health Service with the following four categories of management services: (1) assessment and planning, mainly including assessment of healthcare demand and medical services and design of the medical supply structure; (2) contract signing and procurement: more specifically, signing contracts on behalf of the government, with general and specialist medical service providers; (3) compliance management, dispute resolution, and medical review; and (4) interaction with patients and public relations management. A very important obligation of private insurers that join the FESC is to assess problems in the healthcare system, to provide advice, and to use Internet-based data platforms to analyze data to enhance performance management.

The United States passed the HMO (Health Maintenance Organization) Act in 1973 and the Tax Equity and Fiscal Responsibility Act (TEFRA) in 1982, allowing more private insurers to participate in the management of the public healthcare system. The U.S. government signs contracts with private insurers to entrust a large number of government healthcare projects (such as Medicare and Medicaid) to commercial health insurers which provide information, advice, claims review, benefits payment, financial auditing, and other specialized services. The commercial health insurance entities receive a certain specified percentage in 'management fees,' but they do not bear the risk of the insurance funds. In addition, however, commercial health insurance companies are allowed to increase their operating authority if they do take responsibility for the risk of the funds. Products they design for this purpose must include the basic items of the government-sponsored health insurance programs. Depending on their own circumstances, they are also allowed to add such things as dental coverage, ophthalmic services, disease management, and other special services which customers may choose if they wish. Take Medicare as an example. The Medicare Advantage (MA) plans sold by commercial health insurance companies not only cover all items under Medicare but also offer additional protection from medical costs related to some chronic diseases. In order to increase the attractiveness of the plans, additional items tend to be offered at low prices. Applicants are free to choose between Medicare and MA.[26]

Looking at China's own situation, with respect to enabling commercial insurers to participate in insuring for critical illness, we should make improvements in the following five areas as we build up our systems. (1) Standardize the bidding process and develop a reasonable method for evaluating bids. Curb irrational price competition that drives prices down and makes it impossible for companies to pay expenses, thereby making it impossible for them to adhere to the principle of preserving their capital. Implement an evaluation system that forces insurance companies to pay more attention to quality of service, and foster a market environment that enables standardized and orderly competition. (2) Clarify the way insurance funds should be managed, as well as the corresponding risk-sharing mechanisms and responsibilities, and determine the price of management services based on science-based forecasts and submitted bids. (3) Make use of the professional advantages of insurance companies in aligning them with the basic medical insurance information system so that complete audits of medical expenses can be conducted, medical risk controls can be strengthened, and fraud, waste, and unreasonable expenses can be effectively reduced. (4) Raise the administrative level at which critical illness insurance funds are pooled and managed, formulate standardized contract templates that apply at the provincial level, and prevent fragmentation of the management of critical illness funds. (5) Improve management services, develop a performance evaluation system, and carry out more detailed assessments and management of the regulatory effectiveness of regulatory departments and the managerial effectiveness of commercial health insurance companies.[27]

1.4.3.3 Promote the development of medical professionals and push forward the building of a multi-tiered health services supply system

Healthcare professionals are critical to the health services supply system. If we are to build a multi-tiered health services supply system, change the monopoly position of public hospitals in various medical fields, and encourage commercial health insurance companies to play a constraining role in the provision, supervision, and cost control of medical services, we need to focus on China's human-resource system. We must change the way doctors 'belong to a unit,' rather than belonging to society at large. We must build a new hospital–doctor relationship, so as to release more outstanding medical talent into the system.

In the course of reforming their public hospitals, many countries have adopted a flexible medical practitioner system, and hospitals have gradually been given relative independence in the number of personnel they employ. The administrative layer of the doctor–hospital relationship has basically been removed and the situation is instead moving toward contractual relations. In Germany, for example, most hospitals contract with practitioners for specific services on a part-time basis. This flexible employment arrangement is conducive to balancing resources between the public and private sectors and it more thoroughly mobilizes all medical resources of a country. A 'multipoint practice' has become common in many countries, but the second practice of public hospital doctors is usually limited by a range of measures. First, there are seniority requirements. In the United States, UK, and Germany, new resident physicians are not allowed to go into practice alone. Second, there are restrictions on the place of practice. In the United States, for example, practicing in multiple states requires licenses issued by each of the states in which a physician is practicing. Third, there are time requirements. For example, the United Kingdom adopts a '4 + 1' model to limit the time spent by a physician of a public hospital on his or her second practice. Fourth, there are restrictions on the type of practice. In Singapore, the second practice of public hospital doctors must also be a public hospital, while in the United States a physician who is hired by the federal government is not allowed to practice in other facilities.[28]

1.4.3.4 Create a health insurance big-data platform and promote data sharing within the health insurance industry and between industries

Controlling medical costs and managing them at a more granular level are inseparable from big data and information technology. The mining and use of health-related data will help in regulating the behavior of the healthcare industry. It will help standardize the behavior of institutions, help monitor the quality and safety of medical services, allow insurance settlements to happen across different organizations and different geographic jurisdictions, and will help in fighting insurance fraud. In all these ways, it will become only more important. In addition, the construction of a big data platform for the healthcare system will help promote the innovation and development of insurance actuarial products. Health management data, behavioral data, and environmental data will be fundamentally important in the development of new products. Such data will also help satisfy the need for more differentiated, personalized, and targeted products.

In this regard, the first task is to promote the standardization of information and management systems. Data sharing is central to cooperation among healthcare facilities, health insurance companies, and health services providers. Meanwhile, information and management system standardization is the prerequisite for data sharing and integration. The NHFPC [National Health and Family Planning Commission] has proposed the standardization of four kinds of information that will be highly significant for the standardization of China's medical and health information systems. Those four are diagnosis files, disease coding, operations and procedures coding, and medical terminology. As commercial health insurance companies transition from just handling reimbursements to full participation in health management and medical processes, these four kinds of information will be highly significant to them.

The second task is to set up data sharing mechanisms on a pilot-program basis, to enable the sharing of health and medical information among healthcare facilities, health insurance companies, and health services providers. On the one hand, health insurance authorities and hospitals should speed up the standardization of information systems or information sharing, standardize management and strengthen cooperation to ensure that health insurance funds are used efficiently. On the other hand, we should promote data sharing among health insurance authorities, healthcare facilities, and insurance companies, so that commercial insurance companies can play to their strengths in data analysis and risk control.

Qingdao City, Shandong Province is currently engaged in this kind of experiment. Through the creation of a 'smart health insurance platform,' the insured person can gain access to health management and health security services in a more convenient manner. Health insurance authorities can guide the allocation of healthcare resources more easily, so as to improve service quality and efficiency and reduce medical costs. Commercial insurance companies can make use of the data that is assembled by the information platform, and make use of its attractiveness to insured participants, to develop more diversified insurance products and health services. This will greatly improve convenience and effectiveness for all parties including medical service providers and medical insurance fund managers.

The third task is to push forward legislation that protects medical and health information. Medical and health information is extremely sensitive. As we build a universal electronic health-files system, the question of how to handle patients' health information in ways that protect their privacy will become increasingly important. Based on the commitment to protecting the private health data of patients, we should create constraints on how commercial insurance companies can use that data, and the constraints should be in the form of law.

1.4.4 Create an effective regulatory system that governs commercial health insurance

1.4.4.1 Push for higher-level legislation to build a better external policy environment

We should push for legislation and policy support that is at a higher administrative level, and we should make sure that relevant regulations are updated in a timely manner. Specifically, we may want to improve the *Social Insurance Law* and the *Health La*w to define and position certain concepts in a more detailed way. Those include basic medical insurance, medical services, pharmaceuticals, and commercial health insurance.

In order to provide a sound legal basis for the future development of China's expanded healthcare industry, we should specify the authorities and obligations of each of these as they cooperate with one another. Meanwhile, as required by changing times, we should also revise the *Management Measures for Commercial Health Insurance*, and formulate *Regulations on the Operation and Management of Health Insurance*, so as to regulate commercial health insurance in a more professional way.

Commercial health insurance covers a wide range of business activities. It has many management links, quantities of material to deal with, and highly complex forms of servicing. In addition to 'the insured' and 'the insurer,' its operations involve various medical service providers and various government social security departments. A number of entities participate in the whole process. Regulatory oversight therefore requires the coordinated action of several departments. China has a medical safeguards system that operates over several government levels, and within that system commercial health insurance plays a supplementary role. Its operations are highly influenced by the policies and government structures of the social security and medical and healthcare systems.

Therefore, if China's regulatory departments are to increase regulatory oversight over insurance companies, they must be proactive in communicating with and cooperating with all relevant authorities, including the departments of health and social security. As the regulatory departments guide insurance companies toward effective operations, they must seek to set up a beneficial external environment for the development of the health insurance industry.[29]

Developed countries have highly strict legal and regulatory systems. In Australia, for example, private health insurance must abide by the rigorous provisions set out in nearly 20 relevant laws, including the National Health Act 1953, the Health Insurance Act 1973, and the Private Health Insurance Act 2007, the last of which has gone through multiple revisions after its promulgation. At the same time, the Australian legal system explicitly defines the operating scope of both universal health insurance and private health insurance, in order to ensure that each will be able to continue to develop in a healthy way.[30]

1.4.4.2 Improve supporting policies and encourage commercial insurance operators to participate in the building of the medical insurance and medical service systems

First, we should explicitly set forth in legal documentation the positions and roles of health insurance in handling basic medical insurance, providing medical insurance for critical diseases, and providing supplementary medical insurance plans. This will help us improve the review and approval procedures for market entry of health insurance operators, and it will help us set insurance rates and premium standards. It will enable operations to be conducted according to actual laws, as well as managerial oversight of operations. When commercial insurance companies infringe laws or regulations with respect to basic medical insurance and insurance for critical diseases, or engage in unfair competition, they can be severely punished as according to law. With laws in place, we will be able to preserve sound market order. Meanwhile, we should strengthen supervision over the quality of services, improve information transparency, and voluntarily take in members of the general public as supervisors.

Second, we should put in place policies and regulations that govern the participation of commercial insurance operators in the building of the supply chain of the health industry. The online insurance industry has been growing rapidly in recent years, and we should particularly strengthen supervision over the purchase of online insurance, together with services provided, and claims for reimbursement, in order to protect the rights and interests of consumers.

1.4.4.3 Increase regulatory oversight over the specialized operations of commercial health insurance

First, the relevant regulatory authorities should establish dedicated, separate, departments for health insurance regulation. This will make it easier for regulatory authorities to communicate and work together on a higher level with basic medical insurance, medical, and healthcare departments. It will enable the creation of a more favorable policy environment. It will also help us secure professional teams to provide better guidance and regulation for the industry, in order to promote healthy and orderly development.[31]

Second, we should strengthen controls over access to this sector, strive for a situation where health insurance programs are run by specialized health insurance companies who are in close cooperation with medical institutions. The administration of health insurance is complicated and involves high risk. Health insurance is also greatly influenced by the overall environment of the medical and healthcare sector. There are moral risks and the issue of adverse selection in particular. It is absolutely necessary, therefore, that health insurance programs be operated by specialized health insurance companies with special techniques and tools for risk control. These companies should be closely involved in the processes of providing medical services. Otherwise, it is very easy for losses of insurance companies to mount up. In point of fact, traditional life insurance companies in the United States started to withdraw from the health insurance business as early as the 1980s. Specialized health insurance companies throughout the world, such as Blue Cross and Blue Shield in the United States, are actively engaged in cooperation with medical institutions. They sign strategic cooperation agreements to enhance their intervention in medical service provision and thereby control medical fees and expenditures.

Third, we should move faster to enable commercial health insurance operators to adopt data standards and management systems that are aligned with the medical and healthcare systems. Commercial health insurance covers a very broad scope of activities and its operations involve medical institutions, government institutions, and various other parties. This requires the adoption of unified data management and regulation systems. In order for regulatory authorities to tie in smoothly to medical and healthcare systems, therefore, they should make every attempt to have commercial health insurance companies adopt data management systems that conform to medical and healthcare information systems. The aim is to achieve well-coordinated data collection, storage, and analysis. Also, efforts should be made to form more detailed data codes and standards that are in line with the medical data system of the Ministry of Health.

Finally, we should further improve the systems that are suited specifically to health insurance, including sales, underwriting, risk control, actuarial, and claim systems. They should be differentiated from systems that apply to property insurance and life insurance. This will help us regulate the behavior of market players, and make more professional services available to the general public. To tackle the existing problems of the prolonged claims process and various difficulties in getting reimbursed, the China Insurance Regulatory Commission and various insurance companies should improve their coordination. They should exercise supervisory control and rectification over such behaviors as waste, misuse, and fraud in the claims process. The regulatory authorities may consider drawing up a black list at the national level to keep a record of incidents in which people are cheated. The list would include the relevant individuals and institutions. Meanwhile, measures should be taken to promote the transition towards real-time settlement by commercial health insurance. Currently, the normal procedure for people who have purchased commercial health insurance is for them to pay their medical bills first and then claim back the expenditures from their insurance companies later. Getting a claim approved requires a lot of paperwork and proof of payment. In contrast, for basic medical insurance, patients do not need to pay the part of their bills that is covered by the insurance. That saves them the troublesome process of trying to get reimbursed. If we could achieve real-time settlement of expenditures in the commercial insurance realm, not only would work efficiency be improved but this would increase the feeling among insurance buyers that they were really getting something for their money.

Notes

1 This report is co-authored by Qiu Yue and Guo Pei, with significant input from other members of the research group. CDRF Secretary General Lu Mai and Deputy Secretary General Fang Jin also offered valuable suggestions on the preparation and revision of the report. Our heartfelt thanks go to everyone who has contributed to the research project.
2 *Deepening Medical Reform in China: building high-quality and value-based service delivery.* World Bank Group, World Health Organization, Ministry of Finance, National Health and Family Planning Commission, Ministry of Human Resources and Social Security, 2016.
3 In this volume, Research Topic 3: Role of and development model for commercial health insurance in China.
4 *Blue Book of China's Society,* 2017: Social Situation Report.
5 Analysis. *Research Report on the Outbound Medical Tourism Market in China,* 2016.
6 *Blue Print and Policy Recommendations for the Development of Social Security in China in the 13th Five-Year Plan Period.* Chinese Academy of Social Sciences, 2015.
7 Fang Pengqian. *2014 Report of the Development of the Healthcare Sector in China.* People's Publishing House, 2014.
8 *National Home Elderly Care Survey Report.* China Research Center on Aging, December 2014.
9 This survey was entrusted to the Opinion Poll Center of the National Bureau of Statistics of China. It was conducted during June/July 2017. The respondents were 18–75 years old, living in the surveyed area for more than six months. The survey was designed to collect information on the demographic characteristics, social security participation, and opinions about social security, commercial health insurance purchase, opinions about and future demand for commercial health insurance, and other information of the respondents. Based on data analysis results of the survey, CDRF completed the Survey report on the 'Demand for commercial health insurance in China,' referred to as 'CDRF survey report' in the Main report.
10 Insurance density refers to the ratio of premium to local population (per capita premium), reflecting the level of participation in insurance schemes.
11 Insurance penetration refers to the ratio of total insurance premiums to gross domestic product (GDP), reflecting the status of the insurance industry in the entire national economy.
12 In the narrow sense, the supply of commercial health insurance refers to the supply of commercial health insurance products by commercial health insurance companies. Broadly speaking, the supply of commercial health insurance includes not only the supply of products, but also the participation of commercial health insurance

companies in the construction of the health security system, the healthcare system, and so on. The supply of commercial health insurance in the Main report mainly refers to the supply of commercial health insurance products, including general medical insurance, critical illness insurance, long-term care insurance, as well as the supply of relevant value-added services.

13 Source: Research Topic 3: Role of and development model for commercial health insurance in China.

14 Li Jun. A Study of Policies of Preferential Taxation Treatment for Premiums Paid for Commercial Health Insurance in China. *Labor Security*, August 2011.

15 Research Topic 3: Role of and development model for commercial health insurance in China.

16 Research Topic 2: Researchon the demand for commercial health insurance in China.

17 The data is calculated on the basis of *2016 China Statistical Yearbook on Health and Family Planning, 2015 Bulletin on Human Resources and Social Security Development, 2015 China Statistical Bulletin on Health and Family Planning Development,* and the *2015 Insurance Statistical Report.*

18 Research Topic 5: Impact of comprehensive medical reform on commercial health insurance.

19 Research Topic 4: Policies and regulations relating to commercial health insurance.

20 *Open Up in Chinese Private Health Insurance.* BCG and Munich Re, August 2016.

21 Research Topic 1: Research on the supply of commercial health insurance in China.

22 Research Topic 2: Research on the demand for commercial health insurance in China.

23 Huang Su, Feng Pengcheng. On Stepping up Public Insurance Education in China. *Journal of Insurance Professional College,* 2007(4).

24 Sun Dongya, Fan Juanjuan. What China Can Learn from the U.S. in the Development of Commercial Health Insurance. *China Insurance,* April 2012.

25 Research Topic 5: Impact of comprehensive medical reform on commercial health insurance.

26 Wang Min, Huang Xiao. International Experience and Inspiration on the Participation of Commercial Health Insurance Companies in the Construction of the Health Insurance System [J], April 2015.

27 Research Topic 4: Policies and regulations relating to commercial health insurance.

28 *A Study of China's Healthcare Reform.* China Development Research Foundation, 2016.

29 Research Topic 4: Policies and regulations relating to commercial health insurance.

30 Fan Juanjuan. Regulatory Environment of Private Health Insurance in Australia and What to Learn from it. *Insurance Studies,* 2010 (2).

31 Research Topic 4: Policies and regulations relating to commercial health insurance.

2 Research Topic 1

Research on the supply of commercial health insurance in China

Yu Guifang and Wang Qiguo

Commercial health insurance plays an important role in China's multi-tiered medical security system. It improves levels of health security for China's citizens, spurs innovations in public administration, and furthers social stability and harmony. Since the country is currently entering a 'new normal' in its economic development, and is at a critical moment in its supply-side structural reforms, this is an opportune time for commercial health insurance to develop. The macro-economic situation is stable and moving in a good direction, reform of the insurance system is now releasing real dividends, and people's demand for health safeguards is high. Since resumption of commercial health insurance in China in 1982, the industry has been developing for more than 30 years and has experienced rapid growth in recent years in particular. Nevertheless, an enormous gap still exists between the effective supply of commercial health insurance in China and the demand of people for ways to safeguard their health. Accelerating supply-side structural reforms and expanding the supply of commercial health insurance has therefore long since become a major issue as China engages in deepening reform and furthering innovation. Indeed, this is a difficult issue that has become quite a hot topic and the object of considerable attention by the public at large. It is therefore imperative that we not only carry out research into the supply of commercial health insurance but that we create a supportive environment for its growth and development. We now urgently need to resolve issues that confront the industry. It is time for us to take on this massive and difficult responsibility.

2.1 OVERVIEW OF SUPPLY OF COMMERCIAL HEALTH INSURANCE

The basic scope of 'commercial health insurance' needs to be defined as a prerequisite to carrying out any real study of the subject. In addition, we need to take a thorough look at the current situation of the supply of commercial health insurance in China. This part of our report therefore defines what we mean by 'the supply of commercial health insurance' and looks at the actual practice of such insurance in China since the start of the New Medical Reform. From there, it goes on to analyze the subject on two levels, namely the participation of commercial health insurance in building China's system for medical security (i.e. insurance), and its participation in the building of China's system for medical services (i.e. hospitals and other forms of medical institutions).

2.1.1 Definition of 'the supply of commercial health insurance'

2.1.1.1 Definition of commercial health insurance

Commercial health insurance refers to insurance that provides coverage for such things as critical illness, medical expenses, loss of income due to disability, and nursing care, and that pays out insurance money when these things lead to losses for the insured.[1] Commercial health insurance has played an increasingly major role in China's medical security system since the start of the country's New Medical Reform. Its implications for the country and its influence continue to expand. Because of that, this Report covers not only commercial health insurance as it relates to losses for health and medical reasons, but also to commercial health insurance as it is authorized to 'handle' China's basic medical insurance system and China's critical illness insurance, as well as how such insurance relates to expanding the healthcare industry chain.

Defining the subject in this way allows for the following advantages. First, it goes beyond the basic concept of 'health insurance' in its strictest sense to allow for a richer and broader treatment. Incorporating such things as handling the basic medical insurance system and expanding the healthcare industry chain thereby allow for a wider scope of research. Second, it allows health management and health services to be incorporated as major components in the supply of commercial health insurance. As living standards improve in China and awareness of health gradually increases, people's demand for such things as health management, preventive treatment, management of chronic disease, and rehabilitation is also increasing. These things tie the whole subject of health services firmly in to the idea of health insurance. Instead of just reimbursing for post-event expenses, insurance is changing into something that also covers pre-event prevention, and management processes during an event as well as post-event reimbursement. It is only proper that a study of the supply of commercial health insurance should include new issues that have been emerging since the start of the New Medical Reform.

2.1.1.2 Definition of commercial health insurance supply

2.1.1.2.1 Theoretical basis of commercial health insurance supply

The law of supply and demand naturally governs the supply of commercial health insurance. In order to have an accurate grasp of the connotations and boundaries of commercial health insurance, this report starts by exploring the law of supply and demand as it relates to the insurance market situation in China.

The law of supply and demand is the basic law governing the market economy. Changes in supply and demand in the market affect the prices of goods. The changes in the prices further affect the quantity of a good that is demanded and supplied in the market. As this process continues, supply and demand gradually approach each other until the market reaches equilibrium.

More specifically, supply and demand are economic forces that stand in opposition to each other as they determine market prices. The buyer hopes for lower prices while the seller wants them to go higher. When supply exceeds demand for a product, the price of that product will fall, but lower prices will then lead to rising demand and decreasing supply. When the quantity supplied and the quantity demanded are equal, the market is in equilibrium.

The law of supply and demand is also applicable to the commercial health insurance market. However, in the process of supply and demand interactions, the existence of adverse selection and moral hazard will often lead to aberrations in the supply and demand curve, which will then stimulate a variety of market reactions.[2]

Adverse selection is caused by a situation in which there is asymmetric information. People who buy insurance use any information advantage they can to obtain insurance products at lower prices. That is their intent and their behavior. Where adverse selection exists, however, it may be that the individuals at highest risk are more likely to be insured, while low-risk individuals find it hard to purchase insurance at the desired price. This then results in a net loss in utility. In the case of commercial health insurance, if neither the insurance company or the medical institution are able to share health information regarding the insured, insurance companies can only obtain such information by means of health notifications or physical exam reports. These may not be enough and the insurance company's understanding of the insured may be quite limited. Meanwhile, most people who are buying insurance will purchase products that are beneficial to themselves—this may well create a situation in which those who are frequently sick or have a high probability of getting sick will be most eager to buy health insurance. Affected by adverse selection, the demand for commercial health insurance will keep rising while the supply will keep falling, creating a deviation from normal supply and demand. As that deviation continues to grow, insurance companies will be motivated to increase premiums, thereby worsening the imbalance. So long as this cycle continues, the commercial health insurance market will find it difficult to achieve equilibrium.

Unlike adverse selection, moral hazard includes among other things the tendency for those who are insured to change their behavior after becoming insured. An example is when a person loses the incentive to prevent loss from occurring after he or she has become insured, and also loses the incentive to minimize the extent of the loss once an actual loss has occurred. In the case of commercial health insurance, patients who already possess health insurance naturally seek better and more medical services. In order to make more profits, medical institutions reinforce this—they want patients to choose pricier drugs, more advanced facilities, and longer medical service. Meanwhile, the medical institution must confirm the health conditions of the insured before and after the danger has passed, and the compensated amount must be based on actual medical expenses (this is mainly applicable to medical compensation insurance). The amount paid by an insurance company is therefore not only influenced by factors such as the occurrence of illness and the number of times medical services were received (loss occurrence), but also by the actual amount of medical expenses each time (loss severity). Given the influence of moral hazard, risk management in the commercial health insurance industry is an extremely complicated task. Insurance companies face ever greater operational risks. Generally speaking, insurance companies set prices at a high level, which leads to supply being greater than demand. Meanwhile, high prices then lead to a concentration of subjects that are most susceptible to moral hazard. Under such circumstances, prices will keep rising while the deviation between demand and supply will continue to widen, making it impossible to reach an ultimate equilibrium in the market.

In actual practice in China, the supply of commercial health insurance has shown three main characteristics given the influence of adverse selection and moral hazard. First, the payment of insurance claims is intimately connected to medical services, since supply of commercial health insurance must go through the supply of medical services in order to be realized. Second, commercial health insurance providers face greater operational risks than life insurance providers because, in addition to risks related to the insured, they also face risks from healthcare providers, and these are more difficult to manage and control. Third, due to the complexity of health risks and the difficulty of risk management, commercial health insurance companies face higher operational and management costs and longer profit cycles. To mitigate the risk of adverse selection, insurance companies tend to seek more information on the subject being insured by adding explicit items in their insurance policy forms and skillfully designing their insurance contracts. To mitigate the risk of moral hazard, insurance companies tend to create positive marginal benefits for the insured person so both parties can avoid moral hazard. Those include such things as deductibles, coinsurance, limits on insurance, and premium modification. Ultimately, the aim of the above measures is to restore the normal supply and demand curve for insurance. Only under normal circumstances can the supply side and the demand side make rational choices that maximize their interests as per the law of supply and demand. Only then will the situation ultimately lead to optimal market prices and quantities.

2.1.1.2.2 Definition of the supply of commercial health insurance

In the narrow sense, 'commercial health insurance supply' refers to the total quantity of commercial health insurance products offered by commercial insurance agencies. The situation at present in China is that the country has already established a multi-tiered medical security system that covers both urban and rural residents. 'Basic medical insurance' forms the backbone of the system but is supplemented by other forms of supplementary medical insurance and commercial health insurance. In recent years, China's commercial health insurance business has grown rapidly, with more players joining the market, services constantly being expanded, and more diversified products being offered. Along with the 'Three Medical Reforms' (shorthand for reform of medical institutions, medical insurance, and the pharmaceuticals distribution system), and full implementation of the 'Healthy China' strategy, the status and role of commercial health insurance have risen within the scope of the whole medical system. The definition of 'commercial health insurance supply' in this study therefore goes beyond the mere supply of commercial health insurance products. It extends to 'supplementing' basic medical insurance, 'handling' China's system of basic medical insurance, and extending the health industry chain. In this study, the authors approach the concept from these three perspectives. They carry out a comprehensive and systematic combing through of the subject in these broader terms. More concretely, the supply of commercial health insurance is realized primarily through participation in the development of China's medical security system (social security-type insurance) and its medical services system (hospitals). With respect to the medical security system, commercial health insurance agencies expand the supply of commercial health insurance products, insure for critical illness, and handle basic medical insurance. In doing so, they help improve citizens' medical security. With respect to the medical services system, commercial health insurance agencies actively invest in medical institutions and participate in information technology-based medical reforms, thereby helping extend the industry chain of commercial health insurance.

2.1.2 Supply of commercial health insurance: current situation and actual practice

Commercial health insurance supply plays an important role in deepening China's reform of its medical and healthcare systems and is highly significant in the development of the medical security system and the medical services system. This section of our report discusses the current conditions and practices of commercial health insurance in terms of how its supply contributes to the development of these two systems.

China's commercial health insurance has achieved rapid development since the new medical reform (2009). The supply of this kind of insurance has seen enormous accomplishments. First, the size of the market for commercial health insurance continues to expand and the quality of supply continues to improve, while there has also been a fairly rapid growth of supply. Total income from premiums for commercial health insurance nationwide increased from RMB 57.4 billion in 2009 to RMB 404.3 billion in 2016. This represented an average annual increase of 27.6%. Meanwhile, there are now more suppliers—more than 100 insurance companies have launched a commercial health insurance business.

Service areas continue to expand. Insurance companies are actively insuring for critical illness, they are exploring long-term care insurance, and they are developing high-end medical insurance products that, to a certain extent, are meeting the needs of high-income groups for medical safeguards.

Second, in a staged process, critical illness insurance is being provided for urban and rural residents in order to help prevent 'poverty caused by illness.' Altogether, 11 million people have benefited from the critical illness insurance program that is being undertaken by over ten insurance companies nationwide, that is, in 30 provinces, autonomous regions, and municipalities directly administered by the Central Government. Those who are insured now enjoy medical security that is 10% to 15% better than before on average. Poverty caused by critical illness has effectively been moderated.

Third, commercial health insurance is handling basic medical insurance services in a stable but active way, which is enhancing the efficiency and quality of basic medical insurance. By leveraging its strength in actuarial technology and in professional services and risk management, the industry has taken the initiative in handling this social responsibility. It has accepted the authorization of the government and is actively and professionally participating in the administration and management of all forms of basic medical insurance. From 2010 to the end of September 2015, the insurance industry managed a total of RMB 86 billion of entrusted medical insurance funds and paid out a total of RMB 55 billion in reimbursements. Effective business models have been developed in such places as Jiangyin, Xinxiang, Luoyang, Zhengzhou, and Pinggu.

Fourth, the health industry chain is being extended with innovations that keep expanding the area of services. The insurance industry has been actively exploring new ways to serve China's medical reform by investing in shares of medical institutions and contributing to the reform of public hospitals. The industry has been proactive in applying information technologies to the medical reform, the so-called 'informatization' of the reform. It has leveraged its computer networking and Internet technology to accelerate the development of business information systems, such as information systems for hospitals, medical insurance management systems for government authorities, and social security business management systems for insurance companies. By doing so, it has effectively raised the level of informatization in the medical reform.

Fifth, the industry is being proactive in helping open the market to companies from outside China, which is stimulating greater market vitality. In terms of numbers of entities, by the end of 2016, 56 foreign-invested insurance companies from 16 countries and regions had set up insurance companies in China, while 12 Chinese-funded insurance companies had established 38 insurance business agencies overseas. In terms of market share, the premium income of foreign-funded insurance companies inside China reached RMB 157.7 billion in 2016. The market share of foreign companies was 5.1%, which was 0.3 percentage points over what it was in 2015. Within total premiums, premium income from specifically health insurance products was RMB 24.19 billion, and the market share of this premium income was 6%. Of the total of RMB 24.19

billion, 98.8% or RMB 23.89 billion went to foreign-funded life insurance companies, while 1.2% or RMB 0.3 billion went to foreign-funded property insurance companies. Foreign insurance entities have brought with them new products, effective marketing systems, advanced management practices, and quality services, which provide beneficial examples and inspiration for China's own suppliers of commercial health insurance.

2.1.2.1   Role of commercial health insurance in developing the medical security system

2.1.2.1.1 Supply of commercial health insurance products

Through providing commercial health insurance products, commercial health insurance expands the coverage of China's medical security system and meets its multi-tiered demand for medical security.

In terms of suppliers, as of end-2016, over 100 Chinese insurance entities were qualified to provide commercial health insurance business. Among these, seven were specifically health insurance companies: PICC Health Insurance Co. Ltd., Kunlun Health Insurance Co. Ltd., Hexie Health Insurance, Ping An Health, CPIC Allianz Health Insurance Co. Ltd., Fosun Health (pending), and Ruihua Health (pending).

In terms of the scale of supply, the premium income of commercial health insurance nationwide increased from RMB 57.4 billion in 2009 to RMB 404.3 billion in 2016. This represented an average annual increase of 27.6%, which was much higher than the increase in life insurance premiums during the same period. Of the RMB 404.3 billion of premium income, 25.1% or RMB 101.4 billion went to short-term health insurance, up by 29% for the same period, and 74.9% or RMB 302.9 billion went to long-term health insurance, up by 86.5%. In terms of types of suppliers, the health insurance business of property insurance companies realized RMB 29.4 billion in premiums from original insurance business. This represented 7.3% of their total premium income and was up by

Table 2.1 Comparison of health insurance business of different companies in 2016

	Property insurance companies	*Life insurance companies*	*Specialty health insurance companies*
Premium income (billion yuan)	29.4	374.9	131.82
Annual increase (%)	28.75	71.8	183
Proportion (%)	7.3	92.7	32.6

Notes
1 Excluding life insurance business of China United Insurance Holding Company.
2 Specialty health insurance companies include five companies: PICC Health Insurance Co. Ltd., Kunlun Health Insurance Co. Ltd., Hexie Health Insurance, Ping An Health, and CPIC Allianz Health Insurance Co. Ltd.

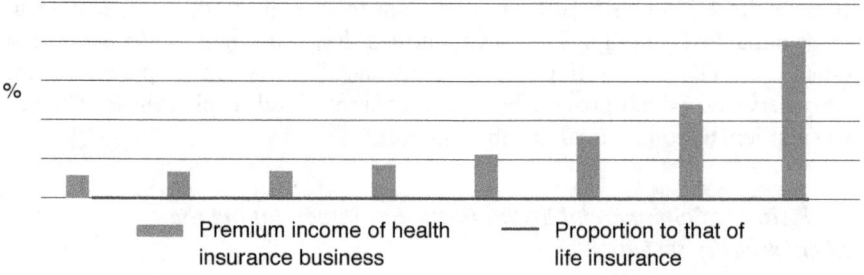

%

Premium income of health
insurance business

Proportion to that of
life insurance

Figure 2.1 Premium income of health insurance business and its proportion to that of life insurance.

28.75% for the same period between 2009 and 2016. The health insurance business of life insurance companies realized RMB 374.9 billion in premium income from original insurance business, which represented 92.7% of total premiums and was up by 71.8%. In 2016, the five existing insurance companies that are specifically oriented toward health insurance contributed 32.6%, or RMB 131.82 billion, of total health insurance premium income.

In terms of levels of security, in 2016 the amount paid out by health insurance for claims reached RMB 100.075 billion. This represented a 31.17% increase over 2015. Of this amount, RMB 23.56 billion or 23.5% was paid by property insurance companies, up by 25.36% from 2015, and RMB 76.515 billion or 76.5% was paid by life insurance companies.

In terms of the number of products supplied, commercial insurance entities have developed more than 2,300 health insurance products. On behalf of residents, they have amassed reserves of more than RMB 350 billion in medical insurance funds in recent years. Short-term insurance products exceed the number of long-term products. Within short-term products, group insurance products greatly exceed the number of individual insurance products. The opposite holds true for long-term insurance products, and the main reason for this is that short-term insurance products are not as attractive as long-term ones—once people are aware of health risks, they prefer long-term protection.

Both the density and the penetration rate of commercial health insurance saw a steady increase in the years between 2009 and 2016. The total population of the Chinese mainland reached 1.38271 billion at the end of 2016, and commercial health insurance payouts or costs in that year came to about RMB 292 per capita, which indicates the degree of density. In terms of insurance penetration, statistics show that China's GDP reached RMB 74.4127 trillion in 2016, of which health insurance accounted for 0.54%.

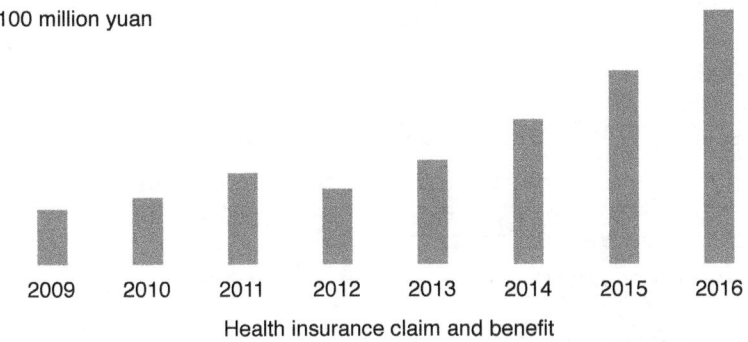

100 million yuan

| 2009 | 2010 | 2011 | 2012 | 2013 | 2014 | 2015 | 2016 |

Health insurance claim and benefit

Figure 2.2 Health insurance claims and benefits and percentage of increase.

2.1.2.1.2 Commercial health insurance companies as providers of critical illness insurance

Critical illness insurance is coverage that is added on top of China's basic medical insurance system, and it provides extra security for patients with serious illness. It is considered an extension and further development of basic medical insurance—it aims to render more effective protection to the insured through institutional arrangements. In August 2012, the National Development and Reform Commission, the Ministry of Health, the Ministry of Finance, the Ministry of Human Resources and Social Security, the Ministry of Civil Affairs, and the China Insurance Regulatory Commission co-issued the *Guidance Opinion on Work related to Providing Critical Illness Insurance for Urban and Rural Residents*, which forms the master plan for business.

In August 2015, the General Office of the State Council issued a further clarification in the form of *Opinions on the Full Implementation of Critical Illness Insurance for Urban and Rural Residents*. This explicitly confirmed adherence to the principle that the government should play the role of leading the process while professional entities should do the actual business of critical illness insurance. It confirmed the role of market mechanisms and the need to make full use of the strengths of commercial insurance entities so as to promote the sound operation and sustainable development of critical illness insurance. This document therefore made explicit the position and role of the insurance industry with respect to critical illness insurance. By now, critical illness insurance has become an important business for commercial insurance entities as well as one important form in which commercial health insurance is supplied.

In terms of suppliers, critical illness insurance currently provides coverage for 1.05 billion urban and rural residents across the country. Such insurance is being provided by more than ten insurance companies throughout China, in 30 provinces, autonomous regions, and the municipalities directly administered by the Central Government. A total of 11 million people have benefited from it.

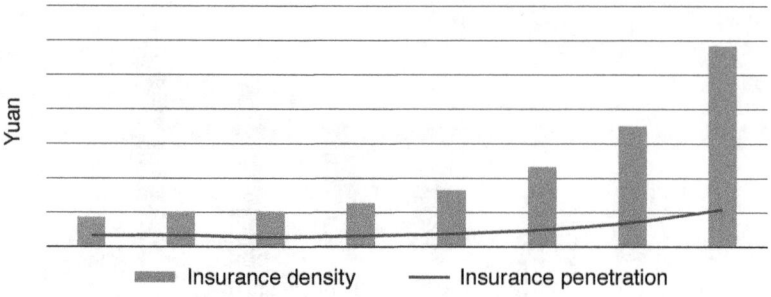

Figure 2.3 Health insurance: density and penetration.

In terms of the size of the business, in 2015, insurance companies took in RMB 25.864 billion for critical illness insurance—that figure includes both premium income and funds that companies were authorized to manage for the purpose. Of this amount, about 95%, or RMB 24.685 billion, was paid out to cover claims. In 2016, patients covered by critical illness insurance enjoyed actual reimbursement rates that were 13.16 percentage points higher than those people covered only by basic medical insurance. The burden of medical expenses that some urban and rural residents faced was dramatically reduced. So far, the largest individual reimbursement amount was RMB 1.116 million.

In terms of the administrative level at which insurance funds were pooled and managed in 2016, 15 critical illness insurance programs were administered at the provincial level, 484 at the city or prefecture level, and 242 at the county or district level. Those administered at the city or prefecture level and at the county or district level accounted for 98% of all the programs.

In terms of the results of implementation, insurance companies detected 860,000 problematic cases in 2015 and 2016 through examination and verification procedures, which saved approximately RMB 5 billion of state funds. As of September 2016, 414 programs that insurance companies managed on behalf of governments had successfully launched one-stop settlement services and another 80 programs achieved the ability to settle claims across jurisdictions. These things enabled patients with critical illness to receive speedy and convenient settlement services. In 2015, 863,700 patients covered by critical illness programs of insurance companies received treatment in cities outside the pooling area of the insurance fund, and the amount of 'outside' claims settlement reached RMB 7.31 billion. In some places, patients with serious illness have been able to enjoy such value-added services as telemedicine and family doctors.

2.1.2.1.3 Commercial health insurance companies as 'handlers' of China's basic medical insurance system

Handling basic medical insurance is another important way for the insurance industry to participate in the development of the country's medical security system. At present, basic medical insurance has become an important business for commercial health insurance entities as well as an important form by which commercial health insurance is supplied.

China has successfully established the world's largest social security network for the world's largest population. This meets basic needs for those who are covered, with a fairly complete range of safeguards and a fairly good level of security. Basic medical insurance has played an important and fundamental role in China's multi-tiered medical security system.

To understand the subject, let us first look at the development of basic medical insurance in China. In 2015, 670 million urban residents were participating in the country's 'urban basic medical insurance' program. Within this figure, 290 million people were covered by the 'urban employees' basic medical insurance (of whom 210 million were still working and 75.31 million were retired). Another 380 million people were covered by the 'urban residents' basic medical insurance' program. In the same year, total income into the fund for the urban basic medical insurance program came to RMB 1.1 trillion while total spending out of the fund came to RMB 931.2 billion. The income figure was 15.5% higher than it had been the year before, in 2014, and the outflow was 14.5% higher. At the end of 2015, the cumulative balance of socially pooled funds for China's urban basic medical insurance program came to RMB 811.4 billion. (This included the balance of funds for urban residents' medical insurance, which totaled RMB 154.6 billion.) At the end of 2015, a total of RMB 442.9 billion was held in individual accounts.

Transforming the function of government in China is of ultimate importance as the country moves further in deepening its overall reforms. In this regard, relevant departments in the government are focusing on using market-oriented mechanisms in the country's medical security system in particular. The commercial health insurance industry has taken the initiative in shouldering this public responsibility, given its advantages in such things as risk management, specialized services, and actuarial science. It has accepted the authorization of the government and is participating in managing the various kinds of basic medical insurance, including the basic medical insurance for rural and urban residents, in a vigorous but stable way.

In terms of the size of the business, from 2010 to the end of September 2015, the insurance industry managed a total of RMB 86 billion of medical insurance funds entrusted to it by the government, and paid out a total of RMB 55 billion in compensation. [In addition,] the commercial insurance business took in RMB 71.1 billion of premium income and paid out RMB 57.5 billion in compensation. It serviced more than 300 million individual cases.

In terms of business models being employed, the commercial health insurance industry is using three main models by which to handle China's basic medical insurance. Those are: entrusted (or authorized) management, as represented by the Henan Luoyang Model and the Jiangsu Jiangyin Model; a contract form of insurance model, as represented by Zhejiang Jiande Model; and a co-insurance and joint management model, as represented by the Beijing Pinggu Model.

Generally speaking, commercial health insurance companies 'handle' China's basic medical insurance in ways that are still fairly limited in terms of size of the business and type of business model. Nevertheless, actual experience so far has proven that the practice of using commercial health insurance companies has reduced operational costs, controlled medical expenses, reduced public-finance spending, and improved the quality and efficiency of basic medical insurance services. In some areas, it has helped address such issues as ballooning medical expenses, ubiquitous use of excessive medical treatments, scarcity of professional service providers, and outdated approaches to regulatory supervision of medicine. It has enabled the provision of better services in a more efficient and professional manner, at lower cost.

2.1.2.2 Role of commercial health insurance in building of China's medical services system

Commercial health insurance is one of the pillar industries in the provision of healthcare services. The strengths of the commercial health insurance industry should be leveraged not only as a way to restructure the health industry chain but also as a way to accelerate the industry's own growth. At present, commercial health insurance mainly participates in China's medical services system in two important ways, namely by investing in medical institutions and by participating in the 'informatization' of China's medical reform, that is, by applying IT technologies to medicine.

2.1.2.2.1 Commercial health insurance companies as investors in medical institutions

Medical institutions represent a combination of various kinds of factors of production—medical staff, diagnostic technology, treatment technology and skills, and so on. With proper institutional (systemic) arrangements, through the means of investment and using capital as the critical bond, commercial health insurance can play an important role in advancing public hospital reform as well as in developing non-public medical institutions.

Let us look first at the investment of capital by insurance companies and the capital requirements of medical institutions. Insurance funds are by nature liabilities, that is, they are indebted capital. They also are by nature long-term and large-scale funds that come from stable sources. These things determine the need to make sure that there is an organic union or balance among the various considerations of security, profitability, and liquidity. The investment of insurance funds should aim for long-term, consistent, stable returns. In contrast, medical institutions, as the main supply platforms of medical services, have quite different characteristics. They require a large initial investment, have a high threshold to entry, are monopolistic in nature, are less likely to be influenced by economic cycles, enjoy abundant cash flow, have stable yields over the long term, and become more profitable as time goes on. Generally speaking, insurance companies and medical institutions are a natural match for one another when it comes to the investment of capital by one and the asset needs of the other.

With encouragement and support from the State, commercial health insurance enjoys a favorable policy environment when it comes to investing in medical institutions. In March 2009, the CPC Central Committee and the State Council issued the *Opinions on deepening reform of the institutional structures that relate to medicine and healthcare*. This called for accelerating the formation of more diversified ways to provide medical and healthcare services. It encouraged the establishment of non-profit hospitals using private capital. In May 2009, the China Insurance Regulatory Commission issued *Opinions for the insurance industry on engaging fully in deepening medical reform by actively participating in the development of a multi-tiered medical safeguards system*. This encouraged insurance companies to explore setting up mechanisms that would allow for negotiated agreements with medical institutions and mechanisms on various kinds of effective payment in order to ensure better regulatory supervision over the payment of medical expenses. It also encouraged them to explore setting up management systems in designated hospitals whereby both hospital and industry would share the risk of the medical institution as well as the profits. By improving reimbursement percentages and providing better services, the idea is to encourage insured people to select such institutions for their medical care. This will allow for better control of medical expenses and better prevention of risks that stem from inappropriate claims. The 2009 *Opinions* aimed to push forward the restructuring of public hospitals by encouraging participation of the insurance industry through investment in medical institutions and furthering cooperation through various capital arrangements. In June 2012, the China Insurance Regulatory Commission issued the *Notice on the plan and implementation program for deepening reform of the medical and healthcare system during the 12th Five-Year Plan period*. This stated that insurance companies should explore the feasibility of and effective ways of setting up medical institutions, and that they should participate in public hospital restructuring so as to extend the health insurance industry chain. In December 2016, the State Council issued the *Plan for deepening reform of the institutional structures that relate to medicine and healthcare during the 13th Five-Year Plan period*. This pointed out that the commercial health insurance industry should make use of its advantages in long-term capital investment to encourage commercial insurance companies to invest in health services organizations including those dealing in medical treatment, care for the elderly, and physical examinations. To sum up the above, with the encouragement and support from the state, commercial health insurance enjoys a favorable policy environment when it comes to investing in medical institutions.

Let us look now at the actual size of insurance funds. By the end of 2016, the total assets of China's insurance industry came to RMB 15.1 trillion and the balance of operating funds totaled RMB 13.4 trillion. Within this amount, 6.9% or RMB 923.36 billion was comprised of stocks, 6.39% or RMB 855.45 billion was comprised of other forms of securities, 9.2% or RMB 1.2 trillion was long-term 'shareholding rights,' and 1.06% or RMB 141.3 billion was in investment-type real estate. At present, there is no accurate data on the size of insurance funds invested in medical institutions, but judging from the types of investment that funds tend to go into, the amount invested in medical institutions is not large.

In terms of how investments are made, commercial health insurance basically follows two main patterns. One is direct investment including full ownership, in which case the investing insurance company sets up its own medical institutions. The other is investing in existing medical institutions (see Table 2.2). In that case, both sides deepen cooperation by adding equity cooperation to operating forms of cooperation.

Here is a typical case. On June 23, 2014, the China Insurance Regulatory Commission announced approval of the investment by the Sunshine Life Insurance Co. Ltd. into the Sunshine Union Hospital Co. Ltd. This marked the official entry of the Sunshine Insurance Group into the medical industry. Sunshine Union Hospital then became the first general hospital in China to be jointly managed through cooperative arrangement with an insurance agency, a large state-owned hospital, and an educational institution. In recent years, many domestic insurance companies have begun investing in medical institutions, creating a very active market (see Table 2.3).

2.1.2.2.2 Participation of commercial health insurance companies in China's medical reform through process of applying IT to medicine and health insurance

Information technology (IT) is a powerful lever that can be used to propel reform of the China's medical and healthcare system. It is also a crucial means to fundamentally resolve the problem of surging medical and healthcare expenses. The participation of commercial health insurance companies in IT-based medical reforms will not only significantly further the development of commercial health insurance, but will also provide a key way to extend the health industry chain.

In terms of the policy environment, the CPC Central Committee and the State Council co-issued the *Opinions on deepening reform of the institutional structures that relate to medicine, pharmaceuticals, and healthcare* in March 2009. This called for the establishment and ongoing development of a medical security information system. It also called for accelerating the building out of a system that allowed for such combined functions as funds management, cost settlement and control, supervisory control over medical behavior, and management services for insured individuals and groups. In May 2009, the China Insurance Regulatory Commission issued *Opinions for the insurance industry on fully engaging in the spirit of deepening medical reform by actively participating in the development of a multi-tiered medical safeguards system*. This too stressed the building up of an information system that both suited the unique management needs of the health insurance business and that could gradually be integrated with the information systems of medical institutions. In June 2012, the China Insurance Regulatory

Table 2.2 Comparison of investment patterns of commercial health insurance in hospitals

	Newly built hospitals	*Private hospitals*	*Public hospitals*
Investment patterns	Rent a building or buy a piece of land for building a new hospital	Equity participation or holding	Acquire all or part of the property rights
Advantages	High standards for hospital hardware environment and advanced operation and management model from the beginning	Traceable business history and certain brand and market resources	No need for relicensing, saved costs of construction, and enjoying brand accumulation and stable customer source
Disadvantages	Difficulty of licensing, long construction period, and long-term market cultivation and investment return	Large investment, difficulty in replicating business models or expanding business in different places, and poorly standardized management	High restructuring costs, rare good investment opportunities, and difficulty in post-investment management

Commission issued the *Notice on the Plan for deepening reform of the institutional structures that relate to medicine, pharmaceuticals, and healthcare during the 12th Five-Year Plan period, and on the program to implement this Plan.* This called for stronger efforts to build a health insurance information system, and it called for a system that gradually standardizes health insurance data so as to allow for a smooth interface among different information systems. It therefore called for a system that enhances the connectivity of medical institutions and social security authorities. This *Notice* also called for greater effort in assembling and analyzing data in order to improve risk management and risk mitigation, so as to lay a solid foundation for the development of health insurance. In November 2014, the General Office of the State Council issued *Various Opinions on accelerating the development of commercial health insurance.* This emphasized the importance of upgrading levels of informatization. It encouraged commercial insurance agencies to participate in the building of a platform for applied use of the population's health data. It supported the necessary sharing of information among commercial health insurance systems and those of China's basic medical insurance and medical institutions. It gave support to having commercial insurance agencies develop health insurance information systems on either a national or regional basis that have comprehensive functions, have high-level security, and are relatively independent. To do this, it called for making use of modern information technology including big data and the Internet, so as to improve the ability to analyze and apply the use of population health statistics and thereby raise levels of 'smart'

Table 2.3 Investment information of insurance agencies in medical institutions[3]

Agency	Ping An Insurance	China Life	Sunshine Insurance Group	NCI	Taikang Life Insurance
Market position	Most innovative insurance group in China	Largest life insurance company in China	A leading domestic insurance group	A leading insurance company in the industry	A leading domestic insurance company in China
Business layout	In March 2015, Ping An announced its Ten Thousand Clinics Plan, i.e. building 10,000 standard Ping An clinics in 10 years, which, combined with Ping An Good Doctor application, will further improve its online and offline medical strength	In 2015, China Life invested in Fosun Pharma and became its second largest shareholder; invested in Town Health (Hong Kong) and became its largest shareholder; and invested in the Beijing Genomics Institute and many other important programs. In 2015, it launched the Big Health Fund program, expected to leverage a total of 50 billion yuan for the creation of a medical service network consisting of 100 hospitals and 10,000 clinics and the Insurance Plus Hospital business model	In January 2015, the China Insurance Regulatory Commission officially approved the launch of the 5 billion-yuan Sunshine Union Medical Care and Health Industry Development Fund initiated by Sunshine Insurance. In 2015, it established Sunshine Union Hospital, the first large comprehensive hospital controlled by an insurance company in Weifang, Shandong	NCI has invested 180 million yuan in setting up fully controlled clinics featuring health management in Wuhan, Xi'an, Qingdao, Yantai, Baoji, Chongqing, Changsha, Chengdu, and Zhengzhou	In September 2015, Taikang Life Insurance decided to launch the health and elderly care project known as Taikang Home in Lvshunkou, Dalian and build a tertiary hospital

Source: yitoubang.com. A Summary of Top 10 Capital Investments in Medical Care [EB/OL]. http://yitougroup.com/a/shuju/221.html.

operations in business. In summary, commercial health insurance enjoys a favorable policy environment when it comes to having the industry participate in information technology-oriented medical reforms.

Let us now look more specifically at how commercial health insurance companies participate in building up the information-technology basis of the industry. Commercial health insurance companies handle China's basic medical insurance, provide insurance for critical illness, and invest in medical institutions—in all of these the industry strengthens its cooperation with social security agencies and medical institutions in terms of developing information systems that contribute to China's medical reform. The industry pushes forward the sharing of health information and actively aims to promote the informatization of medical reform (that is, the application of IT technologies to medicine and healthcare). There is little data at present that quantifies the scale of the industry's contributions in this regard. Nevertheless, contributions to China's medical reform via building up information technologies come in the following three forms.

First, commercial health insurance companies participate in the development of hospital information systems. Such systems use computers and telecommunications equipment to enable hospital departments to improve the ways in which they collect, store, process, extract, and exchange information on diagnosis, treatment, and administrative matters. This helps authorized users to meet the demands of their various functions.

Second, commercial health insurance companies participate in the development of the management systems that pertain to the government's medical insurance. With such systems, the government departments in charge of basic medical insurance (including social security and health departments) provide convenient basic medical insurance management services for civil servants, urban employees, urban and rural residents, farmers, and other groups.

Third, commercial health insurance companies strengthen the building up of business management systems that govern the basic medical insurance business. Such systems are designed and developed specifically for processes related to basic medical insurance and critical illness insurance. They cover each stage of the business, from people's applying for insurance to issuing compensation. They allow for detailed management of basic medical insurance, critical health insurance, and related businesses. In actual practice, commercial health insurance companies have played a very important role in improving levels of healthcare services and lowering medical costs. They have improved managerial productivity and the quality of services, through the use of information systems. They have been proactive in seeking to integrate their information systems with those of hospitals and the medical insurance management systems of government authorities. Their efforts to develop a platform for applied use of data on population health have effectively broken through the problem of a paucity of health-insurance data in China. They have advanced the shared use of sources of health data, leading to the achievements listed above.

Here is a typical example of the many breakthroughs that domestic insurance companies have made as contributors to China's medical reform via use of advanced information technology. In July 2011, PICC Health Insurance Company Limited witnessed the first payment ever made through its independently developed supporting system for casualty insurance in Tianjin. The system supports the payment of claims by the commercial insurance business of PICC Health Insurance, but it also supports such things as advance indemnity payments and confirmation. It thereby facilitates its own in-depth cooperation with social security authorities and it strengthens the company's business capacities in relevant areas. In addition, in recent years, commercial health insurance companies have achieved improved regulatory control over unreasonable medical behavior by using systems they have set up, such as yibaotongapp.com and shebaotong.com, among others. These are used in the course of handling basic medical insurance and critical illness insurance. They are integrated with the information networks of medical services providers and social security agencies and allow for direct settlement of costs.

2.2 FACTORS THAT INFLUENCE SUPPLY OF COMMERCIAL HEALTH INSURANCE

In order to carry out a comprehensive study of the current supply of commercial health insurance in China, it is necessary to look at factors that influence that supply. Due to its unique nature, commercial health insurance is influenced by the usual factors that influence insurance but also by a variety of additional factors. These other factors operate in complex ways, and each has its own form of influence. To facilitate the analysis, this study divides such factors into two categories, namely endogenous variables and exogenous variables.[3]

2.2.1 Variables that are endogenous to the supply of commercial health insurance

2.2.1.1 Product factors

2.2.1.1.1 Price of commercial health insurance products

There is a positive correlation between the supply of commercial health insurance and its price. The higher the pricing, the more insurance providers are willing to offer products, and vice versa. The supply of insurance has two presuppositions. First, the supply at any price can meet the demand at the original price. Second, when the price decreases to equal the marginal cost, further supply stops.

Under the first premise (presupposition), supply is subject to the capacity of insurance companies. Under the second, when the price of an insurance product drops to the critical point or below, supply is subject to the level of return on investment of the insurance agency.[4] However, within empirical studies conducted to date, it has been difficult to find a satisfactory way to measure the pricing of health insurance products. This is because there are many kinds of health insurance products, each with different rate structures, so it is difficult to measure the influence of the product's price on supply by using a unified scale.

2.2.1.1.2 Business capacity of commercial health insurance entities

The 'business capacity of insurance entities' refers to the ability of the entity to provide insurance products. As with 'productive capacity' in other sectors, this is a major factor when determining the supply of insurance products. Business capacity factors include insurance operating costs, size of net premiums, level of professionalism, quality of employees, and efficiency of the insurance industry.[5] In this highly professional and technical business, if other conditions remain the same, the more skilled the insurer is at operations and management, the greater its ability to supply insurance will be.

For a long time, China's commercial health insurance has suffered from a rather weak foundation and a rather low professional level. The business has generally been run by life insurance companies, who rely on their own staff and actuarial methods. Health insurance is distinctively different from life insurance, however. First, health insurance must deal with the dual relationship of both policy holders and medical institutions, so faces greater complexity in dealing with risk. Second, the two types of insurance have quite different actuarial bases. The pricing of health insurance products is based mainly on the incidence of disease and on hospital expenses, while that of life insurance products is based mainly on life expectancy tables. Moreover, commercial health insurance places higher demands on the professionalism of staff. They need to be well versed not only in insurance but also in medicine, finance, statistics, and law. Right now, however, relatively few professionals in the industry have a medical background.[6] Trying to use life insurance models in operating health insurance will therefore not be conducive to improving the quality of the supply of health insurance in China. Although professional levels are gradually improving, commercial health insurance is still in its early stages and has a long way to go.

2.2.1.2 Socio-economic factors

Socio-economic factors mainly influence the supply of commercial health insurance by influencing demand. Assuming other conditions remain the same, the better a country's economic situation, the stronger the purchasing power of its consumers and the greater the demand of its people for insurance. According to the law of supply and demand, more demand for commercial health insurance will lead to greater supply, and less demand will lead to a decline in supply. In China's specific situation, a population that is aging at an accelerating pace is stimulating enormous demand for health insurance—considerations include not only the surging numbers of older people but the way many are old before they make sufficient money to cover their old age. The resulting risk provides a huge incentive for increased demand for health insurance. In 1982, 4.9% of the

Chinese population was aged 65 or above. By now, the figure has already reached 10%. Meanwhile, the working age population is expected to shrink by an average of 7.6 million per year after 2030. By 2050, the working age population will drop to approximately 700 million, down from 830 million in 2030. China's rapidly aging population has also led to many social problems, especially in relation to medical care and care giving for the elderly. With economic and social development and advances in medicine, chronic disease has become a primary component of the burden of disease. Statistics from the fourth National Health Service Survey show that the two-week morbidity rate of China's elderly population is 46.6%, much higher than the national average of 18.9% for people in general. This has led directly to a dramatic increase in medical expenses for the elderly. At the same time, aging also creates demand for long-term care. Under China's current social medical security system, however, which provides for 'low-level broadly-based coverage,' does not generally cover long-term care. Individuals themselves cover a relatively large percentage of medical costs.[7] Therefore, in terms of the potential market for commercial health insurance within China's entire society, an aging population will significantly stimulate the latent demand for commercial health insurance and should spur expansion of supply.

2.2.2 Exogenous variables relating to supply of commercial health insurance

2.2.2.1 *Financial policy environment*

Policies relating to a country's insurance industry depend on the requirements posed by that country's strategy for economic development and by its economic structural reform. Planning for the growth of the industry includes guiding the rational allocation of resources in its direction. Such planning generally falls into the category of medium-term and long-term policies. Such policies impact the supply of health insurance due to their ability to affect the size and quality of supply, but also their ability to define the boundaries of the role that health insurance should play in social and economic life. The social importance of commercial health insurance is intimately related to the guidance of government policy. It can be said that commercial health insurance benefits less from strong economic growth than it does from supportive and stimulating government policies. At present, the majority of OECD countries have passed preferential policies to stimulate their commercial health insurance industries, including such things as financial subsidies and tax incentives.

China too has passed a number of policies granting preferential tax treatment with respect to commercial health insurance, starting with the *Various Opinions of the General Office of the State Council on accelerating the development of commercial health insurance*, issued in November 2014. In May of 2015, the Ministry of Finance, the State Administration of Taxation, and the China Insurance Regulatory Commission jointly issued the *Notice on work relating to a pilot project to implement a personal income tax policy for commercial health insurance* (Ministry of Finance and State Administration of Taxation [2015] No. 56). This vigorously supported pilot projects that allow for preferential personal income tax treatment for individuals who purchase commercial health insurance. In November 2015, the Ministry of Finance, the State Administration of Taxation, and the China Insurance Regulatory Commission jointly issued the *Notice on pilot-project implementation of personal income tax policies relating to commercial health insurance* (Ministry of Finance and State Administration of Taxation [2015] No. 126). This provided more detailed regulations to do with preferential tax for those purchasing commercial health insurance products. The introduction of preferential tax policies has had a positive impact on purchasing behavior. It has stimulated an increase in demand for commercial health insurance and therefore has enlarged the size of the market for commercial health insurance.

2.2.2.2 Level of social security being provided

The level of safeguards under the social insurance system is key to determining how much commercial health insurance is going to be supplied by insurance companies. Regulations governing China's basic medical insurance system have an important impact on the size of the market for commercial health insurance. To a large extent, they also determine its position within the market.

A country's basic medical insurance system affects the supply of commercial health insurance mainly in the following two ways. First, the establishment and expansion of a basic medical insurance system often has a tremendous impact on commercial health insurance. The Nordic countries can serve as an example. With their comprehensive public security program, policymakers of the Nordic countries generally pay little attention to commercial health insurance. Under such circumstances, the commercial health insurance market finds it difficult to expand significantly and, in some cases, the market even shrinks. In Switzerland, for instance, the statutory basic medical insurance system that provides comprehensive protection for citizens was established in 1996. As a result, the commercial health insurance market shrank substantially. Second, the absence or insufficiency of a basic medical insurance system encourages the supply of commercial health insurance. For example, in Ireland, Australia, Denmark, and the United Kingdom, the waiting period, the freedom to choose a doctor, and the relative absence of public security have all become major incentives for an increased supply of commercial health insurance. In the Netherlands, almost all individuals who are not eligible for the public critical-illness funds have bought commercial health insurance, while 90% of those who do participate in social security have purchased additional insurance. To a certain extent, the classic way that commercial health insurance develops is to capitalize on lacunae that exist in the public security system.

In China, the roles assigned to the medical safeguards system and commercial health insurance system over a long period have, to a degree, constrained the supply of commercial health insurance. First, for a long time, commercial health insurance has failed to attract sufficient attention from the government. It has remained in a secondary and supporting position in the overall medical security system. Despite the fact that the State Council issued the *Opinions on deepening reform of the institutional structures that apply to medicine* in March 2009, which explicitly stated that commercial health insurance is an important component of the social security system and its development should be actively promoted, the quality of commercial health insurance supply has yet to improve. Second, there is no clearly defined boundary between basic medical insurance and commercial health insurance. In many cases, the boundaries between the two are indistinct and they have yet to form a beneficial partnership. Under such circumstances, commercial health insurance finds itself in an inferior position, making it hard to achieve fast growth.

2.2.2.3 *Regulatory policy*

Supervisory regulation of the insurance business is mainly achieved through a country's legal system. The legal system affects the supply of health insurance mainly by protecting and preserving market order. The soundness of a country's legal system is of ultimate importance in determining the stability of the industry, regulating the proper behavior of those who run it, and protecting the legitimate rights and interests of consumers. If insurers are seriously insolvent and cannot make payments, if competition becomes vicious, or if other negative forms of behavior undermine the interests of consumers, their confidence in the industry will suffer and the supply of health insurance will decline. In addition, if the legal system fails to address actual issues, this may cause adverse consequences despite the good intentions of the industry.

In China, the legal system governing commercial health insurance has yet to be adequately put in place. First, it has been ten years since the *Administrative Measures for managing health insurance* were adopted in 2006. Given the growth of the industry, these *Measures* are patently inadequate and outdated. They are not conducive to improving the quality of the supply of commercial health insurance. Second, health insurance is not the primary business of property insurance companies and life insurance companies, so irrational forms of competition can easily damage orderly competition in the health insurance business and hurt its operations. Third, concepts relating to regulatory oversight of the health insurance business basically follow methodology that was developed for life insurance. If the uniqueness of health insurance is not recognized, it is hard to regulate risk in the industry effectively, and it is therefore difficult for the industry to meet the needs of the public.

According to China's laws and regulations, property insurance companies, life insurance companies, and specialty health insurance companies can all operate a health insurance business. This leads to rather fierce market competition. In order to expand their business and win over the market, many companies deliberately cut their premium rates, which then sometimes even go below production costs. This blind expansion of business and its resulting vicious competition seriously affect the stability of the companies involved. In addition, the existence of oligopoly in the commercial health insurance market has also exerted an important influence on the quality of supply. Although there are more than 100 insurance companies in China engaged in the health insurance business, the largest market share goes to several major players. Ping An Life Insurance, China Life Insurance, PICC Health Insurance, New China Life Insurance, and China Pacific Insurance hold approximately 70% of market share every year.

2.3 OBSTACLES AND CHALLENGES FACING CHINA'S COMMERCIAL HEALTH INSURANCE SUPPLY

Since the New Medical Reform began, supply of China's commercial health insurance has constantly increased while the quality of supply has also improved. However, this supply is affected by multiple factors. In practice, it has come up against multiple obstacles and challenges. The following section presents problems faced by the supply of commercial health insurance in China from the perspective of growing the industry, having it handle China's basic medical insurance and provide supplementary basic medical insurance, and having it extend the health industry chain.

2.3.1 Obstacles faced by the supply side of China's commercial health insurance

2.3.1.1 Supply of commercial health insurance is heavily influenced by institutional structures that govern China's medical and healthcare systems

First, certain national policies in China define the standing or role of commercial health insurance in ways that affect the scope within which the industry can operate and the spheres within which it can provide services. Meanwhile, changes in the levels of protection offered by the basic medical insurance system and changes in the administrative level at which the system is administered directly affect the supply of commercial health insurance, since it is intimately linked to these things. As an example: if basic medical insurance gradually raises the ceiling on insured costs and the percentage of expenses that can be reimbursed, that will affect the extent to which the commercial health insurance industry can continue to grow, particularly the part that supplements social security. Meanwhile, the rapid expansion of medical safeguards under the basic medical insurance system, and the way the funds are pooled and managed at a higher administrative level, also make it necessary for the insurance industry to improve its capabilities when it comes to both management and services.

Second, reforms to do with the institutional structures that govern China's medicine and healthcare systems have a profound impact on the supply of commercial health insurance. In terms of progress made by these reforms, years of structural reform have not yet resulted in a thoroughly liberalized or 'free' market in the field of medicine. On the one hand, public hospitals still monopolize the core resource, namely physicians. Their monopoly has not yet been broken, which means that doctors are unable to get market-driven salaries, medical services are not offered at market prices, and commercial insurance is kept in an environment in which it cannot operate or indeed exist. On the other hand, the massive amount of public finance that goes into the building of the basic medical insurance system further consolidates the position of non-commercial insurance as the main supplier of national medical security for citizens, leaving little room for commercial insurance to participate in reforms.

In addition, the separation of the management of pricing of medical services and the pricing of drugs should, objectively speaking, make it easier for insurance companies to control medical risks. It should encourage the infusion of social (private) capital into medical and healthcare institutions, and should provide a good investment opportunity for insurance companies as they extend the health industry chain. There is, however, considerable uncertainty about how effective this is going to be. At present, insurance companies have yet to go very far in exploring large-scale cooperation on a fundamental level with medical and healthcare institutions. In the short term, this is detrimental to the ability of health insurance companies to control medical risk. In the long term, it is also detrimental to innovation with respect to health insurance products and services and detrimental to extending the industry chain.

2.3.1.2 It is difficult to control medical risks

One outstanding feature of commercial health insurance is that insurance companies must deal with 'third-party' medical service providers in addition to those they are insuring. As 'those who put up the costs of medical treatment and services,' they also sometimes have to deal with the providers of social medical insurance. The complexity of having various parties involved in the business increases the likelihood of adverse selection and moral hazard. As mentioned earlier, within the current administrative structures that govern China's medical and healthcare systems, insurance companies stand in an inferior position with respect to medical institutions. Their negotiating abilities are particularly limited when they are up against large hospitals that never lack for patients. It is hard to create cooperative mechanisms that 'share risk and also share benefits' between insurance companies and medical institutions, and it is also hard to evaluate, monitor, and control medical risks in an effective way. Moreover, constant advances in medical technology and changes in medical measures have also increased the business risk of health insurance companies.[8]

2.3.1.3 Degree to which health insurance enjoys specialized management is low

At present, China's commercial health insurance still suffers from low or inadequate specialization. The main source of the problem lies in the fact that health insurance companies are not sufficiently aware of the underlying dynamics of health insurance. Many insurance companies in China see health insurance as marginal to their main business and, faced with the pressures of the core business, they either overlook or do not have time to research the laws that govern health insurance. They lack a clear understanding of the concepts that are involved. Given inappropriate business models, insurance companies fail to put the necessary investment into their health insurance business, particularly with regard to the collection and analysis of statistics. This in turn constrains their ability to understand the business as well as their ability to install professional management. Moreover, health insurance is a highly specialized and technical business. It requires professionals who are trained in risk management, medical services, designing of contract clauses, rating of premiums, and medical statistics and analysis. Right now, the industry does not have enough of such people.

2.3.2 Challenges faced by supply side of China's commercial health insurance

2.3.2.1 Role of commercial health insurance in developing China's medical security system

2.3.2.1.1 Supply side of commercial health insurance products

First, there is a significant gap between the supply of and the demand for commercial health insurance products. As a middle class in China emerges and the aging of the country's population accelerates, this gap becomes more and more pronounced. It manifests itself in two main ways. (1) The insufficient supply of health insurance products related to health management services makes it difficult for health insurance to meet any kind of diversified market demand. Right now, most health insurance products on the market are designed to supplement or provide an alternative to basic medical insurance products and are often offered as group insurance or insurance against critical illness. Such products offer fixed-amount payments and short-term benefits. There is a substantial need for insurance that covers large medical bills, long-term medical problems, and nursing care. (2) Products are too homogeneous and the mix of products being offered is unreasonable. Of all the health insurance products on the market, about 98% are for illness or medical services and only 2% are for such things as care giving services or insuring against loss of income due to disability. Products therefore fail to meet diversified needs.

Second, there is a lack of basic data. The lack of empirical data has been a longstanding problem that has hampered the development of health insurance in

China, however. More importantly, insurance companies lack the ability to collect and analyze data. On the one hand, they lack systematically coded data and consistent data definitions. This makes it difficult for them to classify and analyze any data that has been collected. On the other hand, they lack rigorous and effective data management systems so that data is often lost or distorted. In addition, none of the parties involved has set up effective data sharing systems— including the insurance industry, the medical sector, and the social security sector. The design of products and drawing in of preparatory funds is neither scientific nor effective.

2.3.2.1.2 *Commercial health insurance companies as providers of critical illness insurance*

Critical illness insurance is supplementary to China's foundation of basic medical insurance. As an institutional arrangement, it is highly significant in the effort to keep people from falling into poverty as a result of having to pay out high medical bills. This type of insurance is indeed meant to supplement the basic medical insurance and many success stories have emerged, but in actual implementation quite a few problems still need to be addressed as systems are improved. First, the degree of professionalism is still low. In actual implementation, insurance companies are neither sufficiently nor efficiently involved in managing the business. Some companies just follow the business model of life insurance and focus only on premiums and gaining market share. Second, some companies lack any incentive to build a real business and so find it difficult to make a profit, even a meager one. In actual practice, the rights and responsibilities for profits and losses are not given equal standing when it comes to sharing the burden, which increases the risk of losses for insurance companies. Third, the design of mechanisms that can offer real safeguards needs to be improved. In most parts of China, the pooling of funds and administration of insurance programs is done at the municipal level of government, which is too low. Meanwhile, some places have not provided any unified and explicit regulations regarding such things as standards for raising funds, level of deductibles, payment ratios, and other critical issues. This makes it hard to create systems that allow for cross-jurisdiction settlement of claims and for treating critical illness in a different jurisdiction. Finally, there are occasions when improper behavior occurs and outright transgression of laws and regulations. Some companies fraudulently report non-existent expenses; some disregard costs when bidding for contracts, thereby engaging in malicious price competition; some even seek improper profits by fraudulently using the pretext of critical illness cases.

2.3.2.1.3 *Commercial health insurance companies as handlers of basic medical insurance*

Since the New Medical Reform began, commercial health insurance has used its advantages to fulfill its role as the handler or administrative manager of basic medical insurance, effectively improving efficiencies, reducing costs, and expanding the methods by which commercial health insurance is supplied. Nevertheless, in actual practice, a whole series of problems has also emerged.

First, although the New Medical Reform was explicit in giving the orientation and ways in which commercial health insurance should participate in basic medical insurance, in actual implementation, relevant authorities and local governments have not had a very deep understanding of the spirit behind the Reform. They have been insufficiently accurate in defining the scope of government functions. They have not appreciated the role that health insurance should play in setting up a multi-tiered medical safeguards system. Accustomed to handling all types of medical insurance themselves, they have in fact excluded commercial health insurance companies from participating in the business. Objectively speaking, they have occupied the space into which commercial health insurance is meant to grow.

Second, commercial health insurance agencies lack any solid assurance that they will get paid a management services fee when they undertake to administer basic medical insurance. Some companies have no assurance that there is a source of such management fees, which greatly impacts the enthusiasm with which they participate in handling basic medical insurance.

Third, those insurance companies that include commercial health insurance in their business vary considerably in terms of business capacities and levels of professionalism. When they are entrusted with managing various types of medical safeguards, the quality of their services is undermined by the lack of uniform qualifications, operational norms, performance evaluations, and exit systems.

2.3.2.2 Role of commercial health insurance in building China's medical services system

2.3.2.2.1 Commercial health insurance companies as investors in medical institutions

By purchasing shares of medical institutions and actively participating in other forms of investment, commercial health insurance companies have been effective in extending the health industry chain. They have provided customers with a variety of health management services, and thereby improved the control of medical risks and the quality of supply. However, a whole series of problems have been found to exist in the course of such investment and share participation.

First, there are fairly high barriers to access. Medical institutions have to pass very strict government reviews before getting licensed or gaining access to medical technology or facilities. Commercial health insurance companies as investors in medical institutions find it difficult to overcome such barriers to access. The Ping An Insurance company serves as one example. Two years after signing a cooperation agreement with the Longgang District Traditional Chinese Medicine Hospital of Shenzhen, it had to drop out because of its failure to obtain market-entry approval from relevant authorities.

Second, it is hard to recruit professionals. Having a professional medical staff with rich clinical experience is crucial to the quality and competiveness of a medical institution. Under the existing management structure by which medical institutions are administered, the authorities who administer healthcare rarely consider anyone from private medical institutions when they give out promotions or approve participation in academic exchanges and so on. People who leave a public medical institution find themselves at a disadvantage when it comes to career development. As a result, public medical institutions always have the best medical staff. Again, Ping An Insurance can serve as an example. All of the medical institutions that Ping An has invested in suffer from the lack of medical professionals, without exception. Although relevant policies and measures encourage a reasonable flow of medical staff in the direction of private medical institutions, such policies and measures do not include details on how to implement the process. The unequal status of people in private and public institutions remains pronounced and this has become a bottleneck that holds back the flow of human resources.

Third, the return on investment cycle is long. The initial investment required to set up a medical institution is quite sizeable. The construction period is long and it takes a long time to realize a profit. Meanwhile, public acceptance of private medical institutions is still on the low side. For example, in 2015, China had 14,500 private hospitals. They contained 1,034 million beds, which accounted for 19.4% of the total number of inpatient beds nationwide. However, these beds only served 370 million patients that year, about 12% of total inpatients. Less than one-seventh of all patients in China chose a private hospital over a public hospital.[9] Once a medical institution that an insurance company has invested in starts to do business, it generally takes a while to begin to get brand recognition. The time required for a return on investment and the lack of public acceptance severely affect the enthusiasm of commercial insurance companies for investing in medical institutions.

2.3.2.2.2 Commercial health insurance companies as contributors to 'informatization' of China's medical reform

By participating in the process of building up the 'informatization' of China's medical reform, commercial health insurance companies have developed a key path toward improving their own professional capacities, extending the industry chain, and upgrading the quality of supply of health services. Problems these companies face in this process are as follows.

First, there are deviations from the norm when it comes to accurate understanding and operations. In some places, systems are designed as a simple replica of the manual version. After being used for a period of time, users discover that business procedures need to be improved and the software then has to be redeveloped a second time. In other places, inadequate evaluation of demand means that the software cannot meet changing needs in order to handle the health insurance business. In yet other places, the system is designed to accomplish all tasks once and for all, with no consideration given to the ever changing needs of medical insurance, including shifting management patterns, business processes, and organizational structure. In some places, the data and infrastructure of existing systems are simply discarded once a new system is built, leading to duplication of effort and the loss of important data.

Second, information systems are largely isolated from one another, and there is no effective mechanism for the sharing of information. This problem of compartmentalization is quite severe. Hospitals, social security bureaus, health administrations, civil affairs authorities, and other parties involved simply develop information systems of their own. Each party uses a different developer, a unique version of the operating system, and a distinct data type, which makes for problems when it comes to developing an interface and trying to integrate systems. In some places, systems were designed solely for the purpose of medical insurance. They failed to take changes in social insurance into account, with its need to become a single unified system in China. The isolation of such systems adds to operating costs, and leads to enormous waste as a result of redundant building. Moreover, effective ways to share information do not exist among the various entities involved, including among different social security authorities, between social security authorities and the public sector, and between social security authorities and insurance companies. The actual use of software that was developed to handle data is low.

Third, the rate at which historical data is used is low. After years of operation, medical insurance information systems have accumulated a considerable amount of historical data, which could be a valuable asset. At present, historical data is mainly used for two purposes. One is when people who are insured want to know their past history of medical insurance settlements and payments. The other is when authorities need to use statistics for making official reports. In neither case is the true value of historical data fully mined. This means that policy is often made blindly and is no more than the result of just 'scratching the head.'

Fourth, the application of information technology to the health insurance industry suffers from a lack of human and financial resources. First, there are not enough IT professionals. The lack of qualified database managers and operators makes it difficult for the industry to meet business needs, let alone keep up with the fast pace at which 'informatization' needs to be upgraded. Second, there is not enough financial support. At present, financial support for building information technology into the industry mainly comes from funds that are raised locally. Economically disadvantaged areas which are usually limited in financial resources in the first place are left out. They simply cannot meet the funding needs that are required.

2.4 INTERNATIONAL EXPERIENCE OF COMMERCIAL HEALTH INSURANCE AND LESSONS TO BE DRAWN

Each country develops systems according to its own unique characteristics when it comes to commercial health insurance. Nevertheless, evaluating the situation and some specific models around the world can provide China with an effective way to understand the supply side of commercial health insurance. This section of the study seeks to look at the issue from the perspective of actual experience. It presents an in-depth study of the international experience of supplying commercial health insurance, as a way to better guide our domestic practice.

2.4.1 International experience in developing and supplying commercial health insurance

2.4.1.1 Basic development models adopted by international community

The entire world has seen soaring healthcare costs in recent years. Three factors are believed to have played a major role, namely, the aging population, the complexity of medical services (including examination, treatment, and care), and the substantial increase in the price of healthcare related products and services. Given this, some welfare states are finding it difficult to maintain previous levels of medical safeguards. Instead, commercial health insurance is providing more supporting services. Some countries have seen commercial health insurance as a key way to reduce their social security burden and meet the needs of the elderly population for health services. The contradiction between limited levels of funding and the need for greater social security services is growing acute, given rapidly aging societies and an accelerating demand for healthcare. Internationally, governments seek to take advantage of the unique advantages of commercial health insurance—its flexibility in providing safeguards and its wide range of coverage. These things make it an ideal supplement for the inadequacies of social security systems. Commercial health insurance can be better at meeting the diversified demand of the elderly population for multi-tiered health security.

The Organization for Economic Co-operation and Development (OECD) identifies four categories of commercial health insurance, based on four different roles in the healthcare system. These are primary, duplicate, complementary and supplementary.

Primary health insurance. This is the commonly adopted model when commercial health insurance plays a dominant role in or acts in parallel to the healthcare system. It is usually found in countries that have not yet provided all citizens in the country with coverage via the public medical safeguards system. The classic example of this is found in the United States.

Duplicate health insurance, or double-layer insurance. This model allows high-income earners to purchase commercial health insurance if they wish, while also benefiting from public healthcare. The United Kingdom is the classic example of this type of insurance model.

Complementary health insurance. This model allows social health insurance programs to define deductibles, co-pays, and out-of-pocket maximums and requires citizens to pay part of the expenses. In order to cover such expenses, citizens can purchase complementary health insurance products offered by commercial insurance companies. The representative example is Germany.

Supplementary health insurance. This model provides full or partial coverage of items that are excluded or uncovered by statutory health insurance programs. Different countries with different welfare policies offer different levels of compensation. The typical example is found in Canada.

When governments intervene in providing social medical insurance, the 'fairness' aspect of such insurance is relatively greater. In contrast, the 'efficiency' aspect tends to be higher with commercial health insurance, due to market competition. Precisely because of this, all countries try to exploit the strengths of each type of insurance when designing healthcare programs. A survey of social security systems around the world shows that the majority of countries are trending in the direction of diversified welfare systems, as evidenced by such things as the following: use of both administrative and market measures, presence of both governmental and non-governmental entities, close cooperation between for-profit and not-for-profit organizations, sharing of cost burdens among family, household, enterprise, community, and government, and so on. A number of countries are in the process of diversifying their funding mechanisms. They are engaged in structural reforms that allow for multi-tiered and diversified safeguards, which also means that they are transitioning from simply 'treating illness' to 'managing health.' In doing so, they are improving the health of their citizens in a very real way.

Internationally, many insurance companies have actively participated in the building of basic medical safeguards systems as they themselves grew and took advantage of their own business expertise. On the one hand, this has given them more room to grow as they expanded business scope and provided services to more people. On the other hand, it has won them government support since it improved the operating efficiencies and results of safeguards for the elderly. This has allowed them a beneficial environment in which to exist. Focusing particularly on market entry mechanisms has been successful in raising levels of efficiency and services with respect to medical safeguard programs for the elderly. Western countries are increasingly focusing on taking advantage of market mechanisms. They are adopting methods whereby the government procures services which are provided by specialized entities and particularly by insurance companies that operate in the area of health insurance. Such services include medical safeguards for the elderly that are of a social welfare nature. Not only does this employ the technical advantages and services of such companies, and improve the level of medical services to the elderly population, but it allows for medical safeguard programs to be provided on a sustainable basis.

2.4.1.2 International experience in developing and supplying commercial health insurance

In order to take an objective look at the way commercial health insurance has developed and is supplied in other countries, the following selects three countries as case studies. The United States serves as the example for the primary health insurance model, the United Kingdom for the duplicate model, and Germany for the complementary model. We investigate the supply of commercial health insurance in each case with respect to the country's medical safeguards system, its supply situation, existing problems, reforms, and innovations.

2.4.1.2.1 United States

The United States has the world's most advanced commercial health insurance. It is also the only country among OECD countries that does not have health insurance for all citizens. Commercial health insurance plays the dominant role in America's medical safeguards system, while public safeguards are supplementary. As a result, the social and economic position of commercial health insurance is supremely important in American society. The American healthcare system (medical safeguards system) is mainly composed of the following components: social insurance programs sponsored by the government, public medical relief (aid) programs which are not insurance programs by nature, and commercial insurance programs run by private insurance companies.

2.4.1.2.1.1 OVERVIEW OF U.S. MEDICAL SAFEGUARDS SYSTEM

2.4.1.2.1.1(a) Social medical insurance

The U.S. government provides publicly funded medical safeguards only to elderly people, the disabled, the poor, military personnel, children from low-income families, and families who meet certain eligibility requirements. These safeguards not only include payment of medical fees and expenses, but also such things as supplementary income for the disabled and long-term nursing expenses for the elderly. Medical safeguards for other groups of people are managed via the commercial health insurance market.

The publicly funded medical safeguards of the U.S. system mainly include the following.

Medicare. This is a federal social insurance program ('medical care plan') for seniors (generally persons aged 65 and above) and certain disabled individuals.

Medicaid. This program ('medical relief or aid plan'] is targeted at low-income families. It is funded jointly by the federal government and states but is administered at the state level. It represents the 'final payer' in the American health insurance system.

Children's Health Insurance Program (CHIP). This serves certain children and
families who do not qualify for state Medicaid programs but who cannot
afford private coverage. It is funded by the federal government, which provides funding to the government of each state.

Military health benefits, provided through TRICARE and the Veterans Health
Administration (VHA) systems.

Health insurance benefits for American Indians, provided through the Indian
Health Service (IHS).[10]

2.4.1.2.1.1(b) Commercial health insurance

Commercial health insurance is purchased by employees, trade unions, or individuals from private insurance companies. Insurance providers include Blue
Cross and Blue Shield, a federation of health insurance organizations and companies, and other commercial insurance companies. Insurance companies take in
premium income from individuals, employers, and governments. They then pay
out compensation to the providers who have provided services to patients for
whom commercial insurance has been purchased. Healthcare providers are
responsible for providing medical and healthcare services to the insured—such
providers include doctors, health professionals, hospitals, and other medical and
healthcare organizations. These are then compensated for their services by
private insurance companies and by the government. Services include much
more than just standard items such as hospital stays, emergency procedures, diagnosis and treatment by general practitioners, prescription drugs, dental care,
ophthalmic care, physical and general exams, and other primary services; they
can also include a wide range of other things such as mental health services,
maternal and childbirth care, physiotherapy and rehabilitation, and nursing home
care. Coverage can be quite extensive in terms of services, as well as types of
people covered.

2.4.1.2.1.2 SUPPLY OF COMMERCIAL HEALTH INSURANCE IN U.S.

Let us first look at the size of the industry. Health insurance premiums in the
United States reached USD 160 billion in 2015. This represented a decline of
0.9% over the previous year. Within this amount, premiums from group health
insurance accounted for USD 101 billion, which was up by 11.2% over the
previous year, and premiums from individuals accounted for USD 58 billion,
down 13% over the previous year (see Figure 2.4).

Looking next at the reimbursement paid out by insurance companies, in 2015,
the health insurance reimbursements made by life insurance companies came to
USD 115 billion, which was a 1.5% decline over the previous year. Within this
amount, group health policies paid out USD 75 billion, while individual health
policies paid out USD 40 billion (see Figure 2.5).

Next, we look at the level of safeguards. Employer-sponsored group health
insurance and individually purchased health insurance are the two most common
forms of health insurance in the U.S. commercial health insurance market. Let

us first focus on group health insurance. Over 60% of American companies provide employer-sponsored programs, which has contributed to the prevalence of group health insurance in the country. Large employers offer much more generous plans than small- and medium-sized enterprises. All large companies with more than 1,000 employees offer health insurance to their employees, and 99% of employers with over 200 employees offer health insurance. Only 62% of small companies with less than 200 employees provide similar plans. On average, 65% of all employees are covered by group health insurance. Specifically, 66% of people working for large companies and 65% of those working for small enterprises (with 3 to 199 employees) are insured through group plans. According to statistics, about 55.1% of Americans are covered through an employer, while about 9.8% purchase health insurance directly.

Finally, let us look at individual health insurance. The individual insurance market targets self-employed individuals, retirees who are not yet eligible for Medicare, and consumer groups that are not covered through an employer. Policies are managed by insurance companies while individual insurants pay premiums and pay their own medical expenses. In the personal insurance market, risks vary by health status. Therefore, healthy consumers are considered to be low-risk groups who are allowed to pay less, while high-risk individuals need to pay more. Benefits also vary significantly according to the policy and according to the desires and needs of individual insurants.

2.4.1.2.1.3 PROBLEMS RELATING TO SUPPLY OF COMMERCIAL HEALTH INSURANCE IN U.S.

The American model sees health insurance as a special commodity whose supply and demand is regulated by the market. Medical services and insurance products are driven by profits in a free-market-style model. Insurance companies therefore attempt to expand the demand for healthcare in order to bring in more revenue and profits. This has led to an overly fast increase in national medical and healthcare costs, accompanied by constant increases in medical insurance costs. The

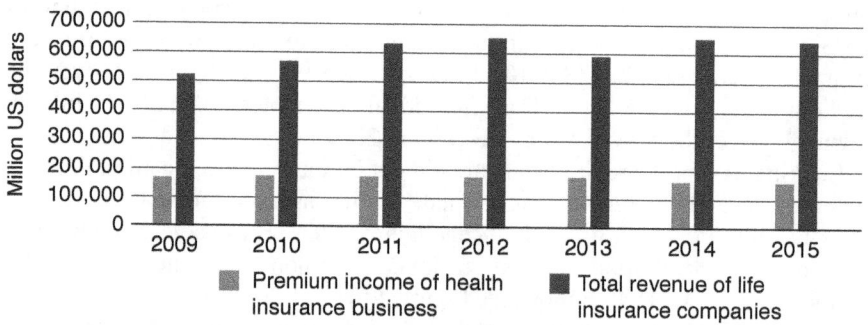

Figure 2.4 Total revenue of life insurance companies and premium income of health insurance business in the U.S. from 2009 to 2015.

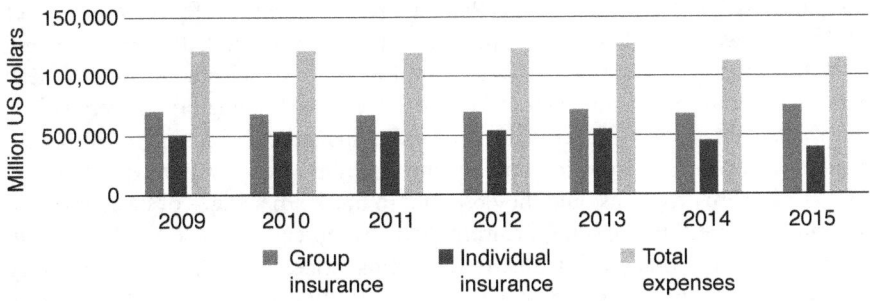

Figure 2.5 Reimbursement payments made by the health insurance business of life insurance companies in the U.S. from 2009 to 2015.

situation now poses a heavy financial burden on the government, on employers, and on individuals. Some employers and individuals have chosen to lower their level of protections in order to curb costs, which has made it ever harder for Americans to receive medical services that are commensurate with the enormously high medical costs of the system.

This model has long been criticized for its expensiveness and lack of fairness. The huge medical expenses form a sharp contrast to the fact that tens of millions of people are left unprotected. The high percentage of uninsured people, the heavy financial burden of hospital visits, and the unfair distribution of medical resources in the society are but some of the prominent social problems accompanying this model. Moreover, the failure to safeguard social fairness and the difficulty that low-income groups have in becoming insured reflect the underlying issues of unequal access to medical services and limited degree of safeguards. Those who are not insured face problems when it comes to the convenience, quality, and timeliness with which they can get medical services. Those who are insured find that premiums and the quality of medical services vary significantly.

2.4.1.2.1.4 REFORM OF COMMERCIAL HEALTH INSURANCE IN U.S.

In order to address these issues, the Obama administration enacted the Patient Protection and Affordable Care Act, often shortened to the Affordable Care Act (ACA) in 2010. This initiated reform of the health insurance system and of healthcare in general. Aspects relating to commercial health insurance included the following. First, basic medical insurance plans could now be offered by private insurers. Private insurance entities could act as third-party purchasers of insurance. They could carry out detailed management and oversight of medical services, which helped with issues that traditional medical care programs were facing such as the lack of preventive healthcare, excessive medical treatment, and the absence of clinical accountability. As a result, they were helpful in controlling inflated medical expenses. Second, mandatory insurance provisions were introduced. According to the Patient Protection and Affordable Care Act [PPACA], passed in 2010, mandatory provisions were added to regulate the basic healthcare transactions between applicants and private insurers. These included requirements on mandatory purchases and mandatory underwriting. Third, the Act set up the creation of health insurance exchanges. These set standard rules for underwriting and pricing. They pushed for standardization of basic healthcare programs, and they brought to market packages of basic medical programs offered by private insurers, which increased market competition. Fourth, the Act adopted mechanisms for setting prices according to community rates when offering basic medical insurance. Putting this into implementation expanded the extent to which healthy people provide support to those who are sick. This was helpful when it came to gaining full coverage for basic medical insurance for everyone in the country.

The implementation of Obamacare resulted in a significant reduction in the number of uninsured people in the low- and middle-income brackets. It also meant that commercial health insurance was now constantly increasing in size and scope of coverage. According to statistics of the U.S. Census Bureau, the number of uninsured people fell from 48.6 million in 2009, or 15.7% of the total population, to below 30 million in 2016, or 8.6% of the total population. However, the reform still faces many difficulties. In 2015, overall healthcare spending reached USD 3.2 trillion and accounted for 17.8% of GDP. Average spending per capita came to USD 9,990, much higher than that of other developed countries. In 2016, the federal government spent more than USD 1 trillion on health insurance, or 28% of total federal expenditures, and this percentage keeps going up. Moreover, because of the stricter regulatory provisions that Obamacare has imposed on insurance companies, many insurers have stopped offering certain programs. This has forced applicants to choose alternative plans that might have higher premiums. Premiums rose by 7.5% in 2016 over 2015, and are expected to rise by another 25% in 2017.[11]

Opponents have long used soaring premiums and increased taxes as the main reasons to attack Obamacare. In essence, however, the real things that have set the stage for the 'failure' of Obamacare have been funding deficiencies and problems with compensation plans. As the U.S. presidential election came to an end, on assuming the Presidency, Mr. Trump targeted his first executive order ('administrative order') at Obamacare. Procedures for repealing the Act have already begun. On March 6, 2017, the Republicans publicly released the *American Health Care Act*, aimed at repealing and replacing Obamacare. This subsequently passed the House Ways and Means Committee and the House Energy and Commerce Committee.

As Trump sees it, the ideal healthcare system is not only 'affordable' but also offers 'options.' To him, the essence of Obamacare lies in placing constraints on the buying side and forcing the public to buy health insurance that has been approved by the government. In Trump's view, this is the wrong direction and Obamacare 'just doesn't work.' Therefore, Trump plans to replace subsidies that primarily benefit low-income households with tax deductions and expanded Health Savings Accounts to increase the purchasing power of individuals so that they can freely choose whatever insurance products they like in the market. However, in actual implementation, these measures face a series of problems as well. For low-income and high-risk groups, it is very difficult to purchase affordable insurance products in a competitive market. Although President Trump was willing to keep parts of Obamacare, including requiring insurers to accept all applicants and charge the same rates regardless of pre-existing conditions, banning annual and lifetime coverage caps on essential benefits, and allowing young adults under 26 to be insured on their parents' policies, in point of fact only people with incomes of over USD 75,000 per year could be expected to enjoy the tax refund policy. Moreover, the new Act allows insurance companies to charge elderly customers up to five times as much as younger customers (while Obamacare only allowed up to three times). The new Act also proposes that federal funds that the national government gives to states as a supplement for Medicaid should no longer be granted on the previous basis of matching funds for anyone who qualifies. Instead, funds would be granted to states on a capped, per-capita basis. This change might well relieve the financial burden on the government but it may also lead to fewer Medicaid beneficiaries.[12]

Generally speaking, given the efforts of the Obama administration, the United States finally, to a certain degree, realized the ideal of universal health insurance that had been sought by eight previous presidents. However, controversy accompanied the reform from the start of the legislation. Trump's open attack has only added further uncertainty to the U.S. health insurance system.

2.4.1.2.2 United Kingdom

The United Kingdom presents the classic example of a 'duplicate health insurance model' or 'double-layer' insurance. The insurance system is mainly financed by national tax revenues. Medical expenses of individuals and medical service institutions are ultimately funded through disbursements from the national budget.

2.4.1.2.2.1 OVERVIEW OF HEALTH SAFEGUARDS IN THE UK

In 1948, England promulgated the *National Health Services Act*. This then created the National Health Service (NHS), which was financed by the government and given responsibility for managing national healthcare. The NHS provides medical coverage for the entire UK population. In the early 1990s, a healthcare reform in the UK introduced commercial capital into the system and the government became both the provider and the purchaser of health services. Although the great majority of services and medicines are provided for free, 12% of the UK population (about 7.3 million people) purchases commercial health insurance so as to enjoy the better medical services offered by private medical institutions.

2.4.1.2.2.1(a) National Health Service (NHS)

The Beveridge Report, first published in 1942, recommended that the UK government establish a comprehensive social insurance system and a national health insurance system to protect every citizen from poverty or the lack of medical treatment due to want, disease, or unemployment. The NHS bill was formally proposed in 1944 and the National Health Service Act was enacted some time later. The UK proceeded to enact the Family Allowances Act in 1945, the National Insurance Act in 1946, and the National Assistance Act in 1948, which enabled the country to set up and continue to develop what was then one of the best social security systems in the western world.

2.4.1.2.2.1(b) Commercial health insurance

Private medical insurance is also known as supplementary voluntary health insurance (VHI) in the United Kingdom. In the 1990s, commercial insurers began to enter this business arena. There are three main types of VHI, namely complementary voluntary health insurance, substitutive voluntary health insurance, and supplementary voluntary health insurance.

Complementary VHI is complementary to the inadequacies of a public health-care system in terms of sufficient coverage or protection. It covers certain medical services that are not included in public healthcare programs. An example would be dental care, which is provided by the public system in the Netherlands and Spain.

Substitutive VHI provides coverage for groups not included in the public health-care system, such as those whose annual income disqualifies them from social security. This type of VHI can be found in Germany, the Netherlands, and the United States.

Supplementary VHI is an optional form of private health insurance. When services in the public health system do not meet their expectations, some people opt for supplementary VHI products to have access to better medical services. This is the most commonly adopted pattern in the United Kingdom. There are many reasons for dissatisfaction with public healthcare safeguards, including low-quality services and long waiting lists. These have spurred the rapid development of supplementary VHI. Different VHI programs offer different services at different levels for premiums that vary in price.

In the United Kingdom, private medical insurance can be further divided into three categories according to the coverage of services, namely, comprehensive policies, standard policies, and budget policies.

As the most expensive type, comprehensive policies offer a wide range of benefits such as outpatient services and other medical services in addition to the normal core services.

Standard policies are less expensive but only offer limited services besides the core benefits. They generally do not cover mental illness, complications in pregnancy and childbirth, ophthalmic care, or emergency treatment. Such policies may also have restrictions on the choice of hospitals and certain hospital charges or inpatient services.

Budget policies are the cheapest and offer a limited range of benefits with possibly more restrictions. Some budget policies add restrictions on expensive medical services, including most inpatient and day care services. Most budget policies limit applicants' choice of hospitals and hospital accommodations.[13]

2.4.1.2.2.2 SUPPLY OF COMMERCIAL HEALTH INSURANCE IN THE UK

Let us first look at the suppliers. Of all the insurers in the private medical insurance market in the UK, 19 offer private medical insurance products, 8 do not offer such products but provide underwriting services for those without independent underwriting capacity, 4 offer both private medical insurance products and underwriting services, and 15 do not have an independent underwriting capacity. Therefore, the entire market has 42 suppliers and most of the major companies are product providers.

Second, we look at the scope of coverage. As the quality of the UK's basic medical safeguards has gradually improved, patients' and insurants' satisfaction with the public system has risen significantly. This has further narrowed the business space for complementary medical safeguards and reduced the coverage of the health insurance industry. Since 2008, there has been a steady decline of commercial health insurance applicants in terms of percentage of the total UK population. In 2012, the figure was only 6.3%. The percentage of health insurance beneficiaries in the total UK population went from 9.01% in 2011, to 8.79% in 2012, and 7.96% in 2013, down by one percentage point in just two years (see Figure 2.6).

Third, let us look at market share. Provident companies and commercial companies each take roughly half the market. At the outset, private medical

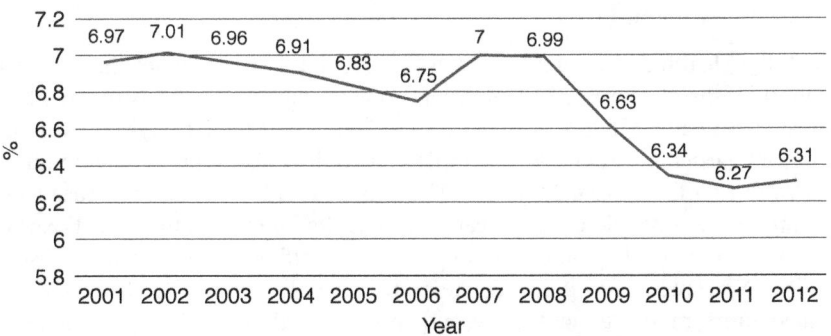

Figure 2.6 UK commercial health insurance applicants as percentage of total population.

insurance was mainly provided by provident companies. The 1990s was an important period for the development of private medical insurance as commercial companies entered the market, initially taking about 9% of the market share. By early 1998, this had risen 22% and by now has reached roughly 50%.

Fourth, we look at methods of supply. Private medical insurance can be sold directly through insurance companies and indirectly through specialized intermediary agencies. The over 100 intermediaries are the major players in the group insurance market, taking 74% of the market share. In the individual insurance market, many private medical insurance providers are capable of providing potential customers with quotations online, using sex, age, and other customer-provided factors as the basis for formulating price quotations. Today there are about 3,000 intermediaries selling private medical insurance in this market—they are mostly general insurance brokers or financial advisers.

2.4.1.2.2.3 PROBLEMS WITH SUPPLY OF COMMERCIAL HEALTH INSURANCE IN UK

The crux of the problem with the UK's supply of commercial health insurance lies in the medical safeguards system. The aim of the UK model was to set up a welfare type of system that provided coverage to all people. A host of problems appeared in the course of actually operating this system, however. First, the cost of healthcare and medical services has risen sharply. A medical system that relies on high tax revenues has become an onerous burden on citizens, particularly as the population ages at an accelerating rate. Second, the allocation of health resources is done through a system that relies heavily on planning as opposed to the market. This limits the role of market mechanisms, reduces the vitality of the healthcare system, and leads to an inefficient supply of medical services and a failure to meet people's needs for medical insurance. Finally, it is difficult to guarantee the quality of medical services provided by the national health insurance system. Medical scandals have become a frequent occurrence.

2.4.1.2.2.4 REFORMS AND INNOVATIONS RELATING TO COMMERCIAL HEALTH INSURANCE IN UK

In 2012, the Health and Social Care Act was signed into law under the impetus of support by the Cameron administration. This provides for what is regarded as the most significant 'Medical Reform' in the UK since the NHS system was set up 60 years earlier. Currently being implemented, it is also seen as a summation of the reforms of the past 20 years. The Cameron administration focused on reforming the supply side of healthcare services. Its intent was to control excessive growth in medical spending by improving the efficiency and quality of services. Specific measures were concentrated mainly in two areas. First, it delegated more budgetary authority and drug-prescribing authority to general practitioners so that they would come up with the most cost-effective treatments. In so doing, it sought to shift risks that the government had previously borne directly onto general practitioners. Second, it incorporated more private service providers into the National Health Service in order to reduce the role that government played in the medical safeguards system. It pushed for a greater separation of authority between providers of medical services and the authorities overseeing the system. The hope is that the introduction of competitive mechanisms will inject vitality into the NHS and help further separate its administration from actual implementation in the medical service system. Moreover, the Cameron administration proposed to establish a National Health Service Commissioning Board that would carry out regulatory supervision of general practitioners as well as health service providers. It also would determine rules and regulations on market entry and exit. Shifting these responsibilities from the government to such a Commission Board is intended to further separate out government administration from actual handling of the business.

2.4.1.2.3 Germany

Germany is the birthplace of the modern social insurance system. In 1883, the Medical Insurance Bill mandated that salaried workers and employees below a certain income threshold automatically had to be enrolled in a critical illness plan, funded by both employers and employees. This marked the formal establishment of the world's first compulsory medical insurance system that carried with it certain aspects of social security. Since then, medical insurance has become a widely accepted concept. In 2012, 11.3% of Germany's GDP was spent on healthcare, the equivalent of USD 4,496 per capita. In terms of the funding of healthcare in Germany, social or publicly funded insurance accounted for 76.5% in 2012, while commercial insurance accounted for 10.3%.

2.4.1.2.3.1 OVERVIEW OF HEALTH INSURANCE IN GERMANY

The overall framework for health insurance in Germany includes statutory medical insurance and commercial health insurance that operate in tandem. The legally mandated type of insurance is primary while the safeguards system that people may choose if they want is secondary. Statutory health insurance is composed of two parts, insurance for critical illness and insurance for nursing care. Commercial health insurance includes four main categories, namely comprehensive health insurance, long-term care insurance, additional insurance, and special insurance. The mandatory system covers 89% of the population, on top of which is the role played by commercial health insurance. The result is that the German system in its entirety provides coverage for more than 99% of the German population.[14]

2.4.1.2.3.2 SUPPLY OF COMMERCIAL HEALTH INSURANCE IN GERMANY

Let us first look at the suppliers. Of all insurance companies in the German market, 47 offer commercial health insurance. Listed in order of premium income, DKV is the market leader, followed by Debeka and Allianz. These three insurers hold over 38% of market share.

In terms of the scale of suppliers, Germany's health insurance market offers a variety of products and large companies sometimes provide a dozen or dozens of programs. The many programs mainly fall under four categories, however, namely comprehensive health insurance, long-term care insurance, additional insurance, and special insurance. According to statistics of German Insurance Association (GDV) (2012), the premium income of commercial health insurance and long-term care insurance reached 34.6 billion euros in 2011, up by 4.2% over 2010. Of this amount, comprehensive insurance maintained a 72.5% share, without any change, while supplementary insurance continued to maintain 19.3%. The figure for supplementary drops to 13%, however, if you include only what is covered by social health insurance.

The rest of Germany's premium income goes to long-term care insurance and special insurance (such as overseas travel insurance), accounting for 6.1% and 2.1% respectively. The reason the overall premium income has risen relates to two factors, namely the growing number of applicants for comprehensive insurance and the slightly slower rate at which premiums are increased. The premium income of long-term care insurance (including common and supplementary long-term care) rose by 0.4%, and has recently surpassed the figure of 2.1 billion euros.

While the premium income rises annually, so do the costs paid out by commercial health insurance. According to statistics of GDV (2012), overall costs paid out by commercial health insurance, excluding long-term care, reached 22.05 billion euros in 2011. This was up by 6.1% from 21.22 billion euros in 2010. Expenditures paid out just for long-term care insurance rose steadily to 720 million euros in 2011, up by 3.1% from 2010.

Let us move to the coverage of health insurance in Germany. Commercial health insurance covers 32% of the population and accounts for 10.3% of health finance in the country. Laws and regulations in Germany require that health insurance be operated separately from life insurance. As independent insurers, commercial health insurance companies may be engaged in any health insurance business that they consider appropriate and profitable as permitted by law.

2.4.1.2.3.3 PROBLEMS WITH SUPPLY OF COMMERCIAL HEALTH INSURANCE IN GERMANY

Various problems in the medical safeguards system are impacting the quality of the supply of commercial health insurance in the country. In overall terms, these are expressed as follows. First, medical insurance funds operate on a system of pay-as-you-go, that is, current income is paid out for current expenses. In the longer term, given the aging of the population, this is creating an insufficiency of reserves and may lead to a potential payment crisis. Second, family members of qualifying employees also enjoy coverage under the employee's policy, which can easily lead to rapid escalation of medical costs. Third, employers are required by law to cover employees, and their constantly increasing costs add to their cost of labor. This puts them at a disadvantage with respect to competitors in the midst of fierce international competition. Fourth, the separation of statutory health insurance and commercial health insurance increases the likelihood that high-income earners are able to evade social responsibility.

2.4.1.2.3.4 COMMERCIAL HEALTH INSURANCE REFORM AND INNOVATION IN GERMANY

First, Germany has adopted mandatory insurance. The 2009 *Statutory Health Insurance Competition Act* includes commercial health insurance companies in the category of 'statutory insurers.' They are obliged to provide basic medical safeguard contracts for all income groups. They provide an inexpensive 'basic rate' to commercial insurance contracts to protect low-income insurants.

Second, Germany has set up a clearing house for statutory health insurance. Starting on January 1, 2009, the German government instituted a 'central healthcare fund' at the national level. This formulates statutory health insurance premiums on a unified basis and thereby increases the coordination and funding cooperation among different critical illness foundations.

Third, Germany has instituted group bargaining between insurers and medical institutions. Representing all health insurance companies in Germany, the Health Insurance Industry Association engages in group bargaining with hospital associations, physicians' associations, pharmaceutical companies, and other interest groups on issues related to the pricing, standards, and quality of drugs and medical services, in order to better protect the interests of policy holders.

2.4.2 Lessons to be learned from international experience

The following lessons can be drawn from our study of the supply of commercial health insurance in the United States, the United Kingdom, and Germany, and from the reforms and innovations adopted by those countries.

2.4.2.1 *Excellent top-level institutional design is prerequisite for improving supply of commercial health insurance*

Healthcare is vital for the wellbeing of the entire population. International practice shows that many countries have come to the same conclusion—the best course is to set up a system with different kinds of medical safeguards that is multi-tiered and has a variety of policies and programs. Commercial health insurance occupies a critical position and plays a key role in this system, whether a given country relies more on publicly funded insurance or on private insurance. It is an effective way to ameliorate the financial pressures being felt by advanced countries in their medical insurance systems, and it also presents a pathway by which developing countries can improve upon their own systems.

The development of commercial health insurance in any country inevitably requires a legal or policy framework that clearly defines the status and role of commercial health insurance and public medical insurance in the national healthcare system as well as the scope of coverage, nature of competition, and policy incentives allocated to the commercial and the public systems. Without such clarity, it is difficult for commercial health insurance and public medical insurance to assume their proper responsibilities and take advantage of their own strengths, while complementing each other effectively and reinforcing each other in the overall system.

2.4.2.2 Specialization is only way forward for commercial health insurance

Health insurance is governed by a unique set of laws in terms of actuarial pricing, product design, underwriting of claims settlement, and customer services, which makes it different from other types of insurance. Meanwhile, health insurance involves a variety of entities including insurance companies, policy holders, medical institutions, and social security authorities. It faces many different kinds of risk: soaring medical expenses, the imbalance of power and information asymmetry between hospitals and insurance companies, the adverse selection and moral hazard incurred by policy holders, and policy changes given the restructuring of the national healthcare system. All of these things mean that health insurance is vastly more challenging than other kinds of insurance, and as a result specialization is an inevitable trend.

In developed countries, general insurance companies are evolving into specialized entities due to fierce market competition. Comprehensive insurance companies gradually divide out into two main types of company, namely life insurance companies and property insurance companies. Life insurance companies cover life insurance, annuities, and health insurance, while property insurance companies cover property and casualty insurance. The growth of life insurance has slowed due to saturation of the market, including the personal financial services market. In contrast, health insurance has maintained consistently rapid growth for some time, due to such things as an aging population and advances in medical technology. As a result, some companies have shifted their main focus to health insurance. Separate from life insurance, annuities, and so on, health insurance has gradually been set up as its own specialized business. As an example, in 2004, the American company Cigna announced a restructuring of its business lines, with the intent to focus on medical and health fields as the core business. Germany has a system in which social insurance is primary, and laws already mandate that only specialized insurance companies are allowed to provide health insurance.

2.4.2.3 Support from fiscal and tax policy is general practice in many countries

Health insurance is globally acknowledged to be a highly difficult enterprise. Problems include risk mitigation, the need for specialized technology, thin profit margins, and long investment cycles. To a certain extent, these things have undermined the sound development and proper functioning of the business.

Because of its nature as a quasi-public good and its irreplaceable role in providing multi-tiered healthcare for the public, commercial health insurance generally enjoys policy support in many countries. The most important method by which such support is realized is through tax policies. Most developed and developing countries, such as the United States, France, Germany, Australia, and South Africa, provide tax incentives for commercial health insurance policy holders and companies. Although tax relief and subsidies may reduce the current fiscal revenues and tax income, in the long run they also alleviate the pressure on a country's basic medical insurance spending. They meet the higher demands on healthcare of some corporate groups and special groups, they facilitate the establishment and development of the national healthcare system, and they serve the long-term interests of a country and its people.

2.4.2.4 *Effective management of and control of medical expenses are key to smooth development of health insurance*

The medical services market has long been considered a place of concentrated risk, with transactions that are highly susceptible to moral hazard and adverse selection. The complexity of medical behaviors poses a great challenge to health insurance risk control. An insurance company, as a third-party payer who is independent of the doctor–patient relationship, must establish mechanisms that constrain the interests of both doctors and patients and must also provide quantitative and qualitative controls over medical services. It can be said that the key links in ensuring smooth growth of health insurance are a sound medical services market but also effective controls over medical spending.

2.4.2.5 *One important part of commercial health insurance operations involves meeting demand of customers for multi-tiered health insurance, in addition to providing comprehensive healthcare services*

The traditional definition of health insurance included such things as safeguards for critical illness, hospital fees, outpatient fees, long-term nursing care, and loss of income due to disability. In recent years, commercial health insurance companies in developed countries have added to that list. They now generally bundle health insurance services together with health management services. They provide comprehensive health safeguards services that include such things as health consulting, faster access to medical attention, management of health funds, and so on. This is aimed at satisfying a multi-tiered kind of demand for health safeguards.

2.4.2.6 Health insurance is important component of health services industry and crucial 'integrator' of the industry chain

In developed countries, commercial health insurance is assigned an important position in the healthcare industry due to its role as the provider of financial support and the link between the supply side and the demand side. A more developed health industry has a key role to play in protecting citizens' right to health, driving economic growth, optimizing the economic structure, and enhancing comprehensive national strength and international competitiveness.

2.5 POLICY RECOMMENDATIONS FOR IMPROVING SUPPLY OF COMMERCIAL HEALTH INSURANCE IN CHINA

As we seek to improve the quality of the supply side of commercial health insurance in China, our most urgent task is to find an operating model that meets China's needs by combining international experience with our domestic situation. The basis for this model will be a general framework that incorporates commercial health insurance into the basic medical safeguards system (social security) and the medical services system (hospitals). That will mean integrating commercial health insurance as a supplement to basic medical insurance and having it 'handle' basic medical insurance. It will require breaking through the obstacles and challenges that commercial health insurance faces in the actual practice of expanding the health industry chain. It will also require making breakthroughs in the legal and regulatory system and the policy system in ways that are feasible, i.e. that have a strong chance of succeeding. Specific recommendations are as follows.

2.5.1 Enduring ways to improve quality of supply of commercial health insurance in China

2.5.1.1 Clarify specific actions by which commercial health insurance can better serve overall medical reform

Top-level design is crucial for improving and expanding the supply of commercial health insurance in China. We must strengthen top-level design in order to make sure that commercial health insurance has a more powerful role to play in the healthcare system. That involves defining the boundary between government and market more explicitly, and making commercial health insurance serve the interests of the overall healthcare reform. Each of those is described below.

2.5.1.1.1 Further strengthen role and positioning of commercial health insurance in medical safeguards system

Improving the quality of the supply of commercial health insurance will require a forceful 'top-level design.' Such design must set up effective coordinating mechanisms that transcend the interests of different departments. It must be proactive, visionary, and systematic in its planning so as to change in a fundamental way the fragmented and compartmentalized way in which the situation is currently developing. The planning should address the role and positioning that commercial health insurance is to play in the future. Commercial health insurance is in no way merely a limited and simple kind of supplement to China's social basic medical insurance. Instead, it must become an essential component of China's medical safeguards system. As such, its role should include the following three aspects: serving as the major provider of supplementary health insurance, serving as the major 'handler' of China's basic medical insurance, and serving as the integrator of the healthcare industry chain. Commercial health insurance companies should become a true 'value creator' in the building of a sound and well-functioning national healthcare system, thereby making its proper contribution to the social and economic development of the country.

2.5.1.1.2 *Further define boundary between government and market and better serve overall healthcare reform*

Expanding the supply of commercial health insurance in China and improving the quality of that supply must be a process that adheres strictly to 'having two hands work together.' In other words, the government and the market must play their respective roles to ensure that publicly funded insurance and commercial insurance complement each other and serve the interests of China's overall healthcare reform. First, this means adhering to the principle that 'government safeguards the basics while the market provides diversity and multitiered options.' This means going further in clarifying that 'the basics' means giving priority to 'fundamental needs' and ensuring 'fundamental standards,' given that social resources are limited for funding basic medical insurance. Through 'marketized' measures, commercial health insurance then must step in to satisfy people's needs for diversified and multi-tiered healthcare safeguards. Second, this means adhering to the principle that 'government ensures fairness, market realizes efficiency.' It means supporting the roles of both social insurance and commercial insurance in ways that allow the power of government actions to be in sync with market measures such that social insurance and commercial insurance cooperate closely. All parties must share the burden of raising funds for healthcare and bearing the attendant risks, including the government, public insurance, commercial insurance, employers, employees, individuals, and households. Third, this means adhering to the idea that efficiencies serve to achieve a higher fairness. By having commercial health insurance entities handle China's basic medical insurance, the aim is to lower operating costs, raise efficiencies and the quality of services, expand the effective use of funds, develop innovative social governance methods, promote a transformation of government functions and, ultimately, achieve a more cost-effective and beneficial healthcare system.

2.5.1.2 Further open commercial health insurance sector to outside investors

2.5.1.2.1 Increase extent to which commercial health insurance sector is open to outside investment

The prerequisite for gradually raising the level of openness in the commercial health insurance sector is better top-level design with a deeply researched master plan that ensures that the commercial health insurance sector opens to the outside world in line with the overall pace of the insurance industry.

2.5.1.2.2 Increase force of innovative reforms in commercial health insurance sector

We should encourage foreign insurance companies to play a bigger role in accelerating reform and innovation in the commercial health insurance sector. This has to do with the key aspects of carrying forward market-oriented reform in general, adopting innovative business models and deepening availability of services. We should also encourage foreign companies to play a bigger role in the development of China's medical safeguards system (insurance) and medical services system (hospitals and medical care).

2.5.1.3 Actively promote professional development of health insurance industry

2.5.1.3.1 Establish specialized health insurance companies

Regulatory authorities should encourage large insurance groups, capital from the healthcare services industry, and foreign health insurance companies to set up specialized health insurance companies in China. These should be encouraged to provide support for the development of different types of specialized health insurers. We should explore the possibility of introducing health management organizations and other innovative organizational forms so as to have a greater abundance of health insurance providers and to upgrade their degree of specialization and high-quality services.

2.5.1.3.2 Formulate systems that apply specifically to underwriting and claims

In terms of underwriting, uniform business standards should be established and applied, including codes for critical illness and surgical procedures, codes for providers of medical services and their specific services, and standards for statistical analysis and information retrieval. A business coding system that applies across the industry should be designed and put into use at the appropriate time. Physical examinations and health examinations should be underwritten to a reasonable degree in order to prevent adverse selection, and in order to reduce the incidence of diseases and improve the stability of the health insurance business. In terms of managing claims settlement, we should explicitly define the authorities of those entities that reimburse claims at different levels of government. We should implement a system whereby those who overstep their authority or try to get around regulations are subjected to a review process. Records on claims should be assembled and recorded, and a system should be set up whereby any large and difficult cases are subject to discussion so as to improve the degree to which claims management is scientific and reasonable.

2.5.1.3.3 Build professional risk control system

In view of the unique reliance of commercial health insurance on actuarial methods, the government should encourage insurers to establish professional pricing and actuarial evaluation systems. Insurers should collect actuarial data promptly so as to determine premiums for health insurance products more accurately and to mitigate risks associated with product development. At the same time, a risk control system should be established that covers the whole process from sales, underwriting, and day-to-day management to claims and customer services. Medical insurance should play the role of the neutral third party in curbing medical overspending and improving operational efficiency.

2.5.1.3.4 Set up professional teams

Human resources are the core competitive strength of any industry as it develops. In the commercial health insurance business, professionals are vital to improving the quality of results. They are also crucial for improving the supply of commercial health insurance. First, insurers should be encouraged to establish their own 'talent incubators' where health insurance specialists are trained through professional programs and rewarded for their professional competence through performance evaluation and promotion mechanisms. Second, we should encourage the establishment of a multi-tiered training system for professionals. In this, relevant educational units, research institutions, and business entities should play the dominant role while specialized management agencies or associations provide assistance. Third, in a targeted way, we should attempt to attract professionals into the health insurance sector from both inside and outside the country.

2.5.1.4 Establish long-term partnerships with medical institutions

Commercial health insurance has to do with three separate parties: insurance companies, those being insured, and third-party medical institutions. Therefore, it is highly significant that we establish solid partnerships between medical institutions and insurance companies in order to improve the supply of commercial health insurance in the country. The partnerships should feature a new form of relationship that involves mutual trust and mutual supervision. The tripartite alliance of medical insurance, pharmaceuticals, and the medical profession should contribute to realizing the goals of China's overall medical reform—this is highly significant in terms of improving the supply of commercial health insurance.

2.5.1.4.1 Encourage third-party payment mechanisms to play bigger role

We should encourage commercial health insurance companies to better leverage their 'group purchase' advantages and expertise, especially as such companies serve as 'handlers' of China's basic medical insurance and providers of its critical illness insurance. As representatives of those who are being insured, such companies should strengthen controls over the fees for medical services and pharmaceuticals. They should increase the efficiency with which basic medical insurance funds are used. They should ensure that limited funds are used more effectively. The government should support commercial insurance companies as they enter into the processes of evaluating and monitoring the quality of hospitals and setting prices for medical services. The aim should always be to improve the quality and lower the costs of medical services.

2.5.1.4.2 Encourage commercial health insurance companies to join in fight against medical fraud

At present, out-of-town (cross-jurisdiction) medical treatment has become a commonly abused arena for medical fraud. The government should encourage commercial health insurance companies to make good use of their national network to strengthen protections against this kind of behavior. Insurance companies should work closely with healthcare authorities to increase punishments for such things as falsifying medical records and creating fake receipts in order to get insurance reimbursements. They should work together to form effective deterrence mechanisms.

2.5.1.4.3 Support participation of commercial health insurance companies in reforms regarding method of payment

Strictly under the premise that standards of service for people being insured must be maintained, the government should support having commercial health insurance companies participate in the reform of how payment is calculated. The aim is to curb soaring medical spending by having the current multiple ways of figuring payment, including by headcount, by type of illness, by days in the hospital, and so on, be combined into a composite form of payment calculation. The aim also is to use reform of payment methods to help transform the behavior of medical institutions. From behavior that is determined mainly by evaluations and external monitoring it should shift more toward internally determined motivations such as forming standard business practices, controlling costs, taking in patients for treatment on a reasonable basis, and referring patients for rational reasons.

2.5.2 Specific measures for improving supply of commercial health insurance

2.5.2.1 With regard to participating in building of healthcare system

2.5.2.1.1 Supply of commercial health insurance products

We should encourage product innovation in order to build a system that meets people's needs for multi-tiered healthcare safeguards. Commercial health insurance should be able to offer products that meet different needs for services, and moreover the rates for those services should accommodate differing abilities to pay. Given that there is a strong tendency toward adverse selection in the demand for health insurance, commercial health insurance products should be designed to target specific groups quite accurately. Premium rates should be determined scientifically, and product offerings should be accompanied by effective risk-control measures.

First, we should encourage commercial health insurance companies to increase their degree of market penetration by offering products that are appropriate for different regions, levels of income, age groups, and social groups. Second, we should encourage companies to formulate product-development strategies that are scientifically based and come up with things that are easily marketable. Companies should develop products that target special-needs medical cases, pharmaceuticals, medical equipment, and examination and diagnostic services. They should offer insurance products that cover adverse reaction to medicines and that cover preventive services. They should develop products that integrate health insurance and health services, such as medical care, nursing care, rehabilitation, and care giving for the elderly. At the same time, products should be upgraded and adjusted in a timely manner, given the changing policy environment for medicine and the likelihood of changing policies regarding medical insurance. Third, we should encourage the creation of a platform that accommodates the demand for diversified services and safeguards in the market. We should also formulate and implement standards that cover healthcare services and that standardize services and processes. The industry should seek to make use of its specialized technology to provide healthcare planning, handling, and management services for corporate groups and social insurance departments (government authorities handling social security).

Further, we should encourage commercial health insurers to strengthen management practices over healthcare and medical costs. Expanding and improving upon the supply of commercial health insurance necessarily calls for better management of healthcare costs, mitigation of business risks, and reduced operational costs for insurers. In the first place, this means strengthening controls over medical institutions. Insurers can strengthen their partnership with medical institutions by such methods as signing cooperative agreements or investing in medical institutions while still controlling their own operating risks. By setting up certain systems, insurers can improve their ability to control healthcare and medical costs—these include systems for monitoring medical services, for overseeing how medical services are being used, for standardizing second-party opinions on diagnosis and treatment, and for providing supervisory oversight of medical institutions. In the second place, this means strengthening management with respect to policy holders. Insurers can improve their ability to control risk by a variety of means, including providing services to policy holders such as health evaluations, health advising, management of chronic conditions, and health education. They can effectively manage the daily health conditions of people who are insured through these means, and thereby reduce the likelihood of high-cost medical events and therefore medical spending. Insurers can implement control measures that evaluate customer quality in terms of the possibility of adverse selection and moral hazard. They can set up 'blacklists' with respect to the honesty of customers, that record those who submit reports that are fraudulent, or who supply false health information, who cheat the reimbursement system, and so on. They can also gradually share this information with others in the industry.

2.5.2.1.2 Commercial health insurance companies as providers of critical illness insurance

Critical illness insurance is an important systemic innovation for dealing with the problem of poverty that is brought on by illness. A large amount of data confirms the success of this approach. In order to be able to take on the task of providing insurance for critical illness, insurance companies must first pay attention to the following aspects. First, they should improve their ability to 'handle' the business of critical illness insurance. We should encourage the industry to go further in improving its actuarial models and establishing reasonable pricing and policy plans. The industry should set up a well-functioning information management system that effectively allows for and integrates customer management, compensation settlement, 'smart' audits, medical behavior monitoring, customer service, statistical analysis, and data mining. This system should be integrated with that of China's basic medical insurance so as to provide one-stop real-time settlement. Insurers should be able to provide critical illness insurance and basic medical insurance through a shared business channel so that the two types of insurance can complement each other and bring convenience to the public through streamlined reimbursement procedures. Insurers should strengthen risk control. Inspection tours, professional auditing, systemic monitoring, and payment reform are some of the recommended measures for curbing dishonest medical behavior and medical overspending, together with independent accounting, strict control of costs and expenses, and proper management of operating profits. Finally, insurers should strengthen their institution building and reduce their institutional costs of handling critical illness insurance. They should constantly seek to improve the mechanisms whereby they provide critical illness insurance. They should standardize the administrative level at which funds for such insurance are pooled and managed. They should set up sound and stable mechanisms for public-finance inputs into the funds, in order to help the industry emerge from the passive position of having to operate at a loss.

2.5.2.1.3 Commercial health insurance companies as handlers of basic medical insurance

We should vigorously promote the major trend to have commercial health insurance play a bigger role in transforming government functions as government turns more toward procurement of services. The insurance industry should further leverage its strengths and advantages, provide more in-depth services for a larger customer base, by handling China's basic medical insurance system. First, insurers should better utilize their comparative advantages. Commercial health insurance companies should fulfill their obligation of monitoring medical behaviors, optimizing the efficiency with which medical resources are used, helping ensure the sound and proper use of medical insurance funds, and improving the management efficiency and service quality of the healthcare system. Second, insurers should improve upon their methods of evaluation. They should set up an evaluation mechanism that combines incentives and restraints so that the procurement of basic medical insurance services is no longer a simple outsourcing business. Instead, by increasing the efficiency with which funds are used, insurers become creators of value and receive reasonable compensation in return. They achieve efficiencies by using their industry advantages, including the ability to make technological innovations, to control risk, to provide services, and to build networks. Third, insurers should expand the scope of their business operations. They currently mainly insure the new rural cooperative medical program. They should expand to such other forms of basic medical insurance as the urban residents' basic medical insurance, the urban employees' basic medical insurance, and the urban and rural medical assistance (aid) program. In addition, they should vigorously pursue discussions with the relevant government departments and local governments to explore expanding their business once pilot programs in suitable locations have assembled enough experience to proceed. Fourth, basic medical insurance and critical illness insurance should be handled in a uniform manner where conditions permit so as to achieve economies of scale and of scope. Fifth, publicity should be strengthened to achieve an exemplary effect. The experience of the Jiangyin Model of the China Pacific Insurance Company, the Luoyang Model of China Life, and other exemplary models should be summed up and advertised in order to build up the image of the industry, increase its influence, and increase communications with others about such models.

2.5.2.2 With regard to participation in development of medical services system

2.5.2.2.1 Commercial health insurance companies as investors in medical institutions

First, we should encourage insurance companies to invest in medical institutions as an important way to advance the reform of the institutional structures that govern China's medical, pharmaceutical, and healthcare systems. We should move further in ensuring the coordinated action of various government departments, including health and social security authorities, to loosen constraints on market access, introduce supporting policy measures, and provide feasible approaches through design of our entire institutional system and regulatory arrangements. At the same time, we should set up platforms by which investment capital and industry can link up effectively, in order for medical institutions to communicate and cooperate with insurance companies.

Second, we should be proactive in creating a favorable environment for investing in medical institutions. (1) In accelerating the reform of medical institutions, public health authorities should create the conditions by which insurance companies can invest in medical institutions. (2) Authorities should refine policies that allow doctors to practice in multiple hospitals. They should explicitly state that public hospitals cannot prohibit doctors from working in multiple locations unless there are special reasons for such prohibition. Meanwhile, doctors should not be required to get permission from local hospital authorities in order to work in multiple hospitals. (3) Authorities should set up a fair and transparent system by which market access is granted to insurance companies to be 'designated' handlers of China's basic medical insurance. Based on the premise that the public should be allowed easy access to medical care, such qualifications as price and quality of medical services should be taken into account in determining the qualifications for 'designated' status, i.e. where basic medical insurance claims can be reimbursed, and equal consideration should be given to both for-profit and not-for-profit hospitals. (4) We should support the applications of insurance companies that want to invest in setting up medical institutions themselves. This should depend on the local plans for developing healthcare. It should help insurance companies gradually build up their own brands.

Third, we should increase the force with which we make sure that supporting policies are actually implemented. We should create documents and revise documents where necessary so as to be explicit about matters relating to non-public medical institutions, including market entry, operations, and regulatory oversight. We should put into effect supporting documentation regarding specific rules that encourage and enable social (private) capital to invest in medical institutions. These should be formulated in line with actual circumstances and should be aimed at eliminating any policy obstacles that prevent insurance capital from investing in medical institutions. The aim is to promote the sound and sustainable growth of non-public medical institutions. At the same time, we should support various ways of having insurance companies invest in public institutions, including via debt instruments or shares, so as to improve their governance structures.

Fourth, we should encourage commercial health insurance companies to participate in the reform of public hospitals via innovative financial instruments. We should support such things as investment via debt instruments, convertible bonds, preferred stock, common stock, and so on. Depending on the different needs of public hospitals, as they reform their systems to become either for-profit or not-for-profit institutions, insurance companies should participate in their reform through a variety of channels. The aim is to create a favorable situation for holding down medical and drug costs and for improving the health of the population.

2.5.2.2.2 *Commercial health insurance companies as contributors to improving use of information technologies in China's medical reform*

One of the key areas in which commercial health insurance can advance the health-industry chain is 'informatization,' that is, applying information technologies to healthcare. This also helps expand the supply of commercial health insurance and improves the quality of that insurance. In this regard, efforts should be strengthened in the following areas.

First, we should improve the regulatory framework within which informatization takes place. The process must go forward in a holistic way, under uniform plans, which requires changing our current approach of setting up different systems in a fragmented way. We must be more forceful in coordinating organizational efforts. Relevant departments should all put forward their working principles and guidance opinions for common consideration. They should then formulate the basic norms for an information system for the New Medical Insurance. They should provide guidance for building a standardized national health insurance information system that contributes to more scientific management, better safeguards, and the sustainable functioning of all regulatory systems.

Second, we should strengthen the integration of information systems. This means addressing and thoroughly resolving the various problems of uneven development of systems in different parts of the country and the phenomenon of information silos and mutually inaccessible systems among units and departments. It means gradually achieving linked-up usage of information systems among social security and health departments, hospitals, and insurance companies. Both government and commercial insurance companies should work together to improve the framework within which a multi-tiered medical safeguards system operates.

Third, we should improve the functions of the information system. (1) This means improving the function of automated real-time verification. It will require renovating the system of real-time settlement and payment by adding a new process of regulatory oversight of automated real-time verification that works together with the process of post-settlement verification and monitoring. (2) It means building a system that is centered on the policy holder. The goal is to have a system that records data on the policy holder for his or her entire life and that manages that person's insurance data and serves that person over a lifetime. The file on the policy holder should include information on the individual, type of insurance, health data, credit data, and so on. (3) The information system should have improved functions that allow for data mining. Based on the idea that it should enable data analysis and data mining, the system should allow for thorough exploitation of the inherent value of historical data. This requires setting up databases and associated systems that support decision making through the restructuring and upgrading of data modules.

Fourth, we should improve the ability to share information. (1) Social security and health authorities should speed up the process of managing or co-administering information and data through standardized systems. They should strengthen cooperation in order to prevent the occurrence of duplicate requests for reimbursement of insurance claims and in order to improve the efficiency with which public finance funds are utilized. The aim is to further the sound development of medical insurance in the society. (2) Social security and health authorities should share their data with insurance companies. Medical insurance data provides the basis for settlements and for pricing. It also provides the basis for improved risk management in the industry. At the policy level, insurance companies should be empowered to extract medical insurance data, and this authority should be made concrete in the process of building information systems.

Fifth, we should speed up legislation on informatization of the industry. Standards relating to medical and health information impact the development of commercial health insurance. For the immediate future, we should have the National Office on Healthcare Reform coordinate the process of setting up binding standards with the main relevant departments. Over the following period, we should actively encourage experts and legal scholars in the various departments to formulate departmental regulations. They should also do the research and preparatory work for enacting national legislation. Over the long term, we should incorporate this effort into the State legislative planning process. Ultimately, we should promote a legal structure that allows for the application of information technologies to China's medical and healthcare systems but that also provides protections for the privacy of patients.

Sixth, we should promote the setting up of standards that allow for uniform exchange of health insurance data. This involves making sure that research into standards is an ongoing and sustainable effort, setting up an alliance for researching cross-industry standards, and making sure that the exchange of medical insurance data is done according to regular standards. Meanwhile, applying information technology standards to medical insurance has an impact on many industries and government departments. In order to ensure that the process is coordinated properly, we recommend that a working team be set up under the National Office on Medical Reform. It can adopt the same model as used by China's Standards Alliance to coordinate all relevant departments and commissions, including social security, commercial insurance, the ministry of finance, and so on, in formulating relevant standards.

APPENDIX

Case study. How commercial health insurance provides critical illness insurance: the Jiangyin and the Taicang Models

The Jiangyin and Taicang Models represent two innovative practices of commercial health insurance companies that are providing critical illness insurance. They can be used as a blueprint in the process of reforming China's medical safeguards system. The following presents the main elements and some specific practices of these two models.

2.A.1 Background for launching critical illness insurance

At present, China has basically established a medical safeguards system that covers the entire population. The coverage rate of the system is over 95%, with more than 1.3 billion people participating in one of the several systems, including the 'urban employees' basic medical insurance,' the 'urban residents' basic medical insurance,' and the 'new rural cooperative medical insurance.' Under the 'urban and rural residents' insurance program,' fiscal subsidies went from RMB 80 per capita in 2008 to RMB 380 per capita in 2015. In recent years, the main threats to human health have changed as a result of economic and social development and changes in the spectrum of disease, so that respiratory, cardiovascular, and cerebrovascular diseases now predominate. Usually either chronic or critical in nature, these diseases have a long course and become extremely expensive in terms of medical costs. They are putting individuals and families at increasing risk, which is expressed as the possibility of being unable to cover the cost of massive medical bills. Although China's basic medical insurance serves the purpose of providing some medical safeguards, its main focus has been ordinary illness. Its ability to provide coverage for critical illness is limited. What's more, it can only reimburse a limited amount of medical expenses and that limit is far below the amount people have to pay to receive medical treatment. As a result, a substantial portion of the population is being either forced into poverty or forced back into poverty due to economic distress. They are unable to cover the costs of critical illness. Against this background, the CPC Central Committee and the State Council have had the vision to launch a major new institutional innovation. In timely fashion, they are putting forward an initiative intended to benefit the country and the people, namely critical illness insurance.

Two landmark events serve to mark the launch of critical illness insurance. In August, 2012, the National Development and Reform Commission, the Ministry of Health, the Ministry of Finance, the Ministry of Human Resources and Social Security, the Ministry of Civil Affairs, and the China Insurance Regulatory Commission issued the *Guidance Opinion on the provision of critical illness insurance for urban and rural residents*. This was a master plan for the endeavor. This *Guidance Opinion* explicitly stated that critical illness insurance should adhere to the basic principle of having the 'government provide guidance while actual operations are handled professionally.' It confirmed that critical illness insurance should take advantage of the professional expertise of commercial insurance entities. The government supports having commercial insurance handle critical illness insurance in order to make use of market mechanisms to improve efficiencies and raise levels and quality of service.

In August 2015, the General Office of the State Council issued the *Opinions on comprehensive implementation of critical illness insurance for urban and rural residents*. This went further in clarifying the principle of having 'government provide guidance while actual operations are handled professionally.' It confirmed that China should make full use of market mechanisms and the professional advantages of commercial insurance entities to further the steady and sound operations and sustainable development of critical illness insurance. The *Opinions* defined the status and role of the insurance industry in the provision of critical illness insurance and stated that, by 2017, the goal was to establish a fairly complete system of critical illness insurance. Meanwhile, the *Opinions* changed the criteria for identifying critical illness—the previous criteria had been defined by type of illness. The standard by which critical illness costs can now be reimbursed is to be defined by the extent of medical expense, specifically, the occurrence of high medical expenses. This was an important institutional arrangement that allowed for the ability to use critical illness insurance as a means to deal with catastrophic healthcare expenditures. This change will play an increasingly important role in China's poverty alleviation policies.

Fundamentally, critical illness insurance is an extension of the safeguards of China's basic medical insurance system. It is a kind of institutional arrangement that goes further in safeguarding people from the high costs of critical illness. It further increases the scope of safeguards and so is a beneficial supplement to basic medical insurance. It takes a critical step forward in terms of China's policy, in that it goes from the idea of merely ensuring basic medical care to the idea of targeting poverty alleviation as the goal of policy. At the same time, in protecting and preserving the healthcare rights and interests of the entire population, it is highly significant in safeguarding public health and deepening China's overall medical reform.

2.A.2 Major approaches

Critical illness insurance works in the following basic way: either a certain percentage of funds or a specific quantity of funds are earmarked for critical illness insurance from the overall funds held by China's existing insurance systems. Those are the urban residents' basic medical insurance, the new rural cooperative medical insurance, and the urban and rural residents' basic medical insurance. Through a bidding process, these systems then use the funds to purchase critical illness insurance from commercial insurance companies that meet certain operating qualifications. In the process of experimenting with actual implementation of this concept, two places have been notable, namely Jiangyin City and Taicang City, both in Jiangsu Province. They have developed unique methods that suit their local conditions.

2.A.2.1 *Jiangyin City*

Jiangyin City has already established a medical safeguards system consisting of the new rural cooperative medical insurance, critical illness emergency relief, and supplementary commercial insurance. The municipal government has set up a committee called the New Rural Cooperative Management Committee that is responsible for overall coordination and arrangements. It is specifically responsible for formulating policy and for administering funds. Under this committee is a General Office that is also affiliated with the administrative offices of the public health authorities. This Office is responsible for drafting working plans, carrying out regulatory oversight of companies, and coordinating the monitoring of medical services. An insurance company (China Pacific Insurance Company) is responsible for the 'new rural cooperative' business of claims and payments, including such specific handling work as reviewing and checking expenses. The municipality's Audit Office and Bureau of Finance are in charge of auditing and regulatory supervision. The China Pacific Insurance Company is in charge of carrying out a system of medical specialists in the new rural cooperative medical program. In principle it assigns one or two people to each designated medical institution. They are responsible for managing the qualifications review of those who participate, for providing policy advice, for checking on payments made for medical treatment carried out in other cities, and for monitoring medical institutions. Any medical issues are reviewed and decided upon collectively by medical professionals who are engaged by the China Pacific Insurance Company.

Jiangyin City began to explore its critical illness relief initiative when the new rural cooperative medical insurance program was just starting. In 2013, the city made major adjustments to the system. It added 20 critical illness categories and also introduced 'major medical expenses' as a criterion for receiving relief and reimbursements. The sources of funds for the critical illness relief system include the new rural cooperative fund, public finance, and civil affairs authorities. These funds are then divided into two categories, outpatient and inpatient services. The inpatient funds cover three types of patients who can qualify for the program: the 'members of the six disadvantaged groups,' people insured under the new rural cooperative system who are suffering from one of the 20 categories of critical illness as determined by the provincial ministry of health, and people under the new rural cooperative system who have major medical expenses. People under the first category receive 100% policy-type compensation—the relief fund covers all hospital expenses that are not covered by the new rural cooperative system. People under the second category settle bills depending on amount, with the new rural cooperative and relief assistance fund together providing up to 70% reimbursement of actual costs. People under the third category have a benchmark figure of RMB 20,000—anyone paying over this amount for

Table 2.4 China's multi-tiered health care system

Medical support systems	Definition	Fundraising	Coverage	Competent authority
Basic medical security	New rural cooperative medical insurance (NRCMI)	Medical mutual assistance system primarily designed for coordinated efforts against critical illness, it is organized, guided, and supported by the government, funded jointly by individuals, communities, and the government, and voluntarily joined by farmers	Personal contributions plus financial subsidies (dominant part)	Farmers	National Health and Family Planning Commission
	Basic medical insurance for urban residents	System that provides insurance for the medical needs of urban residents. Under the guidance of the government, fundraising primarily relies on contributions of individuals or their families and is supplemented by fiscal subsidies. Reimbursements are based on contributions	Personal contributions (dominant part) plus financial subsidies	Urban residents	Ministry of Human Resources and Social Security
	Basic medical insurance for urban employees	Public insurance system established to compensate employees for economic losses resulting from risks of illness	Joint contributions of employers and employees	Urban employees	Labor security and finance

	Description	Funding source	Target population	Regulatory body
Critical illness insurance	Covering the high medical expenses incurred by critical diseases for urban and rural residents, it is aimed to prevent poverty caused by illness, an issue of major concern to the general public. In most cases, the insurance has prevented patients from falling back into economic difficulties	Allocated from funds of basic medical insurance for urban and rural residents	Urban and rural residents (covered by NRCMI and basic medical insurance for urban residents)	Ministry of Health and Ministry of Human Resources and Social Security
Medical assistance	System that provides special help and support for citizens unable to afford treatment, it relies on resources of the country and the public	Social donations	Citizens unable to afford medical treatment	Ministry of Civil Affairs
Disease emergency rescue	Provides support for the very few patients who require emergency rescue but cannot afford it because they cannot be identified or lack economic means	Government subsidies and social donations	Patients suffering from serious injuries or other critical conditions in China who require emergency rescue but cannot afford it because they cannot be identified or lack economic means	Funds managed by the Ministry of Health and monitored by a special monitoring committee
Commercial health insurance	Type of insurance that views the body of the insured as the object of insurance and ensures that the insured person receives compensation for direct or indirect damages incurred by injuries or accidents; commercial health insurance includes sickness insurance, medical insurance, income insurance, and long-term care insurance	Personal contributions	Policy holders of commercial health insurance	China Banking and Insurance Regulatory Commission

items that are within the scope of coverage automatically becomes qualified for Relief Assistance, with no need to make an application. Such a person enjoys the same relief as a member of the vulnerable (disadvantaged) population, with full reimbursement made for any service within the scope of the list of approved items.

The China Pacific Insurance Company has set up a payment system in Jiangyin that can be described as follows: 'prepayment of the full amount + payment according to type of illness + micro-managed oversight and control.' Based on this formula, it holds negotiations with the hospital. It signs a contract and assumes the key responsibility of carrying out payment obligations. The insurance company has also taken on the task of setting up mechanisms for regulatory control over improper behavior relating to the practice of pushing excessive medical treatments, drugs, and equipment. It has also therefore established the new rural cooperative fund's 'safe usage of funds model.' In 2014, Jiangyin City allocated funding of RMB 50 per capita into its critical illness relief fund, and reimbursed RMB 27,1229 million to a total of 3,089 people. The percentage of people who were reimbursed due to 'high medical bills as a result of critical illness' was 54.9%.

2.A.2.2 Taicang City

Taicang City operates its critical illness insurance program according to the guiding policy of 'having government play a leading role while government and insurance company jointly manage affairs, having professional operations and convenient services.' The insurance company, PICC Health (People's Insurance), works together with government departments to develop and manage a platform for operations. This then provides services to those who are insured that are a combined form of both China's basic medical insurance and its new critical illness insurance. The platform provides a kind of one-stop handling for policy holders. The actual design of the platform follows the idea that payments should be differentiated, treatment should be fair, and compensation should be inclined in this policy direction. Every year, the government allocates a certain amount of funds from the basic medical insurance fund with which to purchase supplementary critical illness insurance from PICC Health. The amount is intended to cover all policy holders of basic medical insurance in the city. Between 2011 and 2015, the per-person amount designated for this type of insurance came to RMB 50 per state employee and RMB 20 per resident per year. In 2016, an additional RMB 10 per person was added to that base amount. In 2015, outpatient visits were added to the covered services, at a rate of RMB 20 per both state employees and residents. The medical insurance coordination fund allocated half of this, while the municipal financial department allocated the other half.

The insurance responsibilities for hospital stays involving critical illness are as follows. A deductible of RMB 10,000 yuan must be paid by the patient out-of-pocket before the insurance company covers the remaining costs according to a percentage formula. (The deductible was raised to 12,000 yuan in 2016.) The lowest percentage that the insurance must pay is 53% (for costs between 10,000 and 20,000 yuan). The highest is 82% (for costs over 500,000 yuan). There is no cap on the amount that can be reimbursed in one year.

For outpatient visits, the annual deductible is 3,000 yuan while the percentage covered by the insurance company is between 50% (for costs between 3,000 and 6,000 yuan) and 66% (for costs over 20, 000 yuan).

2.A.3 Main lessons learned from the Jiangyin City and Taicang City case studies

Both cities have chosen to have insurance companies provide their critical illness insurance. This has significantly furthered the allied set of reforms that are aimed at medical insurance, pharmaceuticals, and medical care. It has raised operating efficiencies in terms of managing healthcare safeguards and it has made very apparent contributions to controlling medical costs and improving the results of funds management.

2.A.3.1 Close management has significantly curbed soaring medical expenses

Insurance companies have significantly curbed soaring medical expenses through tighter management controls over medical institutions, while ensuring that levels of medical safeguards for the public are not affected.

In the case of the Jiangyin Model, the insurance company has set up an Internet-based information system which integrates remote review and claims settlement, real-time treatment monitoring, and other useful functions. It has also engaged professional teams to carry out inspection tours. The Internet-based information system is linked to designated medical institutions. Real-time treatment information on insured patients can be transmitted to the company's business management center. Doctors hired by the center can carry out real-time monitoring of treatment and can interfere with any inappropriate behavior in advance. At the same time, monitoring teams make regular visits to designated medical institutions in order to combat any fraudulent medical claims. Meanwhile, the insurance company has been empowered by the Jiangyin municipal government to formulate a plan for reforming the system by which medical and healthcare payments are made. The company has signed service agreements with medical institutions to curb medical overspending through a combination of incentives and punitive measures.

In the Taicang Model, the insurance company participates in the supervision and management of the critical illness insurance fund through the development and standardization of medical inspections, monitoring, early warning checks, expert reviews of medical cases, and systems for claims investigation. Inspection plans are developed on a monthly basis. Through regular visits to medical institutions, the company is able to detect fraudulent patient behavior and, to a certain extent, mitigate medical risks. Through the monitoring and early warning

Table 2.5 Taicang critical illness insurance program between 2011 and 2015 (unit: 10,000 yuan)

Year	Number of insured	Number of beneficiaries	Return rate	Fund raised	Fund reimbursed	Reimbursement rate	Operating costs	Balance
2011	538,472	2,606	0.48	2,167.17	1,565.2	8.299	73.14	432.14
2012	549,567	3,093	0.56	2,277.27	1,792.85	7.83	126.29	249.13
2013	563,211	3,410	0.61	2,410.79	1,996.11	7.72	118.7	182.12
2014	569,023	3,762	0.66	2,413.73	2,216.71	7.38	132.85	−48.84
2015	572,228	4,235	0.74%	3,605.28	2,441.62	6.96%	159.65	467.02

system, the company is able to detect abnormal medical behavior and expenses, arrange timely verification, and properly address misconduct. Incidents of a serious nature are handed over to the healthcare center for further handling. Through the medical review system, the company is able to double check information related to critical illness insurance. The medical review system applies both a systemic review and manual checking procedures. This double-barreled approach effectively improves the accuracy of payments. Meanwhile, the head office, as well as branches, carries out random checks of a portion of cases. This also raises the accuracy of insurance payments for critical illness. In addition, as organized by the Center, the insurance company asks experts to carry out reviews of specific cases which are then written up in document form and presented to the Center. Depending on the results, the Center may use this feedback to punish any medical behavior that goes counter to rules and regulations.

The insurance company is also in charge of investigating serious claims cases. By reviewing records of hospital stays, verifying medical expenses, and looking into actual treatment, the company is able to effectively prevent the occurrence of medical overspending.

2.A.3.2 Professional operations gradually raise operating results of insurance funds for critical illness

Insurance companies use professional techniques and market mechanisms to manage insurance funds, which has improved operating results. First, this saves on the administrative costs of government management. When government brings in an insurance company to participate in a given medical safeguards project, it can make direct use of the management platform of the company and its service network. Government no longer has to add on an agency to handle these things. It does not have to add to its payroll for additional human resources, and it is saved the pressure of funding the expenses of administering the project. This lowers management costs and reduces the amount of fiscal spending required. Second, this allows the public to get convenient, fast, and efficient services. Using the professional management of insurance companies and their market-oriented operations improves the operating results of critical health insurance. Third, government can take advantage of the scale of insurance companies that carry out accounting on a nationwide basis, to improve its own ability to mitigate risk, to raise its level of service, and to expand the effectiveness of safeguards.

In the Taicang Model, PICC Health incorporates a three-in-one management concept into its medical insurance management and services system. The three elements are pre-illness health management, during-illness disease diagnosis, monitoring, and control, and post-illness verification and checking on payment. This process of managing and controlling medical risks includes the entire process of medical care and ensures that insurance funds are used securely and efficiently. Through active monitoring, the company is able to regulate the behavior of both hospitals and patients, and thereby able to reduce unreasonable spending out of the fund. Through active reviewing of reimbursements and analysis of cases, the company ensures that the funds are put to use in a proper way. Over the past five years, the company has discovered approximately RMB 10 million in improper medical costs. This has been effective in raising the efficiency with which funds for critical illness are used.

2.A.3.3 Innovative management reduces incidence of disease

In the Jiangyin Model, the insurance company has relied on years of accumulated medical and health statistics to develop targeted insurance products that have low development costs but high safeguard results. In addition, however, the insurance company has been able, to a certain degree, to reduce the incidence of critical illness. It has done this by analyzing big data using 'Internet-plus' tools, and by studying the external environment for the occurrence of critical illness as well as the lifestyle habits of those who become ill. Through such analysis, the company has been able to make 'health-management' recommendations as a way to prevent illness.

In the Taicang Model, PICC Health incorporated health management services into the basic medical insurance system and the public healthcare system. This enriched the offerings of public services and also raised the consciousness of policy holders about overall health. It added points to the index that Taicang calls its 'Municipal health and wellness index.' Over the past five years, the company has organized 51 lectures on health. It has instituted a new visiting program on top of its existing on-site visits that covers disadvantaged households and patients in need, and has made 88 visits to the former and 179 to the latter. In line with the philosophy that a healthy lifestyle is of primary importance, it has promoted a series of health-oriented videos. These have been shown at 36 forums on health and have been broadcast on 41 television programs. Meanwhile, just in Taicang, PICC Health has sent 76 messages on health topics to more than 14,000 mobile phone users.

Notes

1 See: Administrative Measures for Commercial Health Insurance (Order of China Insurance Regulatory Commission (No. 8 [2006])).
2 Sun Qixiang. *Insurance*. Beijing: Peking University Press, 2015.
3 An endogenous variable is a variable that is determined by the internal structure of the economic model. An exogenous variable is a variable that is not determined by variables in the economic model, but by external factors (such as politics, nature).
4 Cao Xiaolan. *Study on the Sustainable Development of Commercial Medical Insurance in China*. Hangzhou: Zhejiang University Press, 2009.
5 Cao Xiaolan. *Study on the Sustainable Development of Commercial Medical Insurance in China*. Hangzhou: Zhejiang University Press, 2009.
6 Liu Na. *Study on Factors Influencing China's Commercial Health Insurance Development*.Tianjin University of Finance and Economics, 2012, 28.
7 Yan Jianjun. *Direction of China's Medical Reform and Development Path of Commercial Health Insurance*. Beijing: China Financial and Economic Publishing House, 2015.

8 Xiong Zhiguo, Yan Bo, Suo Lingyan. *On the Development Model of Commercial Health Insurance in China*. Beijing: Peking University Press, 2012.

9 xinhuanet.com. China's Private Hospitals Doubled in Five Years. [EB/OL]. http://news.xinhuanet.com/health/2016-06/12/c_129053088.htm.

10 Insurance Association of China. *Country Study Report of Commercial Health Insurance*. Beijing: China Financial Publishing House, 2015.

11 people.com.cn. US Medical Reform: New Administration, Old Problems. [EB/OL]. http://world.people.com.cn/n1/2017/0316/c1002-29148246.html.

12 Suo Lingyan. Trump's Health Care Reform and Inspirations for China. [EB/OL]. http://pl.sinoins.com/2017-03/21/content_226473.htm.

13 Insurance Association of China. *Country Study Report of Commercial Health Insurance*. Beijing: China Financial Publishing House, 2015.

14 Insurance Association of China. *Country Study Report of Commercial Health Insurance*. Beijing: China Financial Publishing House, 2015.

3 Research Topic 2

Research on the demand for commercial health insurance in China

Tao Cunwen, Zhou Hua, and Bai Wenjuan

3.1 INTRODUCTION

3.1.1 Research background and significance

3.1.1.1 Research background

China's people are increasingly concerned about health as their economy improves, and increasingly hoping to enjoy high-quality medical services when they run into health problems. Despite this, most are also finding that excessively high medical costs are an onerous burden. In order to satisfy the demand for health and for medical services, China must now go further in improving its existing medical safeguards system.[1]

The country currently has three types of basic medical safeguard systems which are designed for different groups of beneficiaries: (1) the urban basic medical insurance system, which includes the urban employees' basic medical insurance and the urban residents' basic medical insurance; (2) the new rural cooperative medical insurance system, and (3) the urban and rural medical relief (aid) system. However, all of these three systems are government provided, which means that they are of a publicly funded nature and can only allow for the most basic safeguards. They clearly cannot meet the different kinds of healthcare demand that are coming from various types of people. Because of this, the Chinese government has been vigorously supporting the development of commercial health insurance. It has been attempting to make sure that commercial health insurance plays its proper role in improving China's overall structure of medical safeguards. On May 17, 2009, China published the *Opinions of the CPC Central Committee and the State Council on deepening reform of the institutional structures that govern the medical, pharmaceutical, and healthcare systems* (referred to below as the new medical reform.) The new medical reform highlighted the need to develop commercial health insurance. It gave support to and indeed encouraged commercial insurance companies to develop a diversified range of products that could meet the varying demands of different people for health insurance. It also encouraged them to simplify claims procedures so that people could more fully enjoy high-quality medical safeguards. It stated that insurance companies should set up systems that work together with China's existing social medical safeguards system (the publicly funded system), which focuses on 'broad coverage but low-level safeguards,' in order to create a better overall structure of medical safeguards.

Given this background, the question of whether or not China's commercial health insurance market can indeed grow quickly has become of considerable concern to people. Citizens are increasingly aware of their own health and of risks to their health as medical and healthcare reforms are being promoted throughout the country. It is clear that the role of commercial health insurance in China's overall system is indispensable. Right now, however, the market for such insurance is relatively small in size, not well developed, has high compensation rates, is operating at a loss, and has considerable room to grow.

The U.S. consulting firm McKinsey & Company believed that the market for commercial health insurance in China between the years 2004 and 2008 could have been between RMB 150 billion and RMB 300 billion, as measured in premium income and depending on the granularity of statistics used. The German health insurance company DKV also did research on China's market. It concluded that a conservative estimate of China's health insurance market in 2015 would be 'more than three times what premium income had been in 2009.' It therefore would reach more than RMB 170 billion. The Swiss reinsurance company, Swiss Re, made a forecast of the size of China's market in 2007 that stated the total demand for commercial health insurance in China would reach RMB 500 billion in 2015. (This forecast was made in the sixth issue of the publication *Sigma* in that year.) All of these forecasts were overly optimistic. Through these years, China's health insurance market did not reach anything like these figures. In 2008, premium income in China's commercial health insurance market came to a mere RMB 58.55 billion, far below McKinsey's low estimate of RMB 300 billion. In fact, premium income only broke through the RMB 100 billion level in 2013. Under the impetus of highly favorable policies, China's health insurance market began to grow in 2012, but there is still massive potential as compared to countries in which health insurance is more mature.

3.1.1.2 Significance of the research

The reason for the disparity between effective demand for health insurance in China and the estimates of insurance companies and consulting companies relates to errors in understanding and hence errors in evaluating China's market. It is therefore highly significant that we look into the factors that influence demand for commercial health insurance in China, and that we re-evaluate the potential for growth in the market.

This study identifies, analyzes, and evaluates the factors that influence effective demand for commercial health insurance in China. It then tests factors using an econometric model. Its aim is to enable China's government to have a more fine-tuned analysis of market demand so as to make better forecasts and so as to have a theoretical basis for putting forth policies and regulations that spur growth in the commercial health insurance industry. Its aim is also to provide health insurance companies with material on consumer preferences so that they can more accurately understand demand. This study presents proposals on how to increase the demand for commercial health insurance in China, so that the industry can provide China's population with reliable, convenient, and targeted health insurance services.

This research is therefore significant for the following reasons. It benefits the endeavor to develop commercial health insurance. It benefits the degree to which consumers enjoy health insurance safeguards. It benefits the improvement of the overall structure of health safeguards in China. It improves the efficiency with which China's overall medical resources are put to use.

3.1.2 Purpose and design of the research

3.1.2.1 Purpose

China's new medical reform was launched as a policy initiative in 2006. It then went through years of research, discussion, and revision, and the final version was officially released in April 2009, called the *Opinions of the CPC Central Committee and the State Council on deepening reform of the institutional structures that govern the medical, pharmaceutical, and healthcare systems*. On a policy level, the new medical reform explicitly confirmed the position of commercial health insurance in China's overall system. It set forth the goal of accelerating the establishment and improvement of a medical safeguards system that has China's basic medical safeguards as the central component, but supplemented by various other forms of medical insurance and commercial health insurance. The overall structure of the medical safeguards should cover citizens in both urban and rural areas and should be multi-tiered. The reform program singled out commercial health insurance for special emphasis. It noted that China should actively promote such insurance and it encouraged commercial health insurance companies to simplify procedures for reimbursement of claims and to develop health insurance products that could meet diversified healthcare needs.

On August 10, 2015, the China Insurance Regulatory Commission (CIRC) formally issued the *Interim Measures on the administration of health insurance that enjoys preferential individual tax treatment ('Measures')*. This sets out specific requirements for the design of health insurance products that allow for preferential treatment of individual taxes, as well as requirements on related business conditions. In the *Measures*, various provisions were considered to help in speeding up the arrival of a 'springtime' for the health insurance industry, including such key things as insurance for people with pre-existing conditions, a simplified reimbursement rate of not less than 80%, and allowable pre-tax purchase items.

China currently adheres to the principle of 'broad coverage and low-level safeguards' in its social (publicly funded) medical safeguards system, even as the demand for health insurance among the population is clearly diversifying.

Given this fact, China must be proactive in developing commercial health insurance as a way to provide more complete and higher-quality medical safeguards for its people. At the same time, by taking advantage of market-oriented measures, the country will be able to build a better structure of medical safeguards that saves on public resources and reduces the burden on public finance.

The purpose of this study can therefore be summarized by the following three points:

1 Understand the main problems facing growth of the commercial health insurance industry in China by analyzing its experience to date, then looking at development strategies and operating models that improve upon that experience.
2 Use 'grey-correlation analysis' to ascertain the key factors that influence demand for commercial health insurance, then analyze the extent to which each factor influences demand, and estimate potential demand for commercial health insurance based on the GM (1, 1) model.
3 Gain a more intuitive understanding of the impact of each factor on the development of commercial health insurance in China through qualitative and quantitative analysis and provide recommendations to policymakers on how to promote the development of commercial health insurance in China.

3.1.2.2 Design

Researching the demand for commercial health insurance in China required coming to grips with five linked considerations:

1 analyzing the current demand for such insurance and problems with the existing situation;
2 analyzing and verifying the factors constraining demand;
3 evaluating the massive potential for demand for such insurance;
4 forecasting the speed at which demand for commercial health insurance can grow and the scale of demand;
5 making policy recommendations on how to tap into the potential demand for commercial health insurance in China.

This research study first analyzed demand and existing problems, as noted above. On that basis, the authors then selected the most representative indicators from among factors that influenced demand in three main areas, namely economic, social, and healthcare resources. We then used grey-correlation analysis to rank the degree of correlation between each factor and commercial health insurance. We ranked these in order of correlation and analyzed and interpreted the results. In addition, we used a GM (1,1) model to forecast premium income for commercial health insurance over the next three years. Finally, we proposed reasonable policy recommendations that were guided by the results of our study. These are more specifically as follows.

The first section provides an introduction. The authors first point out the context for doing the study, then elucidate its purpose and its significance, namely, that the purpose of the study is to enable China to take firm hold of policy dividends, to help commercial health insurance companies expand market demand for insurance and thereby emerge from their current difficulties, and to realize fast growth in the industry and thereby ensure that it truly does play the role it should play in the overall structure of China's medical safeguards systems. Finally, the authors describe the structure of the study and its research methodology, and they provide a literature review of related research.

The second section analyzes the current commercial health insurance market in China. It first defines the general concept of demand for commercial health insurance, and it distinguishes between potential demand and effective demand. It goes on to provide more detailed analysis of those two with respect to the market for commercial health insurance in China. On that basis, it comes to the conclusion that potential demand is enormous while effective demand is insufficient, and it points out that the key consideration in transforming potential into effective demand is identifying factors that affect demand. It then gives several fundamental reasons for why China's commercial health insurance industry is being held back.

The third section provides a qualitative analysis of the factors that influence demand for commercial health insurance in China. It summarizes and analyzes three types of factors that influence the effective demand for commercial health insurance in China, namely economic, social, and healthcare resources. It identifies the following nine key factors: personal ability to pay and external assistance, structure of consumer spending, degree of competition among market players, situation regarding R&D being put into health insurance products, supply of healthcare resources, age structure of the population, educational structure of the population, insurance awareness, health status, and attitudes toward health risks.

The fourth section gives a quantitative analysis of the factors that influence the demand for commercial health insurance in China. In this section, we first introduce the grey-correlation analysis approach. We select variables and a model and analyze empirical evidence, and then summarize the results of the empirical analysis. The section ends with a summary of the factors that influence the demand for commercial health insurance in China, and the degree to which they influence demand.

The fifth section estimates the demand for commercial health insurance by type of insurance. The section estimates the demand for commercial health insurance based on the results of the quantitative analysis in the previous section. It constructs an estimation model, makes two adjustments to the model, and conducts a residual test and residual tolerance test. We then use the model to estimate the premium income of commercial health insurance companies in China between 2015 and 2017. At the end of the section, using different perspectives, we estimate the premium income from four major types of health insurance.

The sixth section presents policy recommendations that support the development of commercial health insurance. It mainly combines the theoretical and empirical analysis of the preceding sections in putting forward policy recommendations on how to expand the effective demand of commercial health insurance in China. It notes that the aim is to achieve the rapid growth of the market for such insurance in China.

3.1.3 Literature review

Foreign countries began to research the demand for commercial health insurance fairly early and have therefore assembled a systematic and comprehensive literature on the subject. Research findings are also particularly abundant.

In 1963, Kenneth Arrow published the paper *Uncertainty and the Welfare Economics of Medical Care*, which combines uncertainty and health insurance and which analyzes many of the basic problems in health insurance.[2] In 1974, the economist Mark J. Brown pointed out that an asymmetry of information exists in the market for healthcare services. For example, doctors are in control of more complete information than patients, who are at a disadvantage. Doctors may induce patients to purchase more services than they actually need, which affects the demand for such services.[3] In 1965, M.E. Yaari published *Uncertain Lifetimes, Life Insurance, and the Theory of the Consumer* in the journal *Review of Economic Studies*. This suggests that the uncertain length of lifetimes leads to uncertainty in future income flows based on the life-cycle hypothesis, and this uncertainty will reduce the optimal marginal utility of consumption, which in turn causes consumers to reduce consumption. This paper is considered to be the earliest theoretical study of the demand for health insurance. Pratt (1964)[4] and Arrow (1970)[5] divide attitudes toward risk into risk-loving, risk-averse, and risk-neutral. Because of these different attitudes towards risk, people have different attitudes towards insurance, which directly affects the demand for insurance.

In the United States market for supplementary insurance, Wolfe and Goddeeris (1991)[6] used historical data from retirement surveys and discovered that the healthier people were, the more likely they were to buy supplementary insurance (the data only used valid respondents.) In addition, the more people purchased supplementary insurance, the less they spent on hospitalization, physical therapy, and prescription drugs. In contrast, however, Lillard and Rogowski (1995),[7] Ettner (1997),[8] and Hurd and McGarry (1997)[9] found that there is insufficient evidence to show that health conditions affect the possibility of people buying private insurance.

In 2000, research done by Barry G. Save and Mark P. Douescher[10] points out that the main factors that influence a person's decision to buy health insurance include wealth, income, education level, health status, and whether or not the person is part of a minority group.

Given that health insurance is a kind of product, demand for that product is affected by price, namely premiums, as well as the income level of the consumer. Gruber[11] studied the influence of taxation on insurance coverage (2001) and discovered that tax subsidies from the government could affect corporate behavior in providing insurance, and could therefore raise the coverage of health insurance. Nyman (2002) pointed out that people who purchase a relatively large amount of medical services often have higher income elasticity when purchasing insurance.[12]

In 2006, Y. Machnes[13] studied the demand for private healthcare and supplementary health insurance of migrant workers and self-employed individuals in Israel. As variables, he selected income, age, marital status, health status, place of birth, education, occupation, and job status. He found that self-employed individuals are more inclined to buy private healthcare and supplementary health insurance due to fear of income loss caused by illness.

Among foreign researchers, level of education is also believed to be one of the key factors affecting the demand for health insurance. The level of education often affects such demand by influencing risk attitudes, awareness of the need for medical services, and related knowledge about healthcare and health. Generally speaking, the more highly educated a person, the more that person understands insurance, the higher their income level is likely to be, and the more willing as well as able they are to buy insurance. In addition to the above, there are also foreign studies on the influence of such factors as availability, price, quantity and other healthcare-related factors on the demand for health insurance.

Within China, scholars began to carry out research on the demand for health insurance only once the reform of the health insurance system was launched and as commercial health insurance began to emerge. This research was mainly carried out on two fronts, namely theoretical and empirical. In 2007, Xu Meifang conducted an empirical study on the demand for commercial health insurance in Shanghai, based on data from the *Health and Healthcare Survey of Shanghai Residents 2006*. This survey had been carried out by the Shanghai Academy of Social Sciences. In 2008, Chen Tao[14] pointed out that the key underlying cause of insufficient demand for commercial health insurance in China relates to imperfect supply. Li Qiong (2009)[15] noted that the growth of urban and rural incomes indirectly stimulated the demand for commercial health insurance in China. Zhou Minglai and Shang Ying (2011)[16] summarized the results of the domestic literature on the demand for commercial health insurance and listed four key factors that affect the demand for commercial health insurance in China: health status, average level of education, level of income of consumers, and the mandatory nature of basic medical insurance as provided by the Chinese government. Peng Xiaobo and Sun Qixiang (2012)[17] used grey-correlation analysis to study factors influencing the demand of Chinese farmers for health insurance. Guo Pei (2010)[18] built a panel-data model to run a regression analysis of factors influencing the demand for commercial health insurance which was based on data from the *Yearbook of China's Insurance* and the *China Statistics Yearbook* for 1999–2010. The above are just a few examples. Existing studies mainly verify the strong correlation between premium income of commercial health insurance and influencing factors on the macro level. Most empirical studies use a time series model for quantitative analysis. However, only in 1999 did China begin to collect data on the premium income of commercial health insurance companies. Statistical groups are fairly few, which may affect the dependability of the results of the analysis.

As for research methods, most scholars have used multiple linear regressions, autoregressive hysteretic distribution, VAR, fixed effects, random effects and other models. With regard to data selection, most researchers have used macro time series or provincial-level panel data.

From the above literature review, we can see that most existing studies focus on the macro-economic level. In other words, for explanatory variables, they use the premium income of commercial health insurance or data derived from it, such as insurance penetration and insurance density, in order to analyze the impact of macro-economic factors on premium income. They run a regression analysis and do econometric modeling to explain its significance. However, this only explains that the premium income of commercial health insurance and allied variables do have a strong correlation. It fails to explain purchase decisions from the perspective of individual consumers. In addition, in the empirical analysis, a large part of the existing literature uses a time series model. But China did not begin collecting data on the premium income of commercial health insurance until 1999. The lack of data, combined with too many explanatory factors, undermines the reliability of the model.

3.1.4 Methodology

Based on combining both theoretical analysis and empirical research, this study uses a number of methodologies including comparative analysis, qualitative analysis, quantitative analysis, and grey-correlation analysis to look at the factors influencing the development of commercial health insurance in China.

3.1.4.1 Comparative analysis

This study compares and analyzes several widely used business models in the commercial health insurance sector, and tries to find and summarize useful experience and lessons and select business models suitable for China's commercial health insurance companies.

3.1.4.2 Qualitative analysis

This study divides the factors that influence the development of commercial health insurance in China into different categories, and conducts qualitative analysis on each, which serves as a basis for empirical analysis later in the study. The qualitative analysis supplements factors that cannot be subjected to empirical analysis. At the same time, the study also puts forward some suggestions to promote the development of commercial business in China that are combined with factors relating to China's legal system.

3.1.4.3 *Quantitative analysis*

This study collects a large quantity of data related to the purchase of health insurance, income levels, and healthcare expenditures to truly reflect the status of the commercial health insurance industry in China, and it conducts quantitative analysis to figure out the impact of each factor on the development of commercial health insurance.

3.1.4.4 *Grey-correlation analysis*

This study makes use of grey-correlation analysis of factors that influence the development of commercial health insurance to look at the extent to which each factor is influential. It then puts forward some suggestions to promote the beneficial development of commercial health insurance.

3.2 DEMAND FOR COMMERCIAL HEALTH INSURANCE AND RELATED PROBLEMS

3.2.1 Current effective demand for commercial health insurance in China[19]

3.2.1.1 *Market size*

As shown by the data, China's commercial health insurance is starting from a fairly low point and its growth has been relatively slow. Although income from premiums is continuing to increase, the total sum of premium income is rather small. It was, for example, RMB 57.4 billion in 2009, RMB 67.8 billion in 2010, RMB 69.2 billion in 2011, RMB 86.3 billion in 2012, RMB 112.4 billion in 2013, RMB 158.7 billion in 2014, and RMB 241 billion in 2015. It can also be seen from this that the size of the commercial health insurance market did not change much with the increase in personal insurance, especially life insurance. The growth of commercial health insurance has lagged significantly behind that of life insurance.

Since 2012, the premium income of commercial health insurance has entered a period of rapid growth (see Figures 3.1 and 3.2). Between 2012 and 2015, income from health insurance premiums grew at a compound annual growth rate of 40.86% (over the same period, the compound annual growth rate of property insurance was 14.46%, that of life insurance was 14.14%, and that of casualty insurance was 18.07%). In 2015, the insurance industry as a whole reported total premium income of RMB 2.42 trillion, which represented a 20% increase over the previous year. Of this amount, income from health insurance premiums reached RMB 241 billion, which was a 51.87% increase over the previous year. The growth rate of health insurance premiums was 31.87 percentage points higher than that of total premiums in the insurance industry. Since 2012, health insurance has been the fastest growing segment of the insurance market.[20]

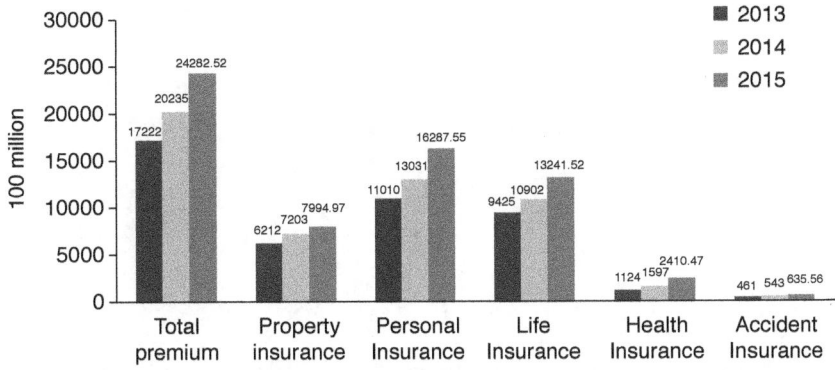

Figure 3.1 Premium income of China's insurance industry.
Source: Statistics column on website of China Insurance Regulatory Commission.

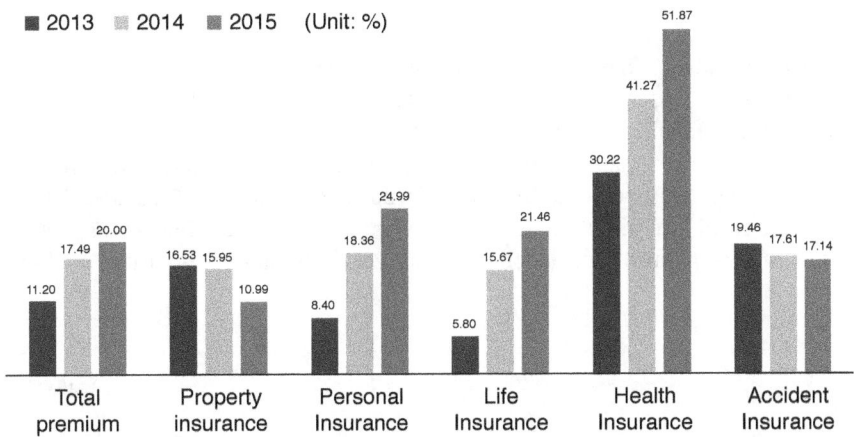

Figure 3.2 Year-on-year growth in premium income of China's insurance industry.
Source: Statistics column on website of China Insurance Regulatory Commission.

In terms of the dynamics of growth, China's commercial health insurance industry grew steadily between 2000 and 2015 and its premium income grew at an acceptable average rate of 30.62% per year (see Figure 3.3). In fact, however, the growth rate of premium income has been extremely volatile. It reached more than 90% in 2002 and 2003 and more than 50% in 2008, then declined to only 1.92% in 2007 and 7.42% in 2004. In 2001 and 2009, the industry even reported negative growth although there has been fairly steady growth since 2012.

In terms of growth relative to other forms of insurance, commercial health insurance occupies a relatively low percentage of all income from personal

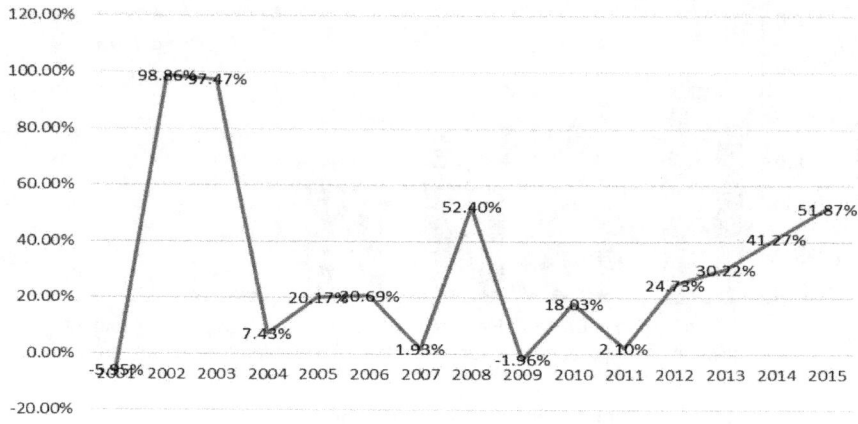

Figure 3.3 Health insurance growth trend in China during 2001–2015.

Source: *Yearbook of China's Insurance 2001–2015.*

insurance premiums. That percentage has also not always grown consistently. As shown in Figure 3.4, between 2000 and 2015, the percentage fluctuated around 8.0% except for the three years from 2012 to 2015.[21]

It should be noted that commercial health insurance rose sharply in terms of its percentage of total personal insurance in 2011. It went from 5.22% to 7.12% in percentage of premium income. This was not, however, due to an actual increase in health insurance income in this year but rather because the China

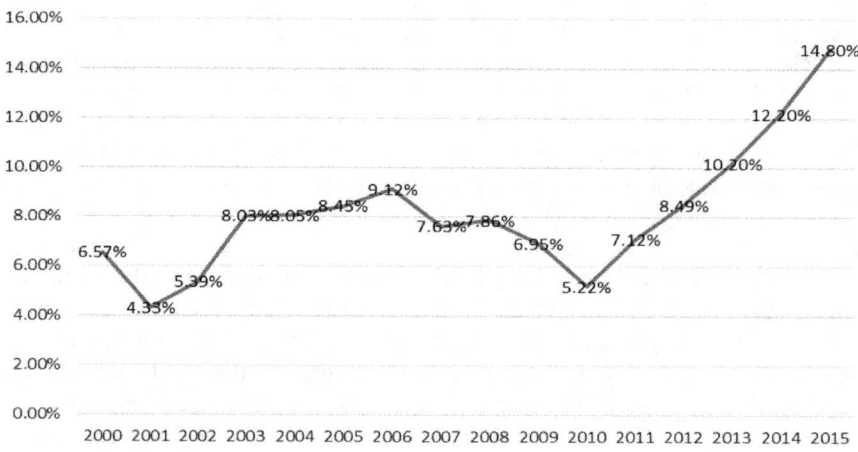

Figure 3.4 Health insurance growth trend in China during 2000–2015.

Source: *Yearbook of China's Insurance 2001–2015.*

Insurance Regulatory Commission changed the way in which it calibrated the statistics. Income from personal insurance premiums dropped sharply due to changes in the accounting for investment-linked insurance and universal (all-purpose) insurance. As a result, income from personal insurance premiums slipped substantially and the percentage of health insurance in all personal insurance therefore rose. In recent years, the share of commercial health insurance in all personal insurance has been rising, but the share remains low when compared to the United States, Japan, and other countries that have more mature commercial health insurance markets. In such countries, the percentage of health insurance stands at around 30%. China's health insurance could be described as at an embryonic stage, but faster growth has become apparent over the past three years.

3.2.1.2 Level of development

In the year 2000, the density of commercial insurance was RMB 5.17 per person. It rose during the years 2000–2014, which was mainly in sync with the rise in income from commercial health insurance premiums.[22] Generally speaking, the rate of increase was substantial, but a closer look at annual figures shows that it was extremely unstable. For example, the growth in commercial health insurance density was high in 2002, 2003, and 2012, low in 2004 and 2007, and negative in 2001 and 2009. In 2012, the density of commercial health insurance was only RMB 63.72 per person, which shows that commercial health insurance was not at all widespread in China. Although it rose to more than RMB 100 per person in 2014, this was still low compared to China's per capita health spending. The conclusion is that effective demand is still preparing for further expansion.

The penetration of commercial health insurance reflects a situation that is even more severe. In 2000, the penetration of commercial health insurance was 0.07%. This shows that the income from commercial health insurance premiums accounted for only a small part of China's GDP. In the national economy as a whole, China's commercial health insurance industry had a very low standing.

After 2000, the penetration of commercial health insurance fluctuated around 0.17%, without any sign of significant growth. Even in recent years during a period of rapid growth, the penetration rate of insurance has been still less than 1%, indicating that the development of the commercial health insurance market is in large part driven by economic growth rather than any self-driven growth of the health insurance market, as shown in Figure 3.5.

As can be seen from premium income, insurance density and insurance penetration, the effective demand for commercial health insurance in China remains low.

3.2.1.3 Coverage and utility

China's basic medical insurance has developed rapidly in recent years. The number of insured people has grown by multiples (see Figure 3.6), but China is still very far from achieving the goal of universal coverage of basic medical

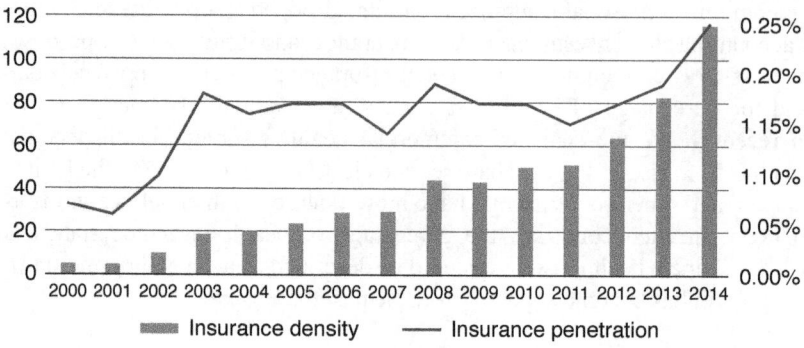

Figure 3.5 Insurance penetration and density in China during 2000–2014.
Source: *Yearbook of China's Insurance 2001–2015.*

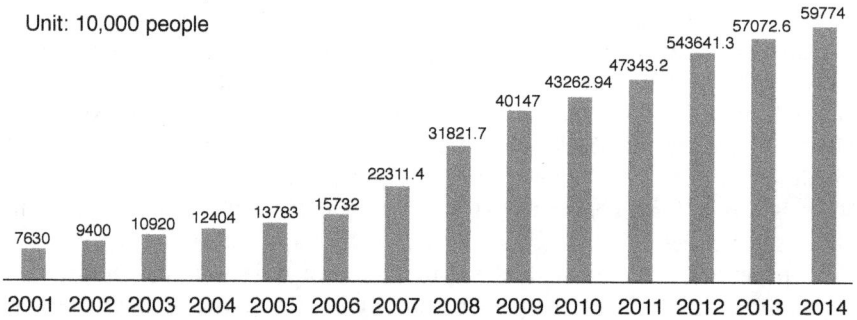

Figure 3.6 Enrollment in China's basic medical insurance program, 2001–2014.
Source: *Labor and Social Security Statistics Report 2001–2007; China Statistics Yearbook 2014.*

insurance.[23] Meanwhile, the country's unique urban–rural dual economic structure and its extreme regional imbalance in economic growth mean that basic
medical insurance cannot fully meet the diverse healthcare needs of different
groups of people in developed regions. For them, purchasing commercial health
insurance is a reasonable way to improve security and expand the scope of their
protections. Developing commercial health insurance in the present circumstances is a viable option for China.

The accomplishments of China's new medical reform can mainly be
described as follows. The problem of 'expensive access to medical help' has
been moderated to a degree. The percentage of out-of-pocket costs in China's
total medical spending dropped from 59.97% in 2001 to 31.99% in 2014 (see
Figure 3.7), and the financial burden of medical care has been significantly
reduced.

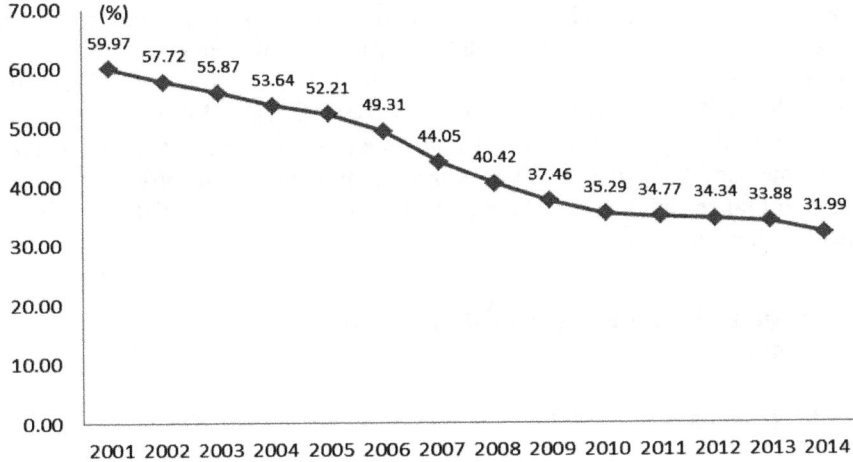

Figure 3.7 Percentage of out-of-pocket costs in China's total medical spending.
Source: *China Statistics Yearbook 2015.*

3.2.1.4 Analysis of effective demand

This study uses sampling data from the China Health and Nutrition Survey for its analysis. This is a collaborative survey project between the Chinese Center for Disease Control and Prevention (CCDC), the University of North Carolina at Chapel Hill, and the National Institute of Nutrition and Food Safety in the United States. It was designed to examine the health, nutrition, and other related conditions of Chinese residents. The project surveyed nine provinces in China: Liaoning, Heilongjiang, Jiangsu, Shandong, Henan, Hubei, Hunan, Guangxi, and Guizhou. The cluster sampling method was used to select the surveyed provinces to ensure they included both northern and southern provinces, economically developed eastern coastal areas and economically underdeveloped areas in the inland, central, and western parts of the country, as well as both urban and rural areas. The data collected in this survey is the highest quality data in any study related to Chinese residents' health and nutrition. The most recent survey was conducted in 2009 and the latest updating was conducted in 2012.

Reports resulting from the survey divide respondents into two groups, adults and minors. There were 9,788 valid adult respondents and 4,786 respondents answered questions related to health insurance. The number of respondents who had purchased commercial health insurance was 194, accounting for 4.05% of the total number of respondents; the number of respondents who had not purchased commercial health insurance was 4,573, accounting for 95.55% of the total. The number of respondents who did not know whether they had purchased commercial health insurance or not was 19, accounting for 0.40% of the total number of respondents. This shows that only 4 out of every 100 Chinese has purchased commercial health insurance, which is very low, especially in comparison with the situation in developed countries such as France and the United States. Even though France has a mature basic medical insurance system under which healthcare is largely government-financed and which covers 98% of the population, 83% of French people still buy commercial health insurance. In the U.S., the health insurance market is dominated by commercial health insurance companies and 95% of U.S. citizens have commercial health insurance. Compared to France and the U.S., the effective demand for commercial health insurance in China is extremely low.

3.2.2 Analysis of the potential demand for commercial health insurance

3.2.2.1 *Looking at the situation from the structure of the national health insurance system*

The main purpose of a medical safeguards system is to provide reasonable financial support for the healthcare of citizens, for treatment of diseases, medical emergency assistance, and other medical services. By establishing a mechanism that is fair but also efficient, such a system helps ensure that resources are allocated effectively. It helps citizens maintain a certain level of health. It compensates for health problems brought on by society's consumption of resources, drives economic and social development, and raises the living standards of the population. A medical safeguards system is an outcome of public choice and it is the result of economic and social development. Its establishment, existence, and reform are defined by specific historical, social, and economic conditions. It also plays a role in keeping society stable and promoting economic growth and social progress and thus is considered an important tool by governments around the world.

Depending on the means of financing, medical safeguards models can be divided into three types: (1) a government-financed healthcare system, as in the UK; (2) a social insurance system mainly financed by public health insurance, as in Germany and Japan; (3) a medical safeguards system mainly financed by private insurers, as in the U.S. However, most countries have a health insurance market that offers both public and private or commercial insurance. The differences among countries lie mainly in the market share of these different options. Most OECD member countries adopt a hybrid system under which public health insurance and commercial insurance coexist. The economic efficiency of the hybrid healthcare system and the interaction between public health insurance and supplementary commercial insurance have consistently been a major focus of research internationally in the field of healthcare economics. In developed countries where health security is ensured largely by public health security and government-financed healthcare, such as Germany, France, Canada, Australia, and the Netherlands, commercial health insurance still has a place in the healthcare financing system. Especially in the past five years, however, the percentage of healthcare financing from commercial health insurance has increased significantly in these countries. They have instituted reform programs designed to improve the status of commercial health insurance, which has meant that the market plays a more forceful role in allocating resources.

We can see from the actual experience of health insurance systems around the world that commercial health insurance is a necessary supplement to basic medical insurance, no matter what model a country adopts for its system. In a multi-tiered health safeguards system, each level should target specific groups for coverage, and should have specific funding standards. In the UK, for example, the National Health Service covers almost every citizen but private medical insurance still operates to meet the medical needs of certain people. What's more, commercial insurance has maintained stable coverage in terms of market size as well as stable income from premiums. In Germany, commercial health insurance is an indispensable supplement to statutory public health insurance. For those with higher incomes, it provides more complete and more elite medical services. In the United States, commercial health insurance is even more central to the medical safeguards system, since the government provides protection only to certain groups of people.

In sum, commercial health insurance is of vital importance. Since it relates to achieving universal coverage of the medical safeguards system in China and to raising the overall level of services, the institutional framework within which the national healthcare insurance system works is creating space within the system into which commercial health insurance is encouraged to grow.[24] China's new medical reform plan has explicitly set forth the directive of strengthening the standing of commercial health insurance within China's overall medical safeguards system. It calls for the government to formulate preferential tax policies in this regard, and to authorize qualified insurance companies to undertake the relevant services.

3.2.2.2 Looking at the situation from demographics and China's base population figure

China has the largest base population in the world. The aging of that population has already become a grave problem and will continue to be a problem confronting the country for the next half century. People over 65 years of age already account for 8.87% of the population, according to the country's sixth national census. By United Nations definitions, this means that the country has entered the stage of an 'aging society.' (If 7% of a population is over 65, or if over 10% is over 60, this qualifies a country or a region to be considered an aging society.) The data shows that China has arrived at this point. Moreover, the life expectancy of people is being extended given better living standards and more advanced medical technology, which means that people have more years to live after they have retired. In addition, the standard model for China's household structure is increasingly what is called the '421 model.' A married couple composed of only-child husband and wife, born in the 1980s or 1990s, will have to bear the responsibility of supporting both sets of parents as they age, as well as raising at least one child. The resulting costs are becoming a tremendous burden on families, and caring for the elderly is becoming a severe problem. China's current social safeguards system can meet just a small portion of the demand for care of the elderly, and the level of protection provided by the system is low. Those who can purchase commercial insurance products are able to provide more comprehensive and higher-level protection for their elders. To a degree, the aging population increases demand for commercial health insurance.

At the same time, the incidence of chronic disease as well as critical illness is greater in old age than at any other stage in life. Older people have a greater demand for medical services and they therefore spend more on those services. Spending on medical costs becomes an important component of daily expenses to the extent that medical costs occupy a high percentage of a person's income.[25] Research conducted by Yan Ping (2009)[26] shows that medical expenses of senior citizens accounted for about 75% of total household medical expenses in 2006. Within this figure, medical costs for people between the ages of 70 and 74 took up the highest percentage of total medical costs, while medical costs of people over 80 were highest in actual amount. As age goes up, average medical costs increase and the burden of those costs inexorably gets heavier. Adding to this problem is the fact that China's current system of basic medical insurance cannot adequately provide safeguards for the medical needs of different ages and levels of seniors, even though it does include certain policies that are intended to help care for the elderly. The socio-economic status of older people also affects their access to healthcare. As medical costs increase, the older population in China is increasingly willing to adopt insurance as a way to reduce that burden.

In short, there will soon be more than 100 million people in China who are over the age 65 and this increase in the elderly segment of the population to a certain degree intensifies the financial and medical burden not just on families but on society as a whole. This has become a grave economic issue. At the same time, the situation presents an opportunity to commercial health insurance companies that are seeking to grow, since it stimulates a whole new source of demand.

3.2.2.3 Looking at the situation in terms of income levels

Income levels affect the demand for commercial health insurance in two main ways. First, a person's income level affects his willingness to purchase insurance. According to Maslow's theory of a hierarchy of needs, once the most basic physical needs are met, the consideration of security appears, and health is a part of that consideration. As incomes rise, and standards of living markedly improve, income becomes sufficient to pay for daily expenses and people begin to focus on quality of life. They want to be able to secure their health. Not only do they have a fairly strong desire to do so, but they are indeed able to purchase insurance in order to satisfy their need for safeguards.

Second, a person's income level affects his ability to purchase insurance. Since incomes were universally low in China in the past, limited purchasing power prevented any consumption of commercial health insurance and there was a tremendous income elasticity of demand for such insurance among the population. As disposable income rises, however, provided prices of health insurance products stay the same, the line of budgetary constraints moves to the right, and the feasible set of purchases that can fall within people's budgetary constraints increases. Commercial health insurance products are 'normal' goods, in that demand for them increases when income increases.

In recent years in China, the standard of living of people has risen on a widespread basis given the growing economy and increase in incomes. The Engel's coefficient, meanwhile, has fallen for households and basic living needs are already being met. Under these conditions, a growing demand for health safeguards has become quite apparent. Purchasing power has constantly improved as well, which means that insurance companies are earning more income from premiums. Purchasing power has a positive effect, therefore, on premium income. The rise in level of incomes in general in China is conducive to an increase in demand for commercial health insurance.

3.2.2.4 Looking at the situation in terms of the operating and management capacities of insurance companies

Improvement in the ability of insurance companies to supply products and services is now providing the basis for their ability to actually meet the demand for health insurance. At the end of 2002, the China Insurance Regulatory Commission issued the *Notice on the Guidance Opinion on accelerating the development of health insurance*. In the form of an official document, this presented the concept of specialized operations for health insurance. The *Notice* encouraged insurance companies to set up specialized operating entities to focus specifically on health insurance as a way to accelerate the growth of the industry. Since 2005, a number of companies that specialize in health insurance have been established, such as PICC Health, Kunlun Health, Ping An Health, and Reward Health (Ruifude Health). To a certain degree, the establishment of these entities is contributing to making the market for health insurance more professional.

To date, more than 100 insurance companies in China have initiated a commercial health insurance business. The statistics in 2011 were as follows: there were 4 insurance companies that dealt in health insurance or dealt only in health insurance, there were 33 Chinese life insurance companies and twenty-eight foreign-invested life insurance companies, and there were 30 property insurance companies. Among all of these, four companies that specialize in health insurance have been actively exploring new business models, business arenas, actuarial technologies, and management tools and have achieved significant success. They are achieving far more professional operations. These are PICC Health, Kunlun Health, Ping An Health, and Reward Health. Between 2006 and 2012, the amount of premium income earned by such specialized health insurance companies increased significantly as a percentage of all premium income in the health insurance industry—it went from 2.5% in 2006 to 9.32% in 2012. PICC Health can serve as an example. In 2012, this company realized RMB 7.5 billion in premium income, which was a 63% increase over the previous year. It did this through its innovative Zhanjiang and Taicang Models, which opened up new business areas for the insurance industry and improved the reputation and brand influence of PICC. At the same time, the company increased its investment in the development of new products and it strengthened internal controls. Meanwhile, in the same year, Ping An Health achieved premium income of RMB 210 million. Reward Health reported premium income of RMB 24.3 million, which was 13.3 times its income in the previous year. In 2012, the premium income of Kunlun Health reached RMB 329.48 million, an increase of 296% over the previous year. These two specialized health insurance companies had breakthrough increases in premium income as compared to the previous several years. (See Table 3.1.)

3.2.2.5 *Looking at the situation in terms of relevant policies*

Commercial health insurance is an important component of the framework of healthcare insurance systems that provide coverage for the entire population. As such, it has consistently been a top priority for the government. On April 6, 2009, the new medical reform was officially launched with the release of the *Opinions of the CPC Central Committee and the State Council on deepening reform of the institutional structures that govern the medical, pharmaceutical, and healthcare systems.* Article 6 of this new round of institutional reform of the healthcare system stressed the need to be proactive in developing commercial health insurance. In 2012, the China Insurance Regulatory Commission issued a *Notice* on deepening the reform mentioned above and also thoroughly implementing it during the 12th Five-Year Plan period. This directed the insurance industry to study and implement the 12th Five-Year Plan for Medical Reform as issued by the State Council.[27] At the same time, the China Insurance Regulatory Commission announced that it would be formulating preferential tax policies, among other things, to encourage both corporations and individuals to participate in commercial health insurance as well as other forms of supplemental insurance. It noted that companies are now encouraged to explore starting up medical institutions and participating in the corporate restructuring of existing public hospitals as a way to extend the supply chain of the health insurance industry.[28] As seen from the current situation, therefore, it should be possible for commercial health insurance to gain gradual recognition and acceptance by people. Even though there is currently a large disparity between sales of health insurance and other types of insurance, there is also tremendous room for growth given the support of government policies.

This can be seen particularly in the constant introduction of tax incentives and other policies that provide a motivation for commercial health insurance companies to realize the existing demand. In recent years, a whole succession of

Table 3.1 Premium income and market share of health insurers in China during 2006–2012 (unit: million yuan)

Year	Company name	PICC Health	Ping An Health	Kunlun Health	Reward Health	Total
		April 2005	May 2005	December 2005	January 2006	
2006	Premium income	888.4	0	0	52.9	941.3
	Market share	2.40%	0	0	0.1%	2.5%
2007	Premium income	2605	2.8	0.5	15.9	2,624.2
	Market share	6.79%	0.007%	0.001%	0.041%	6.839%
2008	Premium income	13,776.4	33.3	19.6	243	14,072.3
	Market share	23.5%	0.057%	0.033%	0.41%	24%
2009	Premium income	6,184.2	66.4	81.7	27.2	6,359.5
	Market share	10.8%	0.116%	0.0142%	0.047%	11.11%
2010	Premium income	2,863.4	62.2	95.5	2.8	3,023.8
	Market share	4.2%	0.092%	0.14%	0.004%	4.44%
2011	Premium income	4,596.4	131.4	83.2	1.7	4,812.7
	Market share	6.6%	0.19%	0.12%	0.002%	6.912%
2012	Premium income	7,499.73	210.75	329.48	24.3	8,064.26
	Market share	8.7%	0.24%	0.38%	0.003%	9.32%

Data source: *Yearbook of China's Insurance 2007–2013.*

policies has tried to support the development of the commercial health insurance market.[29] On May 6, 2015, the standing committee of the State Council decided to use international practice as the basis for attempting a trial run of offering preferential income tax policies to individuals who purchase health insurance. This move was highly significant as a way to stimulate purchase of comprehensive commercial health insurance. On February 16, 2016, the China Insurance Regulatory Commission officially announced the names of the companies that would become the first group allowed to issue products with such preferential tax policy treatment—they were PICC Health Insurance Co. Ltd., Taikang Pension & Insurance Co. Ltd., and Sunshine Life Insurance Co. Ltd. Under the impetus of the lever of preferential tax policies, the commercial health insurance industry is about to enter a period of rapid growth, an era of fast expansion and strategic development.

3.2.2.6 Looking at the situation in terms of people's awareness of how to shift or transfer health risks

Understanding risk and understanding insurance are intimately connected. To a certain degree, awareness of one of these things implies awareness of the other, but the level of awareness relates to a person's level of education, social environment, cultural background, and so on. A number of factors come into play, but the understanding of both these things affects the amount of demand for commercial health insurance.

For one thing, improving people's level of education should have the effect of raising awareness of risk and of insurance. People who are more educated tend to know more about risk and insurance, and they understand the importance of spreading risk. They are fairly able to control the extent of their own personal risk. Commercial health insurance is characterized by the ability to transfer risk, to provide financial security, and to meet the needs of people who want to avoid risk. As a result, people with higher degrees are more willing to purchase commercial health insurance so as to avoid health risks and thereby optimize their own portfolio of assets.

For another, people with higher education generally have higher income. Sun Rong and Wang Xiangnan (2011)[30] show that there is positive correlation between the level of education and expected levels of income. Moreover, people with higher incomes have a greater capacity to transform potential demand for insurance into actual demand. This is consistent with the conclusions in the relevant literature. In addition to increasing peoples' risk awareness and acceptance of insurance products, education also can increase the amount of human capital. In the insurance industry, expected future income is arrived at by estimating human capital. Expected future income is a reasonable measure of insurable assets. The more education a person has, the higher his insurable interest, that is, the more he has something to insure, which makes him more willing to go out and buy commercial health insurance. Sun and Wang also constructed a model based on panel data from 30 provincial administrative regions in mainland China that was collected between the years 2002 and 2009. The results of their study show that higher educational levels spurred the growth of commercial health insurance. To sum up the above, upgrading people's educational level has a positive effect on developing China's commercial health insurance industry.

3.2.3 Major problems relating to the demand for commercial health insurance

The commercial health insurance industry has received a high level of policy concern and support in the form of a succession of policy directives. Those include the *Various Opinions of the CPC Central Committee and the State Council on deepening reform of the institutional structures that govern the medical, pharmaceutical, and healthcare systems, Various Opinions of the State Council on promoting the development of the healthcare industry* (Guo Fa [2013] No. 40), *Various Opinions of the State Council on accelerating the development of modern insurance services* (Guo Fa [2014] No. 29), and *Various Opinions of the General Office of the State Council on accelerating the development of commercial health insurance* (Guo Fa [2014] No. 50). Since 2005, a number of insurance companies have been established, including PICC Health, Kunlun Health, Ping An Health, Hexie Health, and CPIC Allianz Health. Specialized health insurance companies have been actively exploring new business models, business arenas, actuarial technologies, and management tools. So far, more than 100 insurance companies have started up operations to engage in commercial health insurance business. Nevertheless, China's commercial health insurance industry still faces many problems and challenges, particularly with respect to improving the demand side.[31]

3.2.3.1 Some fundamental problems facing the development of commercial health insurance

3.2.3.1.1 The positioning of commercial health insurance within the structure of China's national health insurance systems

At the current stage, the structure of China's medical safeguards is composed of several systems. Those are: basic medical insurance, supplementary medical insurance, commercial medical insurance, and medical assistance (or emergency aid). Public health insurance provides the most basic of medical services. It cannot take into account the specific needs of every participant. Commercial health insurance caters to the special needs of individuals. Some people may prefer public health insurance and some may prefer commercial health insurance. The reality of the situation, however, is that the boundary between commercial health insurance and public medical safeguards is unclear in China. Each locality has its own policies with respect to social safeguards. The lack of unified policies has led to chaos in the market for supplementary medical insurance. Administrative means are being used to keep out market competition—this phenomenon definitely exists, which makes it very hard to design or price commercial health insurance products. The final result is that people's need for medical safeguards cannot effectively be met.

At present, China's public safeguards are gradually expanding to cover a greater scope of items, and the percentage of out-of-pocket expenses that individuals have to pay for total healthcare costs is gradually going down. Objectively speaking, one might assume that this has a certain 'squeezing' effect on commercial health insurance, a negative effect. At the same time, however, government spending can also be seen as a kind of transfer payment. It stimulates consumption and in that sense provides commercial health insurance with more room to grow. What is needed at this point is to define the scope of operations of commercial health insurance in an explicit way, so that insurance companies can make major progress that does not belong to the market space of government transfer payments.

Speaking to this issue from another perspective, the 'positioning' of commercial health insurance has not been clarified. Although the new medical reform defined its position as 'supplementary' to basic medical safeguards, that reform did not delineate the boundary between the two. It did not specify who the operating entities are. In terms of the scope of responsibilities for coverage, it also never clarified who is responsible for amounts above the ceiling on reimbursements. That is, does the insurance company cover these or does the public health agency? In terms of operating entities, the phenomenon of overstepping bounds of authority exists in some public organizations. For example, in some places such entities as trade unions, education bureaus, and hospitals take advantage of their position to carry on a health insurance business, sometimes even forcing their members to purchase insurance. Not only does this give the insured no way out, but it makes the orientation of these entities highly unclear and causes chaos in the health insurance market. This then affects the normal and proper growth of the industry. Moreover, since social medical insurance offers exemption from premiums and preferential rates to some people, this naturally makes consumers think first of social health insurance when they are considering their health-insurance plans. They naturally do not take into consideration commercial health insurance, which is designed to generate profit for private insurers. The positioning of social health insurance as 'basic' in fact has a strong 'crowding-out effect' on commercial health insurance.

Commercial health insurance is the inevitable outcome of the development of a commodity economy. It permeates all social and economic arenas and it affects all aspects of work and life. It can be said that commercial health insurance plays a key role in mitigating risks, promoting economic development, and stabilizing people's lives. These very qualities make it similar to public health insurance in many ways. First, the basic theory behind both is to use the law of large numbers to spread risk, to distribute economic losses associated with the occurrence of critical illness over large numbers of people. Both do this by assembling premium funds from either many economic entities or many individuals and using the assembled money to set up an insurance fund to insure against risk.

Both therefore share the same function of spreading risk and safeguarding health. Second, the large quantity of funds that are collected in the form of premiums can be used on the one hand for investing in and building up the national economy and, on the other hand, for safeguarding the interests of the people who are insured. Third, both make use of their social management functions to participate in health management, medical assistance, and other things that improve the quality of life and the health of China's citizens.

Health insurance has an irreplaceable role in the healthcare system. First, health insurance policies are contracts that set out the rights and obligations of both parties. This allows both to avoid the impact of policy changes or 'interfering behavior' by the government. It thus ensures long-term stability and carries the force of law. Second, private insurers offer a wide range of policies and have networks covering the whole country. They have fairly strong management capabilities, financial resources, a solid foundation, and thereby sufficient ability to expand. Notably, the insurance industry has a strong supporting system in the reinsurance business. It has multiple layers of safeguards when it comes to security. Third, commercial health insurance operates on the premise of voluntary participation. This makes it more acceptable to the public and it becomes easier to avoid unnecessary problems and disputes. Fourth, private insurers have resourceful, high-caliber, teams of professionals who are just in the process of growing in strength.[32] Fifth, publicity about the compensation that people receive, specific reimbursement cases, has had a great impact. This is enormously helpful as the country goes further in broadening awareness of catastrophic loss and the safeguards that insurance provides against catastrophic loss. Sixth, operating mechanisms that are increasingly business-oriented provide a wide range of choices to the insured, in order to meet healthcare needs as much as possible.

3.2.3.1.2 On the issue of how to combine supportive government policies with the role of market-oriented mechanisms

Policies that are relevant to health insurance have been listed above. The question remains, however, about how much of a role these actually play in growing China's health insurance industry. Given the unique context in which China's market operates, the whole issue of how to combine supportive policies with market mechanisms remains a major concern.

On August 10, 2015, the China Insurance Regulatory Commission formally issued the *Interim Measures on the administration of health insurance that enjoys preferential individual tax treatment*. This set out specific requirements for the design of health insurance products that allow for preferential individual tax treatment and related business conditions. In the *Interim Measures*, new provisions regarding insurance for people with pre-existing conditions, reimbursement rate of not less than 80%, pre-tax purchase, and other provisions have been regarded as a way to accelerate the approach of 'springtime' in the commercial health insurance business. The estimate is that implementing this preferential tax treatment policy will provide the industry with a market of some RMB 30 to 50 billion in the initial period.

The *Interim Measures* provide that the insurance company shall offer health insurance products that enjoy preferential personal tax treatment in accordance with long-term health insurance requirements and shall not refuse insurance to someone, or refuse to renew, or cancel an insurance policy solely because of the past medical history of the insured. The principles of product management, which are at the core of the management of health insurance products that enjoy preferential personal tax treatment, are undoubtedly the focus of attention. Among these principles, the 'Shall not refuse to provide insurance' clause has drawn wide attention. It is noteworthy that this provision breaks away from the general rules of commercial health insurance. In the current Chinese health insurance market, most private insurers adopt a prudent strategy when it comes to high risk groups or they avoid high risk groups altogether. This is understandable behavior for profit-seeking private insurers. However, the root cause for such practice lies in the fact that at present Chinese insurers lack the ability to control high levels of risk—their medical data is imperfect enough that actuarial calculations are inaccurate, plus their inability to control risk makes them unable to foster good relations with medical institutions. To ensure profitability, private insurers are bound to take a more prudent approach when it comes to high-risk groups. They either refuse to provide insurance or they raise premiums to a very high rate. To address this problem, officials of the China Insurance Regulatory Commission have pointed out that this principle aims to ensure fairness and the industry should voluntarily take on the social responsibility. After all, preferential tax treatment is in fact a transfer payment to the insurance industry from the government. The insurance industry should therefore do all it can to reduce the burden of medical costs, promote the medical reform, and provide insurance to all who are eligible.[33]

Insurance products that enjoy preferential personal tax treatment should be designed as all-purpose kinds of insurance. For the insurer, such products involve two kinds of responsibility, namely health insurance and the accumulation of value in personal accounts. Not only can such all-purpose insurance serve the function of being an investment, but it can be attractive to young people. Such design therefore 'stimulates the enthusiasm of consumers for the product.' At the same time, the design allows greater flexibility to insurance companies since they can make adjustments in real time depending on the needs of the market.

The *Interim Measures* also provide that the simple loss ratio of a health insurance underwriter shall not be less than 80% and if the simple loss ratio is less than 80%, insurers must issue rebates for the discrepancy to the personal accounts of the insured. This provision has stirred heated debate. Some analysts point out that the requirement means that an insurance company's profit margin is only 20%. Low profitability will have a negative impact on the operations and growth of small- and medium-sized insurance companies.

In addition, the *Interim Measures* also provide that, to offer health insurance products that enjoy preferential personal tax treatment, except for specialized health insurance companies, all other life insurance companies must set up a health insurance department. This should have an information management system that is relatively independent and that is linked in to the commercial health insurance information platform. They should have professional teams—no less than 50% of the staff should have a background in the health insurance business and no less than 30% should have a background in medicine.

From the above analysis, it might be assumed that the preferential tax policy should play a fairly positive role in spurring the development of China's health insurance. However, the specific impact can only be evaluated after a fairly long observation period. Once policies are put in motion, the effect of the 'policy dividend' may only appear after a few years, including, for example, the effect of the 2009 new medical reform. The fifth section of this study will present further analysis of the impact of the preferential tax policy on the market.

3.2.3.1.3 On the issue of the relationship between income levels and people's understanding of how to shift health risks

Risk preferences and the degree of willingness to buy are two factors that affect consumers' decision to buy insurance. Consumers with a high degree of risk aversion are more aware of risk management and thus have a stronger desire to buy health insurance. In contrast, an individual with low awareness of risk management is less willing to purchase health insurance. Different risk preferences lead to different choices when it comes to health insurance. Most people are 'overconfident' when it comes to personal health risks. They believe in their own physical conditions and feel that disease, at least major disease, won't happen to them. This mindset suppresses their need for health insurance. China's urban employees' basic medical insurance program and the urban residents' basic medical insurance program, which particularly emphasize 'broad coverage,' have been successfully rolled out with strong support from the government. The protection from these two programs, coupled with overconfidence, makes consumers feel they are already insured by publicly funded coverage and have no need to purchase further commercial coverage. The result is a mistaken understanding of the functions of public and commercial insurance.[34]

Adequate purchasing power is one of the necessary conditions if potential demand of consumers is to be transformed into effective demand.[35] The possibility of matching up supply and demand can only happen if purchasing power is adequate, and only then can there be any hope of turning that purchasing power into premium income for insurance companies.

We can divide the impact of people's disposable income on the premium income of health insurance companies into three levels. When disposable income is low, potential demand for health insurance cannot be transformed into actual demand. When disposable income reaches a certain level, potential demand can be converted quickly into actual demand. When disposable income exceeds a certain level, however, actual demand for health insurance is inhibited and health insurance is no longer the only option for people, or no longer is it a necessary choice.

In other words, even if a person has an understanding of risk, income constraints may keep that person from turning potential demand for health insurance into effective demand. Another phenomenon exists in real life, however, which is that there may be adequate purchasing power but an insufficient understanding of risk. The unique economic structure of China means that benefits of many State-Owned Enterprises are really quite good. These entities provide welfare benefits to employees, and sometimes even pay medical costs for employees out of corporate earnings. As they see it, they save money that way—since insurance companies are for-profit, if they themselves serve as the insurance company, they can save on costs. Such companies have plenty of purchasing power but they fail to purchase insurance due an inaccurate understanding of insurance.

3.2.3.1.4 On the issue of the profitability of insurance companies and the supply of commercial health insurance products

3.2.3.1.4.1 PROFITABILITY OF INSURANCE COMPANIES

In the decade or so between 2003 and 2014, the loss ratio of health insurance was higher than that of personal insurance. In 2013 and 2014, all of the four major specialized health insurance companies were operating at a loss (Ping An Health, PICC Health, Hexie Health, and Kunlun Health.)

As can be seen from Figure 3.8, over the past decade, the loss ratio of China's health insurance industry has been on the rise. In 2012, the claims paid by the health insurance industry reached RMB 29.817 billion, with a high loss ratio of 34.6%. This amount was 16% of the total claims paid by the personal insurance industry while the premium income of the health insurance industry only accounted for 8% of the total premium income of the personal insurance industry. The ongoing high loss ratio of the health insurance business is holding back innovation in product development and curbing enthusiasm for R&D. As a result, it is holding back the development of China's commercial health insurance in general.

3.2.3.1.4.2 INSUFFICIENT PRODUCT INNOVATION

According to the regulations of the China Insurance Regulatory Commission, any life insurance company, specialty health insurance company, and financial company can enter the market for health insurance once they obtain a license to carry on the business. From this, it can be seen that the threshold for market entry is somewhat low. This is helpful when it comes to increasing the supply of commercial health insurance products and promoting the development of the domestic commercial health insurance market.

In the meantime, China's commercial health insurance industry is still in the very early stages of development, and the potential demand for commercial

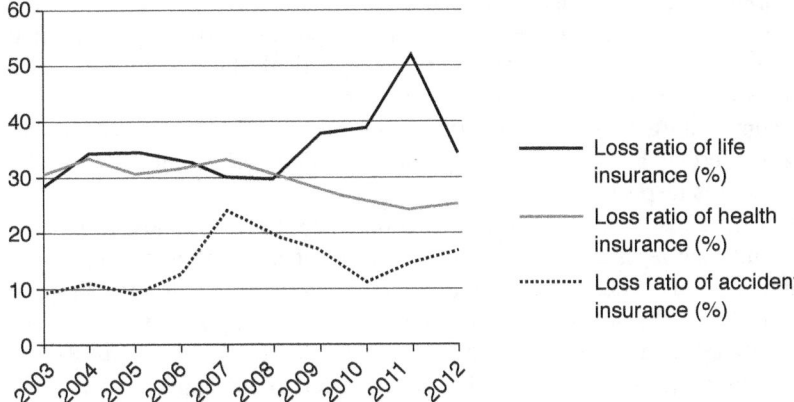

Figure 3.8 Comparison of loss ratios of life insurance, health insurance and accident insurance.

health insurance is huge, while the market is still immature and underdeveloped. Faced with this massive market, all insurance companies are vigorously developing products related to commercial health insurance in order to improve their product offerings, increase their profits, take more market share, and thereby improve their overall competitiveness. Every year, commercial health insurance companies launch several major health insurance products, or sell such products as add-ons, or bundle them with other popular insurance products. Nevertheless, although there are many types of products, the innovative nature of these products, their usability, and their profitability, all have problems. What's more, they do not in fact satisfy the demand of consumers whose needs are diversifying by the day.

First, the homogeneity of commercial health insurance products is striking. There is little difference in the terms of different policies, including terms about liability, exclusion, scope of coverage, and value-added services. This is mainly because the cost of product development is higher than the cost of simply copying, and the cost of real innovation is vastly higher than copying. In order to save on costs, many insurance companies simply copy the products of other companies.

Second, not only are health-insurance policies very similar to one another, but all of them are redundant in many ways with China's basic medical insurance program. Basic medical insurance does have a certain crowding-out effect on commercial health insurance, and at present the differences between the two are relatively minor which magnifies that crowding-out effect. Furthermore, most short-term commercial health insurance policies in China contain age restrictions, leaving senior citizens exposed to health risks. Most long-term health insurance policies also set a cap on the amount of claims. Taking both these things into consideration, at present the protection provided by commercial health insurance products is actually limited.

Third, current commercial health insurance products only cover a limited number of diseases—between 29 and 42 types of critical illness. At this point in China's history, however, the problems of food safety and environmental pollution are contributing to broadening the range of what is considered critical illness. Commercial health insurance products cannot satisfy the demand for safeguards in this respect.

Fourth, China is still in an exploratory period when it comes to loss of income insurance and long-term care insurance. The range of products is small. Only a small number of insurance companies provide such products. Current long-term care insurance products are similar to annuities in design. They are often offered as add-ons, such as Taikang Jixiang Health Scheme (with a Long-Term Care Rider). Such things are frequently bundled with other products. Their supply is insufficient to meet the demand in the market. This too negatively impacts the role that commercial health insurance should actually play in offering protection.

3.2.3.2 Problems that affect the growth of the industry from the perspective of consumers

3.2.3.2.1 Consumers' lack of risk awareness

Risk preferences and the willingness to buy are two factors that affect a person's decision to buy insurance. Consumers with a high degree of risk aversion are more aware of risk management and thus have a stronger desire to buy health insurance. In contrast, an individual with low awareness of risk management is less willing to purchase health insurance.[36]

China's insurance industry generally uses agents to sell insurance, but many of these exaggerate the features of the products they are selling in order to increase their own earnings, or they even make totally false representations. As a result, the insurance industry has a bad reputation in the market. In addition, China's traditional culture is at odds with the conceptual underpinnings of insurance. The culture emphasizes good fortune and chance, whereas insurance emphasizes preparing for risk prior to an adverse event. As the insurance industry promotes its products to the market, it therefore encounters intangible obstacles. There are in fact hundreds of millions of people in China who do not have any social medical safeguards, but due to the prejudice against health insurance in society at large, these people are not inclined to purchase commercial health insurance. During the 2008 earthquake in Wenchuan, the premiums paid by residents in Aba Prefecture, which was the epicenter of the earthquake, accounted for only 0.17% of total premiums in Sichuan, and the amount paid out in premiums for casualty and health insurance amounted to less than RMB 450,000. The total market share of the two cities that were hit worst, Deyang and Mianyang, was less than 10%. It is imperative, therefore, that China increase public awareness of risk management and strengthen education about insurance.

3.2.3.2.2 Lack of understanding about commercial health insurance products

As a unique kind of social commodity, public resources are non-exclusive but subject to competition in how they are used. As a result, they are often used to excess, a phenomenon generally known as the tragedy of the commons.[37] Commercial health insurance products are similarly open to every policy holder. Such products are provided by companies and are offered at a cost to the companies, but the whole system is based on the idea of mutual cooperation among policy holders and the sharing of risk. A policy holder has the right to make a claim for losses that are covered under a policy, but the total amount of compensation sought by the consumer has to be limited. If the amount of compensation paid out for a given health insurance product is higher than its income, that product is unsustainable. Commercial health insurance therefore is also like a public resource in that it is susceptible to the 'tragedy of the commons' phenomenon. When those entrusted with the resources (in this case, consumers of insurance policies) engage in moral hazard behavior, the commercial insurance market can be put in jeopardy.

Some consumers, for example, may know that others have carried out fraudulent behavior with respect to health insurance, and they may also realize that this has a detrimental effect on the development of the insurance market as a whole. Nevertheless, their own policy terms and the underwriting obligations of the insurance company mean that their individual interests are protected if they themselves have a problem. The fraudulent use of insurance resources by others does not impact them, so they are not motivated to organize any regulatory control over the cheating by others. On the contrary, they too hope to earn back their premiums, and more, once they themselves have a health problem. This only goes to increase the overall moral hazard of the group of consumers. The inadequate understanding of the 'tragedy of the commons' nature of the problem is a major factor currently blocking the development of the health insurance industry in China.

3.2.3.2.3 Lack of understanding of relevant government policies

There are actually not that many government policies relating to health insurance in China. The most important ones relate to preferential tax treatment and social security, and these were only recently introduced. China had previously passed other preferential tax policies but they were incomplete and imperfect. In order to support the development of supplemental health insurance, the Ministry of Finance offered a 4% pre-tax deduction for those purchasing supplemental health insurance, but this ran into problems. As Jiang Cai and Ye Xiaolan[38] pointed out in 2008, this tax incentive actually violated the whole purpose of instituting the policy, since it unfairly benefited those less in need while failing to benefit those most in need of the subsidy. This not only affected the fairness of the market for health insurance in general, but the pre-tax deduction also did not significantly increase coverage. Another problem has been that China lacks the kind of accounting items that enable the supplementary health insurance to benefit from such policy initiatives. To a certain degree, this lack of accounting standards constrains not only the willingness of individuals to buy health insurance, but also the willingness of insurance companies to offer health insurance products.[39]

Looking at the situation overall, the imperfections and unreasonable nature of tax policies and social security policies are proving to be a major factor inhibiting the development of the health insurance industry. Meanwhile, consumers who have little understanding of insurance to begin with are put off by the complexities and tedious nature of policies. One course of action in the future therefore must be to improve the effectiveness of government policies as a way to foster the development of commercial health insurance.

3.2.3.2.4 The problem of low income levels of potential consumers

China's residents must have adequate purchasing power if the country is to transform potential demand for health insurance into effective demand. Only adequate purchasing power will provide even the possibility of matching up supply and demand, and only then will there be any hope of transforming that demand into premium income for insurance companies. If consumers have the desire to buy but not the ability, they generate potential but not effective demand. Right now, China's unrealized potential demand is mainly a matter of insufficient purchasing power. The primary reason is that prices of commercial health insurance products are higher than what consumers can pay. Generally speaking, we believe that consumers with higher levels of income have greater purchasing power. In terms of empirical analysis, income is a factor that is fairly easy to quantify.

The situation with respect to China's urban residents is as follows. Average disposable income over a given period increased at an average yearly rate of 11.89%. GDP over the same period increased at rate of 13.89%. Medical expenses, however, increased at the high rate of 52.52%. Given this high rate, not only could disposable income not keep pace, but it did not even keep pace with the increase in GDP. Even if consumers had a strong desire to buy health insurance, they were prevented from doing so by their lack of sufficient purchasing power. They were therefore unable to transform potential demand into the reality of effective demand and their express opinion was that the price of health insurance products was simply too high.

3.3 QUALITATIVE ANALYSIS OF FACTORS INFLUENCING THE DEMAND FOR COMMERCIAL HEALTH INSURANCE

3.3.1 Analysis of economic factors

3.3.1.1 Capacity to pay, by individuals and by external assistance

In line with previous research done on the subject, we can divide the capacity to pay into two components, payment by individuals and payment by external assistance. The capacity of an individual to pay refers to the income level of the person, while the capacity of external payers refers to government expenditures on health.

The capacity to pay has a direct bearing on people's demand for health insurance. Generally, the more economically developed a region is, the more its industries flourish and the same is true of the insurance industry. The demand for insurance relies quite heavily on whether income is high or low, so insurance is a product whose demand is elastic relative to income. Only if income is high will the capacity to pay be high, and only then will people have the possibility of purchasing insurance. Only then can potential demand be transformed into effective demand. As for the capacity of external assistance to pay for insurance, the most important player is the government, with its expenditures on healthcare. Government healthcare expenditures are economic subsidies to consumers with respect to healthcare and medicine. In that sense, they are a way to improve the ability of consumers to pay as well. China's income levels have risen fairly quickly since the start of Reform and Opening Up. Incomes on average have gone from RMB 343.4 in 1978 (per annum) to RMB 28,843.9 in 2014. Lives are increasingly prosperous and the individual's capacity to pay is constantly improving (see Figure 3.9).

Commercial health insurance develops in direct ratio to the quantity of demand for the insurance. That demand in turn comes from both the number of consumers who represent demand for health insurance and those who have the desire and the ability to pay for it. Over the short run, people's inclination to buy insurance is a constant, and the most decisive factor in that respect is

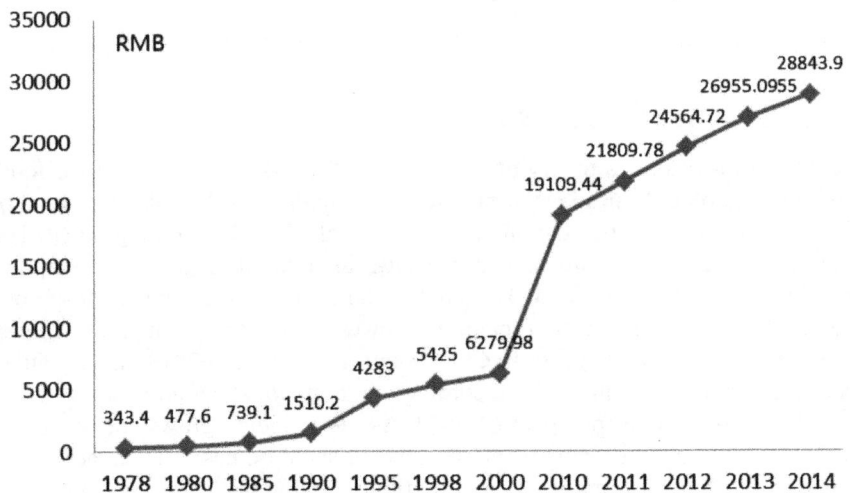

Figure 3.9 Disposable income since 1978.

Source: *China Statistics Yearbook 2015.*

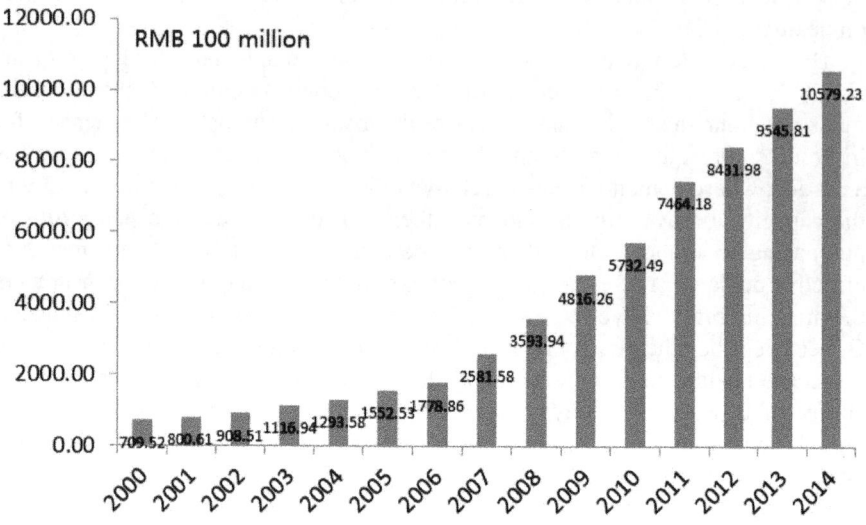

Figure 3.10 Government expenditure on health, 2000–2014.

Source: *China Statistics Yearbook 2015.*

disposable income. As China's economy has grown and its citizens have experienced rising standards of living, their demand for health insurance has grown stronger.

In the meantime, the government has become more forceful in providing public-finance subsidies for people's medical and health needs (see Figure 3.10).

3.3.1.2 Structure of consumption spending

According to Maslow's theory of a hierarchy of needs, once the need for food, clothing, and other basics is met, people turn to higher-level needs. This kind of change in demand can be quantified by what is called the Engels coefficient. The Engels coefficient measures the percentage in a family's total consumption spending that is spent on food. The smaller the coefficient, the more prosperous the family. The larger the coefficient, the lower the family's standard of living. The coefficient among families in China's cities was 35% in 2013, having fallen from a figure of 57.5% in 1978. According to international definitions, this figure of 35% is already at a 'prosperous' level. As the economy grows and standards of living rise, this percentage of family income spent on basics is already much smaller and China's structure of consumption spending is already coming in line with that in advanced countries. In other words, the situation already provides the material basis for buying commercial health insurance for the great majority of people in China.[40]

3.3.1.3 Degree of market competition among the primary players

The pattern of market competition has a direct bearing on the quantity and quality of commercial health insurance products and services that are available. The more market-oriented the situation, the more the market's main players engage in competition. Prices of health insurance products are fairer, services are better, companies are more innovative with respect to both products and services, and all of this is beneficial to the long-term growth of the market. The extent of market competition is generally measured in several ways: by the concentration ratio (CRn), the Herfindahl-Hirschman Index (HHI), the Gini coefficient, and the Lorenz curve. Among these, CRn and HHI are more frequently used in anti-trust market analysis (see Figure 3.11).

3.3.1.4 The situation with respect to R&D of health insurance products

Insurance companies are increasingly faced with the problem of how to satisfy diverse needs among customers while at the same time controlling their own costs. This is due to the fact that today's customers have increasingly diverse kinds of risk, while their preferences, consumption abilities, and customs are all different as well. We can imagine that any insurance product that is personalized to the extent that it satisfies the individual is necessarily a product that will spur demand for health insurance.[41]

Many more choices are now available on the commercial health insurance market, and policies are better targeted at specific needs. Not only are there

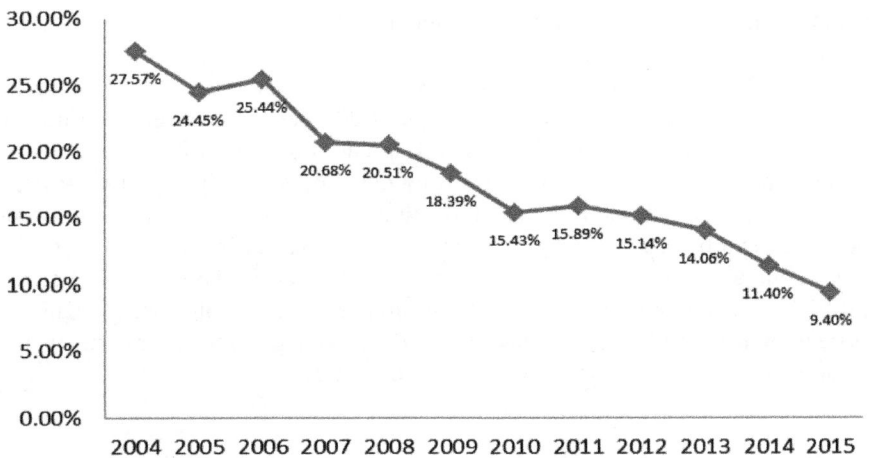

Figure 3.11 HHI of personal insurance in China over the past years.

Source: *China Statistics Yearbook 2015*; data in statistics column of website of China Insurance Regulatory Commission.

products aimed at children, but there are maternity policies for women. Not only are there products aimed at cancer, but there are policies specifically written against the H1N1 influenza virus. There are special products for inpatient services, and care policies for nursing. Nevertheless, compared with what is available in developed countries, where insurance industries are more mature, we still have a very long way to go. We can only truly address our supply-side reform of commercial health insurance by diversifying the products and services that are available to the market.

3.3.2 Analysis of healthcare resource factors

The status of a country's healthcare and medical system is not only an indication of that country's comprehensive strength, but these things are also vital to the welfare of the people. The more abundant the facilities and the more accessible the medical system, the easier it is for people to get healthcare services. The chance of their buying health insurance is also greater. Just imagine, if someone was quite able to pay and indeed would like to buy insurance to mitigate the risk of serious illness, but found it difficult to access medical treatment and difficult to ensure follow-on services, would that person buy insurance? Probably not. According to the 5th National Healthcare Services Survey, among people who should have been hospitalized but were not in 2013, 23.7% believed hospitalization to be unnecessary, 43.2% failed to go to the hospital because of cost, and 11.5% failed to go because they did not have the time. For those who thought it unnecessary or did not have the time, some felt it was too much trouble to see a doctor and some could not manage the travel or stand in line so long. The cost of time and effort was more than the cost of continuing to be sick for these people. The expectation of ever receiving medical services in such a household would naturally decline, which would in turn suppress any desire to purchase commercial health insurance.[42]

Tables 3.2 and 3.3 present the total number of hospital beds in China and the average number of medical technicians per 1,000 people. In overall terms, the numbers are on the rise, but there is still an enormous disparity between these figures and levels in developed countries over the same time period. What's more, the disparity between cities and countryside in China is even more pronounced. The basic situation is that healthcare resources in China are not only scarce but are also unevenly distributed in the country. To a certain degree, therefore, adding commercial health insurance as a supplement to China's systems will contribute to increasing and diversifying healthcare resources and creating a more effective market for those resources.

Table 3.2 Number of hospital beds in China, 2001–2014

	2001	2002	2003	2004	2005	2006	2007
Number of hospital beds	2,469,644	1,686,839	2,358,120	2,008,968	2,595,875	2,661,037	2,721,129
	2008	2009	2010	2011	2012	2013	2014
Number of hospital beds	2,920,916	3,155,048	3,418,173	3,705,118	4,161,385	4,580,045	4,961,884

Source: Statistics from the official website of the Ministry of Health of the People's Republic of China.

Table 3.3 Number of medical technicians per 1,000 people in China, 2003–2013

Year	Number of medical technicians per 1,000 people		
	Overall	Urban	Rural
2003	3.48	4.88	2.26
2004	3.53	4.99	2.24
2005	3.50	5.82	2.69
2006	3.60	6.09	2.70
2007	3.72	6.44	2.69
2008	3.90	6.68	2.80
2009	4.15	7.15	2.94
2010	4.39	7.62	3.04
2011	4.61	6.68	2.66
2012	4.94	8.54	3.41
2013	5.27	9.18	3.64

Source: Statistics from the official website of the Ministry of Health of the People's Republic of China.

3.3.3 Analysis of social and cultural factors

3.3.3.1 Age structure of the population

In 2000, people above 60 years old accounted for 10.33% of the Chinese population (see Figure 3.12). This figure indicates that China has now officially entered the ranks of 'an aged society.' The aging of a population is a symbol of social progress, but it also adds to the economic burden of the society. Caring for the elderly presents a severe challenge to the social security systems of all countries.[43]

Demographic structures include a variety of factors that lead to demand for health insurance that is more diversified and more personalized. They include the intensification of the aging of the society, changes in the distribution of the population, changes in the structure of groups with different income levels, and so on.

First, the aging of the population leads to an increase in demand for services-type health insurance. As the aging of society accelerates, and families become smaller, this gestates a massive demand for such services as critical illness treatment, nursing care, rehabilitation, and so on. This in turn stimulates demand for healthcare products and actual demand for insurance to cover those products.

Second, changes in the overall demographic structure are resulting in demand for increasingly diverse forms of insurance. Population aging and the growth of the middle-income and high-income segments of the population will mean more demand for diverse and personalized health and medical insurance. China's aged

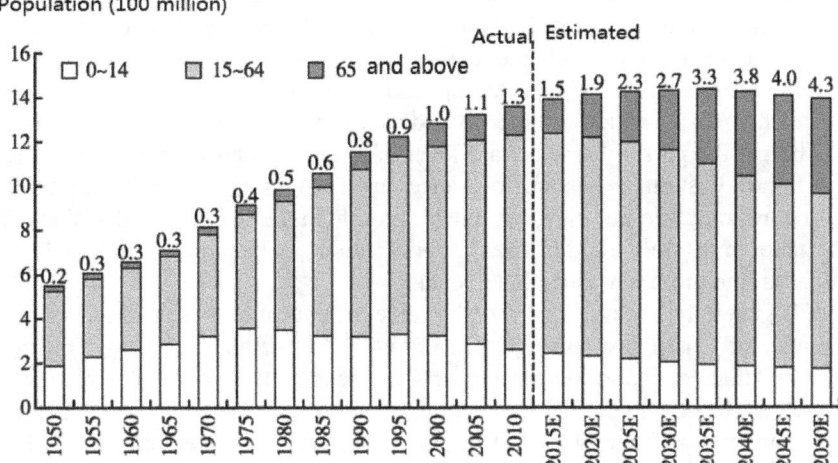

Figure 3.12 Estimation of China's population structure.

Source: *China Population Bluebook.*

population is one of the largest in the world, and the needs of these people are obviously different from others in terms of health insurance. Their spending requirements are different and the greatest uncertainty in what they have to spend relates to medical costs. Beyond social security safeguards, they must carry a certain percentage of the burden of these costs, which means that commercial health insurance can help them lower that burden. The conclusion is that health insurance companies should develop products that are specifically targeted at different age segments of the population.

Third, changes in the distribution of China's population are leading to an increase in the demand for safeguards-oriented insurance. Laborers who have migrated to cities from the countryside have by now changed the distribution of population in China. Most of these people are young or middle-aged and they are mainly covered by the urban employees' basic medical insurance program. Developing products that are aimed specifically at their needs will help broaden the scope and stimulate the growth of commercial health insurance.

Fourth, changes in income structure are driving up demand for more personalized insurance products. As the economy grows and incomes increase, not only are standards of living improving but health conditions are tremendously better than before. People are also more aware of health considerations. In addition to common infectious diseases, non-infectious chronic diseases and some new infectious diseases have become a concern to middle-income and high-income groups. This brings new demand for health insurance and commercial products that offer personalized coverage.

3.3.3.2 Education background

People with higher levels of education tend to want healthier lifestyles, and they are also more likely to invest in their own health. Better educated people are also aware of risks to their own health and the health of their families, so they intentionally mitigate those risks by buying insurance.[44] Insurance is a fairly complex type of financial product. In order to understand and accept this kind of product, it is best if the person has a certain level of education, since another consideration is how insurance is sold. Insurance agents in China and financial entities selling insurance do not play that much of a role in the purchasing decision. The consumer must rely on his own determinations, which places much higher demands, therefore, on educational level.

It is generally believed that a higher level of education will lead to increased demand for health insurance (Duker, 1969;[45] Xu Meifang, 2007[46]). The main reason is that education increases a person's sensitivity to risk (Slovic, 1986),[47] as well as deepening their understanding of health insurance. Degree of education can therefore be used to measure human capital. A higher educational level generally means expectations of higher income. Education can improve a person's ability to manage finances and therefore helps persuade people to incorporate insurance products in their asset portfolio. Higher educational levels also mean longer times in school—this increases the demand for insurance for sons and daughters who have not yet reached adulthood.

3.3.3.3 Understanding of insurance

Having an understanding of insurance and having specialized knowledge about it are indicators of a country's degree of progress and civilization. In addition,

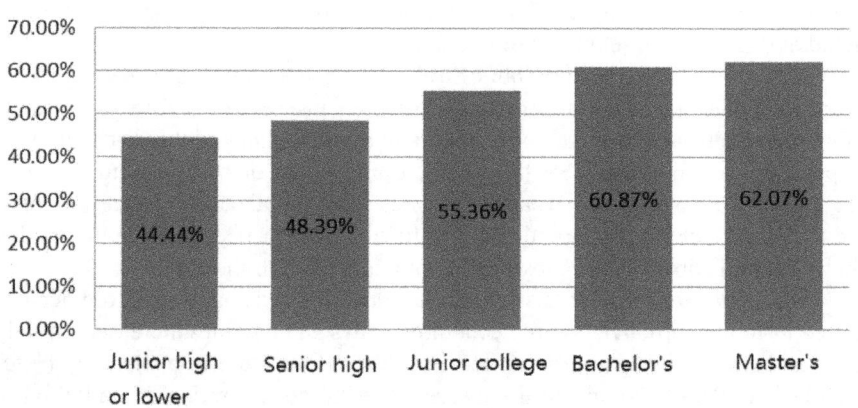

Figure 3.13 Percentage of insurance buyers in population groups with different education backgrounds.

Source: *Research Report on the Financial Capacity of Chinese Consumers 2013.*

these things are a prerequisite for developing that country's insurance industry. Over the past 30 years of Reform and Opening Up, China has pushed forward modernization but its people are also now facing a greater array of risks than they were before. More and more consumers want to truly understand insurance, in order to use it to safeguard their lives from the interference of external risk. Nevertheless, a considerable segment of the population still adheres to traditional ways of thinking. They are conceptually bound by the old ways of countering risk, for example: 'Store away money in the bank for when you might need it,' and 'Have children so that they can take care of you in your old age.' Many middle-age and older people in particular still have the idea that you should mainly rely on the government, family, and friends to counter risk and reduce losses. Quite a few people in China are still unfamiliar with the purpose of insurance and how it operates. They are unaccustomed to using insurance to shift and spread all the many forms of risk in their lives. Not only does this curtail the growth of the insurance industry, but it is detrimental to improving the quality of life of China's population. Naturally, the situation is somewhat better as society and economic conditions have improved. The understanding of insurance has indeed gone up to the extent that a certain portion of consumers will now purchase insurance voluntarily to counter risk. Understanding insurance plays a powerful role in furthering the growth of the industry.

3.3.3.4 Health conditions and attitudes toward health risks

A precondition for any consumer to have a need for health insurance is that there are health risks. Insurance has begun to exert a subtle influence on people as the risk of illness changes and evolves in China, since the most direct reason for buying insurance is the economic impact of having a health problem. The possibility of getting sick therefore directly stimulates demand for health insurance: we see that in the way that people who are in poor health are generally more likely to buy insurance. At the same time, consumers generate new kinds of demand for health insurance as new kinds of health problems arise. This makes companies become more creative in developing new products and services.[48]

Health conditions that are related to people's demand for commercial health insurance mainly fall into objective and subjective categories. The objective health conditions of a person relate to the actual probability of that person's getting sick and the possible seriousness of the disease. The subjective conditions relate the person's own understanding of his health. Zhang Xinmin *et al.* (1995)[49] and others believe that subjective conditions are more closely related to the demand for commercial health insurance. The accuracy with which a person evaluates his own health relates to his level of health literacy and overall education. How healthy a person believes him/herself to be depends on his/her health literacy and education attainment. At its current stage in history, China has a population that in overall terms is poorly educated and does not have a good understanding of health issues. To a degree, this suppresses their demand for commercial health insurance.

3.4 QUANTITATIVE ANALYSIS OF FACTORS THAT INFLUENCE THE DEMAND FOR COMMERCIAL HEALTH INSURANCE

3.4.1 Grey relational (correlation) analysis of factors that influence the demand for commercial health insurance

3.4.1.1 Reason for choosing grey relational analysis

The GM (1,1) model is the most widely applied kind of dynamic prediction model within the overall subject known as 'grey system theory.' The model is composed of a first order univariate differential equation. It is mainly used to fit and predict the 'eigen values' of a dominant factor in a complex system to reveal the changes and the future trends of the dominant factor. This study uses grey relational analysis to examine the impact of factors that influence commercial health insurance. Grey system theory was developed by Chinese professor Deng Julong in the late 1970s and early 1980s. The method is mainly used to study systems in which some information is known and some is unknown. It generates, develops, and extracts valuable information from the known information. As compared with traditional research methods, grey system theory has the following advantages. First, less information is needed to build a model. In general, a model can be established as long as there are more than four pieces of data. Second, prior parameters of the distribution of original data are not required. Third, the model can maintain the characteristics of the original system fairly faithfully and thereby reflect the true conditions of the original system. Fourth, grey system theory combines qualitative analysis and quantitative analysis. Last but not least, its calculation method is relatively simple.[50]

China's commercial medical market has developed extremely rapidly in recent years. Many different factors have influenced its growth, some of which are very hard to measure. Those include the impact of government policies and also changes in the general mindset of the population. Despite the fact that there are so many influencing factors, analysis of the industry generally uses traditional approaches, such as regression analysis, principal component analysis, and variance analysis. These methods have their uses but in this case the authors feel that their data requirements are excessive.

Take the least squares modeling method for example. It has strict requirements for the sample size, correlation between sequences, and sequence stability. In real life, however, these requirements are hard to meet, which undermines the reliability of the results of the regression analysis. In the specific case of commercial health insurance, it is hard to find a typical distribution pattern of relevant data in China, since the country started to develop commercial health insurance much later than in developed countries and the industry has grown so rapidly. Based on the above analysis, the authors hope that the use of grey relational analysis to examine the demand for commercial health insurance in this study will provide inspiration for future studies.

3.4.1.2 *Steps of grey relational analysis*

3.4.1.2.1 *Identify the characteristic sequence that reflects the behavioral characteristics of the system and the comparison sequence that affects the behavior of the system*

A sequence that reflects the behavioral characteristics of the system $X_0 = [X_0(1), X_0(2), ..., X_0(n)]$ is called a characteristic sequence. Sequences that affect the behavior of the system

$$
\begin{bmatrix}
X_1 = [X_1(1), X_1(2), ..., X_1(n)] \\
... \\
X_i = [X_i(1), X_i(2), ..., X_i(n)] \\
... \\
X_m = [X_m(1), X_m(2), ..., X_m(n)]
\end{bmatrix}
$$

are called comparison sequences.

3.4.1.2.2 *Perform dimensionless processing of the characteristic sequence and the comparison sequence*

The factors in the system have different meanings and dimensions, making it difficult to compare data directly. Direct comparison with processing will affect the accuracy of the conclusions. Therefore, before running the grey relational analysis, dimensionless processing should be performed. Generally speaking, nondimensionalization can be achieved through equalization,[51] initialization,[52] and other methods.

3.4.1.2.3 *Calculate the grey relational coefficient of the characteristic sequence and the comparison sequence $\xi(k)$*

Degree of association is essentially the degree of difference between the geometric shapes of the curve of the characteristic sequence and that of the comparison sequence. If a characteristic sequence X_0 has many comparison sequences $X_1, X_2, ..., X_m$, the relational coefficient for each comparison sequence and the reference sequence $\xi(k)$ can be calculated by the following formula:

$$
\xi(k) = \frac{\min\limits_{i} \min\limits_{k} |X_0(k) - X_i(k)| + \theta \max\limits_{i} \max\limits_{k} |X_0(k) - X_i(k)|}{|X_0(k) - X_i(k)| + \theta \max\limits_{i} \max\limits_{k} |X_0(k) - X_i(k)|}
\tag{4.1}
$$

The result is the relational coefficient for the comparison sequence and the reference sequence at each point of the curve, where θ is the resolution coefficient (0, 1). In most cases, $\theta = 0.5$.

Denoted as

$$a = m_i\text{in } m_k\text{in } \Delta i(k) = m_i\text{in } m_k\text{in } | X_0(k) - X_i(k) |$$ (4.2)

which is the minimum difference between two sequences.
Denoted as

$$b = m_i\text{ax } m_k\text{ax } \Delta i(k) = m_i\text{ax } m_k\text{ax } | X_0(k) - X_i(k) |$$ (4.3)

which is the maximum difference between two sequences,
where

$$\Delta i(k) = | X_0(k) - X_i(k) |$$ (4.4)

3.4.1.2.4 Degree of association r_i

Since the correlation coefficient is the degree of association between the comparison sequence and the reference sequence at each point in time, each point on the curve has a correlation coefficient. To compare the degree of association between the comparison sequence and the reference sequence in an easier way, the mean of the coefficients is calculated. The degree of association r_i can be calculated by the following formula:

$$r_i = \frac{1}{n} \sum_{L=1}^{n} \xi_i(k)$$ (4.6)

3.4.1.2.5 Ranking factors according to the degree of association

Ranking factors according to the degree of association, the main factor and the secondary factor in each relationship is calculated.

3.4.2 The selection of grey correlation variables for the factors that influence the demand for commercial health insurance

When selecting factors that affect the demand for commercial health insurance, this study has taken into account how representative each factor is and also how obtainable the data is. It integrates research already carried out and has selected the following nine variables in all on which to conduct empirical research. Naturally there is some subjectivity in the selection of variables, which is one aspect that still needs improvement.

Among economic factors, the indicators that this study has selected are per capita disposable income of urban households, the urban Engels coefficient, the government's healthcare expenditures, and the Herfindahl index of the personal insurance market. These are represented by the symbols DI, EC, GHE, and HHI.[53]

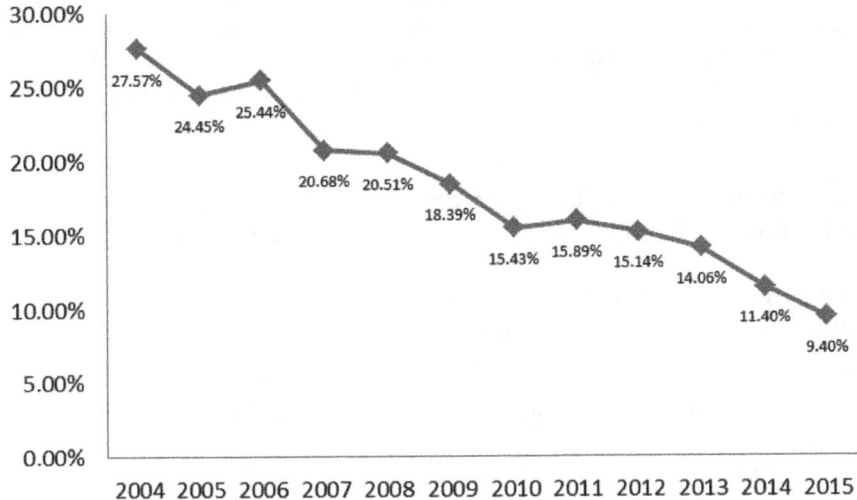

Figure.3.14 Herfindahl Index of China's personal insurance market in recent years.
Data source: Statistics column on website of China Insurance Regulatory Commission.

Among health resources factors, this study has selected the number of health technical personnel per 1,000 people and the income of medical insurance funds. The authors describe the availability of health resources through the number of health technical personnel per 1,000 people, while the income of medical insurance funds reflects the development of social health insurance. These two indicators are represented by HW and SocialIm.

Among social and cultural factors, we selected the percentage of people with a higher education, the old-age dependency ratio, and mortality as representative variables. We chose the percentage of people with a higher education because attitudes towards risk, and awareness of insurance, are both highly related to the level of education. People with higher education levels are more rational and objective about insurance. We chose mortality as one indicator because it can represent the health condition to some extent. The old-age dependency ratio can intuitively show the degree of social aging. These three indicators are represented as EDU, DR, and ODR respectively.

Looking at research done previously on the demand for insurance, we discovered that most studies chose premium income as the indicator that most closely describes demand. This study also uses premium income of health insurance as a characteristic sequence, which we indicate by PREM.

We aimed to select indicators that were as comprehensive as possible and also hoped to find the latest data. However, the updating of the latest statistical yearbook was too late for us to use, so we could not find indicators from 2014. As a result, we selected the indicators from the period 2004 to 2013 for analysis.

The data of DI, EC, GHE, HW, ODR, and DR come from the *China Statistics Yearbook*, the HHI is calculated in accordance with company premium incomes as published in the statistics column on the CIRC website, the EDU is calculated in accordance with the education information in *China Statistics Yearbook*, and the premium income of health insurance is derived from the *Insurance Development Report* of each year.

3.4.3 Empirical analysis of grey correlation for the factors that influence demand for commercial health insurance

3.4.3.1 Selecting the model for the analysis of factors that influence demand for commercial health insurance

Most scholars use a linear regression model for the fixed effects and random effects models to study the factors that influence the demand for commercial health insurance. For example, the linear regression model has an intuitive economic meaning. Through the linear regression model, we can directly see the size and manner of the influence of a variable on the demand for commercial health insurance. This model may not be as accurate, however, because of its high requirements for data and because of the myriad of relationships among all the influencing factors when applied to health insurance. In contrast, grey relational analysis is based on the theory of the grey system, which means we do not need to know the prior characteristics of the distribution of the original data. This gives it certain advantages in terms of accuracy.

3.4.3.2 The grey correlation analysis of the demand for commercial health insurance

3.4.3.2.1 The correlation analysis

Before conducting the grey correlation analysis, we should first determine the correlation between each factor and the demand for commercial health insurance (the correlation analysis results are shown in Table 3.4). The analysis results show that DI, GHE, HW, Sociallm, EDU, ODR, and DR are positively correlated to demand, while EC and HHI are negatively correlated to demand.

The characteristic sequence and related factors are as follows:

X_0=(259.88, 312.30, 376.90, 384.17, 585.46, 573.98, 677.47, 691.72, 862.76, 1123.50)

X_1=(9421.60, 10493.00, 11759.50, 13785.80, 15780.80, 17174.70, 19109.40, 21810.00, 24564.70, 26955.10)

X_2=(37.70, 36.70, 35.80, 36.29, 37.89, 36.52, 35.70, 36.30, 36.23, 35.02)

Table 3.4 Correlation analysis of influencing factors

	PREM	DI	EC	GHE	HHI	HW	SOCIALIM	EDU	DR	ODR
PREM	1.0000									
DI	0.9755	1.0000								
EC	-0.5812	-0.5778	1.0000							
GHE	0.9635	0.9947	-0.5649	1.0000						
HHI	-0.8926	-0.9421	0.5626	-0.9310	1.0000					
HW	0.9757	0.9910	-0.5920	0.9948	-0.9101	1.0000				
SOCIALIM	0.9808	0.9930	-0.5862	0.9920	-0.9029	0.9966	1.0000			
EDU	0.9417	0.9791	-0.6145	0.9872	-0.9040	0.9866	0.9803	1.0000		
DR	0.8006	0.8467	-0.4731	0.8097	-0.9089	0.7802	0.7839	0.7714	1.0000	
ODR	0.9746	0.9962	-0.5961	0.9960	-0.9186	0.9974	0.9966	0.9869	0.8140	1.0000

$X_3 = (1293.58, 1552.53, 1778.86, 2581.58, 3593.94, 4816.26, 5732.49, 7464.18, 8431.98, 9545.81)$

$X_4 = (0.28, 0.24, 0.25, 0.21, 0.21, 0.18, 0.15, 0.16, 0.15, 0.14)$

$X_5 = (3.53, 3.50, 3.60, 3.72, 3.90, 4.15, 4.39, 4.61, 4.94, 5.27)$

$X_6 = (1140.50, 1405.30, 1747.10, 2257.20, 3040.40, 3671.90, 4308.90, 5539.20, 6938.70, 8248.26)$

$X_7 = (5.77, 5.56, 6.22, 6.56, 6.70, 7.29, 8.93, 10.06, 10.59, 11.32)$

$X_8 = (6.42, 6.51, 6.81, 6.93, 7.06, 7.08, 7.11, 7.14, 7.15, 7.16)$

$X_9 = (10.69, 10.67, 10.96, 11.10, 11.33, 11.64, 11.90, 12.30, 12.70, 13.08)$

3.4.3.2.2 Calculation

From the above formula, the grey correlation coefficient is calculated.

ξ_1	1.0000	0.9559	0.9041	0.9922	0.7674	0.8317	0.7672	0.8461	0.7279	0.5660
ξ_2	1.0000	0.8931	0.7920	0.7871	0.6044	0.6059	0.5346	0.5288	0.4470	0.3597
ξ_3	1.0000	0.9992	0.9621	0.7865	0.7840	0.5573	0.5110	0.3802	0.3735	0.3842
ξ_4	1.0000	0.8582	0.7832	0.7237	0.5582	0.5529	0.4822	0.4776	0.4076	0.3333
ξ_5	1.0000	0.9007	0.8158	0.8179	0.6242	0.6486	0.5831	0.5844	0.4982	0.4025
ξ_6	1.0000	0.9843	0.9590	0.7920	0.8220	0.6535	0.6195	0.4648	0.4082	0.3959
ξ_7	1.0000	0.8892	0.8366	0.8481	0.6361	0.6685	0.6429	0.6750	0.5624	0.4468
ξ_8	1.0000	0.9104	0.8303	0.8270	0.6231	0.6329	0.5598	0.5517	0.4636	0.3728
ξ_9	1.0000	0.9036	0.8176	0.8124	0.6151	0.6300	0.5607	0.5578	0.4721	0.3809

3.4.3.2.3 Grey correlation degree

The grey correlation degree is drawn with the above formula, and the sequencing is as follows:

$r_1 = 0.8359, r_2 = 0.6553, r_3 = 0.6738, r_4 = 0.6177, r_5 = 0.6875, r_6 = 0.7099, r_7 = 0.7206, r_8 = 0.6772, r_9 = 0.6750$

Correlation sequence: $r_1 > r_7 > r_6 > r_5 > r_8 > r_9 > r_3 > r_2 > r_4$, the correlation degree of these indicators is all higher than 0.6, indicating that the selected indicator is related to the commercial health insurance demand. Among them, the $r_1 > 0.8$ represents super-high correlation. The analysis results show that the DI is the variable that has the largest influence on the demand for health insurance, followed by EDU and SocialIm, and then by SocialIm HW, DR, ODR, GHE, EC, and the extent of market competition.

3.4.4 Analysis of the results of analyzing factors that influence demand for commercial health insurance using grey relational analysis

3.4.4.1 Per-capita disposable income of urban residents is the primary reason for the growth in premium income

Per capita disposable income has consistently risen with the growth of China's economy. Consumers now have sufficient money to buy what they want. In this study, 'level of economic development' is represented by per capita disposable income. The conclusion that it is the primary driving force behind the growth of China's health insurance is in line with the conclusion that many scholars have made through empirical analysis. We all know that only when consumers are able to afford what they need and want can we truly transform potential demand into effective demand. Yet again, this confirms the scientific conclusion that development is the necessary course to take.

Rapid economic development, growth in per-capita disposable income, and the improvement of people's living standards are major factors that influence the purchase of commercial health insurance in China. As the Engel's coefficient continues to decline in China, consumers are paying more attention to quality of life and the market for commercial health insurance is broadening. However, uneven economic development in China's various regions leads directly to a disparity in purchasing power for health insurance.[54] The disparity is obvious between the most and least economically developed areas, but the disparity is drawn apart even further since insurance companies put less marketing effort and provision of products into places where income levels are low. Uneven development among different parts of China affects the healthy growth of the insurance industry.[55]

For any industry to develop and grow, China's economy as a whole must be thriving. Only when the economy grows and people have more money to spend will consumers be willing to spend time, energy, and money on improving their living standards. Only then will they make long-term decisions about the state of their physical health.

3.4.4.2 The effect of higher education on stimulating demand for commercial health insurance, as well as the effect of income derived from health insurance funds

Since insurance does not have a long history in China and agents are mostly of low caliber, the fraudulent behavior of agents and insurance companies is often in the news. Because of this, the public at large does not have a very good impression of the business. In addition, insurance is a relatively complex form of financial commodity. The mechanisms by which it disperses risk and its functional needs are not easily understood, while health insurance is an even more complex business than other forms of insurance. It is more specialized and the setting of rates and purchasing of policies involve many more factors. People with a higher education can be fairly objective in evaluating how insurance products can be used as a tool to benefit themselves. In addition, given generally higher incomes, people with higher education also have higher demands on their quality of life. They are willing to put more effort into ensuring that their later years are protected.

One indicator of how well China's basic medical insurance system is doing is how much income is being generated by the pool of funds. As this system gets better, people begin to recognize the importance of health, plus they see insurance lowering the cost of seeing a doctor. A portion of the public may begin to have sufficient excess income that they choose to spend on buying commercial health insurance. This in turn satisfies their need for better coverage.

3.4.4.3 Influence of six factors on the demand for commercial health insurance: number of medical technicians per 1,000 people, mortality, elderly dependency ratio, government health expenditures, Engel's coefficient, and market competition

The number of medical technicians per 1,000 people is an indicator measuring the availability of health resources. With economic growth, people are paying more attention to health and China is seeing its health resources grow substantially in both quality and quantity. The phenomenon of not having access to affordable healthcare naturally diminishes when health resources are plentiful. People become more willing to go to a doctor when they fall sick, which indirectly results in higher demand for health insurance. However, looking at the situation from a grey relational analysis perspective, the degree of grey correlation of one medical technician per 1,000 people is only 0.8. This does not describe a high correlation. The authors believe that this stems from China's unique national conditions. China has more people than any other country on earth. Although the state continues to increase its spending on medicine and healthcare, the amount is insufficient to resolve the complexities of how one sees a doctor or gets medical help in the country. Standing in line for a long time is just one of the very real problems. Second, China is still at the position of the 'first stage of socialism.' Its economy continues to advance, but objectively speaking it is still difficult to access medical care. When a person gets hit with major illness, even if they have purchased insurance they still have to pay the portion outside a certain percentage of costs, and that is often difficult to bear. For people like these, the attraction of buying insurance is inadequate, irrespective of any increase in medical and healthcare resources.[56]

Commercial health insurance is intimately connected to the state of a person's health. Every day our bodies are confronted with threats of one kind or another, leading people who are more aware of mitigating risk to purchase health insurance to provide themselves and their families with at least some safeguards. Theoretically, a higher mortality rate should make people more willing to spend money on health insurance products, which should in turn lead to higher income from premiums. It can be seen, however, that the degree of correlation between mortality and insurance demand is also not super high. The authors believe that this is partially due to the way insurance companies try to prevent 'adverse selection.'[57] Generally speaking, people are more willing to buy insurance if they are not well. The goal of insurance companies, however, is to maximize profits, so they do not necessarily want to insure this kind of person. If a person has a hereditary disease, for example, the insurance company may raise premium rates or may simply refuse to insure that person. To take an extreme case, if all consumers of insurance have a high incidence of disease, the income of the insurance company might be quite low—the consumers might indeed be very eager to buy insurance, but the willingness of insurance companies either to raise premiums or refuse coverage ultimately holds down an increase in premium income.

As China's population ages and the total number of elderly increases, as noted above, this population will need more medical services than the younger population. The fact of an 'aging population' therefore generates more potential demand for commercial health insurance. It could be said that the degree of aging spurs the growth of the health insurance industry. However, on the other hand, the great majority of care for elders in China is still carried out by families. When parents get sick, in most cases it is still the sons and daughters who bear the cost of medical treatment, the hospital and drug bills, and so on. As a result, the impact of aging on the growth of the health insurance industry is not as apparent in China as it is in countries where the insurance market is well developed.

As noted above, government spending on health costs is a healthcare form of subsidy to consumers. When such spending goes up, to a certain degree it is equivalent to an increase in a person's spending capacity. This helps turn potential demand into effective demand. However, as a large country with an enormous population, China does increase healthcare spending every year but the amount per capita is miniscule when spread out over the total number of consumers. This consideration does not therefore have any notable impact on increasing demand for commercial health insurance.

As the economy grows, the Engel's coefficient in both urban and rural China gets smaller every year as people's living standards get higher. People begin to think of how to raise their standard of living up another level and some may choose to invest in insurance products. Since Chinese consumers have only a weak understanding of insurance, however, and since China's insurance markets are insufficiently developed, in fact a decline in the Engel's coefficient does not affect the demand for insurance as much as many other factors.

The authors selected HHI as a symbol to measure market conditions in the study. The degree of grey correlation between this factor and commercial health insurance was smaller than any other of the several factors we analyzed. However, it did reach 0.6750, which indicates that the extent of market competition could explain some of the demand for commercial health insurance.[58] As policy restrictions ease in China, the number of insurance companies in China continues to rise, including foreign companies. Compared with the situation several years ago, when just a few giants monopolized the entire market, competition is now becoming quite fierce. Not only is this lowering monopoly-generated profits, and as a result lowering prices, but it is motivating insurance companies to become more innovative in their products and services. Improving the quality of services also stimulates more demand for insurance.

3.5 FORECAST OF DEMAND FOR COMMERCIAL HEALTH INSURANCE BY TYPE OF INSURANCE

3.5.1 Establishing the predictive model for commercial health insurance

Let us suppose that the non-negative original time series $X^{(0)}$ has n observations:

$$X^{(0)} = (x^{(0)}(1), x^{(0)}(2), \ldots, x^{(0)}(n))$$

of which

$$x^{(0)}(k) > 0, \ k = 1, 2, \ldots, n$$

Add these up and we get:

$$X^{(1)} = (x^{(1)}(1), x^{(1)}(2), \ldots, x^{(1)}(n))$$

of which

$$x^{(1)}(k) = \sum_{i=1}^{k} x_i^{(0)}, \ k = 1, 2, \ldots, n;$$

The differential equation of GM (1, 1) is:

$$\frac{dX^{(1)}}{dt} + aX^{(1)} = b \tag{5.1}$$

Let us set $\hat{a}$ as the special parameter vector, $\hat{a} = [a, b]^{y}$, we can get the value of a and b using the Least Squares method:

$$\hat{a} = (B^{y}B)^{-1}B^{y}Y_{N}$$

of which:

$$
B = \begin{pmatrix} -\frac{1}{2}(x^{(1)}(1) + x^{(1)}(2)) & 1 \\ -\frac{1}{2}(x^{(1)}(1) + x^{(1)}(3)) & 1 \\ \vdots & \vdots \\ -\frac{1}{2}(x^{(1)}(n-1) + x^{(1)}(n)) & 1 \end{pmatrix}, \quad Y_N = (x^{(0)}(2), x^{(0)}(3), \ldots, x^{(0)}(n))^\gamma \tag{5.2}
$$

We obtain the predictive model as follows:

$$
\hat{x}^{(1)}(k+1) = \left[x^{(0)}(1) - \frac{b}{a} \right] e^{-ak} + \frac{b}{a}; \; k = 1,2, \ldots, n \tag{5.3}
$$

An inverse accumulated generating operation (IAGO) of

$$
\hat{x}^{(1)} \text{ gets us } \hat{x}^{(1)}(k+1) = \hat{x}^{(1)}(k+1) - \hat{x}^{(1)}(k). \tag{5.4}
$$

By following these steps, we can calculate the future predictive values.

3.5.2 Testing the predictive model for commercial health insurance

3.5.2.1 Residual test of the predictive model

Calculate the residual $\hat{\delta}^{(0)}(k)$ and the relative error $M^{(0)}(k)$ of the original series $\hat{x}^{(0)}(k)$ and the calculated value of the model $\hat{x}^{(0)}(k)$:

$$
\text{Residual } \hat{\delta}^{(0)}(k) = x^{(0)}(k) - \hat{x}^{(0)}(k) \tag{5.5}
$$

$$
\text{Relative error } M^{(0)}(k) = \left| \frac{\delta^{(0)}(k)}{x^{(0)}(k)} \right| \tag{5.6}
$$

Experience shows that when $M^{(0)}(k) < 0.2$, the model passes the residual test.

3.5.2.2 Posterior variance test of the predictive model

Let us first calculate the average of the original series $\bar{x}$ and the residual mean $\bar{\delta}$:

$$
\bar{x} = \frac{1}{n} \sum_{k=1}^{n} x^{(0)}(k), \; \bar{\delta} = \frac{1}{n} \sum_{k=1}^{n} \delta^{(0)}(k)
$$

Then proceed to the variance of the original sequence s_1^2 and that of the residual s_2^2:

$$
s_1^2 = \frac{1}{n} \sum_{k=1}^{n} (x^{(0)}(k) - \bar{x})^2, \; s_2^2 = \frac{1}{n} \sum_{k=1}^{n} (\delta^{(0)}(k) - \bar{\delta})^2,
$$

Variance ratio $c = \frac{s_2}{s_1}$ Small error probability $p = P\left(|\delta^{(0)}(k) - \bar{\delta}| < 0.6715 s_1 \right)$

The accuracy levels of the model are listed in Table 3.5.

Table 3.5 Reference table of accuracy levels

Accuracy level	c	p
Level I (Good)	<0.35	>0.95
Level II (Qualified)	<0.5	>0.8
Level III (Barely)	<0.65	>0.7
Level IV (Unqualified)	≥0.65	≤0.7

3.5.3 Forecasts based on the predictive model for commercial health insurance

3.5.3.1 Forecasting analysis based on the predictive model for commercial health insurance

The authors first selected the premium income of commercial health insurance between 2004 and 2013 as original data. This gave us the original sequence:

$x^{(0)} = (259.88, 312.30, 376.90, 384.17, 585.46, 573.98, 677.47, 691.72,$
862.76, 1123.50).

An accumulation gets us the accumulated sequence:

$x^{(1)} = (259.8771, 572.1790, 949.0817, 1333.2478, 1918.7068, 2492.6843,$
3170.1502, 3861.8714, 4724.6322, 5848.1282).

Applying Equation 5.2, we get:

$$\frac{dX^{(1)}}{dt} + -0.151523X^{(1)} = 249.238833$$

or $a = -0.151523$, $b = 249.238833$.

Substitute the value of a and b in Equation 5.3 and we get the predictive model of commercial health insurance:

$$\hat{x}^{(1)}(k+1) = 1904.772149e^{0.151523k} - 1644.892149 \tag{5.9}$$

It passes both the residual test and the posterior variance test (see test results below).

From Table 3.7, we can see that the relative error of this model is less than 0.2 while the accuracy test shows Level I. In order to test the predictability of this model, we will use Equation 5.9 to predict the premium income of health insurance in 2014 and 2015 respectively and match such values with the actual premium incomes of the two years, which are already known to us.

Table 3.6 Test of predictive model (5.9)

Actual value	259.8771	312.3019	376.9027	384.1661	585.4590	573.9775	677.4658	691.7213	862.7607
Predictive value	259.8771	311.6302	362.6144	421.9399	490.9714	571.2967	664.7637	773.5223	900.0744
Residual	0.0000	0.6718	14.2883	−37.7738	94.4876	2.6808	12.7022	−81.8010	−37.3137
Relative error	0.0000	0.0022	0.0379	0.0983	0.1614	0.0047	0.0187	0.1183	0.0432
Root-mean-square-error ratio	0.1937								
Small error probability	1								

Table 3.7 Prediction of model (5.9)

Actual value	573.9775	677.4658	691.7213	862.7607	1123.4960
Predictive value	573.9775	664.7637	740.7574	895.3619	1082.2341
Residual	0.0000	12.7022	−49.0361	−32.6012	41.2619
Relative error	0.0000	0.0187	0.0709	0.0378	0.0367
Root-mean-square-error ratio	0.167112976				
Small error probability	1				

It can be seen from Table 3.7 that although the model has passed the test and shows quite high accuracy, its predictive strength is still not satisfactory. The authors believe that this is mainly due to the rapid development of the commercial health insurance market and the great changes in its economic and policy environments in recent years. Figure 3.15 captures the rapid changes in the growth rate of the health insurance premium income in recent years. The situation is vastly different from what it was a few years ago. This changing background makes it less desirable to include much earlier data when modeling—despite expanding the same size, such data reduces the accuracy of the model. The grey predictive model, which requires a limited number of samples (five is enough), shows even more obvious advantages. Therefore, in order to build a more realistic model, we only have to include premium income from recent years.

Excluding data of earlier years, we get the sequence:

$$X^{(0)} = (573.977541, 677.465847, 691.721277, 862.760713, 1123.49605)$$

Still applying Equations 5.2 and 5.3, we get the predictive model:

$$\hat{x}^{(1)}(k + 1) = 2936.345415e^{0.189555k} - 2362.367874 \tag{5.10}$$

The model passes both the residual test and the posterior variance test (see test results below).

From Table 3.8, we can see that the relative error of this model is less than 0.2 while the accuracy test shows Level I. In order to test its predictive capability, we will compare the predicted value in 2014 and 2015 with the actual values in those years.

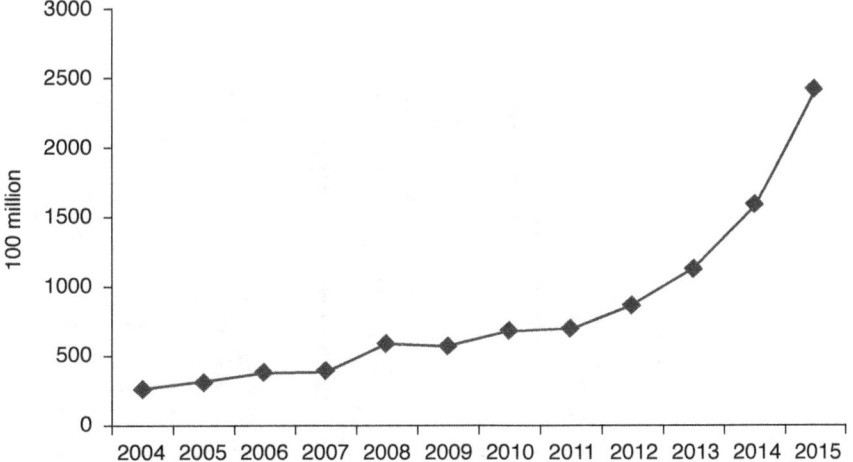

Figure 3.15 Health insurance premium income in China (RMB 100 million).

Source: Statistics column on the website of China Insurance Regulatory Commission.

Table 3.8 Accuracy test of model (5.10)

Actual value	573.9775	677.4658	691.7213	862.7607	1123.4960
Predictive value	573.9775	664.7637	740.7574	895.3619	1082.2341
Residual	0.0000	12.7022	−49.0361	−32.6012	41.2619
Relative error	0.0000	0.0187	0.0709	0.0378	0.0367
Root-mean-square-error ratio	0.167112976				
Small error probability	1				

Table 3.9 Prediction of model (5.10)

	2014	2015
Actual value	1587.1786	2410.47
Predictive value	1308.1087	1581.126
Residual	279.06983	829.34403
Relative error	0.1758276	0.3440591

Test results show that this model is still not sufficiently convincing despite the significantly improved predictive capability. The authors believe that this is attributable to two reasons. On the one hand, the exclusion of data in 2014 leads to the poor performance in predicting the value for 2015 (relative error higher than 0.2) since the closer the data are from now, the more accurately they can be used to predict the future. On the other hand, great policy changes within the short period between 2014 and 2015 led to significant changes in the insurance industry and the public healthcare environment. Such human-generated changes, which cannot be accounted for by any model, lead to the discrepancy between the predicted and the actual value. However, through such tests and corrections, we can still see that the use of information closer to the current time does improve the accuracy of a model. In order to enhance the objectivity and accuracy of the model, the authors included health insurance premiums in 2014 and 2015 and derived a new model:

$$\hat{x}^{(1)}(k+1) = 1805.860189e^{0.359656k} - 1114.138912 \tag{5.11}$$

The new model generated the predictions given in Table 3.10. With its root-mean-square-error ratio being 0.082364 and small error probability being 1, the model passed the residual test and the posterior error test.

3.5.3.2 *The impact of tax incentives on the demand for health insurance*

Our model is unable to predict the degree of influence that preferential tax policies for individuals have, given that policies have only recently been put in

Table 3.10 Prediction of model (5.11)

	Actual value	Predictive value	Residual	Relative error
2011	691.7213	691.7213	0	0
2012	862.7607	781.6427	81.118	0.094
2013	1123.496	1119.966	3.5296	0.0031
2014	1587.1786	1604.729	−17.5506	0.0111
2015	2410.47	2299.315	111.1551	0.0461
2016	–	3294.5430	–	–
2017	–	4720.5424	–	–
2018	–	6763.7669	–	–

place and there is no actual data to use. Nevertheless, given the growth pattern for buying health insurance in recent years, the stimulating effect of this policy should be fairly large. Premium income should therefore show considerable growth. The following discussion summarizes the evaluations of scholars inside China with regard to the impact of this policy on the health insurance market.

Zhu Minglai and Wang Meijiao (2016)[59] point out that tax incentives will increase demand for commercial health insurance through tax avoidance and the demonstration effect. They used data from the sample survey on basic medical insurance policy holders in the Tianjin Municipality to build a 'demand-income' model (Heckoprobit model) for commercial health insurance under preferential tax policies. They forecast the size of the commercial health insurance market after incorporating the stimulus from preferential tax policies and substituting in the wage income distribution of Chinese employees. The results show that the probability of individuals buying preferential-tax-type commercial health insurance is distributed in an inverted U shape relative to income. Middle-income groups are the most eager to buy commercial health insurance, while low-income and high-income groups show relatively lower willingness. The premium that an individual is willing to pay is positively related to income. If the potential demand driven by preferential tax policies were to be fully released, the health insurance premium would see an annual increase of approximately USD 427.6 billion.[60]

In addition, they calculate that the sum of foregone annual taxes will come to RMB 17 billion. This accounts for only about 2.3% of China's total individual income tax and will have little influence on the country's overall tax structure. If China's commercial health insurance continues to develop as it has done in the past three years, its growth rate will reach 25%, 30%, or even 35% in the next five years, bringing in RMB 854 billion to RMB 960.7 billion in premiums by 2020.

According to the estimates of PICC Health, commercial health insurance, driven by a variety of favorable policies, will continue to be the most robust and fastest growing sector in the industry. As it narrows its current gap with property insurance and life insurance, China's commercial health insurance is expected to bring in RMB 700 billion to 1 trillion in premium income by 2020, making it one of the three major business sectors of the industry.

According to professional estimates of Haitong Securities Co. Ltd., under a neutral assumption (see Table 3.11), the implementation of the preferential tax policies is expected to increase premium income for the health insurance industry by RMB 36 billion annually. It is expected to raise the value of new business by roughly 5% per year. In 2011, China had 24 million wage income taxpayers nationwide, according to the data. If each were to spend RMB 2,400 on commercial health insurance each year, and the current tax preferences are fully implemented, the annual sum of health insurance premiums could reach RMB 57.6 billion.

Table 3.11 Estimates of the impact of health insurance tax incentives on industry premiums
and NBV

	Neutral	*Pessimistic*	*Optimistic*
Number of individual income taxpayers (unit: 10,000)	3,000	3,000	3,000
Percentage of the insured	50%	25%	75%
Annual payment (unit: yuan)	2,400	2,400	2,400
Premium increase (unit: million yuan)	36,000	18,000	54,000
Profit rate of products	10%	5%	15%
Industry annual new business value (unit: million yuan)	3,600	900	8,100

Source: Industry research report of Haitong Securities Research Institute.

3.5.4 Consumer-based predictions of the demand for commercial health insurance by type of insurance

Health insurance branches off from personal insurance as an independent category of insurance. It insures a person's physical wellbeing. It provides compensation for losses resulting from medical costs or loss of income due to disability,
as a result of illness or accidental injury. It also provides compensation for such
things as long-term care required for the elderly or as a result of critical illness
or accidents. Health insurance can further be divided into short-term and long-
term categories, and individual and group insurance. Under this kind of categorization, health insurance can be divided into four main types, namely medical,
critical illness, disability, and nursing care.[61]

3.5.4.1 Demand-oriented prediction of the scope of income from premiums for medical insurance

Medical insurance is one of the key components of health insurance. It provides
compensation when the insured person has to pay out for medical expenses. When
the insured person receives medical treatment, he mainly has expenses relating to
such things as outpatient visits, drugs, hospital stays, nursing, miscellaneous hospital costs, operations, and various kinds of examination and treatment costs.

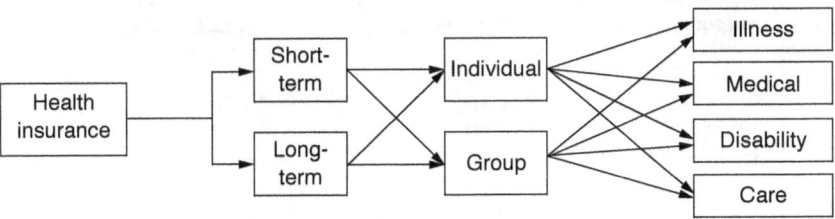

Figure 3.16 Health insurance by type.

In this study, demand for medical insurance=hospitalization rate * total resident population * health expenses per capita.

Based on calculations using the statistics given in Tables 3.12 and 3.13, we can predict the results shown in Table 3.15.

A comprehensive calculation using the method cited above leads to an estimated demand for medical insurance of RMB 314.2 billion in 2014. In contrast, the figure for actual premium income for health insurance in the same year was RMB 158.7 billion. What this shows is that there is massive potential demand for medical insurance in China. It is highly important that we figure out how to fill the gap in the supply of medical insurance more quickly and more effectively. Releasing the potential demand for health insurance in China will provide an opportunity for developing the country's medical and health insurance industries.

3.5.4.2 Demand-oriented prediction of the scale of income from premiums for critical illness insurance

Generally speaking, critical illness insurance entails the payment of benefits once a particular disease is diagnosed. It is not necessary for treatment to have begun for the insurance to come into play. Critical illness insurance is mainly expressed as insurance for specific diseases and covers either a particular disease, a certain type of disease, or several specific diseases. One most common type of critical illness insurance is that for cancer. In the following, we use critical illness insurance as the criterion in predicting the overall scale of premium income, using our demand-oriented analysis.

3.5.4.2.1 Background to putting critical illness insurance into effect

The level of safeguards provided by China's basic medical insurance is still quite low. The system is characterized by 'broad coverage of the population but low safeguards,' and the result is that some people are forced into poverty or forced back into poverty due to high medical costs that they cannot support. For a

Table 3.12 Hospitalization rate and hospital visits per capita covered by basic medical insurance between 2009 and 2014

Year	Hospitalization rate of employees (%)	Hospital visits per employee (%)	Hospitalization rate of residents (%)
2009	11.10	4.00	3.70
2010	11.70	4.10	4.50
2011	12.50	4.40	5.30
2012	13.50	4.60	6.65
2013	14.60	4.90	8.10
2014	15.4	5.20	8.90

Source: *Annual Report on China's Social Insurance Development in 2014.*

Table 3.13 Statistics on health expenditure of urban residents between 2001 and 2014 (yuan)

Year	Overall health expenditure	Government health expenditure	Social health expenditure	Individual health expenditure by cash	Health expenditure per capita
2001	5025.93	800.61	1211.43	3013.89	393.80
2002	5790.03	908.51	1539.38	3342.14	450.70
2003	6584.10	1116.94	1788.50	3678.66	509.50
2004	7590.29	1293.58	2225.35	4071.35	583.90
2005	8659.91	1552.53	2586.41	4520.98	662.30
2006	9843.34	1778.86	3210.92	4853.56	748.80
2007	11573.97	2581.58	3893.72	5098.66	875.96
2008	14535.40	3593.94	5065.60	5875.86	1094.52
2009	17541.92	4816.26	6154.49	6571.16	1314.26
2010	19980.39	5732.49	7196.61	7051.29	1490.06
2011	24345.91	7464.18	8416.45	8465.26	1806.95
2012	28119.00	8431.98	10030.70	9656.32	2076.67
2013	31668.95	9545.81	11393.79	10729.34	2327.37
2014	35312.40	10579.23	13437.50	11295.41	2581.66

Source: Statistics column on the website of the Ministry of Health, People's Republic of China.

Table 3.14 Predictions of the demand for medical insurance by residents (1)

Year	Hospitalization rate of residents (%)	Total population of residents (unit: 10,000)	Health expenditure per capita (unit: yuan)	Medical insurance demand of residents (unit: 10,000 yuan)
2009	3.70	133,450	1,314.26	6,489,355.889
2010	4.50	134,091	1,490.06	8,991,163.596
2011	5.30	134,735	1,806.95	12,903,348.64
2012	6.65	135,404	2,076.67	18,699,096.74
2013	8.10	136,072	2,327.37	25,651,881.14
2014	8.90	136,782	2,581.66	31,428,091.01

number of patients suffering from critical diseases, this is a notable problem. In fact, statistics indicate that over 40% of the number of people defined as impoverished in China are in poverty due to this problem. At present, that translates to roughly 30 million people. Medical insurance has the responsibility to alleviate the risk of critical illness for these people, to prevent the phenomenon of either becoming impoverished or returning to poverty as a result of severe illness. From its strategically advantageous position, the Central Committee of the Communist Party of China (CPC) made the timely decision to include the establishment of a critical and major illness insurance and relief system in the *Report* of the Third Plenary Session of the 18th National Congress of the CPC, as well as the *Decision on some major issues concerning all-round deepening of reforms.* This was to ensure timely prevention and effective mitigation of risks due to major and critical illness among both rural and urban residents.

In 2012, six State departments and commissions issued the *Guiding Opinions on providing critical illness insurance for urban and rural residents,* as an effective measure to reduce poverty caused by illness. These six were the National Development and Reform Commission, the Ministry of Health, the Ministry of Finance, the Ministry of Human Resources and Social Security, the Ministry of Civil Affairs, and the China Insurance Regulatory Commission. Once this document was issued, local (provincial) governments stopped implementing the existing safeguards mechanism, called the Major and Serious Disease Relief Program, and began to implement 'an insurance system for critical illness' on a trial basis. The source of the models for such critical illness insurance came from some local attempts to incorporate commercial health insurance companies in the process. These served as co-providers of a portion of basic medical insurance services. Included among these attempts were the now-famous Zhanjiang Model and Taicang Model.

The Zhanjiang Model derived from the decision in 2009 to integrate the two previously separate types of insurance for urban and rural residents, namely the 'urban residents' basic medical insurance' and the 'rural cooperative basic medical insurance.' As these two systems were 'brought onto the same track' in terms of operations, Zhanjiang City asked a commercial insurance entity to come into the process and co-provide the new basic medical insurance for urban and rural residents. In this system, the pooled funds of the social security system pay for a portion of reimbursements for hospital stays. The portion of expenses that go beyond the cap on those reimbursements is handled by the commercial health insurance company out of its large-sum medical assistance fund, up to the annual maximum payment amount. On the basis of the initial system, in 2012 Zhanjiang set up its large-sum medical assistance and insurance system (referred to by the media as the Zhanjiang Critical Illness Insurance Model). In this, the commercial health insurance company provides a second reimbursement to those who are insured for their hospital stays. This second reimbursement is provided at graduated levels depending on the policy and is for amounts that exceed the annual public reimbursement limits as dictated by healthcare policies.

The Taicang Model was originally designed to address the heavy burden faced by local employees and urban and rural residents in paying out-of-pocket expenses not on the list of items covered by basic medical insurance programs. In 2011, the Taicang government started cooperating with a commercial health insurance company. It allocated a specific percentage of the surplus amount in the basic medical insurance fund for people who held insurance policies and also had high out-of-pocket costs. The government authorized the insurance company to manage these funds using a model described as 'basic + second reimbursement.'

After the six State authorities issued the *Guiding Opinions*, what had originally been local practices were promoted as models for others to follow. The 'critical illness insurance models' began to be advertised and, by 2013, there were already similar pilot programs in 28 provinces. Now, the critical illness insurance system is being implemented throughout the country. The results of implementation, however, are far from satisfactory. In applying the model to new locations, various places adopted the principle of universal benefit. That is, all people received the same percentage of reimbursements, no matter how rich or poor they might be. This meant that policy holders who truly confronted the risk of critical illness could not in fact receive adequate safeguards. Meanwhile, the simplistic way of rigidly copying over the Zhanjiang and Taicang Models made the models inappropriate for some parts of the country. Many places did not in fact have a surplus in their basic medical insurance fund. Allocating a portion of the fund to a commercial health insurance company meant that funds that were tight to begin with became even tighter. For basic medical insurance, this simply added a proverbial layer of frost on top of the snow. On July 22, 2015, the State Council announced that a fairly well formed and complete critical insurance system was to be put in place by the year 2017. Its aim was to prevent families from facing catastrophic medical expenditures and to significantly improve the fairness of medical safeguards for urban and rural residents. Nevertheless, whether or not the current critical illness insurance system can meet this purpose remains to be seen.

3.5.4.2.2 *Basic components of critical illness insurance*

Critical illness insurance includes the following four key features. First, policy coverage: it covers a certain percentage of the out-of-pocket medical expenses of all policy holders that exceed the reimbursement cap of basic medical insurance. Second, fundraising: its sole sources of funds are the basic medical insurance for urban residents and the new rural cooperative medical insurance in the countryside. Third, management: social security authorities and commercial insurance companies, which are selected through a bidding process, enter into partnerships to provide the desired services. Fourth, principles: the system is guided by the principle of 'balancing accounts and preserving principle while aiming for modest profits.' Social security authorities share risk with commercial insurance companies and allow them to make a small profit.

The coverage that the critical illness insurance system provides includes two aspects. One relates to the composition of policy holders: anyone covered by the basic medical insurance for urban and rural residents is automatically covered by critical illness insurance as well. The coverage is therefore very broad and the system is mandatory—the result is safeguards that are of a universal nature. The second aspect relates to levels of reimbursement. After the cap on reimbursements from the basic medical insurance system is reached, critical illness insurance reimburses for a policy holder's out-of-pocket medical expenses at a fixed percentage rate. The higher the sum of expenses, the greater the percentage that the system will reimburse. No distinction is made among types of illness or income level of the insured.

Zhanjiang City of Guangdong Province can serve as an example. In 2014, if a person's out-of-pocket medical expenses for the year exceeded RMB 20,000, and were within the scope of basic medical insurance policies, then the portion above RMB 20,000 could be covered by critical illness insurance at varying percentages, depending on amount. The insurance paid for 50% of the policy holder's out-of-pocket expenses if they were between RMB 20,000 and RMB 50,000; for 60% of the expenses that were between RMB 50,000 and RMB 80,000; for 70% of the expenses that were between RMB 80,000 and RMB 100,000; and for 80% of the portion of expenses that exceeded RMB 100,000 (see Table 3.15.)

3.5.4.2.3 Forecast of premium income from critical illness insurance that is based on the 'major illness insurance system'

We sum up the following equation, based on the above introduction to the subject:

Residents' demand for illness insurance = $\sum$(Out-of-pocket medical expenses *Reimbursement ratio of critical illness insurance)* Total population* Incidence of critical illness.

Through calculations based on the statistics as described above, we can predict the following results:

Table 3.15 Reimbursement ratio of critical illness insurance in Zhanjiang (2014)

Out-of-pocket medical expenses (unit: 10,000 yuan)	Reimbursement ratio of critical illness insurance (%)
20,000–50,000	50
50,000–80,000	60
80,000–100,000	70
Over 100,000	80

Source: Developed by author based on data provided by PICC Health Zhanjiang branch

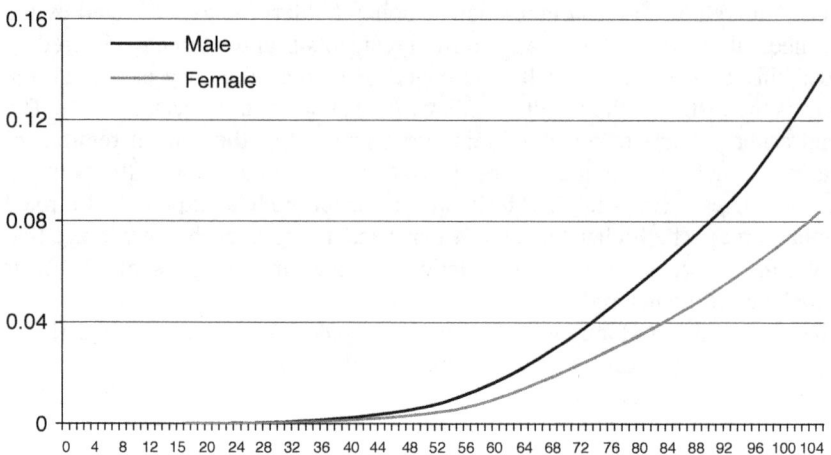

Figure 3.17 Statistical chart of incidence of 25 major critical diseases.

Source: http://insurance.hexun.com/2013-11-14/159694790.html.

Residents' demand for illness insurance = $\sum$(Out-of-pocket medical expenses* Reimbursement ratio of critical illness insurance)*Total population*Total population = (3.5*50% + 6.5*60% + 9*70% + 10*80%)/4*1367820000*3.12% (Weighted average income) = 2128464.702 million yuan

Using the above methodology, a comprehensive calculation arrives at a figure of RMB 2,128.5 billion for estimated demand for critical illness insurance in 2014. This can be compared to the smaller figure of RMB 158.7 billion in actual premium income from health insurance in that year, and with the even smaller actual premium income from critical illness insurance. Obviously, the greatest discrepancy between the predictive and actual demand is for that of critical illness insurance. Faced with the massive potential demand in China for critical illness insurance and, on top of that, the accelerating incidence of major critical diseases every year, it is tremendously important that we quickly and effectively figure out how to increase insurance supply.

3.5.4.3 Demand-oriented prediction of the overall scale of income from premiums for disability insurance

Disability income insurance is a form of insurance that insures the beneficiary's earned income against the risk of a disability caused by illness or accidental injuries as agreed to in the insurance contract. Also known as disability insurance or income protection, it mainly aims to provide economic security for policy holders against the risk of income loss or reduction due to disability.

Residents' disability income insurance demand=Number of days on sick leave from work per thousand people*Total population/1000*Average daily wage of urban residents.

Based on these statistics and through calculation, we can get the following predictions shown in Table 3.18.

Using the above methodology, a comprehensive calculation arrives at the figure of an estimated RMB 19 billion of demand for disability income insurance in 2014. The reality, however, is that disability insurance is still in the early stages of development. Premiums from this insurance account for a very low percentage of all health insurance premiums. The enormous potential demand for this insurance, however, makes this a 'blue-sky' kind of opportunity, one whose development is still to be realized. Insurance companies should pay close attention to this as they manage their health insurance portfolios, and should focus on putting their resources in this direction.

3.5.4.4 Demand-oriented prediction of the overall scale of income from premiums for long-term care insurance (nursing care insurance)

Long-term care insurance is an insurance product that helps pay for the cost of those who require long-term care due to old age, illness, injury, or disability. It can be divided into several categories. Single responsibility insurance covers only long-term care. In other words, as long as policy holders receive quality care services during the valid period, the insurance company has to pay benefits in accordance with the provisions. Comprehensive care insurance adds benefits of survival and death to general care responsibilities. Extended disability income insurance requires insurers to provide policy holders with benefits equal to disability income compensations if such policy holders have a disability and bought long-term care insurance before retirement.

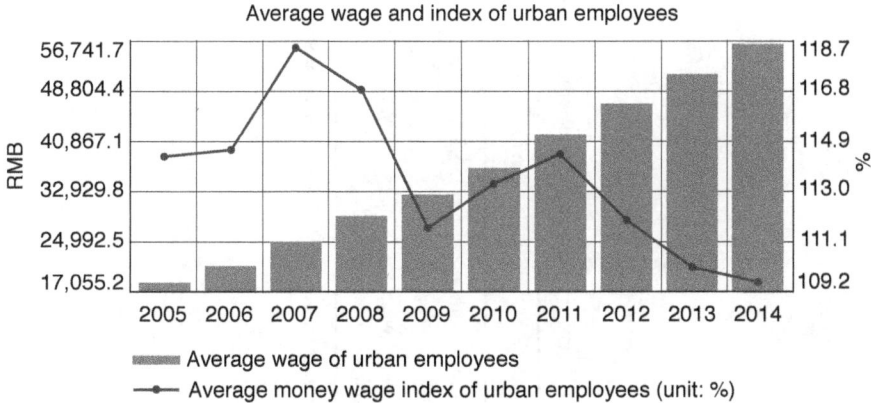

Figure 3.18 Statistical chart of average wage of urban employees in China (2005–2014).

Source: Official statistics on website of National Bureau of Statistics.

Table 3.16 Average wage and index of urban employees (unit: yuan)

Index	2014	2013	2012	2011	2010	2009	2008	2007	2006	2005
Average wage of urban employees	56,360	51,483	46,769	41,799	36,539	32,244	28,898	24,721	20,856	18,200
Average money wage index of urban employees (%)	109.5	110.1	111.89	114.4	113.3	111.6	116.9	118.5	114.59	114.32

Source: Statistics on website of National Bureau of Statistics.

Table 3.17 Two-week prevalence of illness among residents in the survey area in 1998, 2003, and 2008

		Weighted average	Urban	Rural
1998	Number of sick days per 1,000 people	1,257	1,646	1,125
	Number of days on sick leave from work per 1,000 people	308	153	347
	Number of days on sick leave from school per 1,000 people	89	68	95
	Number of days on bed confinement per 1,000 people	113	95	119
2003	Number of sick days per 1,000 people	1,093	1,238	1,043
	Number of days on sick leave from work per 1,000 people	194	84	218
	Number of days on sick leave from school per 1,000 people	50	35	54
	Number of days on bed confinement per 1,000 people	170	175	169
2008	Number of sick days per 1,000 people	1,537	1,842	1,428
	Number of days on sick leave from work per 1,000 people	90	59	97
	Number of days on sick leave from school per 1,000 people	44	29	48
	Number of days on bed confinement per 1,000 people	185	164	193

Source: Statistics on website of National Bureau of Statistics.

Table 3.18 Predictions of demand for medical insurance by residents (2)

	Total population (unit: 1,000)	Average annual wage (unit: yuan)	Number of days on sick leave from work per 1,000 people	Average daily wage (unit: yuan)	Demand for disability income insurance (unit: 10,000 yuan)
2009	1,334,500	32,244	90	88.33972603	1,061,004.279
2010	1,340,910	36,539	90	100.1068493	1,208,108.478
2011	1,347,350	41,799	90	114.5178082	1,388,660.12
2012	1,354,040	46,769	90	128.1342466	1,561,490.057
2013	1,360,720	51,483	90	141.0493151	1,727,357.616
2014	1,367,820	56,360	90	154.4109589	1,900,857.58

Wei Hualin (2012)[62] did the first dynamic estimate of China's demand for long-term care insurance. The prediction covered the years between 2010 and 2050, and utilized a population predictive model and a product actuarial model. In terms of absolute value, long-term care expenses grow at an astonishing rate, and in terms of relative value, they take up a constantly rising share of gross national product. What this means is that spending on long-term care costs will be putting an increasing severe economic burden on society as a whole. In addition, Wei also conducted a dynamic estimate of the supply of insurance for long-term care in the years between 2010 and 2050. The results showed the feasibility of using a combination of individual funding mechanisms and the government's ability to provide safeguards as a source of funds for long-term care costs (see Table 3.19). It even looked somewhat feasible to cover costs based completely on individual paying capacity.

3.6 CONCLUSIONS AND RECOMMENDATIONS

3.6.1 Conclusions about the factors that influence demand for commercial health insurance in China

The demand for health insurance at present in China is still insufficient. A so-called insufficient demand for health insurance refers to two things, not buying enough insurance and not buying any insurance. In the market for health insurance in the United States, Ahking *et al.* analyzed demand by dividing people's reasons for not buying commercial health insurance into five categories. Those were being uninsured for voluntary reasons, due to 'friction,' for structural reasons, for cyclical reasons, and for substitution-type reasons. Voluntary reasons for not being insured included such things as changes in economic environment—for example, the price of insurance goes up or a person's income goes down. Some people would then decide not to purchase commercial health insurance or they would choose insurance with minimum coverage. Frictional reasons for not being insured occur when people are temporarily without health insurance due to asymmetry of information. Because of the mismatch in information, consumers have to take a long time to find the right policy, whereas insurance companies also are required to spend time looking for the appropriate group of customers. Structural reasons relate to people not being provided with the opportunity to be insured due to chronic illness or pre-existing conditions. That is, commercial insurance companies and such people do not yet match up properly. Cyclical reasons for not being insured arise when such circumstances come and go in a cyclical manner. Substitution occurs when publicly funded insurance (social security-type insurance) reduces the number of people in the population who purchase commercial insurance.[63]

One important reason for insufficient demand for commercial health insurance in China's early period lies with the issue of income. The higher the disposable income of a person, the greater their capacity to pay premiums on insurance.

Table 3.19 Dynamic demand measurement of long-term care expenses in China (unit: 100 million yuan)

Year	Low estimates		Medium estimates		High estimates	
	Long-term care expenses	Long-term care expenses/GDP (%)	Long-term care expenses	Long-term care expenses/GDP (%)	Long-term care expenses	Long-term care expenses/GDP (%)
2010	1,999.21	0.50	1,999.21	0.50	1,999.21	0.50
2020	6,769.17	1.04	8,174.86	1.04	9,838.02	1.04
2030	18,854.89	1.77	27,498.79	1.77	39,826.12	1.77
2040	48,947.8	2.82	86,211.97	2.82	150,262	2.82
2050	112,635.1	3.99	239,581.28	3.99	502,529.66	3.99

Zhang Xinmin *et al.* (1995)[64] note that income levels are not uniform in China. The great majority of farmers have low enough income that commercial health insurance for them belongs to a 'first state' category, that is, an unaffordable product. The income level of most urban workers and coastal farmers is between subsistence and moderately prosperous. For them, commercial health insurance may belong to a 'second state' category, that is, a luxury. Finally, there are a minority of people who 'got rich first,' and for them commercial health insurance may belong to a 'third state' category, namely a necessity. The first and second categories clearly produce very little demand for insurance, while the third category constitutes only a small share of the population. The inevitable result is insufficient demand for commercial health insurance in China. However, Wei Hualin and Li Jinhui (2009)[65] take the opposite point of view. They say the real reason for inadequate demand does not lie with people's inability to purchase insurance. Instead, they provide three alternative reasons, based on a survey conducted in three cities in China's central region. First, people are not very aware of risk, or they don't understand it. Second, the supply of insurance is 'improper.' Third, social security-type insurance can be used as an alternative. The second reason, improper supply, is in fact brought on by the frictional and structural reasons mentioned above. In the survey, respondents evaluated China's commercial health insurance in the following terms: some felt there was no suitable insurance available for their needs, some felt that commercial health insurance was unstable (not reliable), some felt that insurance companies had a poor reputation and would not reimburse claims, and so on. People based their decision not to buy insurance on these objective reasons, and instead self-insured using their own methods. Getting to the heart of the matter, the products that insurance companies supply do not meet the needs of the public. They need to be tailored more to individuals and made more specific. The mismatch of the supply side and the demand side has also generated the 'friction reason' for not being insured.

Right now, China's health insurance companies are wary of insuring people with a high probability of illness, or they refuse to insure such people altogether. They cannot be blamed for this, given that their goal is to make money. However, if we look further into the causes of this problem, it relates to their current inability to control risk, to the lack of sufficient medical data to use as the basis for decisions, and to imperfect corporate management and controls, which in turn leads to lack of coordination with medical institutions. From the perspective of their own operations, therefore, such companies must in fact adopt a conservative posture toward high-risk groups of people as they evaluate their own risk. This leads to structural causes for the lack of insurance among high-risk people.

At the end of the day, however, the main reason right now for insufficient demand for commercial health insurance in China is that people rely on social insurance. The relationship between publicly funded social-type insurance and commercial health insurance is unclear. For some time now, the two have shared an indistinct 'positioning' and vague 'division' of tasks due to the fact that commercial health insurance began only recently while at the same time social health insurance was not very good. One phenomenon that is quite apparent right now, however, is that people feel they do not need to invest in commercial health insurance if they already pay into the social-type health insurance. As a result of this, the scope of their coverage is fairly limited and the level of safeguards is not very high. Others go to the opposite extreme, however—having bought various kinds of health insurance, they then discover that some aspects are redundant, given their existing social health insurance.

Social health insurance and commercial health insurance are both forms of insurance designed to address people's physical wellbeing, but they have distinct differences. They are dissimilar in their very nature—one is mandatory and the other is voluntary. They also differ in their purpose and the entities that operate them. One is run by government and is not-for-profit, the other is run by companies and is for-profit. The levels of safeguards that they provide are also different—one is mainly for basic security while the other has higher levels of security. All of these distinctions make it clear that one form of insurance cannot simply substitute for another. Even if people already have social health insurance, it is altogether reasonable for them to purchase commercial insurance for those things that social insurance cannot provide, such as diversity of policies and higher levels of safeguards. In sum, the key position of commercial health insurance must not be disregarded. Commercial health insurance is an effective supplement to social health insurance. It fills the 'empty zone' that currently exists in social health insurance. Moreover, it has already become an organic component of a multi-tiered medical safeguards system in China.[66]

3.6.2 Recommendations on how to develop commercial health insurance in China

3.6.2.1 Recommendations made from the perspective of the government

3.6.2.1.1 Increase the forcefulness of policy support

Policies that extend preferential treatment to commercial health insurance have come out regularly in recent years, giving people inside the industry as well as scholars a measure of hope. Before this time, China rarely initiated preferential tax policies that targeted commercial health insurance. Now, with the implementation of such things as the health-insurance exemption of business tax for one year or more (for companies) and the preferential tax policies for individuals, we can clearly recognize the importance that the government places on the commercial health insurance market. Nevertheless, China's policy support for the industry is vastly insufficient, particularly as compared to the situation in countries with relatively well developed insurance markets.

Right now, the health insurance-related preferential tax policy for individuals says that each person can deduct RMB 2,400 from before-tax income in calculating taxes. As per the empirical findings of the authors as noted above, this raises the spending capacity of the consumer and is indeed a way to encourage people to purchase health insurance. However, the amount is too small— RMB 200 per month is not enough to make a difference. In Taiwan back in the 1990s, the preferential tax consideration was already RMB 4,800 per person for the year. As China adheres to preferential tax policies in the future, therefore, in line with economic development it should raise the amount of income given preferential tax treatment. In order to encourage units (entities) to purchase commercial health insurance, China should also extend preferential tax treatment to non-corporate entities to encourage them to buy supplementary health insurance.

3.6.2.1.2 *Continue to develop social health insurance*

The income of medical insurance funds is a very significant factor among the factors that have a grey correlation with commercial health insurance. Moreover, it is positively correlated with spurring demand. This indicates that the mutually supportive effect between social health insurance and commercial health insurance goes beyond just the substitution effect.

Both of these kinds of insurance are important components of China's medical safeguards system. Not only has the growth of social health insurance raised social welfare standards and quality of life in China, but it has given people a sense of wellbeing. It has also been significant in spurring the growth of commercial health insurance. First, the development of basic medical insurance within the system has made the public at large pay more attention to taking care of health, and it has helped consumers understand more about risk mitigation. Second, due to its nature, social health insurance cannot in fact provide safeguards for all medical needs, so if someone needs more complete services, they have to consider buying commercial health insurance. That is to say, the development of social health insurance has propelled growth in the potential demand for commercial health insurance. Third, the expansion in coverage of social health insurance and improvement in level of safeguards is equivalent to reducing consumers' expenditures and raising purchasing power. Because of this, a portion of those who seek a higher quality of life will choose to purchase commercial health insurance.[67]

It could even be said that accelerating the growth of social health insurance is an effective way to promote commercial health insurance. The government may want to consider introducing market mechanisms into the management of social insurance, in order to reduce the negative influence of inefficiency and lack of enthusiasm among some government personnel. On the one hand, this will raise the work efficiency of these social insurance entities, and improve the quality of services, and on the other hand it will play a role in making government affairs more open (transparent). This should strengthen the public's confidence in the government. Meanwhile, government departments can continue to strengthen cooperation with insurance companies. They should use the inherent advantages of insurance companies in terms of their services and management abilities to raise the professionalism of social insurance work. As for insurance companies, they can collect more meaningful information (data) by working through the vast platform of social insurance departments. This will help them improve the quality of their services and allow them to carry out targeted innovations with their products and services.[68]

3.6.2.1.3 Speed up the opening of the insurance market, both internally within China, and externally, to the outside world

We know from the results of grey relational analysis that market competition plays a role in spurring the growth of commercial health insurance. In comparison to the situation some years ago, China's insurance market is already fairly open—but the government should continue opening up the market and promoting competition.

'Opening to the outside' refers to lowering barriers to market access for foreign-invested insurance companies. This has profound significance for China's insurance markets. Insurance companies in countries where insurance is fairly well developed have over 100 years of history. In terms of operations and services, they have a wealth of experience that China's local insurance companies can learn from. By opening to the outside, domestic and foreign insurance companies can compete with each other and measure their respective strength, which will greatly facilitate the standardization and development of China's insurance market. Opening internally and opening to the outside will both help regulate the pattern of China's market, by spurring competition and reducing the extent to which monopoly profits play a role in the business. In this process, however, the government should focus on certain problems that may arise. This may lead to disorderly competition and indeed vicious competition. This not only would destroy the image of the insurance industry in the eyes of consumers, for example if it led to a price war, but it would have a detrimental effect on the long-term growth of companies as well as the economic growth of the country. It will also increase pressures on the country's regulatory departments. As problems of many different kinds emerge in the process of opening up the market, this will undoubtedly be a challenge to regulatory departments since China's legal and regulatory systems are still imperfect. Government departments should therefore strengthen their regulatory supervision of insurance markets as these open up, in order to create a favorable environment for competition.

3.6.2.1.4 Set up a data-sharing platform

Social medical insurance in China is in possession of a fairly complete data platform. This is an extremely bountiful resource when it comes to medical statistics on illnesses, patient information, drug information, diagnosis and treatments, and so on. In the meantime, such a database that has been specialized for the purpose of insurance can provide powerful support for the development of commercial health insurance. It can strengthen the industry's ability to control risk and it can help make the industry's operations more convenient and professional. For these reasons, the government should set up a data sharing system as soon as possible between China's social medical insurance and its commercial health insurance systems. Commercial health insurance companies should also set up and improve upon their own information systems as soon as possible. The importance of setting up such a data sharing platform lies in the following. First, it helps commercial health insurance make use of social medical insurance data quickly, which raises its level of professionalism, strengthens its ability to compete, and allows it to realize fast growth. Second, it enables the information and data assembled by the social medical insurance system to be put to use and thereby avoids wasting the information. Third, it helps commercial insurance companies carry out stronger regulatory oversight and management of medical institutions, as these companies participate in the process of providing medical services. Fourth, it helps make social medical insurance and commercial health insurance more complementary to each other, which enables consumers to make convenient use of both in protecting their own health.

3.6.2.1.5 Adjust the mindset regarding supervisory management

Commercial health insurance holds an extremely important position in China's overall system of multi-tiered medical safeguards. Unlike normal insurance, not only does it provide insurance products for policy holders but it takes on a certain social responsibility as well. In order to improve upon building the framework behind China's multi-tiered medical safeguards system, the government must make necessary and appropriate adjustments in the need for supervisory management of commercial health insurance. Government should incorporate the social responsibility aspects of commercial health insurance into the scope of supervisory management. Since commercial health insurance is an insurance product, government should conduct evaluations of the market conditions of the industry, and the government's supervisory management should apply to such things as the size of the business, premium income, spending on compensation, operating conditions, and the security of insurance funds. At the same time, since commercial health insurance assumes a certain degree of social responsibility, the government should investigate and test its role in such things as strengthening the force of medical safeguards, expanding the scope of medical safeguards, upgrading the quality of healthcare management services, holding down the growth of medical costs, and improving the overall health conditions of the population.

3.6.2.2 Recommendations made from the perspective of enterprises

3.6.2.2.1 Improve upon the system of health insurance products, and upgrade the quality of services

China's commercial health insurance is at different stages of development in various parts of the country. Substantial differences exist among different provinces and regions. The land mass of China is enormous and the different climates, lifestyles, and eating habits also lead to differences in health conditions. At the same time, economic development varies by region so that people's consumption habits and ability to consume also vary. Because of this, insurance companies must suit the different needs of specific localities and design products and services that satisfy local customers.

Meanwhile, there is a strong homogeneity to health insurance products currently on the market. Policies provided by all the insurance companies are basically very similar. Insurance companies should, therefore, focus on product innovation and attempt to meet the needs of their customers as much as possible. They should attempt to design targeted and individualized products.

No matter what form such innovation takes, however, it must be confessed that insurance products are extremely easy to copy. It is therefore hard to root out the problem of homogeneity. However, it takes a long time to cultivate the ability to provide high-quality service and to sustain that level of service. That is something competitors find hard to duplicate. As a result, insurance companies should focus their efforts on setting up excellent service systems and on building their brand. For example, in the event of sudden changes of weather and increases in infectious diseases, service personnel of insurance companies should remind customers in a timely fashion to dress for the weather as one way to prevent illness but at the same time they should offer preventive medicines at a preferential price. Not only will this win the respect of customers and improve the consumption experience but it may play a certain role in controlling moral hazard. This can become an effective risk mitigation mechanism for the insurance company.

As the expectations for quality of life rise, insurance companies should put thought into innovative services to meet those expectations. They may want to develop distinctive services for targeted customers. For those who buy long-term insurance policies, the insurance company could offer specialized physical exams depending on the customer's gender, age, and work. They may carry out regular forums on health, or address questions that people have about health issues. At the same time, they can set up Internet-based forums and a consultation platform that provides customers with medical knowledge on all kinds of subjects. Company publications should be sent regularly to customers to provide them with information on health and beauty to make sure customers have a sense that the company is concerned about their welfare. Customers will gain an understanding of the company's products from all of these things, which will in turn increase potential demand. Companies with substantial resources might want to organize recreational activities for VIP customers, or parent-child activities, or they might provide them with fitness facilities. While companies enrich their services, they should focus on the quality of key links in their operations, including underwriting and claims settlement. These key aspects of the business are of great significance for the profitability of the company and in terms of mitigating risk. The professionalism and efficiency of the company's underwriting, claims settlement, and other services will not only help the company defend against moral hazard and adverse selection, but it will also allow customers to experience the value of the company's service. This will improve their degree of trust in the company and help establish a positive word-of-mouth reputation.[69]

3.6.2.2.2 *Identify the focus of market development*

From theoretical and empirical analysis, we can see that urban residents have greater demand for commercial health insurance than rural residents, and residents with higher educational levels have greater demand for commercial health insurance than those who are less educated. Therefore, in developing the commercial health insurance market, insurance companies should focus on urban residents and residents with higher levels of education. First, these two kinds of residents have relatively high income and greater capacity to buy health insurance. Second, these two have greater risk management awareness and are more willing to purchase commercial health insurance. Insurance companies can only target the correct customer groups if they have a firm grasp of their market development strategy and only then can they ensure their own growth.

3.6.2.2.3 *Improve the ability to control risk*

The rate of claims in the field of commercial health insurance is much higher than it is in other personal insurance fields. This is one of the reasons many insurance companies are less than enthusiastic about going into health insurance. To address this higher rate of claims, insurance companies must improve their procedures for controlling risk and also raise their ability to control the cost of reimbursing claims. Currently, China's commercial health insurance adopts a post-payment model for managing claims. That is, it uses the reimbursement system. Once the insured person receives medical services at a medical institution, he pays the associated medical costs himself. Then, based on a receipt that he gets for paying the bill, he applies to the insurance fund for reimbursement. The insurance company and the policy holder have a compensation relationship that is formalized in a contract. At the same time, the medical institution provides medical services to the insured. However, the insurance company itself has no constraining relationship with the medical institution. All it can do is review the receipts for bills as supplied by the institution to the insured in making its calculations and trying to control costs and risks. This kind of post-event risk-control method makes it hard for the company to hold down the cost of claims and achieve the goal of limiting risk. Because of this, the insurance company should adopt pre-event risk-control systems as well as mid-event control systems rather than just post-event risk control methods. It should emphasize optimizing its risk-control processes, such as conducting health-risk management of those it insures, offering education about health and consulting about critical illness. It also should cooperate with medical institutions so as to strengthen controls over the costs that are incurred when a policy holder receives treatment. The key to whether or not an insurance company can shift from a post-event mode of risk control to a mid-event mode depends on whether or not it can find methods by which to cooperate with medical institutions. Insurance companies must therefore establish win-win models by which to cooperate with medical institutions. Both sides need to benefit from the process. Only then will the problem of excessive insurance claims be resolved in any fundamental way. Through a competitive process, the insurance company can select designated hospitals and can sign cooperation agreements with medical institutions that are willing to work together with it. Without harming the interests of the insured, by this means the insurance company can increase the number of consumers that use a particular medical institution, so that the institution benefits from the arrangement, while the company can use the professional expertise of the hospital in order to reduce unreasonable spending on medical costs and reduce the cost and rate of claims. Both sides win.

3.6.2.2.4 *Focus on building up good faith*

A crisis of credibility appeared at one point in the development of China's insurance industry which, to this day, exerts an influence on people's opinion. We should absorb lessons from this event. The trustworthiness of insurance has a direct bearing on the sound growth of the industry. It also has a bearing on the operating behavior of the insurance company and business results. The products and services of health insurance are a kind of promise. They are a promise to make good on the future risk of consumers of the insurance, which requires that they follow the principle of utmost good faith. To consumers, the trustworthiness of an insurance company is vitally important. Once an event occurs, what is the possibility that the insurance company will keep its promise, and what is its capacity to do so? The answer determines the purchasing decision of the consumer. Credibility is expressed in the course of sales in particular. It is necessary to give serious thought to whether the sales methods and channels are reasonable or not. Companies should also consider whether or not the consumer has sufficient financial ability and purchasing power, and whether or not their understanding of health and health insurance is rational.

3.6.2.2.5 *Strengthen cooperation with other relevant institutions*

We can see from the successful experience of foreign countries that some large insurance companies directly participate in cooperation with hospitals by acquiring them. Not only does this enable them to upgrade services, and win the trust of consumers, but it is a way to accumulate data in order to meet the goal of controlling risk. Moreover, an insurance company can also cooperate with such government departments as social security and pharmaceutical development and production. By sharing information, they build a health management platform that belongs to their own company. We live in an information age and big data is necessarily becoming the key to victory in the competition among corporations. For this reason, it is imperative that insurance companies apply information technologies to their business as soon as possible, so that information can become a company's core competitive advantage in its early stages.

3.6.2.2.6 Intensify publicity efforts

We have discovered in the analysis presented above that awareness or understanding of insurance plays a role in furthering the growth of the industry. In grey relational analysis, we have found that the level of education has a pronounced effect on the demand for commercial health insurance. People with relatively high levels of sophistication generally also have a fairly high understanding of insurance. In China, the populace at large, and especially the older generation, knows extremely little about insurance. Insurance is therefore not a means by which they choose to counter the possibility of economic loss. Even though these people have the financial capacity to pay for insurance and are indeed encountering the risk of losses, they have not generated demand for insurance.[70] The insurance company, therefore, should bear the responsibility for making knowledge about insurance more widespread in the population. Not only will this improve the status of insurance in the minds of the public at large, and provide customers with an effective way to reduce economic losses, but such publicity will also spur people to take measures to mitigate all kinds of risks. This is the most fundamental way to help prevent and reduce the occurrence of economic losses.

Notes

1 Song Fuxing. Commercial Health Insurance Contributes to the Implementation of the 'Healthy China' Strategy. *Financial Times*, December 2, 2015.
2 J.K. Arrow. Uncertainty and the Welfare Economics of Medical Care [J]. *American Economic Review*, 1963 (5).
3 M.J. Brown. Evidence of Adverse Selection in the Individual Health Insurance Market [J]. *Journal of Risk and Insurance*, 1992 (1).
4 J.W. Pratt. Risk Aversion in the Small and in the Large. In P. Diamond, M. Rothschild (Eds.), *Uncertainty in Economics* (pp. 59–79). Academic Press, 1978. https://doi.org/10.1016/B978-0-12-214850-7.50010-3.
5 K.J. Arrow, R.C. Lind. Uncertainty and the Evaluation of Public Investment Decisions. *American Economic Review*, 1970, 60(3): 364–378.
6 J.R. Wolfe, J.H. Goddeeris. Adverse Selection, Moral Hazard, and Wealth Effects in the Medigap Insurance Market. *Journal of Health Economics*, 1991, 10(4): 433–459. https://doi.org/10.1016/0167-6296(91)90024-h.
7 L. Lillard, J. Rogowski. *Does Supplemental Private Insurance Increase Medicare Costs?* RAND Labor and Population Program, 1995.
8 S.L. Ettner. Adverse Selection and the Purchase of Medigap Insurance by the Elderly. *Journal of Health Economics*, 1997, 16(5): 543–562. https://doi.org/10.1016/S0167-6296(97)00011-8.
9 M.D. Hurd, K. McGarry. Medical Insurance and the Use of Health Care Services by the Elderly. *Journal of Health Economics*, 1997, 16(2): 129–154. https://doi.org/10.1016/s0167-6296(96)00515-2.
10 Barry Saver, Mark Doescher. To Buy, or Not to Buy. *Medical Care*, 2000, 38: 141–151. doi:10.1097/00005650-200002000-00004.

11 J. Gruber. The Wealth of the Unemployed. *ILR Review*, 2001, 55(1): 79–94. https://doi.org/10.1177/001979390105500105.

12 J.A. Nyman. *The Theory of Demand for Health Insurance*. Stanford University Press, 2002.

13 Y. Machnes. The Demand for Private Health Care under National Health Insurance: The Case of the Self-Employed. *European Journal of Health Economics*, 2006, 7(4): 265–269.

14 Chen Tao, Xie Yang. Internal Factors Affecting the Development of Commercial Health Insurance in China and Countermeasures [J]. *Insurance Studies*, 2008 (11).

15 Li Qiong. Analysis of Factors Affecting Premium of Commercial Health Insurance, Based on Comparison of Commercial Health Insurance Markets in Hubei, Beijing and Shanghai [J]. *South China Finance*, 2009 (7): 55–59.

16 Zhou Minglai, Shang Ying. Review of Theoretical and Empirical Studies of the Demand for Commercial Health Insurance [J]. *Chinese Journal of Health Policy*, 2011 (11).

17 Peng Xiaobo, Sun Qixiang. Gray Relational Analysis of Factors Influencing Chinese Farmers' Demand for Health Insurance [J]. *Insurance Studies*, 2012 (10).

18 Guo Pei. *Analysis of Factors Influencing Effective Demand for Commercial Health Insurance in China* [D]. Master's thesis of Jiangsu University, 2010.

19 Sherman Folland, Allen Goodman. *The Economics of Health and Health Care* [M]. Renmin University of China Press, 2002.

20 Guo Pei. Analysis of Factors Influencing Effective Demand for Commercial Health Insurance in China [D]. Master's thesis of Jiangsu University, 2010.

21 He Jingjing. *A Study of the Supply-Demand Gap in China's Commercial Health Insurance Market* [D]. Chengdu: Southwest University of Finance and Economics, 2009.

22 Chen Tao. *Health Insurance* [M]. Chengdu: Southwest University of Finance and Economics Press, 2002.

23 Cheng Xiaoming. *Health Economics* [M]. Beijing: People's Medical Publishing House, 2003.

24 Liu Jingsheng. *A Study of the Development of Health Insurance in China* [M]. Beijing: China Social Sciences Press, 2011.

25 Li Yuquan. *Report on the Development of China's Health Insurance Market (2010)* [M]. Beijing: China Economic Publishing House, 2012.

26 Yan Ping. *A Study on the Medical Cost Burden of the Elderly in China* [D]. Beijing: Renmin University of China, 2009.

27 Chen Tao, Xie Yang. Internal Factor Affecting the Development of Commercial Health Insurance in China and Countermeasures [J]. *Insurance Studies*, 2008 (11).

28 Zhang Xiao. *Commercial Health Insurance* [M]. Beijing: China Labor and Social Security Press, 2004.

29 Yan Bo, Ma Yanwei. A Study of Tax Policies Related to Commercial Health Insurance [J]. *China Finance*, 2012 (3).

30 Sun Rong, Wang Xiangnan. Comparison of Influencing Factors of Life Insurance Demand and Health Insurance Demand in my Country [A]. *Selected Articles of Academic Annual Meeting of Chinese Insurance Society*, 2011.

31 Chen Tao, Zhao Xiao. A Study of the Development Trend of Commercial Health Insurance Business Models in China [J]. *Health Economics Research*, 2010 (7).

32 Wei Sibo. *A Study of Solutions to Problems in the Development of Commercial Health Insurance in China* [D]. Hebei University of Economics and Business, 2012.

33 Wan Min. Exploration of China's Commercial Health Insurance [J]. *Modern Business Trade Industry*, 2008 (7).

34 Sheng Min. *Economic Analysis and Empirical Study of Insurance Purchase Decisions in China* [D]. Tongji University, 2006.

35 Xiao Hongwei. A Study of the Impact of Economic Development on Basic Medical Insurance in China [J]. *Insurance Studies*, 2012 (9).

36 Wang Yingcheng. *A Study of Adverse Selection of Commercial Health Insurance in China* [D]. Northeast Normal University, 2011.
37 Wang Xinguo. Analysis of the Current Commercial Health Insurance Sector in China and Development Suggestions [J]. *Business Culture*, 2007 (9).
38 Jiang Cai, Ye Xiaolan. The Effect of Tax Incentives on the Demand for Commercial Health Insurance. *Finance and Economics*, 2008, 000(011), 86–87, 44.
39 Yan Jianjun. Further Giving Play to the Role of Commercial Health Insurance in Medical Reform in China [J]. *China Finance*, 2010 (15).
40 Zhang Yao, Zhang Shuling. Learning from British Commercial Health Insurance. *Insurance Studies*, 2010 (2).
41 Zhang Yao, Zhang Shuling. Learning from British Commercial Health Insurance. *Insurance Studies*, 2010 (2).
42 Xu Meifang. Analysis on Determinants of Demand for Health Insurance in China: A Case Study of Shanghai 2006. *World Economic Papers*, 2007 (5).
43 According to international convention, a society is aged when people above 60 account for over 10%, or people above 65 account for more than 7% of the population.
44 Zhu Minglai, Shang Ying. Review of Theoretical and Empirical Studies on Demand for Commercial Health Insurance. *Chinese Journal of Health Policy*, 2011 (11).
45 Jacob Duker. Expenditure for Life Insurance among Working-Wife Families. *Journal of Risk and Insurance*, 1969, 36: 525. doi:10.2307/251159.
46 Xu Meifang. Analysis of Determinants of China's Health Insurance Demand: Taking the Shanghai Insurance Market in 2006 as an Example. *World Economic Culture Exchange*, 2007 (5).
47 P. Slovic. Informing and Educating the Public about Risk. *Risk Analysis*, 1987, 6(4): 403–415.
48 Zhu Kun, Zhang Xiaojuan, Liu Chunsheng. History of the Japanese Health Insurance System and What to Learn from It. *Chinese Journal of Health Policy*, 2012 (3).
49 Zhang Xinmin, Zhou Haiyang, Shen Jie. Calculation and Evaluation of Inpatient Insurance Rate in Medical Social Insurance [J]. *Chinese Journal of Hospital Administration*, 1995 (08): 457–460, 511.
50 Peng Xiaobo, Sun Qixiang. Grey Relational Analysis of Factor Influencing Chinese Farmers' Demand for Health Insurance [J]. *Insurance Studies*, 2012 (10).
51 Equalization is a process of dividing all the values of a sequence by the mean of the sequence to obtain a new sequence (equalized sequence).
52 Initialization is a process of dividing each value in a sequence (except the first value) by the first value of the sequence to obtain a new sequence (initialized sequence). Since equalization results are the simple arithmetic means of numerical values in the time series, their ability to reflect the growth trend in a sensitive manner is low, and using the initialization method can more fully reflect the dynamic impact of changes.
53 Liu Hong, Wang Jun. Studies on Chinese Residents' Medical Insurance Purchase Behavior: from the Perspective of Commercial Health Insurance. *Economics*, 2012 (11).
54 Liu Xuening. Empirical Study on the Influence of Income on the Demand for Insurance. *Insurance Studies*, 2012 (11).
55 Yan Jianjun. Giving Better Play to the Role of Commercial Health Insurance in China's Medical System Reform. *China Finance*, 2010 (15).
56 Li Xiaodi. *Study on Influencing Factors of Commercial Health Insurance in Chongqing*. Chongqing University, 2011.
57 Wang Yingcheng. *Study on Adverse Selection in Commercial Health Insurance in China*. Northeast Normal University, 2011.
58 Jeffrey M. Woodridge. *Introductory Econometrics*. Beijing: Renmin University of China Press, 2010.
59 Zhu Minglai, Wang Meijiao. Research on the Incentive Effect of Tax Incentives on Commercial Health Insurance [J]. *Insurance Research*, 2016, 0(2): 47–58.

60 Zhu Minglai, Shang Ying. Summary of a Theoretical and Empirical Study of Commercial Health Insurance Demand [J]. *China Health Policy Research*, 2011 (11).
61 Wan Min. Reflections on the Development of Commercial Health Insurance in China [J]. *Modern Business Industry*, 2008 (7).
62 Wei Hualin, He Yudong. Research on the Potential of China's Long-term Nursing Insurance Market [J]. *Insurance Research*, 2012 (7): 7–15.
63 Zhang Lingyu, Xue Gang. Situation and Enlightenment of the Development of Commercial Health Insurance in Germany [J]. *Shanghai Insurance*, 2009 (12).
64 Zhang Xinmin, Zhou Haiyang, Shen Jie. Calculation and Evaluation of Inpatient Insurance Rate in Medical Social Insurance [J]. *Chinese Journal of Hospital Administration*, 1995 (8): 457–460, 511.
65 Wei Hualin, Li Jinhui. *A Study of Demand for Life Insurance* [M]. Beijing: China Financial and Economic Publishing House, 2009.
66 Chen Tao, Zhao Xiao. A Study of the Development Trend of Commercial Health Insurance Business Models in China [J]. *Health Economics Research*, 2010 (7).
67 Li Yuquan. *Report on the Development of China's Health Insurance Market (2010)* [M]. Beijing: China Economic Publishing House, 2012.
68 Yan Jianjun. Further Giving Play to the Role of Commercial Health Insurance in Medical Reform in China [J]. *China Finance*, 2010 (15).
69 Liu Fangfang, Wang Xiuhua, Bian Hu. An Empirical Study of Factor Influencing the Development of Commercial Health Insurance in China [J]. *Chinese Journal of Health Policy*, 2010 (9).
70 Wan Min. Exploration of China's Commercial Health Insurance [J]. *Modern Business Trade Industry*, 2008 (7).

Bibliography

Ahking, Francis W., Giaccotto, Carmelo, Santerre, Rexford E. The Aggregate Demand for Private Health Insurance Coverage in the United States [R]. *Journal of Risk and Insurance*, 2009 (1).
Arrow, J.K. Uncertainty and the Welfare Economics of Medical Care [J]. *American Economic Review*, 1963 (5).
Chen Lei. *A Study of Factors Influencing the Demand for Long-Term Care Insurance* [D]. Fudan University, 2012.
Chen Tao. *Health Insurance* [M]. Chengdu: Southwest University of Finance and Economics Press, 2002.
Chen Tao, Xie Yang. Internal Factors Affecting the Development of Commercial Health Insurance in China and Countermeasures [J]. *Insurance Studies*, 2008 (11).
Chen Tao, Zhao Xiao. A Study of the Development Trend of Commercial Health Insurance Business Models in China [J]. *Health Economics Research*, 2010 (7).
Cheng Xiaoming. *Health Economics* [M]. Beijing: People's Medical Publishing House, 2003.
China Health Statistics Yearbook 2000–2015.
China Statistics Yearbook 2000–2015.
Cui Wenwei. Analysis of Factors Influencing Demand for Commercial Health Insurance in China [D]. Master's thesis of Southwestern University of Finance and Economics, 2014.
Deng Zulong. *Basis for Grey Theory* [M]. Wuhan: Huazhong University of Science and Technology Press, 2002.
Ding Caixia. Health Insurance Reform and Health Care Reform [J]. *Estate and Science Tribune*, 2008 (3).

Du Liqing. Coordinated Development of Public Health Insurance and Commercial Health Insurance in China [D]. Master's thesis of Shanxi University of Finance and Economics, 2010.

Fischer, S.A. Life Cycle Model of Insurance Purchase [J]. *International Economic Review*, 1973 (14).

Flanders, Sherman, Goodman, Allen C., Stano, Miron. *The Economics of Health and Health Care* (Tu Jan, Meng Qingyue, Trans.) [M]. Beijing: Renmin University of China Press, 101–145.

Geng Jinjuan, Liu Jin. Analysis of Macro-Factors Influencing Demand for Long-Term Elderly Care Insurance in China [J]. *Productivity Research*, 2014 (1).

Guo Pei. *Analysis of Factors Influencing Demand for Commercial Health Insurance in China* [D]. Master's thesis of Southwestern University of Finance and Economics, 2010.

Guo Pei. *Analysis of Factors Influencing Effective Demand for Commercial Health Insurance in China* [D]. Master's thesis of Jiangsu University, 2010.

He Jingjing. *A Study of the Supply-Demand Gap in China's Commercial Health Insurance Market* [D]. Southwest University of Finance and Economics, 2009.

Huang Junjie. An Empirical Study of the Relationship between Public Expenditure and the Health of Residents in China [J]. *Productivity Research*, 2007 (18).

Huang Zhanhui, Wang Hanliang. *Health Insurance* [M]. Beijing: Peking University Press, 2006.

Insurance Association of China, Task Force of Chinese Academy of Social Sciences. *Report of Health Insurance Development in China* [M]. Beijing: China Financial and Economic Publishing House, 2009.

Lewis, F. D. Dependents and the Demand for Insurance [J]. *American Economic Review*, 1989 (9).

Li Bairu. Analysis of factors influencing demand for commercial health insurance in China [J]. *Journal of Insurance Professional College*, 2011 (2).

Li Qiong. Analysis of Factors Affecting Premium of Commercial Health Insurance, Based on Comparison of Commercial Health Insurance Markets in Hubei, Beijing and Shanghai [J]. *South China Finance*, 2009 (7): 55–59.

Li Xiaodi. *A Study of Factors Influencing the Development of Commercial Health Insurance in Chongqing* [D]. Chongqing University, 2011.

Li Yuquan. *Report on the Development of China's Health Insurance Market (2010)* [M]. Beijing: China Economic Publishing House, 2012.

Liang Laicun. Empirical Analysis of Demand for Life Insurance in China [J]. *Journal of Quantitative and Technical Economics*, 2007, 24 (8): 80–89.

Liang Tao. *Report on Regulation and Development of Life Insurance in China* [M]. Beijing: People's Daily Press, 2011.

Lin Yuming. *The Development of a Multi-Pillar Endowment Insurance and Health Insurance System: A Long-Term and Emergency Response Solution for the Population Aging Crisis* [M]. Beijing: Intellectual Property Publishing House, 2009.

Liu Fangfang, Wang Xiuhua, Bian Hu. An Empirical Study of Factors Influencing the Development of Commercial Health Insurance in China [J]. *Chinese Journal of Health Policy*, 2010 (9).

Liu Hong, Wang Jun. A Study of Chinese Residents' Purchase Behavior of Commercial Health Insurance [J]. *Economics*, 2012 (11).

Liu Jingsheng. *A Study of the Development of Health Insurance in China* [M]. Beijing: China Social Sciences Press, 2011.

Liu Na. *Factors Influencing the Development of Commercial Health Insurance in China* [D]. Tianjin University of Finance and Economics, 2012.

Liu Xuening. An Empirical Study of the Impact of Income Level on the Demand for Insurance [J]. *Insurance Studies*, 2012 (11).

Liu, Gordon G., Wu, Xiaodong, Peng, Chaoyang, Fu, Alex Z. Urbanization and Health in Rural China [J]. *Contemporary Economic Policy*, 2003, 21(1): 11–24.

Mankiw, N.G.. *Macroeconomics* [M]. Beijing: Renmin University of China Press, 2010.

Nyman, John A. *The Theory of Demand for Health Insurance* [D]. Stanford, CA: Stanford University Press, 2002.

Pan Changgang. Factors Affecting Health Insurance Demand [J]. *Journal of Guangxi Economic Management Cadre College*, 2008.

Pei Guang, Xu Wenhu. *A Study of China's Health Insurance Statistics System* [M]. Beijing: China Financial and Economic Publishing House, 2009.

Peng Xiaobo, Sun Qixiang. Gray Relational Analysis of Factor Influencing Chinese Farmers' Demand for Health Insurance [J]. *Insurance Studies*, 2012 (10).

Pissarides, C. The Wealth-Age Relation with Medical Insurance [J]. *Economics*, 1980 (47).

Pong Hao. *Econometrics* [M]. Beijing: Science Press, 2010.

Samuelson, Paul A., Nordhaus, William D. *Macroeconomics* [M]. Beijing: Posts and Telecom Press, 2004.

Sheng Min. *Economic Analysis and Empirical Study of Insurance Purchase Decisions in China* [D]. Tongji University, 2006.

Song Fuxing. Commercial Health Insurance Contributes to the Implementation of the 'Healthy China' Strategy [N]. *Financial Times*, December 2, 2015.

Sun Dongya, Fan Juanjuan. Lessons Learned from the Commercial Health Insurance Sector in the U.S. [J]. *Insurance Studies*, 2010 (2).

Sun Dongya, Fan Juanjuan. Inspirations from the Development of Commercial Health Insurance in the U.S. for its Development in China [J]. *Insurance in China*, 2012 (4).

Sun Yugang. A Study of Gray Correlation Analysis and Its Application [D]. Master's thesis of Nanjing University of Aeronautics and Astronautics, 2007.

Wan Min. Exploration of China's Commercial Health Insurance [J]. *Modern Business Trade Industry*, 2008 (7).

Wang Debao. Development Opportunities Brought by New Medical Reform to Commercial Health Insurance in China [J]. *Insurance in China*, 2009 (6): 12–17.

Wang Junzhe. A Study of the Integration between Public Health Insurance And Commercial Health Insurance [D]. Master's thesis of Shanghai Jiao Tong University, 2014.

Wang Xinguo. Analysis of the Current Commercial Health Insurance Sector in China and Development Suggestions [J]. *Business Culture*, 2007 (9).

Wang Yingcheng. *A Study of Adverse Selection of Commercial Health Insurance in China* [D]. Northeast Normal University, 2011.

Wei Hualin, Li Jinhui. *A Study of Demand for Life Insurance* [M]. Beijing: China Financial and Economic Publishing House, 2009.

Wei Sibo. *A Study of Solutions to Problems in the Development Of Commercial Health Insurance in China* [D]. Hebei University of Economics and Business, 2012.

Wooldridge, Jeffrey M. *Introductory Econometrics* [M]. Beijing: Renmin University of China Press, 2010.

Wu Jiangming, Lin Baoqing. Empirical Analysis of China's Insurance Demand Model [J]. *Fujian Forum*, 2003 (10).

Xiao Hongwei. A Study of the Impact of Economic Development on Basic Medical Insurance in China [J]. *Insurance Studies*, 2012 (9).

Xiong Zhiguo, Yan Bo, Lock Lingyan. *A Study of Commercial Health Insurance Development Models in China* [M]. Beijing: Peking University Press, 2012.

Xu Meng. A Study of Commercial Health Insurance in China [J]. *Cutting Edge Theory*, 2009 (7).

Yaari, M.E. Uncertain Lifetime, Life Insurance, and the Theory of the Consumer [J]. *Review of Economic Studies*, 1965, 32 (2): 137–150.

Yan Bo, Ma Yanwei. A Study of Tax Policies Related to Commercial Health Insurance [J]. *China Finance*, 2012 (3).

Yan Jianjun. Giving Further Play to the Role of Commercial Health Insurance in Medical Reform in China [J]. *China Finance*, 2010 (15).

Yang Jiong, Tian Peng, Ye Jianhua. Empirical Analysis of Factors Affecting Life Insurance Demand in China [J]. *China Soft Science*, 2005, (3).

Yang Xia. *An Empirical Study of the Demand for Insurance in China* [D]. Wuhan University, 2009.

Yearbook of China's Insurance 2000–2015.

Zhang Xiao. *Commercial Health Insurance* [M]. Beijing: China Labor and Social Security Press, 2004.

Zhao Guiqin. Testing of Factors Influencing the Insurance Market in China [J]. *Journal of Zhongnan University of Economics and Law*, 2006 (1).

Zhou Minglai, Shang Ying. Review of Theoretical and Empirical Studies of the Demand for Commercial Health Insurance [J]. *Chinese Journal of Health Policy*, 2011 (11).

Zou Hong, Liu Bending, Luo Yanjie. Empirical Study of Regional Disparity in Insurance Demand in China [J]. *Insurance Studies*, 2011 (6).

4 Research Topic 3

Role of and development model for commercial health insurance in China[1]

Shi Xiaojun, Wang Aoran, and Feng Pengcheng

4.1 THE CONTEXT FOR DEVELOPING CHINA'S COMMERCIAL HEALTH INSURANCE

4.1.1 Policy changes, the 'new normal,' and significance

4.1.1.1 Remarkable achievements of China's new medical reform, and policy changes relating to commercial health insurance

4.1.1.1.1 Achievements of the healthcare system reform and prospects for the Healthy China initiative

Reform of China's healthcare system has made astonishing progress since the start of the new medical reform in 2009. The *Outline of the 13th Five-Year Plan for National Economic and Social Development* dedicates a separate chapter to 'pushing forward the development of Healthy China.' It sets forth three explicit targets relating to comprehensive deepening of the reform of the institutional structures that govern China's medicine and healthcare systems.

First, China realized universal coverage of medical insurance. By the year 2015, the number of the participants in the urban basic medical insurance program reached 666 million, while 670 million were insured under the new rural cooperative medical system. Over 1.3 billion, or 95% of Chinese, were covered by the various types of basic medical insurance. In 2015, the funding for the basic medical insurance programs came to RMB 1,102.4 billion. The critical illness insurance program already covers close to one billion people in urban and rural areas.[2] An effective emergency aid system for critical illness was also set up so that Chinese people no longer have to feel helpless.

Second, government inputs have increased dramatically. In 2009, government expenditures on healthcare came to RMB 481.626 billion, which was 27.5% of the country's total spending on healthcare. By 2014, the figure was RMB 1059.07 billion, accounting for 29.9% of the total and up by 119.89% over the figure in 2009. The percentage that individuals spent on their own account for healthcare went down, from 35.29% to 30%, which is the lowest level it has been for the past 20 years.[3]

Third, breakthroughs were made in medical reform work at the grassroots level. With the increase in government spending, nearly every village has a healthcare room, every township has a clinic, and every county has a standard hospital. Eighty percent of Chinese residents are now able to reach a medical center within around 15 minutes.[4] Urban and rural residents enjoy 45 basic public health services in 12 categories at no cost, which basically cover the person's entire lifetime. Seven major public health service programs are being implemented that provide benefits to close to 200 million people.[5]

4.1.1.1.2 Policy changes and the current situation of commercial health insurance

4.1.1.1.2.1 POLICY CHANGES

4.1.1.1.2.1(a) Early stages: prior to 1994

From 1949 to the eve of Reform and Opening Up, China had three separate systems that addressed healthcare in the country: the labor protection medical care system for employees of State-Owned Enterprises, the publicly funded medical care system for staff in Party and government institutions, and the rural cooperative medical care system. Funds to cover medical expenses for individuals in these three systems were provided by the State, enterprises, and collectives. Commercial health insurance was initiated only after the start of Reform and Opening Up. In 1982, the Shanghai Branch of the People's Insurance Company of China started medical insurance for employees of Shanghai cooperatives on a trial basis. This marked the birth of health insurance in China. Between 1985 and 1993, personal health insurance products gradually increased but the size and scope of coverage was limited due to the fact that people had low income levels and did not really understand insurance, which meant that demand stayed low. Commercial health insurance was therefore sold as a kind of supplementary insurance.

4.1.1.1.2.1(b) Picking up the pace: 1994–2002

China's social medical insurance underwent a transformation from old to new systems after 1994. In 1998, insurance coverage for urban employees was initiated and commercial health insurance gradually began to grow. In 1995, China incorporated critical illness insurance into its systems. By 2002, there were around 150 types of health insurance products on the market, accounting for a large percentage of the total health insurance business. Demand from the public began to rise and health insurance did grow rapidly, but effective supply remained inadequate and claims settlement and underwriting technologies were weak.

4.1.1.1.2.1(c) Professional development: since 2003

China began to reconstruct a social medical insurance system after 2003. In that year, pilot programs were set up throughout the country to test the new rural cooperative medical system, and an emergency medical assistance program was set up to cover both urban and rural areas.

In 2007, the program calling for urban residents' insurance was established. In 2009, the policy directive known in short as the *Opinion on the new medical reform* called for 'vigorous development of commercial health insurance.' This presented a tremendous opportunity for the industry to grow. In 2012, the government set forth 'guidance policies' on critical illness insurance. Starting in 2015, pilot programs began that allowed for preferential tax treatment for individuals who purchased health insurance. Between 2003 and 2015, income from premiums grew at an average annual rate of 22.4%.[6] By now, insurers in China are gradually setting up systems that incorporate the idea of 'health insurance + health management.' Nevertheless, the structure of their product offerings has problems and, as before, their effective supply of insurance is inadequate.

4.1.1.1.2.2 CURRENT SITUATION

In recent years, China has put major effort into getting the commercial health insurance industry to participate in the building up of the country's medical and healthcare systems. The government has encouraged commercial health insurance to launch insurance for critical illness and to participate in 'handling' the country's basic medical insurance programs.

First, the industry is indeed broadly participating in critical illness insurance and basic medical insurance. Sixteen insurance companies in the country are providing policies for critical illness insurance, which provide coverage for 920 million people in 31 provinces. From January to September 2016, actual claims from patients with critical illness insurance increased by 13.85% on top of the level claimable from basic medical insurance.[7] As of the end of 2014, the insurance industry served a total 320 million people who purchased various forms of medical insurance, took in newly authorized funds (to manage) of RMB 18.92 billion, and paid out reimbursements totaling RMB 13.52 billion to 36.116 million people.[8]

Second, commercial health insurance is able to provide a diversity of safeguards. The industry has grown rapidly since 2012. Income from premiums has gone from RMB 86.3 billion to RMB 241.047 billion in 2015,[9] with a rate of increase that is faster than that of premiums in the insurance industry overall. Insurance coverage is constantly being expanded and has gone from simply reimbursing costs and providing economic compensation to a more comprehensive approach to health management that provides coverage for services before, during, and after illness.

4.1.1.2 China's commercial health insurance is now confronting a new normal

4.1.1.2.1 Dramatic changes in the spectrum of diseases, decline in the death rate, and the emergence of chronic diseases as the primary cause of death

As China's population ages and as the pattern of disease in the country changes, chronic illnesses have become a severe threat to health. According to the *2015 Report on nutrition and chronic illness in Chinese*, in 2012, the prevalence of hypertension among the population over 18 was 25.2%, while the prevalence of diabetes was 9.7%. Both of these have exhibited a rising trend since 2002.

In 2013, the incidence of cancer was 235 out of 100,000. In 2012, the mortality rate of chronic diseases was 533 out of 100,000. In other words, 86.6% of the number of deaths in the country was due to chronic diseases. Moreover, a broader variety of people are suffering from chronic diseases and the age of such people is getting younger.

4.1.1.2.2 Decline in the rate at which the economy grows and fiscal revenues increase

In 2015, China's GDP grew at a rate of 6.9%. In the first quarter of 2016, the rate was 6.7%,[10] showing a downward trending situation. The target for GDP growth of the 13th Five-Year Plan is 6.5%. It may well be that long-term economic trends are of an 'L-type,' with growth in fiscal revenues slowing down. The government is already finding it hard to maintain the high spending put into the basic medical insurance program since the start of the new medical reform. The financial sources of the basic medical insurance program are in trouble and confronting a grave situation.

4.1.1.2.3 Pressure from medical costs due to the acceleration of population aging and the acceleration of urbanization

In 2014, the percentage of China's population that was over 65 broke through the 10% mark for the first time, reaching the high figure of 138 million people.[11] China's aging situation is characterized by some unique factors. Older people are often impoverished and they reach old age before getting on a sound financial footing or becoming part of China's urbanization process. The prevalence of diseases is high among the elderly population and medical costs are consequently also extremely high. These things pose a massive challenge to the supply of medical services and to medical and healthcare resources.

*4.1.1.2.4 Rapid increase in total healthcare expenses, with individuals
still bearing a heavy load*

As standards of living rise and medical technology improves, the twin trends of
an aging population and higher rates of chronic illness are intensifying the rise in
medical costs. Total healthcare expenses went from RMB 1,998 billion in 2010
to RMB 3,537.9 billion in 2014. They rose at an average annual rate of 13%.
Meanwhile, individual healthcare spending went from RMB 705.1 billion to
RMB 1,174.5 billion in these years, rising at an average annual rate of 12.4%
(see Table 4.1). By the year 2015, total healthcare expenses are expected to
reach RMB 4,058.77 billion, and individual spending on healthcare will reach
RMB 1,216.4 billion, a figure that accounts for 29.97% of the total.

*4.1.1.2.5 Medical insurance funds at risk of long-term deficit: growth
in spending higher than growth in income*

Spending of China's medical insurance funds has gone up constantly since the
start of the country's new medical reform in 2009. By 2013, the increased pace
of spending out of the urban basic medical insurance fund had already exceeded
the increases in income. In 2014, the disparity in rates increased further with
spending growing at 19.6% and income growing at 17.4%. This trend of
increased costs of medical insurance is very hard to turn around in a short period
of time (see Table 4.2; also Table 4.3).

4.1.1.3 The importance and urgent imperative of developing commercial health insurance in China

It will be hard to control the rising trend of medical costs during the 13th Five-Year
Plan period, which means that the funding for the basic medical insurance program
is facing dire straits. Measures associated with the new medical reform require a
relatively long time to take effect in order to have the desired result of 'curbing the
outflow.' Because of that, we have made the judgment that safeguards provided by
the basic medical insurance program should maintain their current level during the
period of the 13th Five-Year Plan. That therefore means we must increase the
power of commercial health insurance. On the one hand, commercial health insurance provides a secondary form of compensation for the portion of claims that are
self-paid. This lowers the financial burden on individuals. On the other hand, the
combined forces of basic medical insurance and commercial health insurance will
be able to reduce improper behavior of medical institutions such as excessive
medical procedures, and should thereby lower spending on medical costs.

4.1.2 Development trends of China's commercial health insurance

First, medical insurance will grow at a fast pace. The favorable effects of critical
illness insurance and preferential tax treatment for individual health insurance,

Table 4.1 Total and individuals' healthcare expenses in 2010–2014 (RMB 100 million)

Year	Total healthcare expenses	Growth rate (%)	Individual healthcare expenses	Growth rate (%)	Individual vs. total (%)
2010	19,980.4	12.2	7,051.29	7.31	35.29
2011	24,345.91	17.93	8,465.28	20.05	34.77
2012	28,119.0	13.42	9,656.32	14.07	34.34
2013	31,868.95	11.77	10,729.34	11.11	33.67
2014	35,378.9	9.92	11,745.3	9.47	33.20
2015 (forecast)	40,587.7	14.72	12,164.0	3.56	29.97

Source: *China Healthcare and Family Planning Yearbook (2011–2015)*. Data for 2015 come from http://field.10jqka.com.cn/20160722/c591902965.shtml.

Note

In 2014, the expenditure decreased mainly because the number of covered residents dropped from 802 million in 2013 to 736 million in 2014 due to the policy on integrating urban worker medical insurance, urban resident medical insurance, and new rural cooperative medical system.

Table 4.2 Revenue and expenditure of urban basic medical insurance (RMB 100 million)

Year	Revenue	Expenditure	Revenue growth (%)	Expenditure growth (%)
2009	3,672	2,797	20.8	34.2
2010	4,309	3,538	17.3	26.5
2011	5,539	4,431	28.6	25.2
2012	6,939	5,544	25.3	25.1
2013	8,248	6,801	18.9	22.7
2014	9,687	8,134	17.4	19.6
2015	11,193	9,312	15.5	14.5

Source: *Statistics Bulletin of Human Resources and Social Security Development (2009–2015).*

Table 4.3 Funding and expenditure of new rural cooperative medical system (RMB 100 million)

Year	Funding	Expenditure	Funding growth rate (%)	Expenditure growth rate (%)
2009	944.29	922.92	20.4	39.4
2010	1,308.93	1,187.84	38.55	28.7
2011	2,048.47	1,710.19	56.49	44.06
2012	2,483.43	2,408.0	21.3	40.8
2013	2,972.13	2,909.2	19.6	20.8
2014	3,025.3	2,890.4	1.8	−0.60

Source: *China Healthcare Statistics Yearbook (2010–2015).*

Note

In 2014, the expenditure decreased mainly because the number of covered residents dropped from 802 million in 2013 to 736 million in 2014 due to the policy on integrating urban worker medical insurance, urban resident medical insurance, and new rural cooperative medical system.

plus the release of demand for multi-tiered medical safeguards, will contribute to this fast growth.

Second, the trend known as 'health insurance + health services' will become apparent. Large insurance companies are actively extending their value chain of health services to create what they call a 'mega health industry' that covers not only health insurance but also health services, medical services, and nursing care for the elderly. They are providing comprehensive health safeguards and health services that cover the entire lifespan of a person.

Third, the demands of regulatory management on the industry will increase. The China Insurance Regulatory Commission is putting its hand to revising the *Administrative Measures for Health Insurance*. This will put forth more detailed regulations and oversight procedures that relate to major illness insurance. The entire commercial health insurance industry will now be incorporated into stand-ardized regulatory procedures that are within the purview of the legal system.

Fourth, the application of new technologies will speed up. In the context of the Internet, big data, and the Internet of Things, the application of technologies allows the accelerated development of such things as personalized, scenario-based, public-benefit, and mutual-assistance type insurance products.

Fifth, cross-jurisdiction competition will become more intense. BAT and other Internet giants are investing heavily in the health industry, and they are bound to gain access to the health insurance sector, while meanwhile the giants in the health industry are waiting for approval to establish health insurance companies. Some medical information-technology companies are cooperating directly with government in order to launch programs aimed at controlling costs, so they too are becoming competitors to insurance companies by crossing over industry and jurisdictional boundaries.

Sixth, professional requirements are rising. Professional competence and high-quality service will become key criteria by which government chooses insurance companies and by which customers choose companies. Insurance companies will have to establish their own competitive advantages by improving systems and the professionalism of their staff. They will have to adopt models that emphasize technology and risk control.

4.1.3 The statistical foundations of China's commercial health insurance must be improved as well as the application of information technologies to the industry

Commercial health insurance is a data-intensive business and has relatively high information-technology requirements. China needs to improve in both of these respects. In the following section, we first present maps showing China's critical illness and chronic disease distribution, based on the relevant statistics. We then present an overview of the status of building up China's medical information systems.

4.1.3.1 Maps of critical illness and chronic diseases in China

Deaths due to illnesses that turn into chronic disease are on the rise in China, and the trend is apparent. Nationwide data from 2010 shows that the top three causes of mortality were cerebrovascular disease, ischemic heart disease, and chronic lower respiratory tract disease. Chronic diseases have already gradually become the primary cause of death in China (see Figure 4.1). The distribution of critical illness as well as chronic disease shows dramatic variation among regions. The death rate from chronic disease is highest in Tianjin (0.537%), Heilongjiang (0.401%), and Shandong (0.397%).

The distribution of chronic diseases leading to the top three death rates also varies by region. The highest rates of mortality from cerebrovascular disease were in Northeast China, North China, and Central China, specifically in Tianjin (0.216‰), Jiangsu (0.154‰), and Liaoning (0.151‰).

With specific reference to ischemic heart disease, the highest numbers of deaths were in Northeast China, North China, and Central China. Specifically, the top three locations with highest death rates from this disease were Tianjin (0.225‰), Beijing (0.143‰), and Heilongjiang (0.133‰).

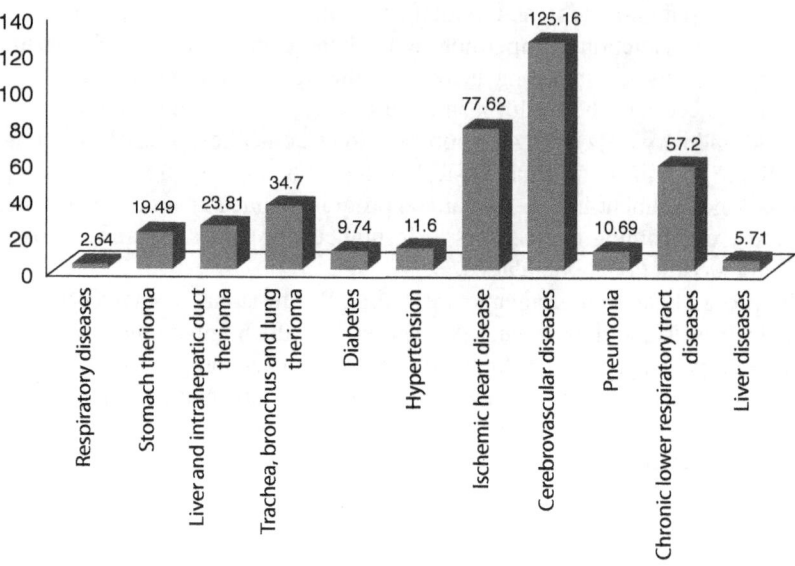

Figure 4.1 Top ten average death rates nationwide from critical illness and chronic disease.

Source: Public Health Science Data Center.

Note
Figures indicate average mortalities per 100,000 persons in 2010.

With specific reference to chronic lower respiratory tract disease, the places where numbers of deaths were fairly high were in Southwest China (excluding Tibet) and Northwest China. Specifically, the places with highest death rates from this disease were Chongqing (0.113%), Yunnan (0.103%), and Sichuan (0.092%).

Pneumonia and respiratory diseases lead to fairly high numbers of deaths in China (Figure 4.1). Fairly high death rates from pneumonia are found in Southwest China in particular. The top three places in terms of death rates from this illness were Yunnan (0.029‰), Guangdong (0.023‰), and Tianjin (0.019‰).

4.1.3.2 Management of medical information and the application of information technologies

Management of medical information includes such management by medical institutions as well as by public healthcare systems. A broader definition of 'medical informatization,' however, also includes Internet-based remote medical care, the 'cloud hospital,' mobile medical care, and the mining of medical big data.[12] Under the impetus of all kinds of policies relating to the new medical reform, the application of information technologies to medicine is booming. According to IDC statistics, China spent a total of RMB 17.076 billion on IT applications to its medical system in 2012, and will invest RMB 33.653 billion in 2017.[13]

China's Hospital Information System (HIS) uses Electronic Medical Records (EMR) as the core data. It collects and processes hospital management data and clinical data which results in the digitization of a patient's information including treatment procedures. According to a CHIMA survey, over 60% of Grade Three hospitals in the country are equipped with EMR systems, as well as close to 40% of hospitals under the level of Grade Three.[14]

Internet-based medicine includes three separate components, namely pre-treatment, during-treatment, and post-treatment care. Websites, smart hardware, APP, and wearable devices are the medium by which this takes place. Services provided to users via these means include health consulting and examinations, online diagnosis, payment services, chronic-disease management, and so on.[15] According to a Special Report published by BOC International [Bank of China], on the *Informatization of the Medical and Pharmaceutical Industries in China*, based on estimates of 10% to 20% Internet penetration rate of medical services, the size of the market of Internet-based medicine in 2012 was between RMB 56.54 billion and RMB 113.08 billion.[16]

Remote medical care makes use of doctors in large hospitals who consult with grassroots medical institutions in less developed regions on difficult and uncertain cases. In 2012, the market for distance medicine in China was just RMB 2.16 billion. As new technologies begin to be applied and as the legal and policy context improves, in 2017 the market may break through RMB 12.5 billion and may exceed RMB 20 billion in 2020.[17]

The 'cloud hospital' is being jointly developed by medical IT enterprises and top-class or renowned hospitals. By sharing data, it allows for two-way referrals and remote diagnosis. Mobile medical care mainly uses smart hardware, APP, and wearable devices to provide effective support for health management. This is able to help patients with chronic diseases monitor their conditions over an extended time period as well as have periodic checkups.[18] In 2014, the size of the market for mobile medical care reached RMB 3 billion. The estimate of *Analysts* is that it will reach RMB 20 billion in 2017, which would give it a growth rate of over 80%.

4.2 THE EGG-WHITE MODEL OF CHINA'S COMMERCIAL HEALTH INSURANCE, WITH CHALLENGES IT IS FACING AND CAUSES OF THE PROBLEMS

4.2.1 The egg-white model

4.2.1.1 Basic structure of the model

Since the start of the new medical reform in 2009, China has established a 'basic medical insurance system' that is characterized by broad coverage of people but low levels of protection. By 2016, this insurance system covered 95% of China's people, which made it a form of universal coverage. Even though healthcare and medical services in the country have constantly improved, a massive number of Chinese are still not covered by the healthcare financing system, however. These individuals and families have to carry the burden of medical costs by themselves. The financial system that applies to healthcare as it currently exists at this stage of China's history is like an egg in terms of structure. It can be divided into three levels: the yolk, the egg-white, and the shell (see Figure 4.2 and Table 4.4).

4.2.1.1.1 Yolk level

The yolk level of the system provides basic social security and various kinds of supplementary medical insurance. In a narrow sense, it includes the lowest level of medical emergency assistance and basic-level social insurance (the urban basic medical insurance system, the new rural cooperative medical system, critical illness insurance, and so on.) The scope of safeguards and degree of coverage of all of these are limited. In a broader sense, this yolk level includes various kinds of supplementary medical insurance and the insurance that enjoys preferential tax treatment, but the scale of those things is small.

4.2.1.1.2 Shell level

The shell level of the system provides commercial health insurance. This shell is extremely thin, and the amount of reimbursement of healthcare costs is actually minimal. In 2014, compensation from China's health insurance came to a mere 1.61% of total healthcare costs. In contrast, in 2013, the average in OECD countries was 6.3%. The figure was 13.9% in France, 9.3% in Germany, and 34.9% in the U.S. (see Figures 4.3 and 4.4). The shell level is not comprised purely of commercial health insurance but also includes the cooperation and interaction between commercial insurance and social insurance, that is, the participation of commercial insurance in handling the basic medical insurance program and other activities.

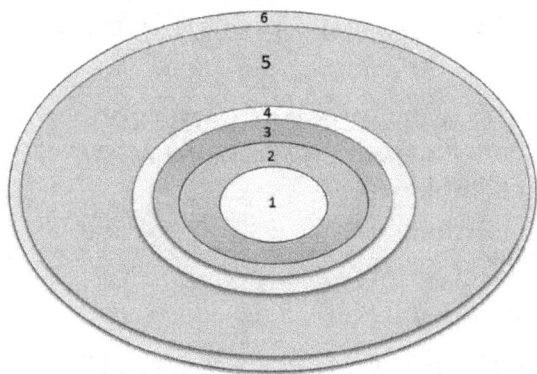

Figure 4.2 The egg-white model.

4.2.1.1.3 Egg-white level

The egg-white layer of the system is an empty zone that lies between the shell and the yoke. It is covered neither by commercial health insurance nor by social insurance. This is the portion of the system that requires that individuals and families pay for medical costs themselves. This zone is enormous. In 2015, the portion of medical bills that families paid themselves came to 29% of total healthcare expenses in the country. In OECD countries, the average percentage is roughly 19.4% (see Figures 4.3 and 4.4).

4.2.1.2 Main features of the egg-white zone

4.2.1.2.1 Financing of healthcare: self-paid expenses of individuals are fairly high

4.2.1.2.1.1 ABSOLUTE AMOUNTS: MEDICAL COSTS KEEP BALLOONING

Between 2010 and 2014, China's total medical expenses increased from RMB 1,998 billion to RMB 3,537.89 billion, which represented an average annual growth of 13.04%. Individual spending on healthcare went from RMB 705.129

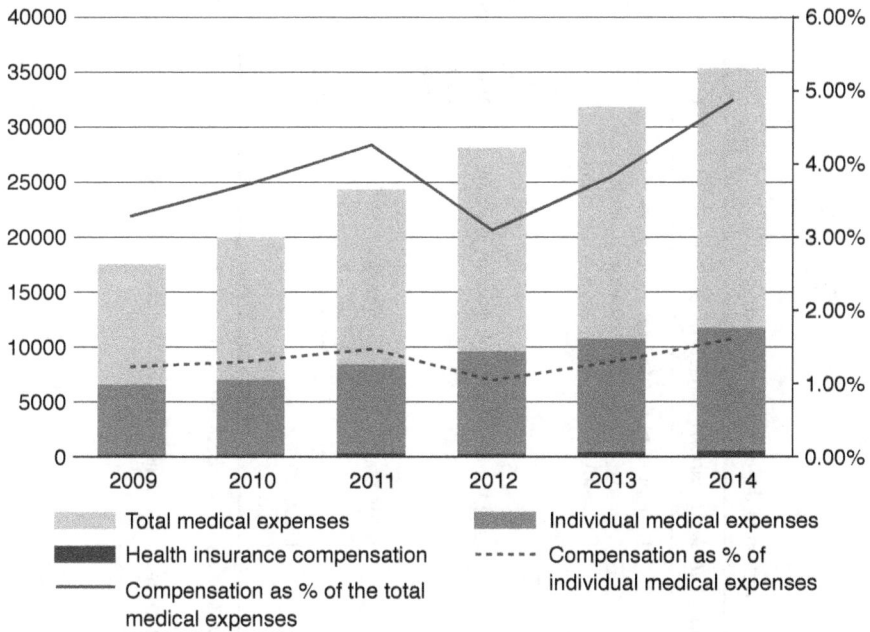

Figure 4.3 Health insurance compensation (RMB 100 million) as % of total medical expenses.

Source: *China Insurance Yearbook 2006–2015.*

Table 4.4 Description of the egg-white model

Classification	Subclassification		Security/insurance	Coverage and scale (in 2015)
Yolk	1	Bottom level	Medical aid from civil administration authorities	Expenditure RMB 21.457 billion, 0.5%
	2	Basic level	Basic medical insurance	New rural cooperative medical system: expenditure RMB 299.35 billion, 7.3% of total Urban resident medical insurance: expenditure RMB 178.06 billion, 4.3% Urban worker medical insurance: expenditure RMB 753.15 billion, 18.4%
	3	Supplement	Supplementary medical insurance	Various supplementary medical insurance, including medical allowance for public servants, subsidy for healthcare incurring heavy expenditure, corporate supplementary insurance, worker mutual medical insurance, commercial supplementary medical insurance, etc.
	4	Addition r	Tax-preference health insurance	Introduced in 2016
Egg-white	5	Uncovered layer	Individual payment	RMB 1.199265 trillion, 29.3%
Shell	6	Outer layer	CHI	RMB 76.3 billion, 1.9%

Source: *China Statistics Yearbook* (2016); *Statistics Bulletin of Health and Family Planning (2015)*.

Note
In 2015, the total medical expenses amounted to RMB 4097.464 billion, and the above percentages indicate how much the expenses account for total healthcare expenditure.

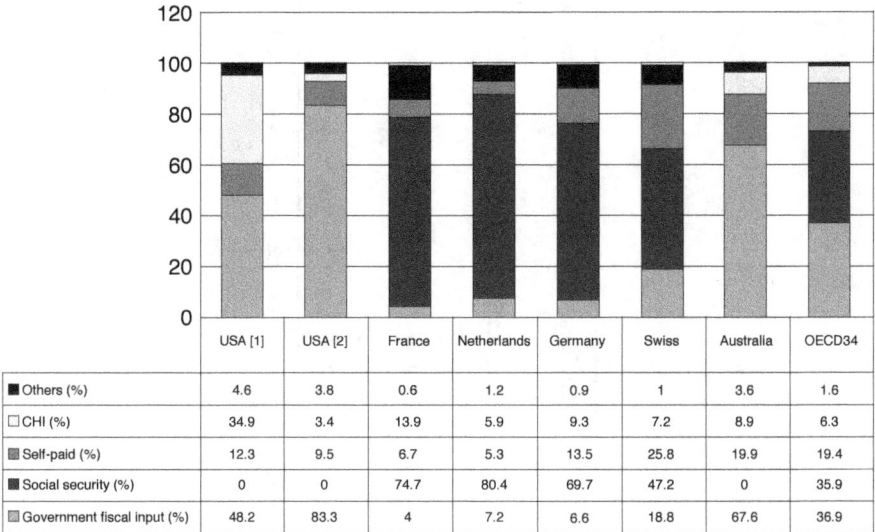

	USA [1]	USA [2]	France	Netherlands	Germany	Swiss	Australia	OECD34
■ Others (%)	4.6	3.8	0.6	1.2	0.9	1	3.6	1.6
□ CHI (%)	34.9	3.4	13.9	5.9	9.3	7.2	8.9	6.3
■ Self-paid (%)	12.3	9.5	6.7	5.3	13.5	25.8	19.9	19.4
■ Social security (%)	0	0	74.7	80.4	69.7	47.2	0	35.9
▨ Government fiscal input (%)	48.2	83.3	4	7.2	6.6	18.8	67.6	36.9

Figure 4.4 Sources of financing of medical care in OECD countries in 2013.

Source: OECD Health Statistics 2015.

Notes
1 In the U.S., social security is financed by the government.
2 Total medical expenses=current medical expenditure+capital formation.
3 In the Netherlands, the mandatorily allocated portion of medical insurance and special medical expenses are covered by social security.

billion to RMB 1,174.53 billion, which represented an average annual growth rate of 12.4% (see Figure 4.5). Costs of diagnosis, treatment, and drugs rose as medical technologies advanced and economic levels rose, which led to rapid inflation of medical costs in general. The aging of the population and spread of chronic diseases further intensified this trend. In China, the medical system is centered primarily on public hospitals—as a result, the social insurance and commercial insurance systems are impotent when it comes to curbing costs. Ultimately, the ballooning of medical costs means that the egg-white zone in which individuals must self-pay for healthcare continues to expand.

4.2.1.2.1.2 RELATIVE AMOUNTS: PERCENTAGE SELF-PAID BY INDIVIDUALS IS ON THE HIGH SIDE

Since the start of the new medical reform in 2009, the percentage of spending by individuals did go down slightly but was still around 33% in 2014. At the same time, however, total spending continued to rise to the extent that it reached RMB 1,174.53 billion in 2014 (see Figure 4.6). In OECD countries, the average percentage paid out by individuals is 17.4%, which is roughly half of the figure in

Table 4.5 Data on medical expenses and health insurance, 2010–2015

Year	Total medical expenses (RMB 100 million)	Out-of-pocket expenses (RMB 100 million)	Percentage of out-of-pocket expenses (%)	CHI premium growth (RMB 100 million)	CHI compensation (RMB 100 million)	CHI compensation rate (%)
2010	19,980.4	7,051.29	35.29	677.47	264.02	38.97
2011	24,345.91	8,465.28	34.77	691.72	359.67	52.00
2012	28,119	9,656.32	34.34	862.76	298.17	34.56
2013	31,868.95	10,729.34	33.67	1,123.5	411.13	36.59
2014	35,378.9	11,745.3	33.2	1,587.18	571.16	35.99
2015	40,587.7	12,164	29.97	2,410.47	762.97	31.65

Source: (2011–2015) *China Healthcare and Family Planning Yearbook*; *China Insurance Yearbook*; data on 2015 medical expenses comes from http://field.10jqka.com.cn/20160722/c591902965.shtml; 2015 insurance data comes from CIRC website.

Table 4.6 Indicator estimate, 2016–2020 (RMB 100 million)

Year	Total medical expenses	Out-of-pocket expenses	CHI compensation (RMB 100 million)
2015	40587.7	12164.00	762.97
2016	46768.39805	13827.05	988.612849
2017	53890.29326	15717.48	1280.98793
2018	62096.71123	17866.37	1659.83083
2019	71552.80314	20309.04	2150.71377
2020	82448.86946	23085.68	2786.77179

Source: Author.

China. Taking out isolated instances, such as Beijing, Shanghai, Qinghai, and Hainan, where the percentage of self-pay is around 25%, in most provinces the percentage is over 30%. In Hebei, Jilin, Heilongjiang, and Hunan, it even exceeds 40% and the burden of medical costs on families is extreme (see Figure 4.7).

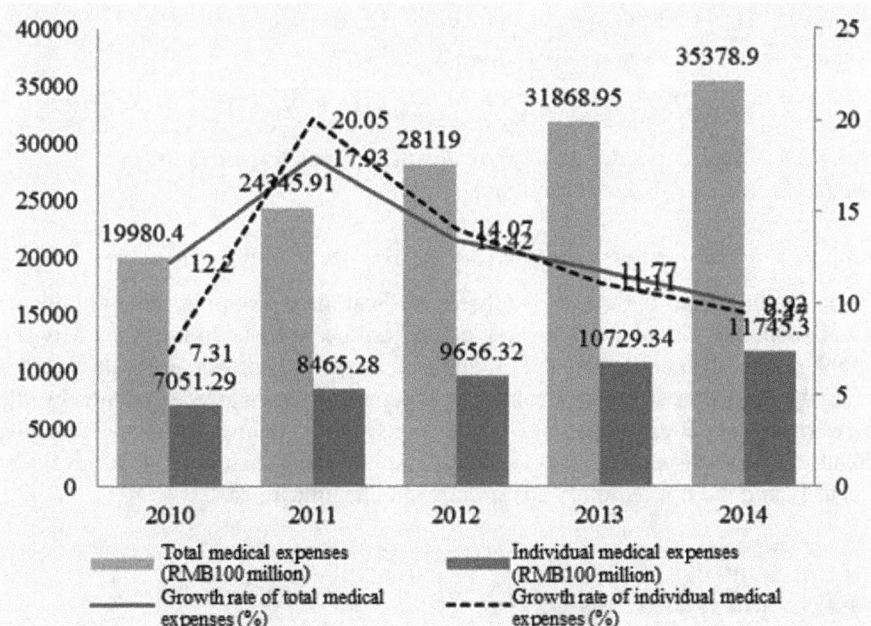

Figure 4.5 Total medical expenses and individual medical expenses, 2010–2014.
Source: *China Healthcare and Family Planning Yearbook 2011–2015.*

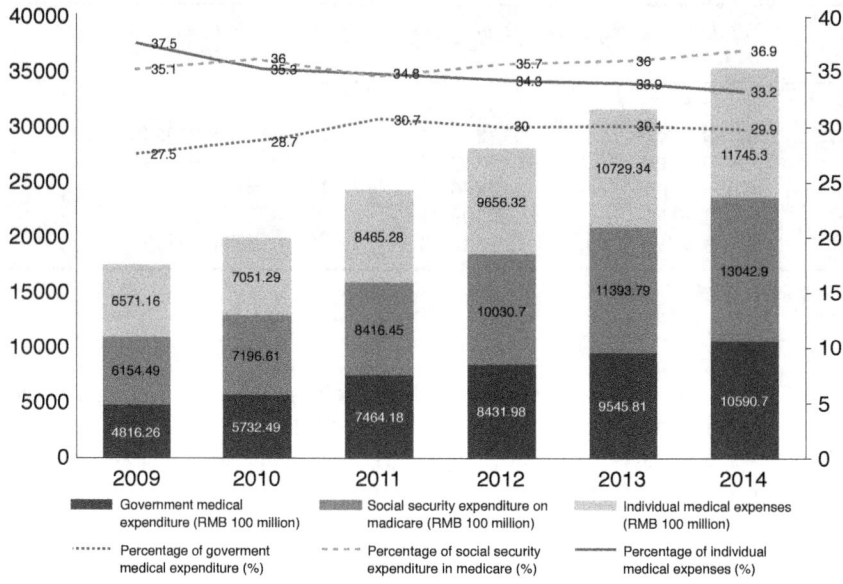

Figure 4.6 Total medical expenses and sources of financing in 2009–2014.

Source: *China Healthcare and Family Planning Yearbook 2014.*

4.2.1.2.2 Coverage: safeguards provided by the (publicly funded) medical insurance program are limited

4.2.1.2.2.1 SOCIAL MEDICAL INSURANCE PROTECTION IS INADEQUATE

The spending from both the urban basic medical insurance program and the new rural cooperative fund are below per capita healthcare costs. In the years between 2009 and 2014, spending by the urban basic medical insurance program stood at roughly 50% of per capita healthcare expenses. Even worse, spending by the new rural cooperative program stayed consistently below 15% of per capita healthcare expenses (see Figure 4.8). Both of these exhibited low levels of security and did not remotely cover per capita healthcare costs.

4.2.1.2.2.2 THE URBAN-RURAL DUALITY SHOWS AN EGREGIOUS DISPARITY IN MEDICAL INSURANCE

The process of integrating medical insurance for China's urban and rural areas continues to be pushed forward. Despite this, the dual structure of the system still persists. A certain gap remains between the provisions of the urban basic medical insurance program and the new rural cooperative insurance program, whether measured in terms of items of coverage or levels of compensation. In

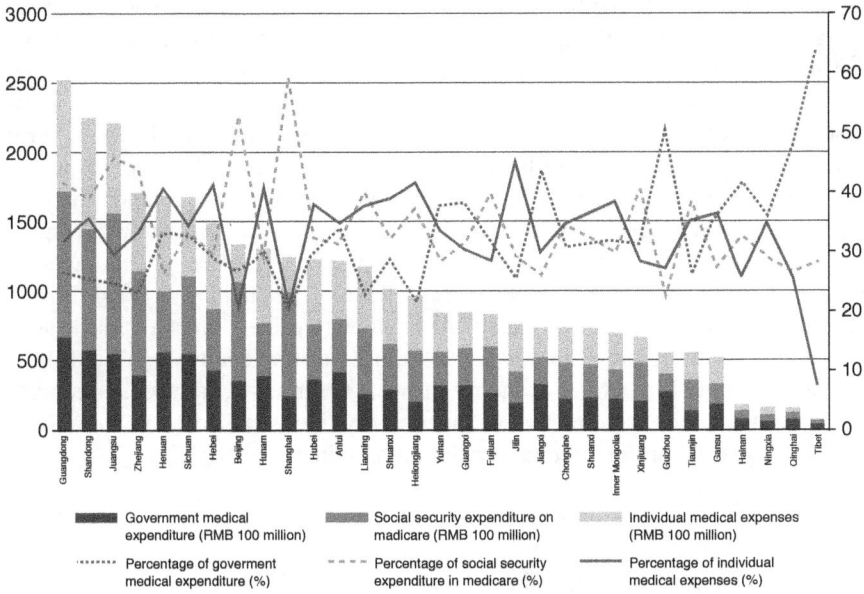

Figure 4.7 Total medical expenses and sources of financing in 2013 (RMB 100 million).

Source: *China Healthcare and Family Planning Yearbook 2015.*

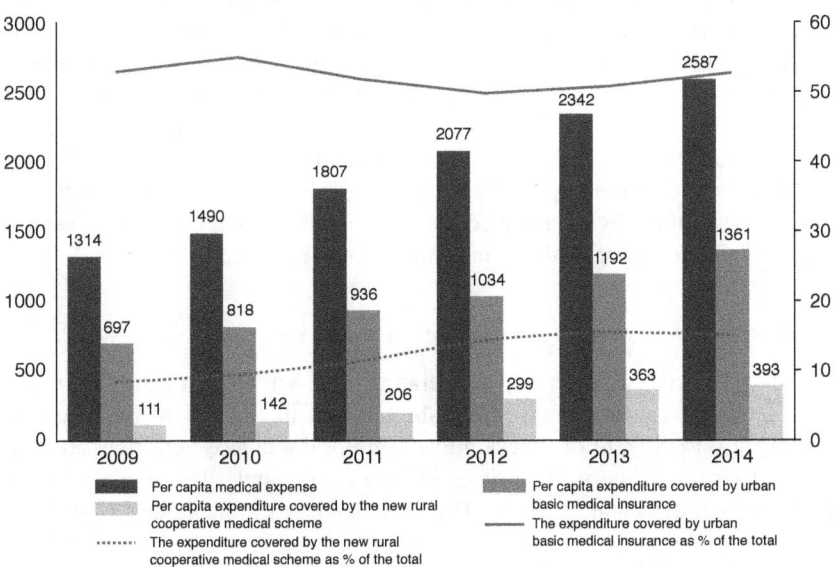

Figure 4.8 Per capita medical expenses and expenditure covered by medical insurance (RMB).

Source: *China Healthcare and Family Planning Yearbook 2010–2015; Statistics Bulletin of Human Resources and Social Security Development 2010–2015.*

2014, the urban basic medical insurance paid out an average of RMB 1,361 per person (in particular, funding levels of the urban employee's basic medical insurance were relatively high), whereas the new rural cooperative insurance paid out a mere RMB 393 on average per person. These two programs paid 52.61% of an urban individual's costs and just 15.19% of the costs of a rural person. In recent years, the level of spending per capita of the new rural cooperative fund has consistently stayed at less than one-third the spending per capita of the urban fund (see Figure 4.8). China needs to improve upon the protections provided by the new rural cooperative program, particularly with respect to acute diseases and treatments requiring hospitalization. The rural population of the country is enormous—still 45.23% of the total population in 2014. Ensuring that this group of people has adequate healthcare protection is a major task if we are to meet the policy directives of 'building a new countryside' and 'promoting social stability as the economy grows.' Meanwhile, large-scale population movements are continuing as the country industrializes and urbanizes. Health safeguards for the migrant population remain a challenge.

4.2.1.2.2.3 INSURANCE FOR CHRONIC DISEASES DOES NOT EXIST

Chronic non-infectious diseases have become a grave threat to people's health as the country urbanizes and ages and as the spectrum of diseases shifts. In 2012, the death rate among people with chronic diseases nationwide was 5.3%. Deaths from chronic disease accounted for 86.6% of total mortality. Cardiovascular disease, cancer, and respiratory-system diseases are the leading cause of death and constitute 79.4% of all deaths. The statistics indicate that the number of older people suffering from chronic disease is rising swiftly and indeed broke through the astonishing figure of 100 million in 2013. The figure is expected to increase to 300 million by 2050. Hospital visits to get treatment currently number 1.35 billion, and that figure will increase to 3.68 billion by 2050. The course of disease is quite long for those suffering from chronic illnesses. China's traditional forms of medical insurance, as represented by social insurance, cannot provide effective forms of health management for these people.

4.2.1.2.2.4 NURSING CARE FOR THE ELDERLY IS HARDLY COVERED

China's population is aging at an accelerating rate, which is posing enormous challenges to medical and healthcare resources and the supply of medical services. Not only is the rate of illness higher among the elderly, but they are less able to care for themselves. There is an enormous demand, therefore, for health management and daily nursing care. The latest statistics indicate that 87.46% of the elderly population handles daily activities completely on their own, 10.54% are disabled to a moderate degree, and 2% are severely disabled. In 2014, according to the report of the *China National Committee on Aging*, 40 million older people in China were disabled to a degree. Within this figure, around 4.44 million were severely disabled, people who need help from family members or long-term care services from society. Nursing care for the elderly is a long-term service and needs whole-process monitoring. At present, however, China's social insurance systems lack any safeguards for such assistance. Meanwhile, nursing care-type products account for only 16.42% of commercial health insurance. There is essentially a great void in safeguards when it comes to care for the elderly in China.

4.2.1.2.2.5 COMMERCIAL HEALTH INSURANCE SAFEGUARDS ARE WEAK

Commercial health insurance suffered from inherent inadequacies from the start, and its market remains tiny. Currently, only five companies are dedicated to health insurance, which indicates that the degree of specialization in the industry is low. It also lacks definite strategies to open up markets and develop products. The health insurance market suffers from double imbalances in terms of both products and distribution. The phenomenon of overly-homogeneous products is severe and products are clearly made to resemble life insurance policies. Meanwhile, the range of items that are insured is quite narrow and the business cannot provide whole-lifespan coverage.

4.2.2 Main problems of China's commercial health insurance business from the perspective of the egg-white model

4.2.2.1 Small market

As noted above, commercial health insurance in China suffered from inherent problems from the start and its market remains tiny. Its ability to provide compensation for healthcare costs remains limited. Although income from premiums is increasing rapidly, the industry is still in early stages.

Between 2005 and 2014, income from commercial health insurance premiums rose from RMB 31.2 billion to RMB 158.718 billion, with an annual average increase that went from 21.4% to 41.27% (see Figure 4.9). Income from commercial health insurance also increased as a percentage of life insurance income—by 2014, it had reached the figure of 12.51%. This was still far lower than the level in advanced countries, however, where the figure is 30%.[19] In 2014, the penetration rate of commercial health insurance was 0.25%, and its density was RMB 116.04. In the United States and Germany, the equivalent figures for density in 2013 were RMB 16,800 and RMB 3,071. In terms of compensation, reimbursements made by commercial health insurance come up to just 1.61% of total healthcare costs. In such advanced countries as Germany and France, the average level is over 10%, while in the United States it reaches 35%. In terms of the scale of premium income and penetration and depth of insurance, we can see from these comparisons that the market for commercial health insurance in China is tiny. It has not even begun to serve its proper functions in providing healthcare safeguards.

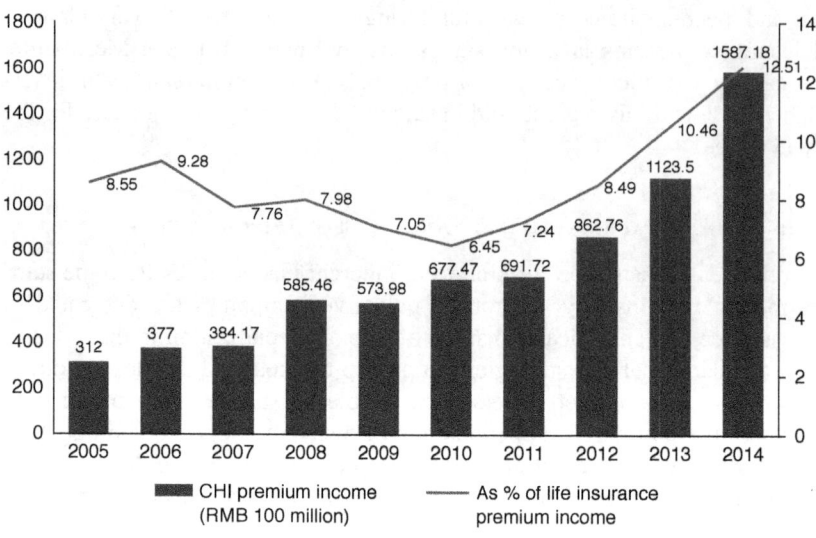

Figure 4.9 CHI premium income and its proportion in life insurance premium income, 2005–2014.

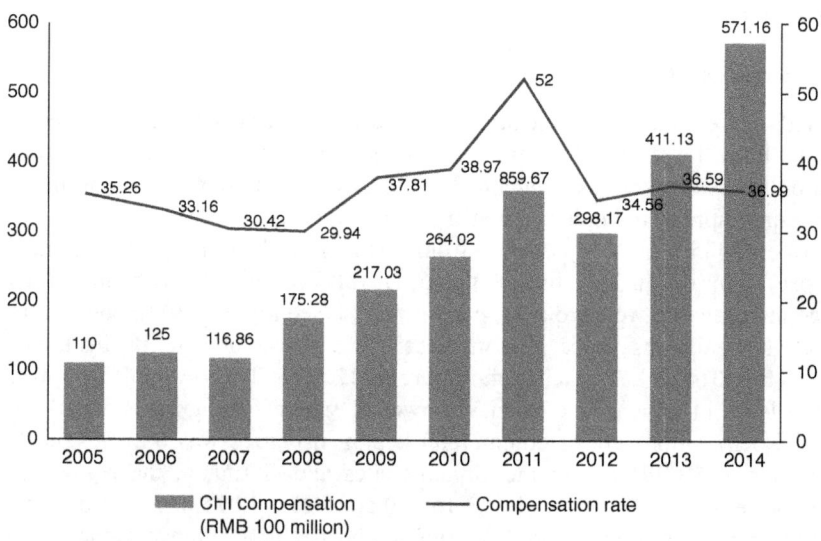

Figure 4.10 CHI compensation and compensation rate.

Source: *China Insurance Yearbook 2006–2015*; *China Statistics Yearbook 2006–2015*.

4.2.2.2 Structural imbalances

The composition of products that are offered by China's commercial health insurance is unbalanced due to limited diversity and lack of innovation. Insurance for critical illness and medical insurance are dominant while the supply of policies for nursing care and disability are severely inadequate. The data shows that premium income from critical illness products in 2015 came to RMB 114.121 billion and represented 47.1% of total premiums. Medical insurance represented 36.11% of the total, while insurance for nursing care was around 17.1%. Policies for loss of income due to disability represented a mere 0.13% (see Figure 4.11). According to publicly available data provided by the China Household Finance Survey of 2013, health insurance products being purchased by respondents also showed a similar composition. That is, critical illness insurance 'sold briskly,' while disability and nursing care insurance 'sold poorly' (see Figure 4.12). Healthcare insurance products are overly uniform. Not only is their homogeneity striking, but there is a severe lack of products that actually provide any real protection.

4.2.2.3 Regional bias

From macro-data, we can see that premium income along China's coastal regions is on the order of RMB 10 billion per province—Beijing, Shanghai, Jiangsu, and Shandong among other provinces reported this level of premium income from commercial health insurance in 2014. This was distinctly higher than premium income in China's central and western regions. The Beijing municipality stands alone as leader in terms of insurance premium density and penetration. The developed provinces within the Yangtze River delta and Pearl River delta areas also rank in the forefront of the health insurance market (see Figure 4.13). The uneven regional development of the health insurance market is influenced by a number of social and economic factors, including level of

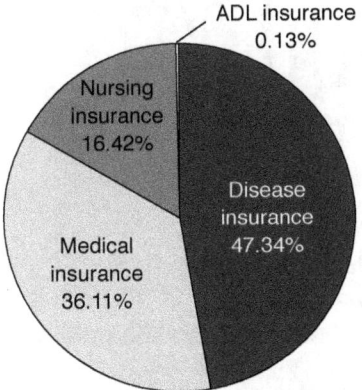

Figure 4.11 CHI products and market shares, 2015.

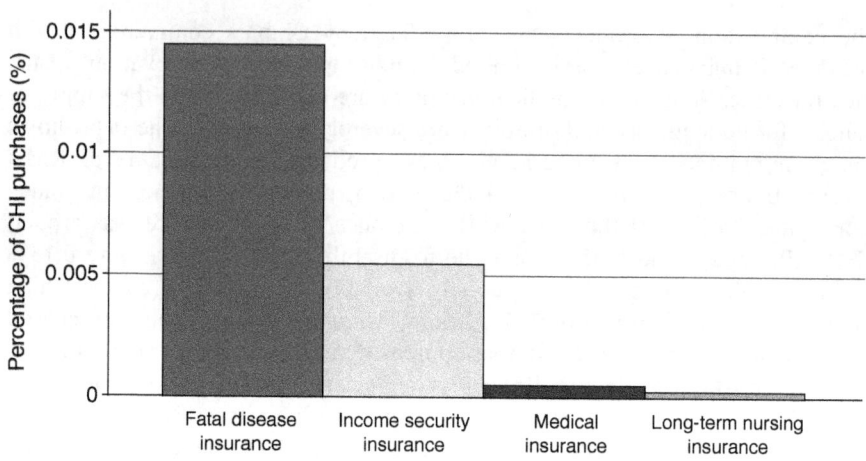

Figure 4.12 CHI purchasers.

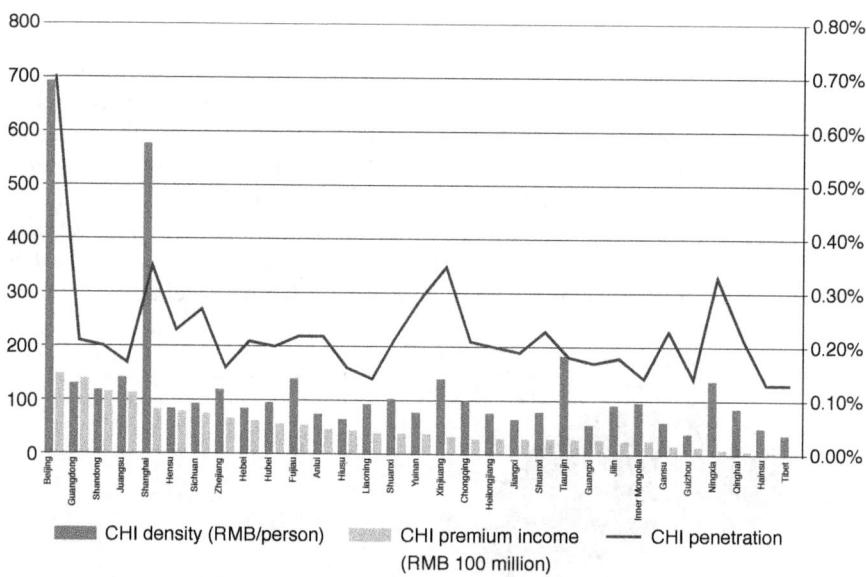

Figure 4.13 CHI markets at the provincial/municipal level in 2014.

Source: *China Statistics Yearbook 2015*; *China Insurance Yearbook 2015*.

economic development, life expectancy of the population, level of education, level of urbanization, and so on. It is also intimately related to the uneven distribution of medical and healthcare resources and social security.

4.2.2.4 *Narrow range of product offerings*

China's commercial health insurance products are dominated by critical illness insurance and medical insurance, which together take up 83.44% of the market (see Figure 4.14). The thinness of the product offerings and the limited scope of safeguards, the lack of products that target different income levels or that segment needs by social status and age mean that there is a disconnect between supply and demand. Insurance for critical illness only includes a limited number of diseases that are pre-specified in contractual form. This form of insurance cannot provide adequate coverage for diseases that are not included in the 'catalogue' of basic medical insurance. Medical insurance is, in contrast, mainly for reimbursing costs of hospital stays and outpatient visits. It only provides for post-event compensation. It does not cover ongoing evaluation and management of the course of a disease over a long period. Products that cover long-term nursing care and the management of chronic diseases are extremely thin in the market. A complete spectrum of products that provides safeguards for various risks has yet to materialize, that is, one that compensates for medical costs on the left side, for management of chronic illness and long-term nursing care in the middle, and for critical or fatal illness on the right side (see Figure 4.14). Along with demographics and diseases that are changing in the direction of chronic illness and aging, the traditional model for insurance, 'reimbursement+compensation,' cannot meet the needs of preventive care, health management, and long-term nursing.

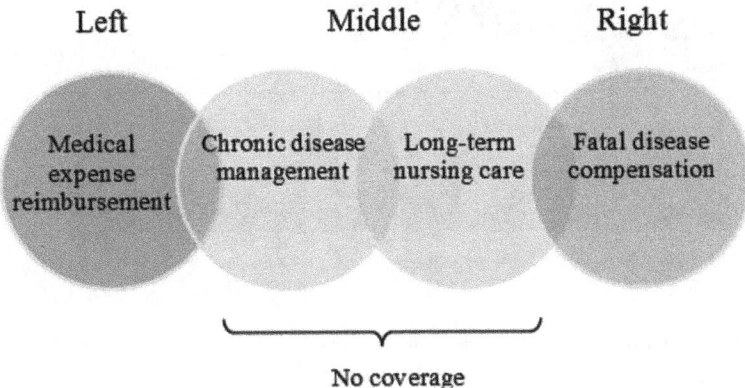

Figure 4.14 Health risk coverage spectrum.

4.2.2.5 *Coverage over the entire lifespan*

A complete system of health insurance products should not just meet the needs of treating illness and managing health, but should also be closely integrated with other life insurance products. The result should be a protective system that covers an individual's entire lifetime. Health insurance is a kind of investment in a person's human capital. In that sense, it is linked with and supplementary to life insurance, casualty insurance, and pension insurance. It can preserve and enrich a person's human capital. Figure 4.15 shows the demand for safeguards that apply to different stages of a person's lifetime, and the supply conditions for those products. A range of insurance products are available, including life insurance against the risk of death, annuity insurance in case of long life, whole life-span insurance against the risk of untimely death, and investment-linked insurance to meet the demand for investment. Among these, life insurance and annuity-type insurance are plentiful and indeed have diversified into a whole product system. Health-insurance products that deal with chronic illness, old-age nursing care, and loss of income due to disability are either overly uniform or lacking altogether. The spectrum as a whole does not meet the needs of an individual for safeguards at each stage of life.

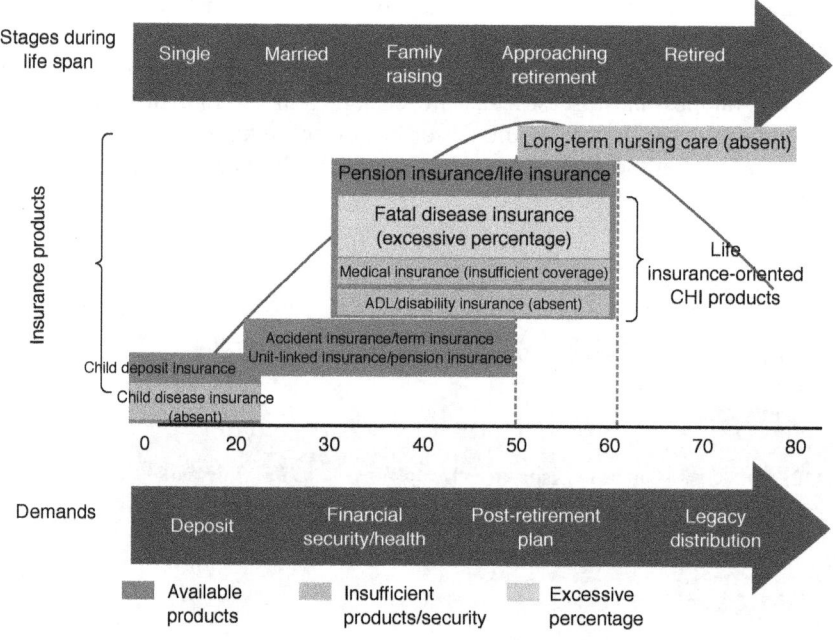

Figure 4.15 CHI in China does not cover whole life span.

4.2.3 Causes of problems in China's commercial health insurance market

4.2.3.1 Two-way adverse selection

Arrow (1963) and Akerlof (1970) point to the problem of information asymmetry leading to adverse selection.[20] Such adverse selection is particularly apparent in the health insurance market. As compared to the companies that sell them, the people who buy insurance policies are more familiar with their own personal risks. Insurance companies can only rely on averages to determine risk pricing. People at low risk tend to pull out, leaving the market to a greater concentration of high-risk policy holders. The research of Rothschild and Stiglitz (1976) makes it clear that pooled equilibrium does not exist in a competitive insurance market. Separate equilibriums may exist but they do not always exist (when the percentage of high-risk groups is small, separate equilibriums also do not exist), while low-risk policy holders do not gain safeguards that are commensurate with what they have paid.[21]

To prevent adverse selection, insurers carry out risk evaluation according to policy holders' age, gender, history of disease, and so on. They then exclude high-risk groups from the market, or they force such groups to accept very high premiums and harsh terms. Meanwhile, there is no specific risk to insure in the case of people suffering from chronic disease, while low-income people lack the ability to pay for premiums. This creates what is known as the 'skimming effect.'

Empirical studies have provided certain evidence for the existence of adverse selection. In their analysis of the Chinese health insurance market, Wang Jun and Gao Feng (2008) discovered the phenomenon of having positive and adverse selection at the same time.[22] According to CHFS household micro-economic data (see Figure 4.16), it was not the case that the healthier a person was, the more likely he was to buy commercial health insurance. Relative to groups with poor health, the healthiest people were actually less likely to buy commercial health insurance—the probability of their buying actually declined. What cannot be denied, however, is that the least healthy people, and the groups least able to pay for insurance, have the least likelihood of buying commercial health insurance.

Commercial health insurance companies that are fully market-oriented are powerless to deal with adverse selection or risk selection problems. When the risk pool is small, there is no way to disperse risk effectively. Low insurance coverage of the low-risk group makes it hard to maintain the risk pool over the long term and impossible to contend with the trends of aging and the spread of chronic diseases. China's commercial health insurance is therefore limited in its ability to compensate for healthcare costs, while the existence of adverse selection makes commercial health insurance fail to perform the role it should play in providing safeguards. With unbalanced product structure and a limited spectrum of products, not only does commercial health insurance not meet the needs of consumers effectively, but these things prevent the market from growing in an orderly fashion.

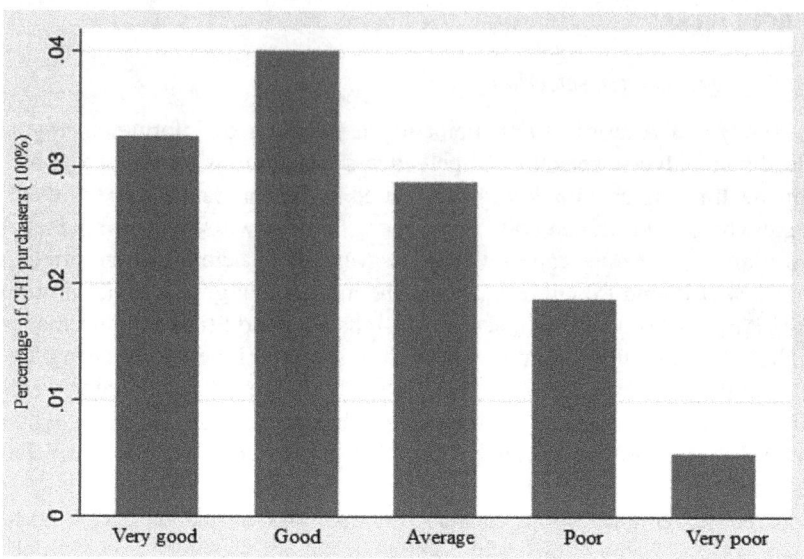

Figure 4.16 Health condition vs. CHI purchase.

Source: *China Household Finance Survey 2013.*

Note
The samples are, as designed in the questionnaire, those aged 21 and above who have reported their health conditions. This figure is based on 12,680 samples.

4.2.3.2 *Twofold moral hazard*

The pre-event moral hazard behavior of insurance buyers increases insurance risks, disturbs actuarial-based pricing, increases the operating cost of insurers, and leads to low market efficiency (Arrow, 1963; Pauly, 1968).[23] Buyers may also commit fraudulent behavior. Once an insured incident has occurred, they may take the easy route of adding costs to their claims that are not within the scope of reimbursable insurance, for drugs or treatments, for example (Wang *et al.*, 2010).[24] Or they may directly cheat the insurance company (Li, 2015).[25] The low efficiencies in the market caused by moral hazard lower the enthusiasm of insurance companies for developing new products and providing them to the public. Ultimately, this leads to an impoverished range of insurance products and an insufficiently developed market.

Meanwhile, the regional distribution of medical resources is uneven in China. Large public hospitals occupy a monopoly position in the medical services system. Insurance companies lack the ability to deal with them on equal terms. They find it hard to have negotiated prices for medical services and drugs, and hard to insert themselves into the process of diagnosis and treatment in order to carry out regulatory oversight of behavior. A number of problems have exacerbated the moral hazard of the hospital side of the equation, including such things as 'using sale of drugs to support the hospital,' and the distortion of price-setting mechanisms for medical services. These things are severe enough to have kept the cost of medicine unreasonably high and this has distorted the allocation of resources. The empirical research of Wang Jun, Gao Feng, and Leng Huiqing *et al.* (2010) makes it clear that moral hazard does indeed exist in the market for health insurance in China. Moreover, the moral hazard associated with regular health insurance is more severe than that associated with insurance for critical illnesses. This research has also proved that moral hazard is an important reason for structural imbalances in the market for insurance products, as well as an important reason for the absence of real safeguards and for the tendency to make health insurance policies resemble life insurance policies.

4.2.3.3 *High transaction costs*

In his book, *The Problem of Social Costs*, Coase defines transaction costs as 'the price you have to pay for obtaining accurate market information, as well as the costs of negotiation and regular covenants.' In the sphere of health insurance, transaction costs may be summarized as (1) contract costs: the time, effort, and money required for several rounds of discussions between the insurance company and the person buying insurance, that is, costs required to sign and execute an insurance contract, and (2) communication costs: the costs that the insurance company incurs surrounding the conclusion of 'a transaction' by communicating with regulatory agencies, intermediaries, and other organizations.[26]

The complex and specialized nature of commercial health insurance ensures that the necessary underwriting and claims settlement processes are indispensable. The high rates of risk, high rates of compensation, large claims settlement workload, and distribution of risk among different types of policies determine the fact that the demands on operating technologies are high and the cost of regulatory management is fairly large.[27] For example, in the early period, an insurance company has to put large sums into underwriting costs so as to do everything possible to minimize the influence of adverse selection. When an insured incident occurs, it has to have a medical institution check the facts and pay only once they are confirmed in order to guard against being cheated. At its current stage, China has few channels through which to sell domestic insurance products, so health insurance products are mainly sold through the channel called Bancassurance, which leads to enormous upfront marketing costs. Moreover, generally speaking, medical institutions and the basic medical insurance system have not yet established ways to interface with insurance companies, or mechanisms by which to share data. Claims therefore still need to be settled in the old-fashioned way, which makes it hard for insurance companies to monitor and control both medical procedures and costs. In addition, insurance companies must record data that comes from paper medical receipts during the claims settlement process, which is expensive and leads to high claims settlement costs.

4.2.3.4 Low level of trust

Trustworthiness is the level of faith that consumers have in suppliers that they will honor their commitments in the course of a transaction.[28] Wang Guojun (2013) believes that insurance is an industry based to a large extent on the trust of the consumer, since the purchase of insurance, the underwriting, the actual insuring, and the settlement of claims are all based on the good faith of both sides.[29] Mutual trust is at the core of insurance. The individual must have personal trust in the insurance company and the extent of that trust affects his ultimate purchasing decision. The people at large must have public trust in the insurance company, and the extent of that affects the growth and development of the entire industry.

Dranove (2015) has noted that the three dimensions of trustworthiness (in the insurance industry) include: faith in impartiality, faith in the competency of a supplier, and faith in the ability of the supplier to control and coordinate resources. The performance of the insurance industry on these three counts affects the way consumers evaluate the industry.[30] First, China's health insurance market has been late to develop and has been subject to turbulence as the country transformed its economic system from one type to another, while the market has also been subject to changes in the structure of society. As a result, the phenomenon of disorderly competition has accompanied the development of the insurance industry.[31] The behavior of insurance companies, who have gone after immediate profits, has caused a decline in both the trust of the individual and the trust of the public. People's desire to purchase insurance has therefore suffered. Second, the number of professional health insurance companies in China is miniscule, levels of expertise and management capability are low, and all products tend to be the same and also lack any real safeguards—this means that they cannot satisfy a consumer's need to get reimbursed for medical expenses. Finally, the commercial health insurance industry as a whole is in a weak position when it comes to dealing with public hospitals. This prevents it from having sufficient ability to provide healthcare protection, it prevents it from being able to control costs, and it limits the way it should be able to supplement and substitute for social insurance. All three of these considerations have led to a fairly low degree of trust on the part of consumers towards the insurance industry. Meanwhile, the dominant position of social insurance has in the health insurance system also has made the public accustomed to going through public medical insurance to resolve problems. This means that commercial health insurance is left with inadequate effective demand.

4.2.3.5 Major institutional obstacles

China's commercial health insurance industry is held back by having to operate within an imperfect market-economy environment. However, it is also blocked by the institutional structures of medicine and healthcare in the country as well as the institutional structures that handle the social safeguards system.

Public hospitals have a monopoly advantage within the system of medical services. Insurance companies are at a disadvantage in the course of doing transactions with this system since they lack the ability to insist on negotiated prices for medical services. Astronomical prices for drugs are the fundamental cause of the problem of expensive access to medical care. Meanwhile, China's control measures in this regard are ineffective, funding by the state is inadequate, and prices for medical services are undervalued as hospitals hike up drug prices to cover their costs. All of this has created a situation in which China's spending on medical costs rises by the year while insurance companies see the cost of their claims settlement soar.[32] The uneven allocation of medical resources is another problem behind the phrase about how hard it is to see a doctor. As public institutions, public hospitals operate within the '*bianzhi*' system in terms of personnel (that is, the staffing quota that applies to public institutions and that is registered as a quota in the government budget). Meanwhile, the reimbursement system requires that all claims for medical insurance be submitted through 'designated' hospitals. These considerations, plus the lack of different grades of medical assistance, mean that the great majority of high-quality doctors concentrate in Grade Two and Grade Three hospitals. Since public hospitals monopolize the best doctors, they also monopolize patients, and commercial health insurance companies have no alternative but to acquiesce in accepting their soaring medical costs.[33]

The social safeguards system also contends with the problem of unfair allocation of social insurance resources. Levels of reimbursement are different, not only among different provinces and between cities and countryside but also among different medical insurance systems. Zhou Qin *et al.* (2016) carried out an empirical analysis of the fairness of benefits to participants in the urban basic medical insurance program. They found that high-income participants benefited more than low-income participants.[34] Xu Ling and Jian Weiyan (2010) did a comparison among China's three large medical insurance systems and discovered that the degree of inequitable treatment in the new rural cooperative medical system was highest.[35] It can be seen from this that at the present time China's levels of compensation within the basic medical insurance system are regressive. The target groups for commercial health insurance, therefore, are problematic—middle- and high-income levels of people lack the interest in products while low-income levels are unable to access sufficient medical safeguards. Problems that are structural or institutional in nature block any intent of insurance companies to be impartial and fair. They lead to waste of resources and they hold back demand from people who really need commercial health insurance. This blocks the proper growth of the commercial health insurance industry.

4.3 EVALUATION OF THE POSITION, FUNCTIONS, AND OVERALL SCALE OF COMMERCIAL HEALTH INSURANCE WITHIN CHINA'S SYSTEMS OF MEDICAL INSURANCE

4.3.1 Relationship between commercial health insurance and the basic medical insurance system: theory, boundaries, and mechanisms

4.3.1.1 Theory

Assuming that high-risk and low-risk consumers exist in the market, and social medical insurance and commercial health insurance provide consumers with medical security, I_S is the security level of social medical insurance and I_P that of commercial health insurance. Assuming that commercial health insurance satisfies the demand of full-amount insurance, I_P is the degree of loss.

Sole reliance on social medical insurance makes it hard to meet the demand for high security. In Figure 4.17, OS is the supply line of social health insurance. Due to its mandatory nature, this kind of insurance does not differentiate between people with high or low risk. It collects fixed-amount premiums that are the same for all and it provides compensation for medical costs that are also the same for all, with a level of safeguards that are at a fairly low level—I_S. Since I_S<medical expenses I_P, it cannot satisfy the demand for full coverage among consumers. Social insurance as a system 'insures the basics,' and is unable to provide for higher-level safeguards.

Sole reliance on commercial health insurance makes it hard to remedy the loss of efficiency due to adverse selection and moral hazard. OP_1^H and OP_1^L

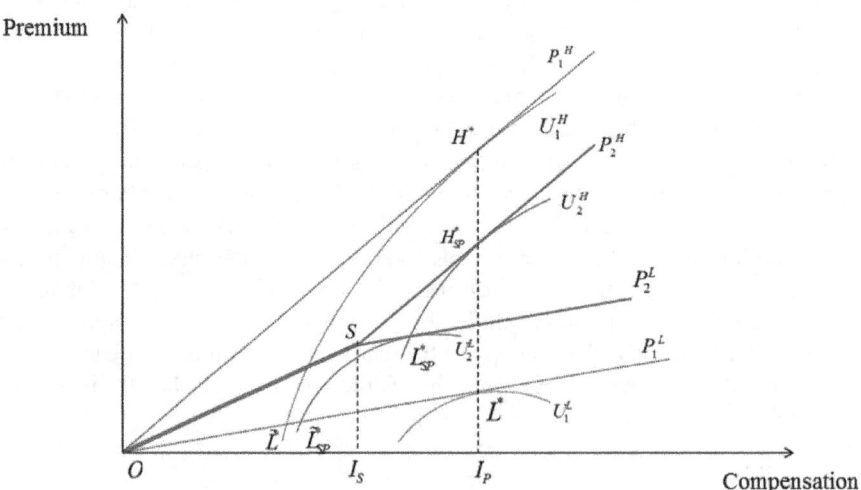

Figure 4.17 Market equilibrium of supplementary CHI.

Source: By the author.

represent the insurance supply lines for high-risk and low-risk consumers in a market that is operated purely by commercial health insurance. Assuming there is no adverse selection or moral hazard, commercial health insurance provides products at the optimal levels H^* and L^*, but the high-risk consumers have to pay higher premiums. As compared with social security s, low-risk consumers enjoy higher security at lower premiums, and the utility is better (the indifference curve U_1^L in Figure 4.17); since high-risk consumers are subject to higher premium rates, their levels of utility fall (the indifference curve U_1^H in Figure 4.17).

When adverse selection and moral hazard do exist, the '$S - H^* - L^*$' equilibrium cannot be maintained. High-risk consumers are motivated to buy products of higher utility, and eventually the commercial insurance companies have to provide low-risk consumers with product $L\%$ (the intersection of the indifference curve U_1^H of the high-risk consumers and the supply line OP_1^L for the low-risk ones), resulting in utility loss for the low-risk consumers. When there are a number of commercial insurance companies, some seek to provide the low-risk consumers with better products—other insurance companies then face the problem of losses brought on by an increasing concentration of high-risk customers. The existence of a 'lemon market' and a 'death spiral' then further worsens competition in the commercial health insurance market, and may force commercial health insurance to withdraw from the insurance market altogether.

Supplementary commercial insurance will elevate security levels and improve utility for consumers. Social security provides basic security I_S. On top of that foundation, commercial health insurance provides customized products for different target groups. In Figure 4.17, OSP_2^H and OSP_2^L are the 'social security + commercial health insurance' supply lines for high-risk and low-risk consumers respectively. Despite adverse selection and moral hazard, the security levels of products L_{SP}^* and H_{SP}^*, when reaching the ultimate equilibrium, are higher than that of I_S of social security and are no lower than those of pure CHI $L\%$ and H. According to the indifference curves, the utility levels for the low- and high-risk consumers, at L_{SP}^* and H_{SP}^*, are higher than that of exclusive social security s. As the premium drops, the utility for the high-risk consumers is higher at H_{SP}^* than at H. When the low-risk consumers find high risk intolerable, product L_{SP}^* brings greater utility than that at $L\%$ (L_{SP}^* is on the right of $L\%$). Social security covers a large population, and the policy design of a supplementary commercial insurance system can effectively use the resulting information advantages of social security to minimize the negative impact of adverse selection and moral hazard. Because of this, the market for commercial health insurance may be sustainable.

Types of commercial health insurance that are cooperative and undertake certain tasks for social insurance can reduce the cost of safeguards and improve utility. Commercial health insurance has actuarial and management advantages, and by exploiting these it can lower the operating costs of social insurance. Surplus balances of (social) medical insurance funds can ultimately be used to subsidize premiums, which improves the quality of medical services and lessens the financial burden on consumers. In Figure 4.18, when OS^{**} rotates to the

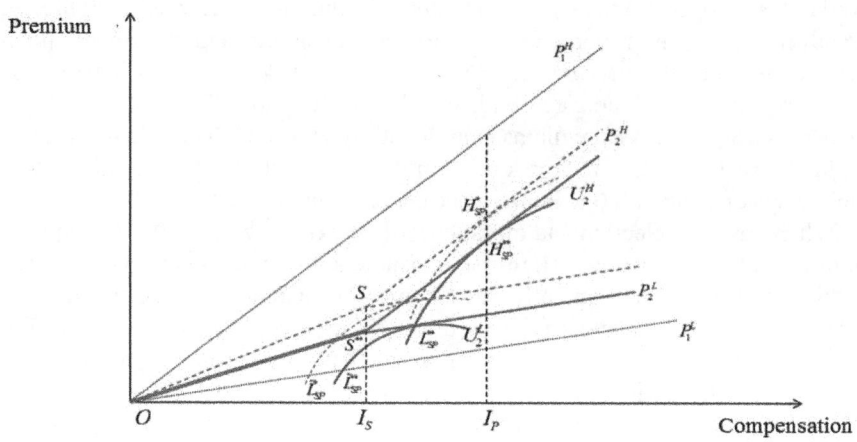

Figure 4.18 Market equilibrium of undertaking and cooperative CHI.
Source: By the author.

lower right of *OS*, consumers can gain comparable levels of social security by paying a lower premium. At the same time, commercial health insurance may provide the same scope of safeguards while collecting a lower premium. In Figure 4.18, the premiums corresponding to the new equilibrium points L_{SP}^{**} and H_{SP}^{**} are lower than those corresponding to the original equilibrium points L_{SP}^{*} and H_{SP}^{*}. The utility is higher at the new equilibrium points. Generally speaking, commercial health insurance that is of a cooperative and participatory kind may not necessarily improve safeguards but can improve consumer utility.

A substitutive type of commercial health insurance may lead to inefficiency of the entire medical safeguards market. This type forms a competitive relationship with social insurance. When the market is out of order and ceases to function properly, each type of insurance operates in its own interests and the competition of the two leads to inefficiency of the entire medical safeguards market. In Figure 4.17, under equivalent levels of security, substitutive commercial health insurance collects the lowest premiums from low-risk consumers and the second lowest premium is charged by social insurance. The highest premiums are paid by high-risk groups to commercial health insurance. The principle of 'voting with your feet' would apply, in that all consumers would concentrate on purchasing commercial health insurance targeted at low-risk groups. The supply of OP_1^H and OS, and eventually OP_1^L would be hard to maintain because of excessive losses.

The way in which China's medical insurance system developed has determined the fact that social medical insurance forms the cornerstone of 'broad coverage,' while commercial health insurance, with its ability to meet personalized and multi-tiered demand, cannot play this role. It cannot substitute for social medical insurance in providing basic types of safeguards.

4.3.1.2 Boundaries between commercial health insurance and basic medical insurance

4.3.1.2.1 Defining the overall boundary

Commercial health insurance in China supplements rather than substitutes for basic medical insurance. The health market is characterized by information asymmetry. Because of this, commercial health insurance cannot exist in isolation from basic medical insurance—any 'substitution' of one for the other would worsen market competition and lower market efficiency. Instead, having commercial health insurance supplement basic medical insurance is an effective way to spur innovation, raise efficiency, and improve market structure.

4.3.1.2.2 Boundaries with respect to the spectrum of products

Basic medical insurance provides basic medical safeguards and its emphasis is on broad coverage of the population. Commercial health insurance should, instead, aim to fill in the gaps in the spectrum of products available. It should bridge various periods of a person's life and put its emphasis on being multi-tiered and diversified. In terms of filling in gaps, commercial health insurance should extend its focus to such things as major illness, chronic diseases, nursing care for the elderly, and so on.

4.3.1.2.3 Boundaries with respect to the health industrial chain

Basic medical insurance enjoys advantages in the medical industry. In contrast, commercial health insurance can build on its existing base of business to merge health insurance with the overall industrial chain of the insurance industry. It can extend its business lines to preventive medicine and post-illness recovery and can provide comprehensive health management as well as services for the elderly. These things can thereby form a complete deployment of products for the health industry as a whole.

4.3.1.2.4 Boundaries at the institutional level

The institutional structures of markets for commercial health insurance and basic medical insurance are different and correspond to a 'market institutional structure' and an 'administrative institutional structure.' If each functions on its own, this causes both market failure and government failure. This means that both structures must have 'a division of labor as well as a combination of forces.' Both must work together in a reinforcing kind of synergy. For example, commercial health insurance may be able to make use of the mandatory nature of social insurance to moderate the problems of adverse selection and moral hazard, while basic social insurance may rely on the market mechanisms of commercial health insurance to realize improved efficiency.

4.3.1.3 Ways in which commercial health insurance and basic medical insurance can cooperate

In the process of building a medical insurance system in China, commercial insurance can strengthen the stability of the basic medical insurance system, improve efficiencies, and deepen safeguards by cooperating, sharing, and being symbiotic with basic medical insurance. Depending on its relationship with basic medical insurance, commercial health insurance can cooperate in three different ways that could be described as 'undertaking certain tasks (or 'handling'-type cooperation),' 'cooperating,' and 'supplementing.' The last could be further divided into two main types, namely 'mutually supplementary' and 'adding supplements.'

4.3.1.3.1 Undertaking certain tasks (entrusted model)[36]

This form of cooperation expresses the key principle that 'the regulator should be separate from those being regulated,' that is, government (administration) should be separate from actual business. In this form of cooperation, commercial insurance companies are authorized or 'entrusted' by social insurance government departments to undertake certain tasks of social insurance, namely payment and supervision. 'Payment' refers to paying the costs of medical services and paying compensation to those who are insured. 'Supervision' refers to investigating whether or not patients are pretending to be someone other than themselves or are committing fraud, whether or not improper or excessive medical treatment is being performed, and so on. The aim is to control unreasonable ballooning of medical spending. At present, the models to follow can be found in Jiangyin, Zhanjiang, and Luoyang.

4.3.1.3.2 Cooperating

This form of cooperation can also be called the 'risk model.' It refers to sharing premium income and co-assuming risk. It operates at the level of basic medical insurance and involves commercial health insurance working together with government departments that handle social security. In concrete terms, social security authorities purchase risk coverage from commercial insurance companies, using a portion of the basic medical insurance premiums they have collected. In return, commercial insurance companies assume the responsibility of paying reimbursement compensation for basic medical insurance at the same percentage. In addition, the government may use financial incentives—when the fund has a surplus or deficit, government may either reward or punish commercial insurance companies with bonuses or fines. At present, the most representative model of this practice is in the Pinggu district of Beijing.

4.3.1.3.3 Supplementing

This form of cooperation includes two types, complementary and supplementary. The mutual reinforcement type, or complementary, refers to having government departments of social security purchase insurance from commercial insurance companies. This incorporates basic medical insurance into the scope of safeguards, but is also appropriate for insuring health risks that generally fall under the commercial health insurance model, such as major illness. At present, the Taicang Model and Zhanjiang Model are representative cases. The supplementary or 'additional' type of cooperation refers to having commercial insurance companies cover health risks that are beyond the coverage of basic medical insurance, in order to expand safeguards for people and extend the degree to which risks are covered. In this case, commercial insurance companies independently provide coverage for more health risks, plus they provide higher financial compensation and higher quality services to people who are insured.

4.3.2 The positioning and role of commercial health insurance in China's overall system of health safeguards

4.3.2.1 Commercial health insurance is a beneficial supplement to the medical safeguards system

As described by the egg-white model of China's healthcare funding system, commercial health insurance mainly supplements China's medical insurance system with respect to medical expenses and medical services.

4.3.2.1.1 Medical expenses

Commercial health insurance is one of the financing sources of healthcare expenses. In the future it will play an important role in compensating medical expenses. Commercial health insurance reimburses the individual expenses and the outpatient and hospitalization expenses that are below the reimbursable line of social medical insurance and above the reimbursement ceiling of social medical insurance. In this way, commercial health insurance lowers the percentage that individuals and households pay on their own, it improves the structure of funding for healthcare, and it raises the degree of safeguards within the medical safeguards system.

4.3.2.1.2 Medical services

Commercial health insurance is a beneficial supplement to the medical safeguards system. It can help make up for the 'empty zone' in safeguards for medical services. It provides coverage for drugs and treatments that are not on the approved list. It provides coverage for management of chronic diseases and for health maintenance practices, it offers insurance for nursing care for the elderly, and loss of income due to disability. It expands the scope of safeguards under the basic medical insurance program, and in general provides for more comprehensive medical security.

4.3.2.2 Commercial health insurance improves the efficiency of the medical safeguards system

Commercial insurance companies can upgrade the results of China's medical insurance system and the quality of its medical services by taking advantage of their own technical expertise and organization platforms.

4.3.2.2.1 Cost efficiencies

Introducing commercial health insurance into China's overall medical safeguards system is an example of introducing market mechanisms into the system. This is the key to controlling medical costs and optimizing the allocation of resources. The insertion of commercial insurance into the system improves the efficiency with which insurance funds are used. It also improves operating efficiencies and the allocation of industry resources.

4.3.2.2.2 Business efficiencies

Commercial health insurance lends strength to the medical safeguards system. If the two have a system of sharing data and information that is fully interconnected, this should also improve the business results of commercial insurance companies. It should improve the efficiencies of taking on insurance and getting underwriting, as well as the efficiency of settling claims and managing risk.

4.3.2.3 Commercial health insurance provides vital forces as China builds up its medical safeguards system

Since the start of the new medical reform in 2009, China has consistently emphasized the role of commercial health insurance in China's overall system of medical safeguards. In 2012, the relevant ministries and commissions released a series of policies in support of having the insurance industry launch businesses related to the new rural cooperative medical system and critical illness. In 2014, the *Various Opinions of the State Council on accelerating the development of a modern insurance industry* recommended using commercial insurance as a 'key pillar' of the social security system. Also in 2014, the *Various Opinions of the General Office of the State Council on accelerating the development of commercial health insurance* pointed out the role that commercial insurance should play: 'Commercial health insurance is a vital force for deepening reform of the institutional structures that govern the medical, pharmaceutical, and healthcare systems. It is a vital force for developing health services, and raising economic performance and efficiency.' Commercial health insurance represents an important approach to integrating resources that relate to medical services and to building an extensive health industry chain. In another regard, it is also a vital force for deepening reform of the institutional structures that govern medical and healthcare systems in the country and for pushing forward the building of China's medical safeguards system.[37]

4.3.3 Ways to develop the 'new public-benefiting insurance'

4.3.3.1 Theoretical basis: theory of benefits

4.3.3.1.1 The concept of goods described as 'benefits,' and their characteristics

The theory of benefits was first put forward by Musgrave (1957), who defined it as follows in his book *Theory of public finance* (1959): 'a commodity that society feels belongs to the class of things that are beneficial to consumers, even though consumers do not recognize the need for them and are therefore unwilling to buy them, or buy them in insufficient amounts.'[38] Since people's preferences can be unreasonable, government must intervene by countering those individual preferences. The unreasonableness of people's preferences can be caused by externalities[39] and by information asymmetry.[40] 'Benefits' are both 'public' and 'private' in nature, and have the following characteristics. (1) Benefits are financed jointly by government, enterprises, and families, and therefore have a certain 'public' nature to them.[41] (2) They are both competitive and exclusive in nature. (3) They can be turned down by consumers who do not want them. Consumers have a certain freedom of choice in terms of quantity and features of the benefits. (4) Benefits have a positive externality, that is, if people rely solely on their private supply, the consumption of benefits will be lower than what is optimum for society as a whole.

4.3.3.1.2 Methods of providing benefits: the synergy of joining the efforts of five different parties

The unique nature of benefits mandates that five parties must join forces in supplying them, namely the government, the market, society at large, companies, and households. Only then will a balance of supply and demand be achieved and will society at large reach its optimum level.

Looking at the supply side, benefits must be a cooperative effort on the part of all players. Sole reliance on the government, the market, or society will lead to failure. First, supply of benefits that is completely delivered by government may lead to low efficiency, waste of resources, and inability to satisfy consumer's needs and therefore may lead to government failure to perform properly. This can stem from the possibility of inaccurate government policies, low efficiency of bureaucratic entities, rent-seeking behavior by bureaucracies, and the innate tendency of bureaucracies to expand. Second, supply that is completely delivered by the market and by price-based distribution may exclude individuals who cannot afford benefits. It may lead to consumption that is below the optimal level for society. This may be due to externalities and insufficient information. Third, supply that is completely delivered by social forces faces multiple defects. Such organizations rely on donations from the public, government assistance, and the voluntary help of public-minded people. The available resources are insufficient but also lack professionalism. Over the long run, they exhibit tendencies to become like corporations, or bureaucracies, or interest groups. This leads to a 'failure of society' due to low efficiencies and ineffective supply (see Figure 4.19).[42]

From a demand perspective, the primary consumers of benefits are households and enterprises. Their resources and capabilities are not enough to be self-sufficient, so they must purchase benefit-type products from outside. Due to incomplete information, the existence of externalities, and the irrational nature of personal preferences, households and enterprises may engage in short-sighted decisions when it comes to consumption of insurance. This may lead to a lower level of benefits being purchased than what is optimum for society at large.

To reach the optimum level, the government should stimulate the consumption of benefits by intervening in personal preferences and by guiding demand. It can do this through such things as subsidies and preferential tax policies that increase an individual's ability to pay. At the same time, intervening in personal preferences is not the same as denying personal preferences. Government should respect the rational consumption demands of individuals and should use market mechanisms and social forces to supplement government measures when those are inadequate. On the basis of providing a basic level of safeguards, government should make every effort to satisfy the diversified needs of individuals.

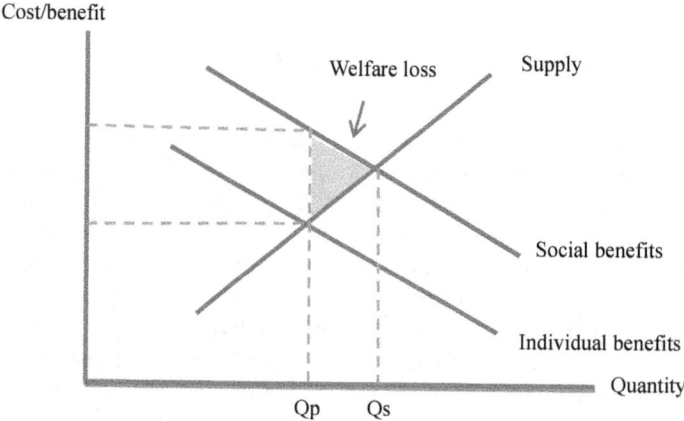

Figure 4.19 Welfare loss caused by inadequate consumption of merit goods in private provision.

4.3.3.2 The concept and key considerations behind the new public-benefiting insurance

The new public-benefiting insurance has two key features: it benefits the public and it is 'new.' If you were to describe China's medical insurance system as a flat pancake, this new public-benefiting insurance would be a process that adds substance or depth to the existing pancake. The 'new' part of the new-benefiting system refers to the way it unifies three aspects: public benefits, special benefits, and long-term benefits. It breaks through the basic medical insurance coverage and reimbursement limits, it provides value-added services, and it provides sustainable security that covers the entire life span. In plain language, it gives more benefits to the public and gives people a sense that they are really getting something. On top of the foundation of broadly based coverage of a given range of safeguards, it allows for the possibility of satisfying multi-tiered demand while ensuring sustainable operation of the system.

The new public-benefiting insurance falls within the scope of being a beneficial good. Building this system necessarily relies on the combined efforts of government, the market, society, households, and enterprises, in order to realize the goals of broadly based coverage, strong safeguards, and sound and secure sustainability (see Figure 4.20). The core factors include front-end, middle, and rear-end considerations.

4.3.3.2.1 Front end

4.3.3.2.1.1 FINANCING

The new public-benefiting insurance consists of three layers: mandatory supplementary health insurance, expanded-type health insurance, and add-on health

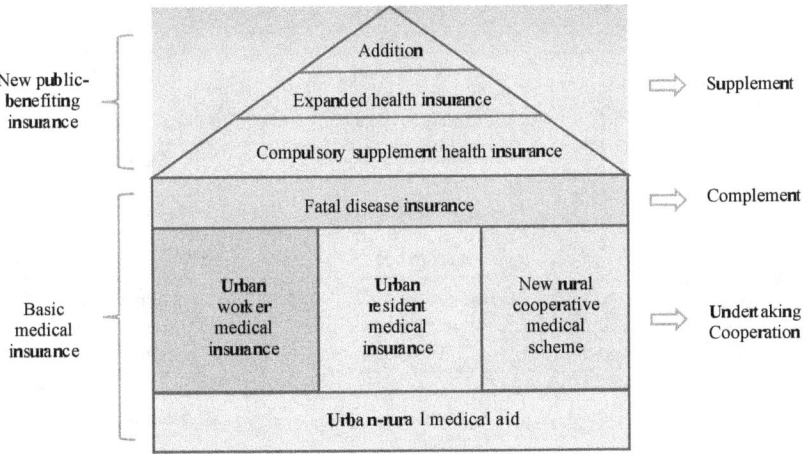

Figure 4.20 Structure of China's new public-benefits medical insurance.

Source: By the author.

insurance. Among these, the first is the most typically described as 'benefits.' Its financing method adopts the formula 'sharing by members of the public + limited amounts of subsidy.' Government subsidies improve the ability of the lowest income-earners to pay, in order to stimulate the consumption of mandatory supplementary health insurance. The second and third layers are more commercial. Through appropriate degrees of tax incentives, the government urges consumers to buy insurance and thereby satisfies the demand of high-end customers.

4.3.3.2.1.2 PRICING

The new public-benefiting insurance adopts a pricing model that uses the formula 'public pricing + risk pricing.' Of the three layers, the mandatory supplementary insurance requires participation in insurance and pricing that is set by the public. All those who are eligible, who meet the conditions for being insured, must participate, and insurance companies set the insurance rates according to similar insurance. No consideration is given to the health conditions of the person buying insurance. The second and third types of insurance, expanded health insurance and add-on insurance, are not obligatory. Consumers can participate on a voluntary basis. Insurance companies set pricing according to risk, which is determined by the health conditions of the insured.

4.3.3.2.1.3 PLATFORM

The administrative unit by which this new insurance is administered is the province (Figure 4.21). The 'platform' through which to purchase insurance is a Health Insurance Exchange that is set up in each province. With respect to the

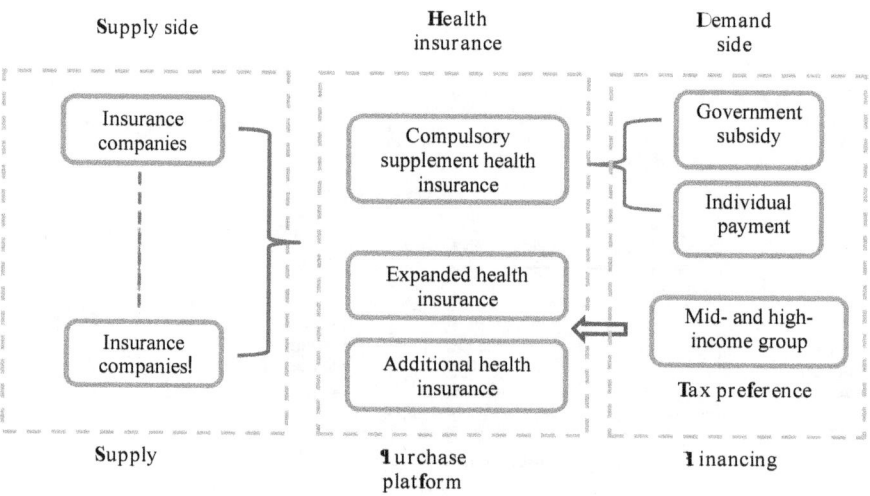

Figure 4.21 Supply and financing of new public-benefiting insurance.
Source: By the author.

mandatory supplementary health insurance, insurance companies must provide a 'basic safeguards package' that is standardized according to the requirements of each Exchange. With respect to the second and third types of insurance, companies may provide services that meet the standard but have differentiated safeguards. The Exchanges carry out reviews and evaluations of products that are put on the market within each Exchange to make sure they meet qualifications. They ensure that policy terms are standardized and easily understood. They strengthen the information disclosure provisions of products and they provide consulting services to the public. Given sufficient information, consumers can make their own decisions about insurance companies and insurance products.

4.3.3.2.2 Middle

4.3.3.2.2.1 POLICY COVERAGE

The new public-benefiting insurance seeks to address two main defects of the egg-white model, namely high out-of-pocket expenses and insufficient coverage. It reimburses expenses paid out by individuals that are below the starting amount at which social insurance reimburses as well as amounts above the ceiling. It thereby reduces the financial burden on individuals and their medical spending in the event of emergencies. It covers items not included in the catalogue that applies to basic medical insurance, including chronic disease, long-term nursing care, health management, and high-end medical needs.

4.3.3.2.2.2 EXPENSE CONTROL

The new public-benefiting insurance creates ways by which hospitals and insurance can have mutually shared interests (Figure 4.22). This serves to break down

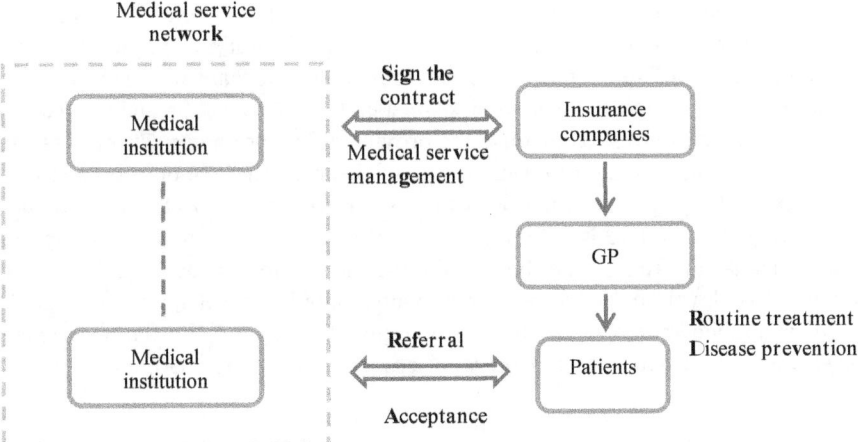

Figure 4.22 Managerial medical service model.

Source: By the author.

the barriers between the two industries and creates a new form of 'insurance-managed medicine.' This is based on the sharing of medical data and medical cost data. The insurance company becomes a third-party payer, representing the patient in negotiating prices with medical and pharmaceutical suppliers. It actively enters into the process of overseeing, monitoring, and controlling the quality of medical services. It curbs unreasonable use of drugs and poor treatment practices. By adopting diversified payment methods, it lowers medical costs. It uses general practitioners as 'gatekeepers' who guide patients toward correct treatments and toward reasonable allocation of medical resources.

4.3.3.2.2.3 RISK MANAGEMENT

The complexities and specific nature of health insurance require a high degree of risk awareness among people in health insurance companies. Once the new public-benefiting insurance is set up, it will attract large numbers of high-risk customers and the ability of insurance companies to control that risk will become of paramount importance. Insurance companies must be able to mine health data and use that data to set up advance-warning systems and create programs to counter risk. They must establish scientifically sound underwriting and claims settlement systems, and should focus on prevention of adverse selection and moral hazard. They should strengthen management of capital adequacy ratios, and improve internal control systems and systems for risk appraisal and management.[43]

4.3.3.2.3 Rear end

4.3.3.2.3.1 RISK ALLOCATION

Setting up a new public-benefiting insurance system that is sound and sustainable, has strong safeguards and all-round coverage, is going to require a corresponding system of reinsurance and risk balancing mechanisms. This will be required to balance and to disperse risk. In specific terms, risk balancing mechanisms should be established that use the provincial level of administration as the basic unit and that are based on incidence of disease. These should be continuously updated. They should apply to the 'public setting of prices + compulsory insurance' methods used by the basic medical insurance and mandatory supplemental health insurance that lie within the new public-benefiting insurance system. Two levels of reinsurance companies should be set up for the entire health insurance market, namely at the regional level and the national level. These are to achieve a spatial dispersal of excessively high risk (Figure 4.23).

4.3.3.2.3.2 INSURANCE REGULATION

Given the unique nature of health insurance and the risks it entails, China should set up agencies and systems that are solely responsible for regulating

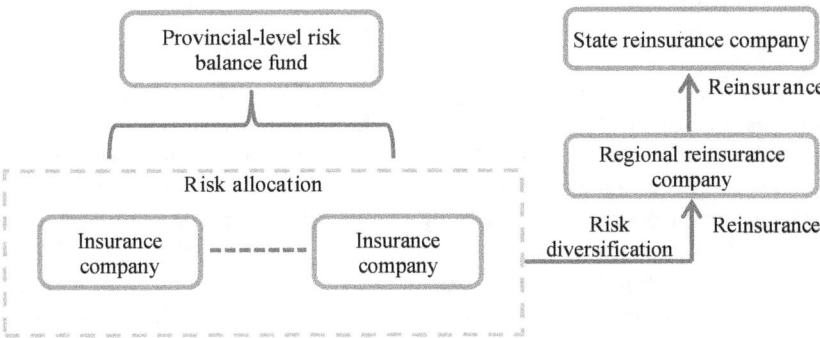

Figure 4.23 Risk allocation system.

Source: By the author.

health insurance. It should also go further in refining the standards that define market entry and operating requirements. In terms of market entry, we should pursue reform of the licensing system that applies to health insurance agencies, be explicit about market-entry standards, and, to the appropriate degree, open up the market. In terms of formulating standards that apply to operating procedures, on the one hand we should improve the statistical systems that apply to the health insurance industry, as well as the financial and accounting systems. We should work out incidence of disease tables and occurrence of loss tables.[44] On the other hand, we should push forward a system for regulating compensation rates in health insurance, and define limits on medical compensation.

4.3.3.2.3.3 MEDICAL SUPERVISION

As the process of implementing managed medicine (managed care) proceeds, to a certain degree insurance companies and medical providers will have mutually shared interests. There will gradually be stronger incentives for hospitals to cut costs for medical services. In this regard, we should set up departments that are specifically responsible for conducting continuous monitoring and supervision of hospitals, as well as making periodic assessments. They should look at the quality of services as well as operating conditions and compliance with regulatory requirements. In addition, in order to ensure reasonable use of drugs and medical procedures, government departments may set up websites that disclose information on commonly used drugs and common medical procedures, and they may also want to set up consumer hotlines in each region so as to make it more convenient for consumers to inquire about related information.

4.3.3.3 Role and functions of the new public-benefiting insurance

4.3.3.3.1 Broad coverage

Coverage of the new public-benefiting insurance is broad in two senses, which could be defined as horizontal and vertical. Horizontal coverage applies to the range of people that are covered. Relative to basic medical insurance, the new public-benefiting insurance applies to the entire body of residents but is adapted to market-oriented operations. It thereby goes further in raising the universal nature of health insurance in China. Vertical coverage refers to the scope of safeguards. The new public-benefiting insurance fills in the blank areas in China's existing medical insurance system by allowing for multi-tiered levels of insurance. It provides safeguards that cover the entire lifespan of a consumer.

4.3.3.3.2 Provision of products: multi-tiered approach

The new public-benefiting insurance and the basic medical insurance complement one another. While they provide universal-type basic safeguards for consumers, they also meet the needs of personalized services for special groups and high-end consumers. Mandatory supplementary insurance provides a layer of basic safeguards on top of the basic medical insurance. The 'expanded' and 'add-on' types of health insurance then are aimed at meeting high-end demand as well as insuring specifically defined risks.

4.3.3.3.3 Operating systems: sustainability

The new public-benefiting insurance goes further in improving the stability and sustainability of China's overall health safeguards systems. It does this by coordinating the relationships among three parties, namely commercial insurance companies, social insurance agencies, and the government. At the level of funding, the new system safeguards the sources of funds and the stability of income by adopting the principle of 'public sharing of the burden and limited subsidies' with respect to the mandatory supplementary health insurance. At the level of spending, the system makes full use of the role of 'managed medicine' in that it encourages commercial insurance to get involved in treatment processes and hold down improper medical spending. At the level of risk allocation, the system strengthens the sustainability and soundness of operating procedures by setting up risk-balancing mechanisms and reinsurance mechanisms.

4.3.4 An estimate of the overall size of China's commercial health insurance business

4.3.4.1 Scenario 1: forecast that uses the existing rate of growth

Health insurance premium income went from RMB 31.2 billion in 2005 to RMB 241.047 billion in 2015. The rate of growth experienced considerable volatility during this period, but the highest rate of growth was in 2008, at 52.4%. The lowest was in 2009, at a negative 1.96%. In the last five years, however, premium income has shown a stable rate of growth (see Figure 4.24).

Given the uneven rate of annual growth, this study adopts geometric average growth rates to carry out its calculations. We measured the growth rates in three different time segments, namely ten years (2005–2015), five years (2010–2015), and three years (2012–2015), and calculated growth rates in health insurance corresponding to those years of 23%, 29%, and 41%. Figure 4.25 shows future income from health insurance premiums based on the different growth rates. From these calculations, income from health insurance premiums will be roughly in the range of RMB 600 billion to RMB 1,400 billion.

4.3.4.2 Scenario 2: forecast that uses the percentage of an individual's out-of-pocket medical expenses

The market space into which commercial health insurance will grow lies in the portion of out-of-pocket health-care expenses paid by individuals. According to the *Outline of the Plan for Healthy China 2030*, the goal is to reduce such

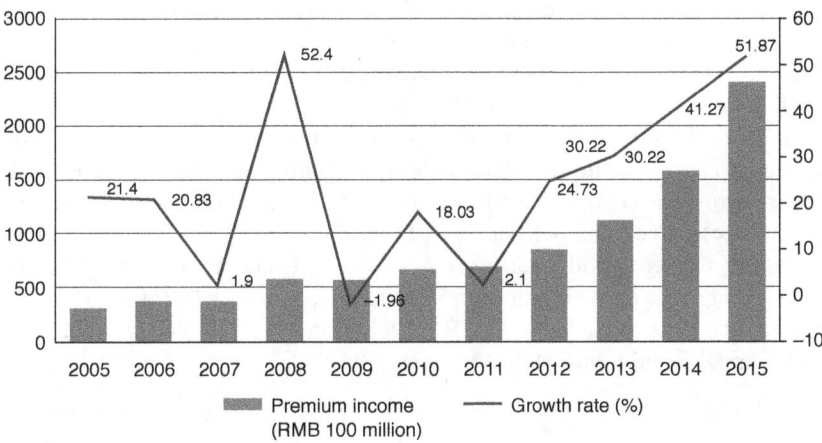

Figure 4.24 Premium income and growth rate over the years.

Source: *China Insurance Yearbook 2006–2015.*

Note
The growth rates are year-on-year growth rates.

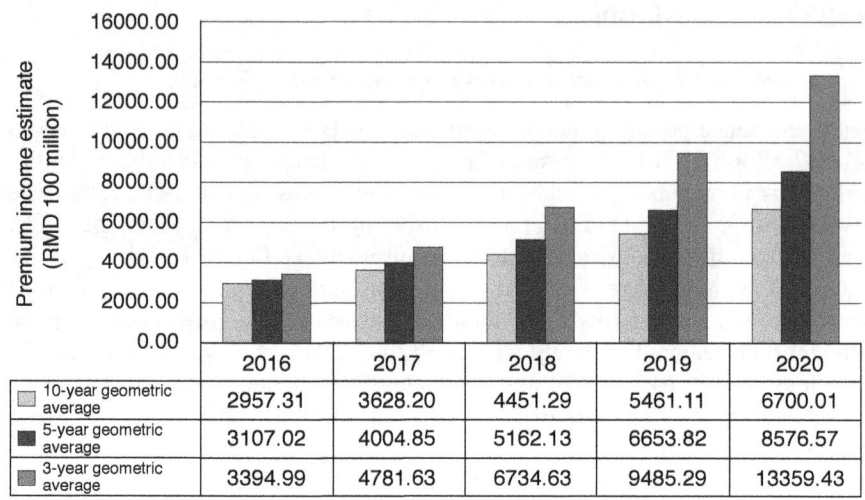

	2016	2017	2018	2019	2020
10-year geometric average	2957.31	3628.20	4451.29	5461.11	6700.01
5-year geometric average	3107.02	4004.85	5162.13	6653.82	8576.57
3-year geometric average	3394.99	4781.63	6734.63	9485.29	13359.43

Figure 4.25 Premium income estimate (as per growth rate).

Source: By the author.

individual payments to 28% of the total by 2020. That is, the percentage self-paid by individuals must drop by 2% between the years 2015 and 2020. During this period, the level of security provided by both social insurance and commercial insurance will need to rise correspondingly. If we make the assumption that commercial insurance contributes three-quarters of this, that is, 1.5%, then reimbursements paid out by commercial health insurance will ultimately represent 3.38% of the total (in 2015, roughly 1.88% of the total). According to estimates of the geometric average growth rate between 2010 and 2015, total healthcare costs will grow at a rate of around 15.22% to reach the figure of RMB 8,244.887 billion in 2020. Assuming that commercial health insurance holds 3.38% of that figure, reimbursement compensation made by commercial health insurance will come to roughly RMB 278.677 billion. In 2015, the compensation rate (reimbursement rate) of commercial health insurance was 31.65%. Taking this into consideration, we set hypothetical rates of 30%, 50%, and 80% for purposes of calculating and came up with premium income of (commercial) health insurance in 2020 in the general range of RMB 340 billion to RMB 940 billion. (See Tables 4.5 and 4.6 and Figure 4.26.)

Table 4.5 Data on medical expenses and health insurance, 2010–2015

Year	Total medical expenses (RMB 100 million)	Out-of-pocket expenses (RMB 100 million)	Percentage of out-of-pocket expenses (%)	CHI premium growth (RMB 100 million)	CHI compensation (RMB 100 million)	CHI compensation rate (%)
2010	19,980.4	7,051.29	35.29	677.47	264.02	38.97
2011	24,345.91	8,465.28	34.77	691.72	359.67	52.00
2012	28,119	9,656.32	34.34	862.76	298.17	34.56
2013	31,868.95	10,729.34	33.67	1,123.5	411.13	36.59
2014	35,378.9	11,745.3	33.2	1,587.18	571.16	35.99
2015	40,587.7	12,164	29.97	2,410.47	762.97	31.65

Source: (2011–2015) *China Healthcare and Family Planning Yearbook*; *China Insurance Yearbook*; data on 2015 medical expenses comes from http://field.10jqka.com.cn/20160722/c591902965.shtml; 2015 insurance data comes from CIRC website.

Table 4.6 Indicator estimate, 2016–2020 (RMB 100 million)

Year	Total medical expenses	Out-of-pocket expenses	CHI compensation (RMB 100 million)
2015	40587.7	12164.00	762.97
2016	46768.39805	13827.05	988.612849
2017	53890.29326	15717.48	1280.98793
2018	62096.71123	17866.37	1659.83083
2019	71552.80314	20309.04	2150.71377
2020	82448.86946	23085.68	2786.77179

Source: Author.

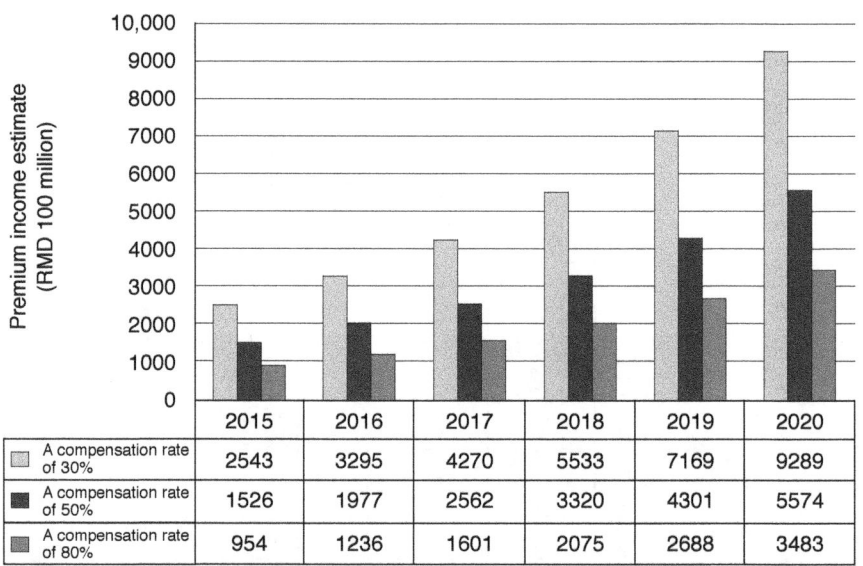

	2015	2016	2017	2018	2019	2020
A compensation rate of 30%	2543	3295	4270	5533	7169	9289
A compensation rate of 50%	1526	1977	2562	3320	4301	5574
A compensation rate of 80%	954	1236	1601	2075	2688	3483

Figure 4.26 Premium income estimate (percentage of out-of-pocket expenses drops to 28% in 2020).

Source: By the author.

4.4 RE-EVALUATION OF THE DOMESTIC AND INTERNATIONAL EXPERIENCE FROM THE PERSPECTIVE OF THE NEW PUBLIC-BENEFITING INSURANCE

The 'public-benefiting' aspect of the new insurance refers to its breadth of coverage. The 'new' part refers to two things—the way it satisfies multi-tiered demand and the way it is sustainable. That is, not only must this insurance bring benefits to the maximum number of people possible but it must guarantee that these benefits are sustainable and for the long term. In terms of economic theory, however, and both breadth and depth, it is hard to satisfy both conditions of short-term satisfaction of demand and long-term sustainability. Therefore it is necessary to strike an enlightened balance among the three objectives: broad coverage, satisfaction at many levels, and sustainability. This section revisits the experience of other countries as well as China from a public-benefiting perspective, in the hope of providing lessons as China builds up its health safeguards system.

4.4.1 Experiences of developed countries

Commercial health insurance in developed countries can be divided into three types, with respect to their relationship with basic medical insurance. These are: complementary, supplementary, and substitutive. The complementary type is most common. On top of statutory (mandatory) insurance, this provides greater financial compensation or a greater scope of coverage. The systems in the UK, the United States, and the Netherlands are prime examples. The supplementary type of commercial health insurance provides safeguards that are equivalent to those of statutory insurance but with higher-quality services and more choices. Switzerland is a typical example. The substitutive type of commercial health insurance operates in tandem with statutory insurance and provides coverage for people who are excluded from or who choose not to be included in statutory health insurance. Germany is an example.

4.4.1.1 Complementary: UK, U.S. and Netherlands

The UK, United States, and the Netherlands are the most representative examples of healthcare systems where commercial health insurance has a complementary relationship with basic medical insurance. In the UK, the government takes the lead. In the United States, the market is the driving force, while a combination of government + market operates in the Netherlands. In terms of medical reform in these three countries, however, a development model that combines the forces of both commercial and medical (basic) insurance is the goal, since sole reliance on either a government model or a market model is not conducive to growth of health insurance markets.

4.4.1.1.1 UK

In the UK, the National Health Service (NHS), a publicly funded medical system for the entire population, is dominant, while commercial health insurance holds a very small percentage of the market. The NHS is operated by CCGs (Clinical Commissioning Groups) which are responsible for specific operations. The NHS also cooperates with commercial health insurance through the Framework for Procuring External Support for Commissioners (FESC) (see Figure 4.27). After reforms, the extent of nationalized medicine is gradually diminishing and the country is transitioning from purely state-run

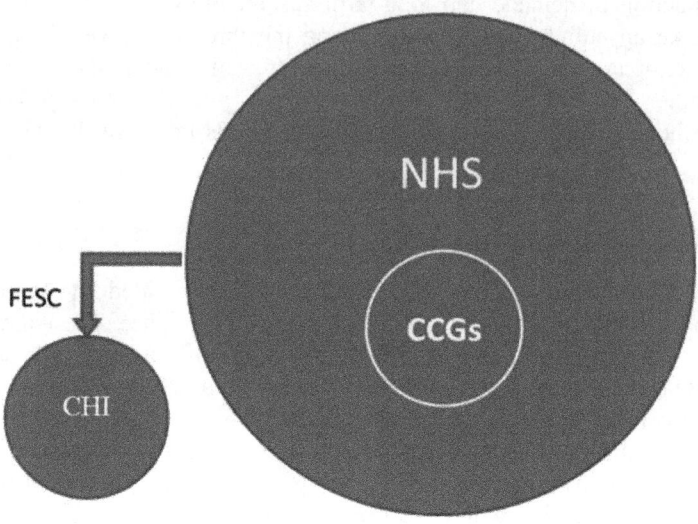

Figure 4.27 UK medical insurance system.

mechanisms to an intermediate system. Market mechanisms have become an effective way to raise efficiency.

A balance is achieved between breadth of coverage and diversification by having fiscal revenues support the National Health Service while commercial insurance satisfies the demand for complementary safeguards. In the UK's system of medical insurance, the government allocates funds for basic medical safeguards for the entire population, which includes coverage for emergency treatment and nursing, general medical services, dental services, drugs, ophthalmology, hospitalization, rehabilitation, community health services, and psychological health services. Since publicly funded medical care holds the commanding position, commercial health insurance only provides complementary safeguards for high-end consumers and meets individualized insurance demand for such things as critical illness, private care, and long-term nursing. It is mainly used to improve the experience of medical care.

The NHS is operated by CCGs who use 'managed care' to strengthen internal market competition. This allows for a balance between the public-benefit nature of the services and sustainability. After medical reforms launched by Prime Minister Cameron, CCGs became core operators of the National Health Service, and establishing an 'internal market' became the guiding philosophy. Providers of medical services within the NHS were separated from the buyers of medical services. CCGs represent patients in buying services. They in turn pay hospitals and specialists but they also monitor and supervise them. General practitioners are the 'gatekeepers' of the NHS. They are authorized by CCGs to help patients decide on treatment and on whether or not to be referred to specialists. Their compensation is determined by their number of registered patients. By adopting internal competition and a managed care model, the NHS has improved efficiencies and lowered costs, which has helped make the public-benefit nature of the NHS more sustainable. (See Figures 4.28 and 4.29.)

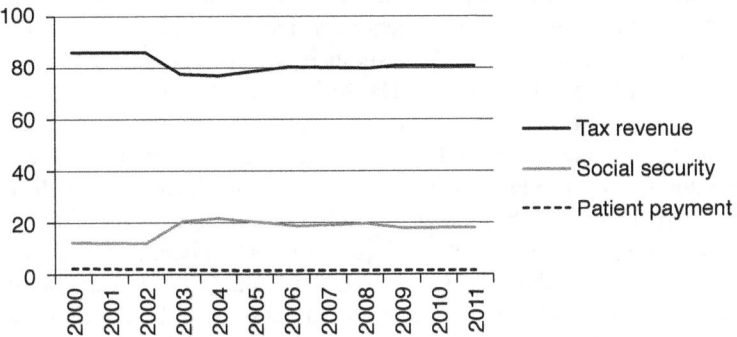

Figure 4.28 NHS financing sources.

Source: *OHE Guide to UK Health and Health Care Statistics*, 2013.

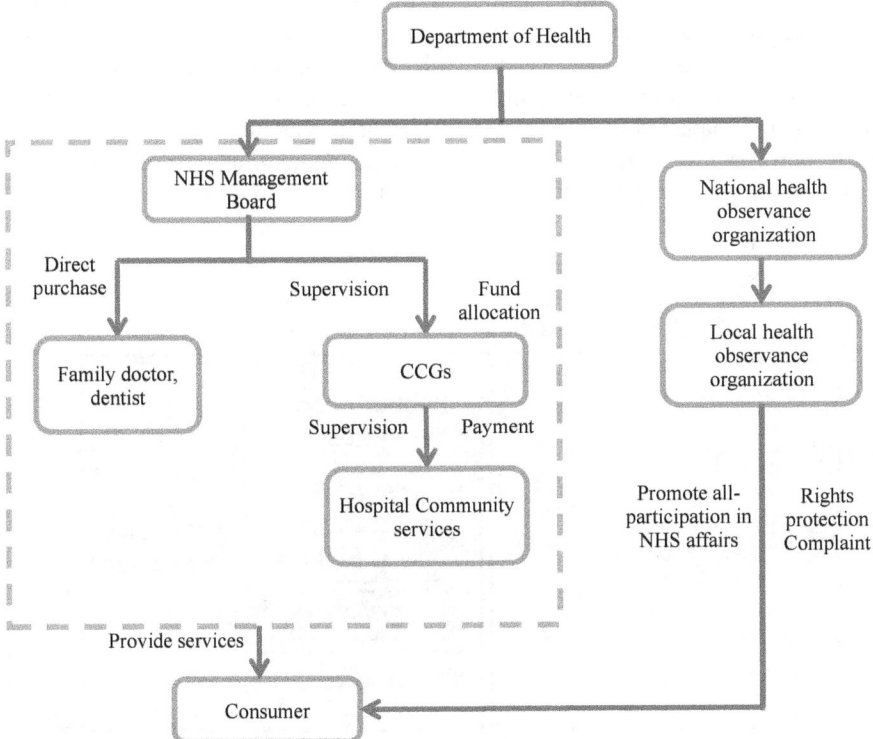

Figure 4.29 NHS operation.

4.4.1.1.2 U.S.

Obamacare, the reform adopted by President Obama in the United States, incorporates uninsured people into the medical insurance system by requiring compulsory private insurance. The plan set up health insurance exchanges which provide a diversity of insurance plans thereby achieving the aim of balancing broad coverage with diversified options. Generally speaking, the system in the U.S. is dominated by commercial health insurance with the public safeguards system as a supplement (see Figure 4.30). The former mainly serves companies while the latter provides services to older people, low-income families, children, and retired military personnel (veterans). The health insurance exchanges in each state provide standardized products to people who are not insured as well as employees of small companies. Such plans are divided into four levels that are based on actuarial pricing, called copper, silver, gold, and platinum. Each has specified deductibles and reimbursement percentages. Policy holders can get tax benefits for paying premiums as well as cost-sharing subsidies. In addition, the exchanges protect the rights and interests of consumers by monitoring products and ensuring information disclosure. When taken together with other safeguards, the Obamacare plan meets the goal of providing coverage for all people in the country.

Universal coverage is achieved in the United States by having the government mandate that insurance companies take on underwriting while the public determines pricing. The system adopts diversified risk-balancing plans in order to allocate risks among private insurers, which guarantees the sustainability of the system. 'Managed care' uses market-oriented operations. The use of third-party purchasing, a referral system, health management, and so on helps keep costs down while ensuring better services. Moral hazard and also expenditures

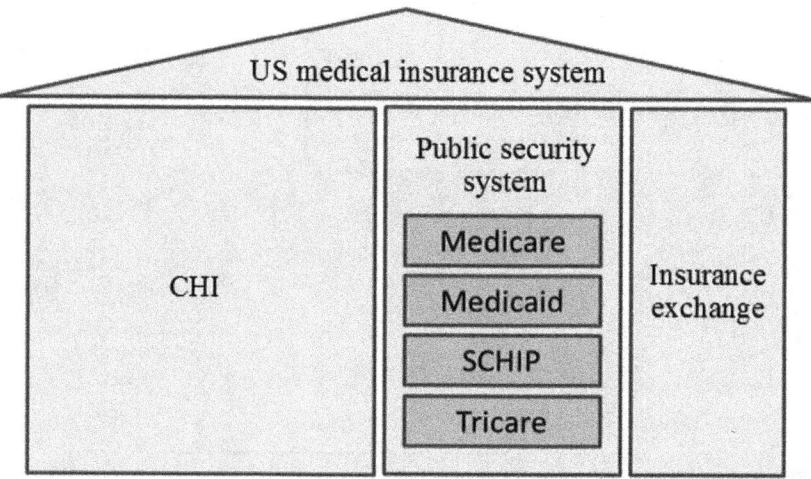

Figure 4.30 U.S. medical insurance system.

are effectively reduced by raising the amount of deductibles and regulating the percentage of co-payment required. The popularity of consumer-directed health plans indicates that the managed-care style of medicine is gradually becoming more accepted. The trend is toward a greater awareness that consumers them-selves are able to control costs. Figure 4.31 shows the basic situation in the U.S. health insurance market.

4.4.1.1.3 *Netherlands*

In the Netherlands, mandatory health insurance and complementary health insur-ance supplement one another, thereby achieving a balance between broad coverage and diversified demands. All citizens of the country must participate in statutory health insurance. Private insurance companies provide standardized basic medical insurance packages, and people themselves may choose different levels of deductibles. Statutory (mandatory) health insurance is priced by the public. The premium consists of nominal and income-related parts. The former is decided by the deductibles, and the latter is a certain percentage of income. Low-income people are granted government subsidies to pay the premium. These mandatory measures result in some 99% of people in the country having insurance coverage. The statutory form of insurance is divided into statutory (mandatory) private health insurance coverage and long-term nursing care insur-ance. Together, these cover nearly all basic medical services as well as preven-tive and long-term services. Complementary health insurance is optional and priced according to risk. In purchasing such insurance, the policy holder can enjoy safeguards beyond the coverage of statutory insurance as well as better services. On top of the foundation of broad coverage, this therefore improves the depth and diversity of a person's insurance options.

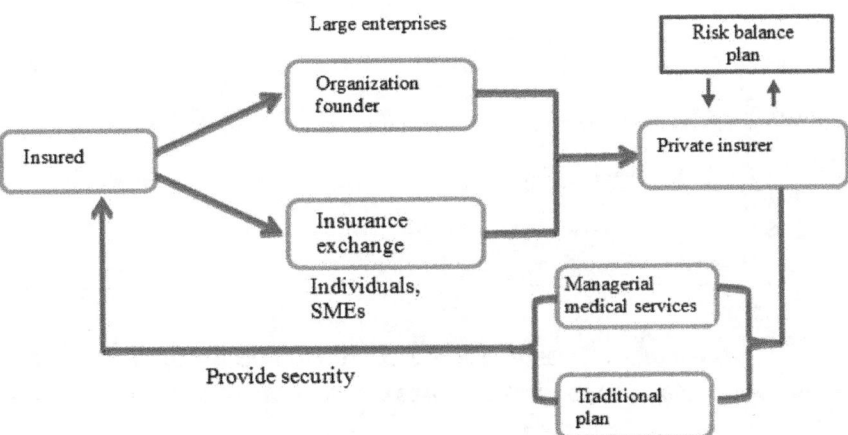

Figure 4.31 U.S. health insurance market.

The combination of good risk-balancing mechanisms and managed-care services achieves a balance between the public-benefiting nature of the system and sustainability. The risk-balancing mechanisms in the Netherlands include pre-event risk adjustment as well as post-event compensation. Pre-event risk adjustment takes such risk factors into account as age, gender, source of income, geographic location, cost of diagnosis, and cost of drugs in calculating risk compensation discrepancies, so as to allocate the 'risk-balancing fund' among insurance companies and balance out the medical expenditures among them. The post-event compensation is used to make up for inadequacies of the pre-event adjustment. These risk-balancing mechanisms iron out the concentration of risk caused by public pricing. They satisfy the need for profits on the part of private insurance companies, and they are essential in ensuring the sustainability of mandatory health insurance. (See Figures 4.32, 4.33, and 4.34.)

4.4.1.2 Supplementary: Switzerland

Supplementary health insurance seeks to strike a balance between broad coverage and the need for diversity by providing 'supplements' to mandatory health insurance. In Switzerland, all citizens must participate in statutory health insurance. Private insurance companies provide standardized health insurance benefits packages and individuals may themselves choose among different deductibles. The government of each canton in the country issues subsidies to low-income people. Statutory health insurance allows each company to set its own prices, but premiums can only be related to deductible levels that the insured person has chosen. The age group of that person and his canton are also

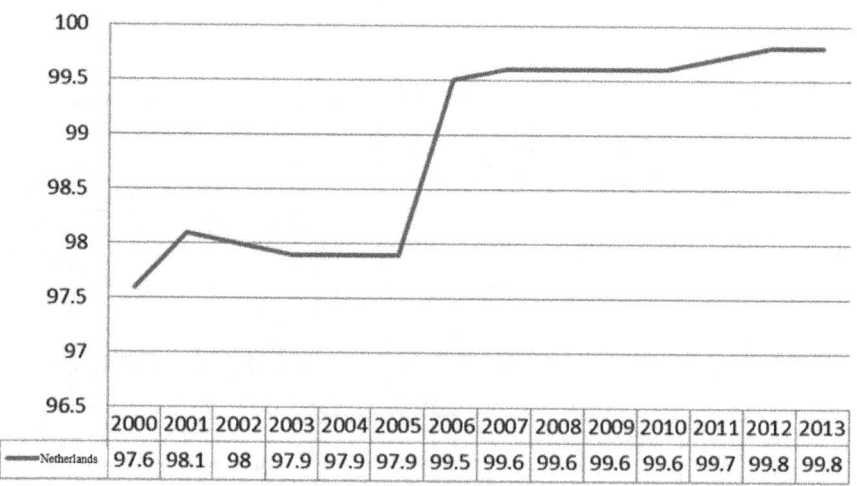

	2000	2001	2002	2003	2004	2005	2006	2007	2008	2009	2010	2011	2012	2013
Netherlands	97.6	98.1	98	97.9	97.9	97.9	99.5	99.6	99.6	99.6	99.6	99.7	99.8	99.8

Figure 4.32 Penetration rate of mandatory health insurance in Netherlands.
Source: OECD.Stat.

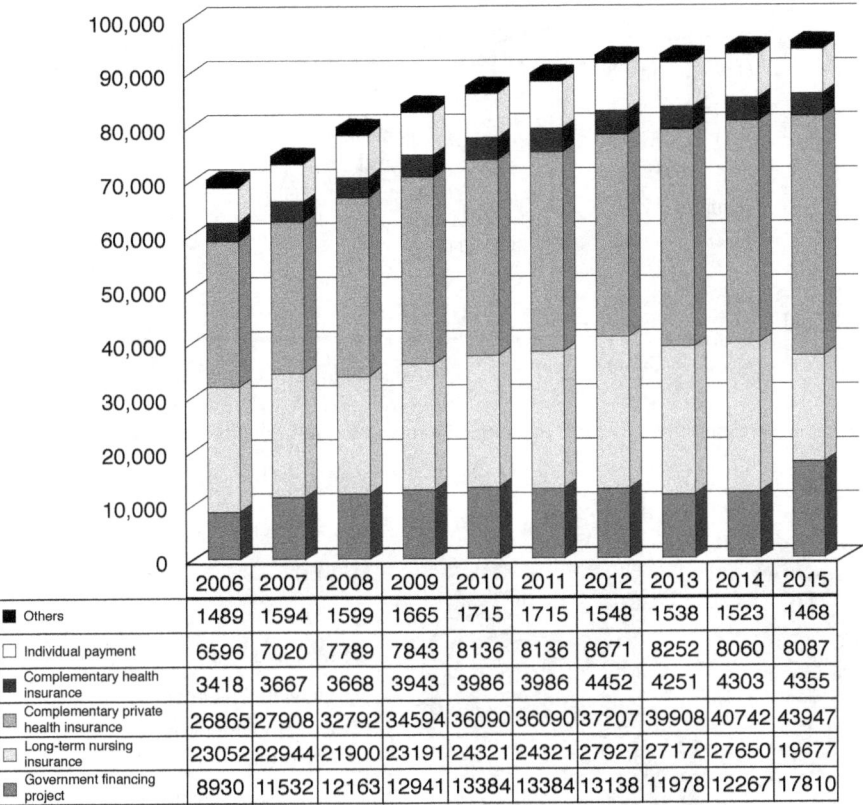

	2006	2007	2008	2009	2010	2011	2012	2013	2014	2015
■ Others	1489	1594	1599	1665	1715	1715	1548	1538	1523	1468
□ Individual payment	6596	7020	7789	7843	8136	8136	8671	8252	8060	8087
■ Complementary health insurance	3418	3667	3668	3943	3986	3986	4452	4251	4303	4355
▨ Complementary private health insurance	26865	27908	32792	34594	36090	36090	37207	39908	40742	43947
□ Long-term nursing insurance	23052	22944	21900	23191	24321	24321	27927	27172	27650	19677
■ Government financing project	8930	11532	12163	12941	13384	13384	13138	11978	12267	17810

Figure 4.33 Financing channels of medical expenditure in Netherlands (millions euros).
Source: CBS, StatLine.

related, and nobody can be denied insurance. These mandatory measures have meant that the rate of participation in insurance plans is over 99%. Supplementary health insurance is optional for both the person being insured and the insurance underwriter, and pricing is not controlled. It operates mainly as a layer on top of the basic statutory health insurance. It offers higher quality services and a broader range of choices, in order to allow for greater depth and greater diversity (see Figure 4.35).

The combination of the cost-sharing mechanism, price competition among insurers, and managed medicine, results in a balance between broadly based public benefit and sustainability. At the level of the insured, Switzerland's three cost-sharing mechanisms are effective in curbing excessive use of medical services. Those are the deductibles, the system of mutual insurance, and a bonus for no claims. At the level of the insurance company, Switzerland requires that any given insurance company must adopt publicly determined pricing for any given

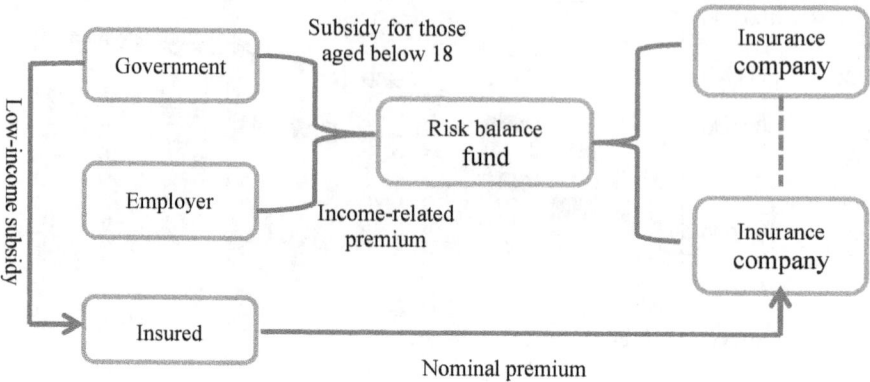

Figure 4.34 Compulsory health insurance financing in Netherlands.

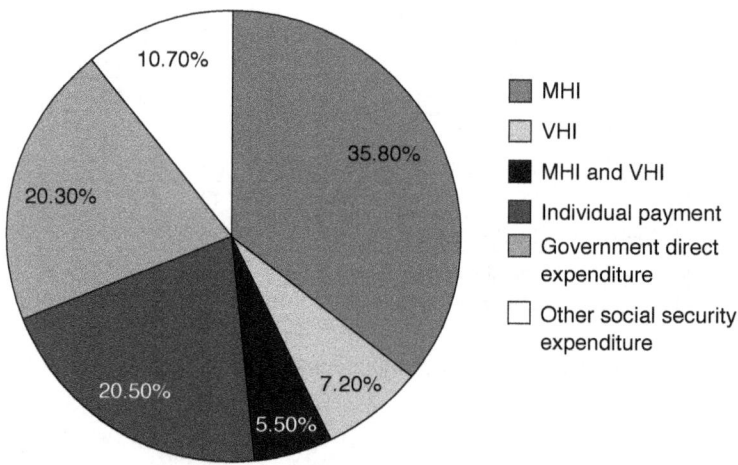

Figure 4.35 Financing sources of healthcare spending in Switzerland.

Source: *Switzerland: Health System in Transition*, 2015.

policy, but the country does not place any other restrictions on how insurance companies set their prices. This encourages price competition among insurance companies and has pushed down their operating costs. In addition, Switzerland has promoted the use of managed medicine, which includes three types of organizations, namely Health Maintenance Organizations, Independent Practice Associations, and gatekeepers. Insurance companies can also hire certified physicians to perform similar functions.

The mandatory cost-sharing mechanisms of deductibles, the system of mutual insurance, and a bonus for no claims have been effective in curbing excessive use of medical services. Meanwhile, insurance companies have relative freedom to set pricing for basic medical insurance, and managed medicine practices are widespread—all of these have also helped keep down medical spending. They have strengthened the sustainability of Switzerland's health insurance system.

4.4.1.3 Substitutive: Germany

In this model, commercial health insurance and basic medical insurance are in competition with each other, which is what achieves a balance between broad coverage and the demands of diversified policy offerings. Germany's health insurance system is operated to a large degree by social organizations, which are self-regulated. All citizens of Germany, or foreign nationals who have lived for a long time in Germany, are required to purchase either statutory health insurance or private insurance that is of a 'substitutive nature.' Statutory health insurance holds the dominant position and is operated by 'critical illness foundations.' The system achieves universal coverage via the mandatory insurance as well as subsidies from public finance. It provides basic medical services to the insured as well as long-term nursing care. Premiums are related solely to income levels. In order to control medical costs, Germany's statutory health insurance has gradually incorporated optional deductibles and mutual-payment mechanisms. It also provides a bonus for no claims.

Commercial health insurance includes the two layers of substitutive-type insurance and supplementary-type insurance. Premiums are mainly determined by the age and health conditions of the insured and the scope of coverage. The substitutive-type of insurance within this system is further divided into three

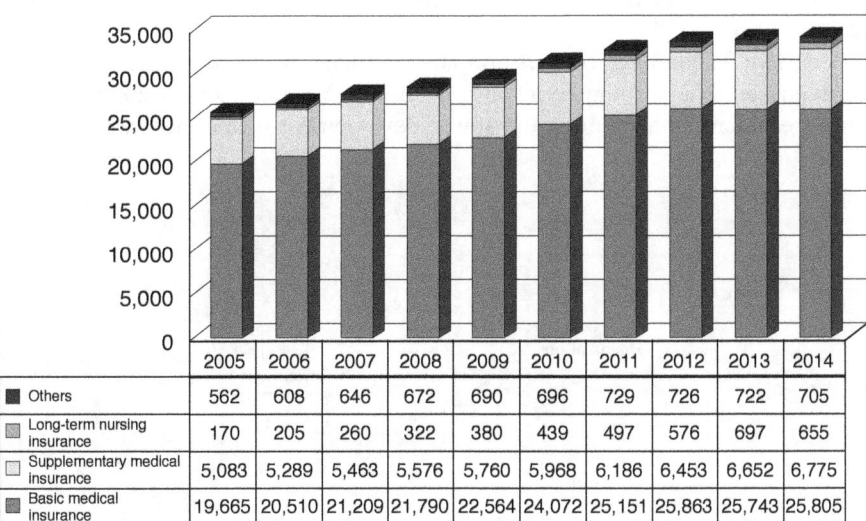

	2005	2006	2007	2008	2009	2010	2011	2012	2013	2014
Others	562	608	646	672	690	696	729	726	722	705
Long-term nursing insurance	170	205	260	322	380	439	497	576	697	655
Supplementary medical insurance	5,083	5,289	5,463	5,576	5,760	5,968	6,186	6,453	6,652	6,775
Basic medical insurance	19,665	20,510	21,209	21,790	22,564	24,072	25,151	25,863	25,743	25,805

Figure 4.36 Premium incomes of health insurances (millions euros).

Source: *Statistical Yearbook of German Insurance 2015.*

kinds, namely basic, standard, and 'comfortable,' with safeguards increasing at each level. The scope of safeguards cannot be less than what is provided by statutory health insurance and premiums for the basic level cannot be higher than the highest premiums under the statutory health insurance. Supplementary health insurance mainly provides coverage beyond what is offered under statutory health insurance and there are no restrictions on how to price those products. Critical illness foundations compete with each other and at the same time carry on competition with insurance companies. This motivates both to meet diversified demands that are above and beyond the needs of broadly based coverage.

Risk is dispersed through both horizontal and vertical mechanisms—horizontal being dispersed by risk balancing mechanisms, and vertical risk being dispersed by the old-age critical illness reserve funds. In this way, a balance is achieved between the public-benefits nature of the system and its sustainability. Premium rates for statutory health insurance are determined in a unified way by the central healthcare funds administration (Central Health Foundation). These funds are allocated by risk-balancing mechanisms on the basis of incidence of diseases. Age, gender, and incidence of disease are the three risk factors by which the fund carries out pre-event transfer of funds to critical illness foundations. This is to prevent critical illness foundations from having either profits or losses that are due to differences in the groups of people being insured. (see Figure 4.37). The old-age critical illness reserve fund is an important risk-balancing mechanism for individuals as a way to insure health across different periods of life. It is a key way to ensure that health insurance can continue to grow even as the society is aging. It can effectively mitigate the accumulation of risk caused by an individual's aging and changes in physical condition.

Germany encourages competition among social insurance organizations and between social and commercial insurance organizations, which contributes to higher efficiencies as well as the sound development of the medical insurance

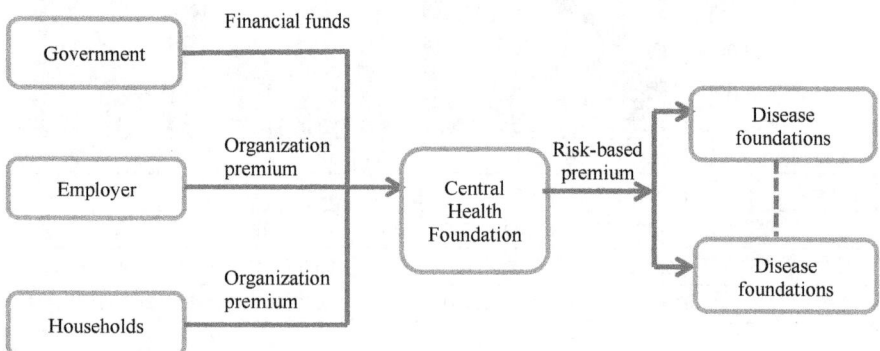

Figure 4.37 Risk balance mechanism of Germany.

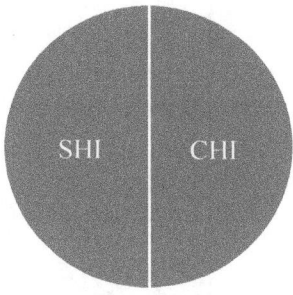

Figure 4.38 Medical insurance system of Germany.

system. The risk balancing mechanisms and old-age critical illness reserve funds allow for two-way risk dispersal. These thereby create the conditions for both 'public benefits' and sustainable growth.

4.4.2 Lessons that can be drawn from developing countries

In 2005, WHO adopted a resolution on 'Setting up sustainable funding systems in order to advance universal coverage and social health safeguards.' Since then, Mexico, India, and many other developing countries have been able to realize universal health coverage, and the safeguards of all countries are constantly being improved. In terms of buying medical services, some Asian and African countries have begun to transition from subsidizing the supply side to subsidizing the demand side. The most representative countries in this regard are Kenya, Indonesia, and the Philippines. In terms of the forms that safeguards take, Asian and African countries have creatively used community-based insurance, with small-sum insurance plans. These have been a useful lesson for low-income countries as they set up pre-payment programs.

However, as medical spending rises, healthcare funding faces severe challenges in developing countries that mainly rely on government spending and the self-funded spending of individuals. That is, developing countries are facing the need to make changes in the structure of their healthcare funding. Both extent of coverage and sustainability are inadequate, with Africa being the worst. Generally speaking, extending the reach of healthcare insurance has been slower in developing countries due to their limited levels of economic development. Basic medical insurance is limited when it comes to real public benefits and to sustainability, while commercial health insurance is at a rudimentary stage. Among developing countries, Mexico and India do somewhat better in terms of public benefits, but they need to improve upon the sustainability of their systems (see Table 4.7).

Table 4.7 Medical financing around the world in 2013 (%)

Place	Government expenditure/total health expenditure	Out-of-pocket expenses/total health expenditure	External financing/ total health expenditure	Actual payment/ total health expenditure	Social security expenditure/total health expenditure	Individual pre-payment program/ total health expenditure
World	57.7	42.2	0.5	22.4	34.6	15.5
America	49.2	50.8	0.1	15.7	35.1	28.9
Europe	75.3	24.4	0.1	19.5	40.2	5.7
Southeast Asia	39.2	60.8	1.8	50.8	3.3	2.4
Africa	49.5	50.5	10.4	31.7	4.7	13.8
Western Pacific	62.9	37.1	0.1	28.6	43.5	3.8
Middle East	49.4	50.6	1.0	43.6	8.8	3.5

Source: WHO database.

4.4.2.1 Mexico

Social insurance in Mexico has mostly accomplished universal coverage. The balance between breadth of coverage and diversified needs is realized by reliance on multi-tiered service packages and supporting funds. The 2003 medical reform in Mexico created a 'Public Insurance System' that drew unemployed people into the scope of safeguards, as well as people with no formal employment. In 2012, this system achieved universal coverage. The system allows for voluntary participation by individuals, with premiums being covered jointly by the federal government, state governments, and the individual (see Figure 4.39). Low-income families are subsidized. The federal government allocates funds to states according to how many people have enrolled. It uses a 'Democracy-driven Budget' to motivate states to improve the quality of their medical services and expand the coverage of safeguards. The Public Insurance System provides for basic services and comprehensive services, and it also has a major illness fund to balance healthcare spending among states and their varying degrees of risk. Commercial health insurance covers just 7% of the population. It mainly targets high-income groups and is used to meet their more diversified and in-depth needs.

The fragmentation of healthcare systems in Mexico lowers their fairness and efficiency, however, while public finance often has limited staying power. This makes it hard to cover the need for both short-term universality and long-term sustainability. Mexico has three main systems of social security, namely Instituto de Seguridad y Servicios Sociales de los Trabajadores del Estado (ISSSTE; aimed at public servants), Instituto Mexicano del Seguro Social (IMSS; aimed at formally employed people), and Seguro Popular (aimed at the unemployed and those with irregular employment). All of these have independent medical systems, and policy holders in one system can only access doctors within that system. Each system has its own ways of handling reimbursements. The funding of healthcare relies heavily on inputs from public finance. State (local) governments have little enthusiasm for spending on social insurance and it is always hard to get funding in a timely fashion. With respect to costs and spending, methods of payment have not noticeably improved in

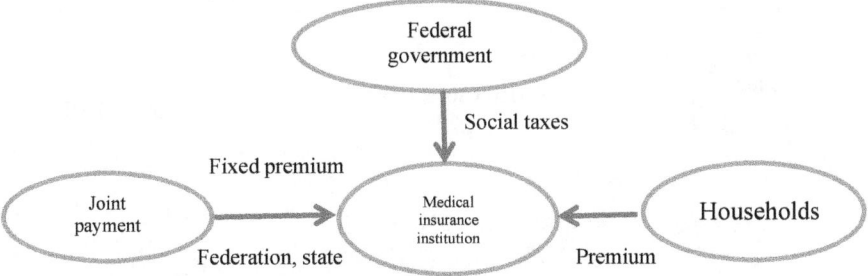

Figure 4.39 Financing sources of Mexico's public insurance.

Mexico, and the medical profession lacks any incentive to control costs. The volatility of government spending and the rise in healthcare costs mean that the continued functioning of the entire medical insurance system faces severe challenges.

4.4.2.2 India

India implements a system of free medical care for the entire population. It encourages the development of private hospitals as well and so balances the two aspects of broad coverage and diversified needs. India's government has funded the establishment of an urban public hospitals system as well as a network of rural medical care, which together provide free basic medical services to both urban and rural populations. Low-income groups get medical attention primarily in public hospitals, which means that subsidies from public finance are weighted in the direction of vulnerable groups of people. This secures the public-benefit nature and fairness of the medical insurance system. Commercial health insurance is primarily for high-end groups of people, while poor people mainly participate in the government insurance plans or those of not-for-profit organizations. They have medical safeguards that are relatively low in terms of both premiums and coverage (see Figure 4.40).

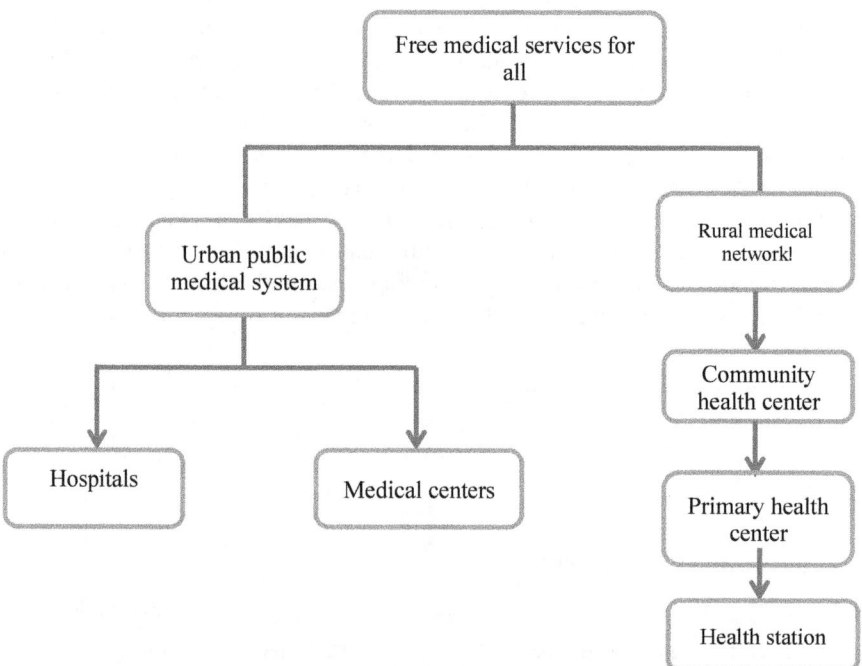

Figure 4.40 Public medical system of India.

India's public medical system relies primarily on inputs from public finance. However, the level of healthcare spending by the government is extremely low. It is only about 1.29% of GDP (2013). The main source of funding for healthcare costs is still the individual, and poor people have quite a low level of security. In addition, public hospitals lack any incentive to control costs, they are extremely inefficient, and their number of patients is disastrous given the lack of medical facilities and also the lack of drugs. Any long-term public benefits of the system will be hard to maintain, given the heavy burden on public finance and the lack of control over expenses.

4.4.3 Summary of the global experience

Any country needs a synergistic combination of policies in order to institute broadly based coverage, mandatory insurance, public-finance subsidies, and publicly determined pricing. Any country, whether in the developed world or the developing world, needs to ensure sustainability. It also needs to have risk-balancing mechanisms to regulate risk and balance spending and it needs to have competition and managed medicine in order to control costs. In order to satisfy different levels of demand, it must rely on a coordinated relationship between basic medical insurance and commercial health insurance. Countries can only rely on their own experience and realities in making decisions about the importance of each of these. Given the fundamental need to respect the circumstances of individual countries, the cooperative model will vary by each place, that is, the extent of cooperation between government and market, commercial health insurance and social insurance, and the extent of public-benefit versus diversified offerings. What's more, the experience of developing countries makes it very clear that growing a commercial health insurance industry must rely fundamentally on a given country's economy. Not only must commercial health insurance take advantage of basic medical insurance to help it open up markets, but commercial health insurance must be an effective supplement to basic medical insurance. The two must cooperate, share interests, and co-exist.

4.4.4 Domestic experience

China has basically addressed the issue of broad coverage, but the safeguards under its system are low. The goal now must be to achieve a healthcare and medical security system that has universal coverage and also strong safeguards. China's experience in trying to do this to date can be described by three model examples. These represent three types of solutions as defined by the relationship of commercial insurance to social insurance—in abbreviated form, those types are described as 'handling,' 'cooperative,' and 'supplementary.' The following goes into more detail on each, in trying to answer the question of how to achieve strong safeguards.

4.4.4.1 Handling (or undertaking): by which commercial insurance undertakes to handle China's basic medical insurance

This solution, which could also be called the 'authorizing or entrusting model,' refers to having government departments who handle social insurance authorize commercial insurance companies to handle the work of basic medical insurance, including the payment of compensation and supervisory tasks. This is one major manifestation of the policy goal of separating out government from business, separating administration from the actual handling of affairs. The prime examples of this are the Jiangyin Model and the Luoyang Model.

4.4.4.1.1 Jiangyin: outsourcing of services

Jiangyin is a prime example of a public-private partnership (see Figure 4.41). The government purchases services from commercial insurance companies. A new 'surveyor's pole,' i.e. a new way to handle affairs, is set up at the county level in the form of 'public–private cooperative handling.' The breakthrough in this new model has come from reform of the payment system. Through intensive and meticulous work, the links in the management chain that deal with the front end, middle, and end of the process are seamlessly connected. Once this foundation of cooperation between social and commercial insurance is mature, policies are designed to promote supplementary health insurance. This allows for a greater degree of safeguards on top of the basic medical insurance and thereby forms a medical insurance system that is strong, steady, and sustainable.

4.4.4.1.1.1 THE RESULTS OF THE JIANGYIN MODEL IN ACTUAL PRACTICE, AND KEY CONSIDERATIONS

Starting in 2001, the Jiangyin Branch of Pacific Life began to participate in the general services of the new rural cooperative insurance initiative by building a 'rural medical safeguards system' that was now multi-tiered. On its part, the local government, in adhering to the principle of separating out government from handling of affairs, authorized the insurance company to be a 'third-party entity' in managing medical services. This was achieved through reform of the payment system for those services. Inserting such a third party into the system held down excessive medical costs and various forms of deceptive and fraudulent behavior. On top of the new rural cooperative plan, which 'insures the basics,' people who wished to participate in higher forms of insurance could voluntarily purchase supplementary commercial health insurance. This broke away from the limited catalogue of things that could be insured under basic medical insurance. It raised actual reimbursement to patients who had large out-of-pocket expenses by almost 10%.[45] In addition, the new system provides remote consultation to participants, which reduces the number of times they must travel to see a doctor and which effectively resolves the difficulty and high cost of seeing a doctor. Meanwhile, the new system has radically lowered administrative costs and improved the performance of the funds.

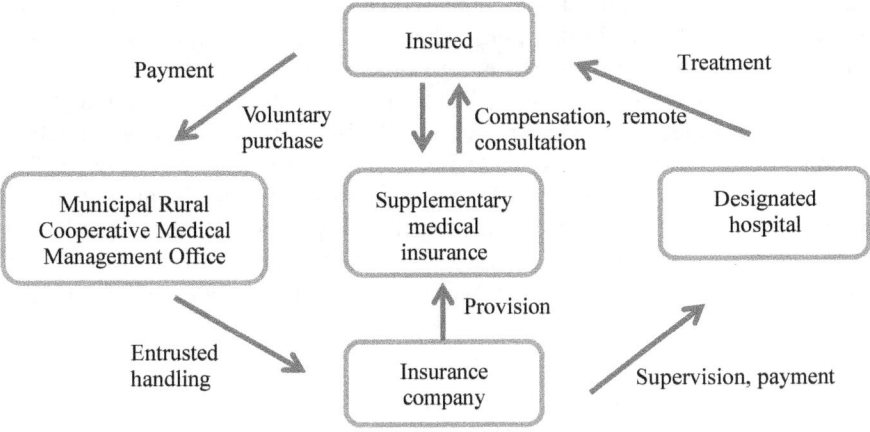

Figure 4.41 Jiangyin model.

4.4.4.1.1.2 FRONT END: SUSTAINABLE FINANCING

The Jiangyin Model retains the original new rural cooperative insurance program, but it is now funded jointly by government, collectives, and individuals. Those who cannot pay the individual portion are subsidized by the municipal and township governments. Economic entities owned by township and village collectives also provide support for the new rural cooperative insurance program as their conditions permit. 'Administered towns' that have the financial means to do so are also encouraged to provide subsidies for the self-payment portion on behalf of people who are solely engaged in farming. On top of this, a new supplementary insurance has been added that carries a premium costing RMB 90 per capita. This is paid by the individual insured. This policy change in the system has in reality become a mandatory kind of health insurance and it has basically achieved universal coverage. In 2014, the per capita GDP of the permanent population in Jiangyin reached the high figure of RMB 169,000,[46] so RMB 90 is an acceptable amount to pay. What's more, since the amount is completely self-paid, the new insurance does not put any new pressures on public finance. The funding for the Jiangyin Model is therefore sustainable.

4.4.4.1.1.3 MIDDLE: EXPENDITURE CONTROL

As a commercial health insurance company, Pacific Life has been able to use its actuarial expertise and its information advantages to strengthen and tighten up controls over management. It has effectively kept costs from rising as a result. Reform of the payment system, meanwhile, has ameliorated the inequitable relationship between commercial insurance and hospitals and has forced hospitals to take the initiative in controlling expenses. Pacific Life has carried out R&D to develop an information system that applies to the new rural health insurance. This ensures that the payment of claims settlements out of funds is more impartial and more efficient. In addition, it helps with real-time monitoring of and intervention in hospital diagnosis and treatment procedures. Depending on the results of the monitoring of funds, Pacific Life also manages the catalogue of drugs and treatments, it manages outpatient visits, and it formulates medical insurance plans—all of these provide assurance that funds are being used safely and efficiently. Pacific Life provides actuarial analysis of the rural cooperative insurance plans and in the fourth quarter of each year makes recommendations to the township governments regarding policy formulation. This provides assurance that the overall system can adapt to changes in the environment and continue to improve on an annual basis.

4.4.4.1.1.4 REAR END: SUPERVISION AND AUDITING MECHANISMS

Jiangyin City authorized the commercial insurance company to review and investigate its medical practices, but in addition it established a full set of supervisory and auditing mechanisms. These oversee medical institutions and staff and also audit the use of funds in order to ensure that funds are being properly employed. A three-level audit system includes the following: a commissioner who resides in the hospital, a new rural cooperative medical insurance administration center (professional insurance company), and the municipal administrative center (the Department of Health). These three levels take allied action in conducting audits. A report goes to each designated hospital at regular intervals. This includes the performance review of the new rural cooperative insurance system, any excessive expenditures, and withdrawals of funds. Any improper expenditures are to be returned back to the system. A 'blacklist' program ensures that the supervisory oversight extends to individuals in the medical system. The administration centers review documentation on cases—if there are medical personnel who have violated rules for two consecutive months, the centers revoke the ability of such people to work in the hospitals designated under the new rural cooperative insurance system. They also control the ability of such people to use any of the pharmaceuticals or equipment that fall under the purview of the new rural cooperative system.

The Department of Health regulates the activities of commercial insurance companies and carries out overall coordination. The Auditing Department audits the use of the funds, so as to ensure the safe use and operation of funds at the rear end of the process.

4.4.4.1.2 The Luoyang Model: separating out government administration from the handling of business under the 'entrusting and handling' model

Luoyang is also a representative case of having commercial insurance take on the handling of basic medical insurance (see Figure 4.42). The list of things it

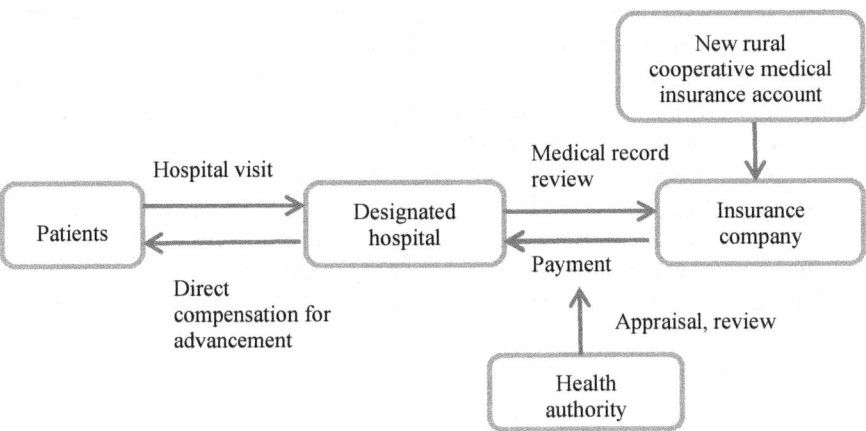

Figure 4.42 Luoyang model.

'handles' covers the entire scope of basic medical insurance tasks. By having commercial insurance carry out vertical management, Luoyang has de facto realized the management of insurance funds at the municipal level. The funds for social insurance still reside in a special account in public finance, which ensures their safe application. By using the direct-payment platform of commercial insurance, however, the settlement of claims can be achieved from other locations including such cities as Beijing and Shanghai. This is in the forefront of the effort to enable medical access anywhere (without needing to have insurance settled in the same place), through the cooperation between social and commercial insurance.

4.4.4.1.2.1 MAIN COMPONENTS OF THE MODEL AND RESULTS IN
ACTUAL PRACTICE

The core aspect of the Luoyang Model is the way it authorizes or entrusts handling of the business to commercial insurance. In 2007, the Luoyang Branch of China Life began to get engaged in services relating to the new rural cooperative medical insurance plans of the five counties and seven districts that make up Luoyang. By 2015, it had achieved universal coverage by being authorized to carry out the following activities: medical emergency assistance for vulnerable groups in urban and rural areas, the new rural cooperative medical insurance, urban residents' basic medical insurance, insurance against medical disputes, insurance for major illness for residents in both urban and rural areas, and urban employees' basic medical insurance. Local governments procure services from the insurance company. These include such non-core activities as initial review of medical records, payment of fees, and so on. Public health administrative departments are responsible for carrying out supervisory management of medical institutions and health insurance agencies.

In addition, by using the network of its parent company, the Luoyang Branch of China Life has built a direct compensation platform. Insurance bills under the Luoyang urban employee plan and the critical illness insurance plan can be settled in any one of more than 20 cities throughout China, including Beijing, Shanghai, and Tianjin. This makes Luoyang a pioneer in exploring ways to pay for medical treatments that do not physically take place where the insurance is issued.[47] Meanwhile, the insertion of commercial insurance into the process of handling social (publicly funded) insurance has made social insurance more transparent and more professional. Government is able to focus its efforts on formulating regulations and on supervisory management. The system has allowed for full utilization of the advantages of both social insurance and commercial insurance.

4.4.4.1.2.2 FRONT END: SUSTAINABLE FUNDING

The Luoyang Model is an example of a public–private partnership that out-sources services. The social security funds are managed in two lines: the government collects premiums and ensures that funding is stable while the insurance company does initial reviews of medical records and handles such things as payment of compensation. In this way it saves an enormous amount on the costs of labor and financing the operation. The management fees it receives for its services are allocated from a line-item account of public finance. This means that sources of social security funds are not compromised and it also allows for sustainable operations.

4.4.4.1.2.3 MIDDLE: CONTROL OVER SPENDING

The main tasks of the insurance company are to do initial reviews of medical records and to pay costs of medical expenses. The Luoyang Branch specifically set up a health department for these tasks, with related entities at each level of administration, municipal, county, and township. These carry out vertically integrated management. Medical institutions are paid via the commercial insurance company. The funds are pooled and managed at the county level and claims are settled within each county. Within that primary framework, the insurance company uses the advantage of vertical management of its organizations, people, and networks at the municipal and county level to carry out overall planning at the municipal level.[48] Patients only have to pay the self-pay portion of their bills. Due to the double-management model of 'direct-compensation reserves' and 'post-event payment,' what patients pay does not affect any auditing results.[49]

The insurance company is involved in medical processes in that it reviews the records of patients and conducts on-site checks on actual diagnosis and treatment. The social insurance authorities review the audited material of insurance companies in order to keep down any improper spending. Those authorities also organize specialists to re-examine any medical records that are doubtful or in dispute. Expenses that violate regulations must be paid by either the hospital or the physician in charge; expenses that are acceptable are disbursed to the institution the following month. At the same time, the administrative office (supervisory management) of the new rural cooperative medical insurance program conducts audits of 30% of certificates of evidence (bills) that have already been audited by the insurance company. As an incentive to the insurance company to do a good job, it holds back a 10% management fee as a guarantee that contract provisions will be carried out as agreed upon.

4.4.4.1.2.4 REAR END: MECHANISMS FOR SHARING RISK

In order to ensure the safety of the social security funds, they remain in a dedicated account of the public finance department of the Luoyang municipal government. This respects the principle of 'having government play the leading role while operations are handled by industry, in order to separate out administration from actual operations.' The insurance company is merely responsible for auditing expenses and paying compensation. Funds are disbursed from the account dedicated to the 'new rural cooperative' fund. They pass through a designated account at the Luoyang Branch of China Life before being disbursed to the main accounts of designated hospitals. On an annual basis, any left-over funds and interest are repaid back into the account of public finance. Funds are not maintained in the account of the insurance company, and the company also does not assume any risk in managing the funds.[50]

Given its advantages in knowing how to apply information technologies to management, the insurance company is able to curb medical costs and prevent improper increases in the spending of public funds. By analyzing historical data and information on hospital stays, the insurance company is able to provide statistical data that helps in formulating policies and adjusting payments and reimbursement percentages, as a way to mitigate risk.[51] The Luoyang Branch of China Life also takes on the insuring of Luoyang's emergency aid to vulnerable groups of people. In 2014, it launched a supplementary medical insurance program for the new rural cooperative insurance program—this allows for risk-sharing between social and commercial insurance. The commercial supplementary insurance is a secondary source of compensation which also alleviates problems in the event of an overdraft of social security funds.

4.4.4.2 The cooperative type of relationship between social and commercial insurance

The cooperative type of relationship works by having insurance companies share premium income as well as risk with the basic medical insurance level of social insurance. The result is 'co-insurance' and the representative model for this is the Pinggu Model. Pinggu was first to put into effect this form of proportional co-insuring whereby both parties share insurance and also have a defined way of working together. Under this model, the company is authorized to inject its management controls into medical institutions by adopting the authority and prestige of government authorities. By evaluating the quality of services and checking up on diagnoses and treatments, the insurance company can also amass a large amount of risk data. In turn, government relies on the technical expertise and human resources of the insurance company to improve the results of its funds management, to lower administrative costs, and to ensure a win-win situation among all parties, including government, insurance company, hospitals, and the public.

4.4.4.2.1 Primary components of the model and actual results

Pinggu took the lead in practicing (an earlier form of) the co-insurance model in 2004. By 2010, Pinggu's new rural cooperative fund already had an overdraft of RMB 24.97 million.[52] To address this overspending problem, the district government of Pinggu and the Beijing branch of PICC (People's Insurance Company of China) signed a cooperative agreement: the government would purchase risk-insurance services from the insurance company in the form of premiums that equaled 50% of the funding amount of the program. Both the district government and the insurance company agreed to respect the principle of 'sharing risk, profits, and also losses.' The company therefore assumed 50% of the responsibility for making reimbursements under the new medical cooperative insurance program. If the fund for this program had a surplus, that surplus would be entered into the government's medical-fund account. Using other channels of funds, the district government would pay the insurance company 50% of the amount as a bonus (see Figure 4.43). The success of controlling costs has been quite apparent since setting up this Pinggu Model. Between 2011 and 2013, spending out of the new rural cooperative fund rose at an average annual rate of just 2.2%, which is far lower than the average annual rate in Beijing of 13.3%.[53]

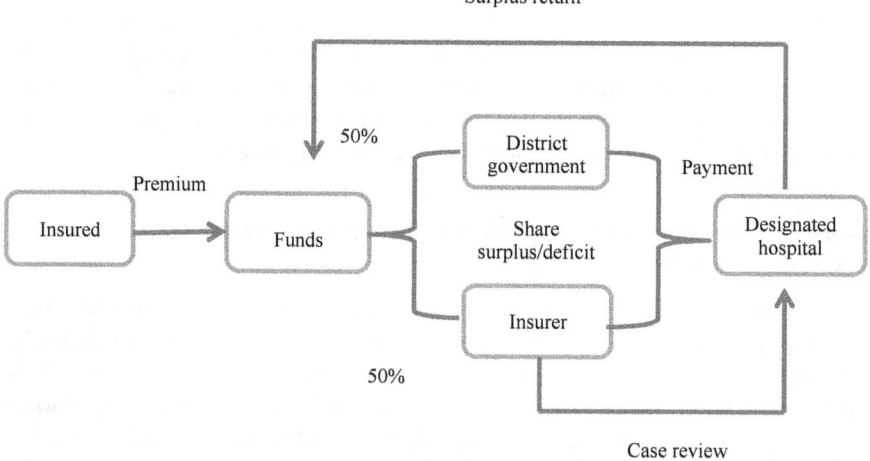

Figure 4.43 Pinggu model.

This has allowed the new rural cooperative program in Pinggu to operate in a stable manner.

4.4.4.2.2 Front end: sustainable financing

The Pinggu Model is essentially 'proportional co-insuring,' where the government purchases insurance from the insurance company and the insurance company underwrites the risk of (the government's) social basic medical insurance. Both parties share risks and losses. The premiums paid by the government to the insurance company come from the income of the new rural cooperative medical insurance. These funds are inherently secure and sustainable. The government's premium expenses account for just 50% of the amount it funds, but the government also shifts away half of its unpredictable spending risks. In this way, the leverage of insurance is brought into full play to improve the effectiveness with which funds are used and to raise the results of funds management.

4.4.4.2.3 Middle: control over costs

The Pinggu Model uses an 'allied forces' method of controlling the costs that arise in the course of managing services and paying for medical expenses. The Beijing Branch of PICC and the New Rural Cooperative Insurance Center of the district (Pinggu administration) set up a joint effort to supervise and regulate any improper behavior by medical personnel. At the same time, this Joint Office set up working teams inside hospitals to carry out on-site investigations. People in the teams carry out an audit of the 72-hour medical record when a patient enters the hospital. They confirm the patient's ID information, carry out a dynamic medical records review and, before the patient is discharged, review medical records once again. In this way, hospital personnel are subjected to 'whole-process' supervisory management. The government and the insurance company have also set up mobile inspection platforms and a supplementary system for auditing medical treatments. This is linked to the hospital's HIS system for whole-process and on-site dynamic overseeing of treatments. The supplementary system for auditing treatments is able to automatically analyze patient information in real time. This has proven extremely effective in screening out irregular behavior and has improved the overall results of audited cases. Meanwhile, the district government has set up a system for reporting on visits to doctors who are outside the district, as well as a hotline for regulating such visits to non-local Grade Three hospitals. In addition, the Beijing branch of PICC works closely with the new rural cooperative insurance team to carry out publicity and educational activities on how to stay healthy.

4.4.4.2.4 Rear end: risk sharing mechanisms

Under the proportional co-insuring model, the government and the insurance company each bears the burden of 50% of the risk of compensation. In contrast to full-coverage insurance, this model puts a limit on the amount of compensation the insurance company is responsible for paying. This prevents the company from suffering massive losses due to excessive risk exposure. It also helps keep the funds in balance. For the purpose of regularly monitoring and controlling the funds, the Pinggu government has set forth quotas that control the total amount of funds that can be used and the total number of people who can be inpatients at the hospital. The way funds are being used is reported on at each monthly meeting. The extent to which each hospital's total figures are meeting the quotas is discussed, as well as any questions that are discovered in the course of normal investigations and audits by the Joint Office. Punishments for violations help keep risk within a controllable range. The co-insuring model is set up on the basis of actuarial balances. Since the insurance company assumes a portion of risk, this motivates the company to be proactive in using its strengths in risk management to prevent the excessive spending of funds in real time.

4.4.4.3 The supplementary type of relationship between social and commercial insurance

Supplementary insurance refers to situations when the insurance company agrees to provide coverage of certain health conditions on behalf of social insurance departments (government)—these are already included in the scope of coverage by basic medical insurance but they are more suited to being insured by commercial insurance than by publicly funded insurance. An example would be coverage for the risk of contracting a major disease. The two representative models in this instance are the Taicang Model and the Zhanjiang Model.

4.4.4.3.1 Taicang: secondary compensation based on actuarial balance

The Taicang model is based on integrating the three types of urban and rural insurance into one (see Figure 4.44). It uses the principle of maintaining an actuarial balance. By purchasing reinsurance, the model creates a secondary compensation mechanism for major illness. Systemic modifications allow the insurance company to make accurate predictions about spending on major disease—such things include being allowed to insure for things outside the list of items covered in regular policies, and eliminating the ceiling on compensation. The ability to share risk in a reasonable way is what ensures that major-disease insurance will move forward in a steady and stable way.

4.4.4.3.1.1 MAJOR COMPONENTS AND ACTUAL RESULTS IN PRACTICE

The Taicang model is an example of a private–public partnership which grants specific authorization for handling certain kinds of business. In 2011, the Department of Human Resources and Social Security and PICC Health signed a cooperative agreement by which the Department would purchase insurance from

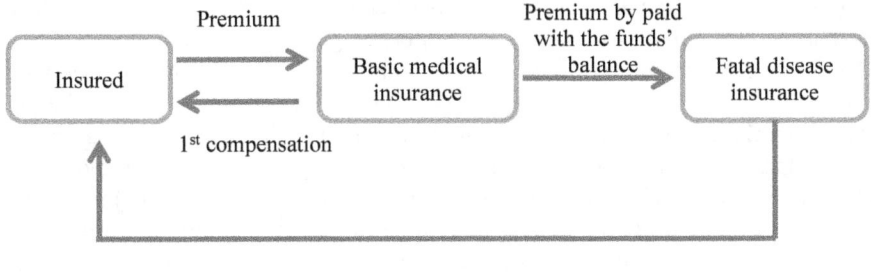

Figure 4.44 Taicang model.

PICC Health for items that fall outside the coverage of the basic medical insurance. The insurance was for major disease and hospitalization and was supplementary to social medical insurance—hospitalization expenses would receive secondary compensation. The deductible was set at RMB 10,000, and the percentage of reimbursable expenses after that was between 53% and 82% of costs, with a higher percentage the more the patient self-paid in costs. There was no ceiling on the amount.[54] The coverage breaks through the list of things that are reimbursable with respect to both drugs and treatments at the Suzhou Municipal Hospital. The only things that are not reimbursed are drugs outside the scope of the *Pharmacopoeia of the People's Republic of China*, and ten items such as artificial organs that exceed the price limits of social insurance.[55] In 2015, outpatient expenses were included into the coverage, for which the deductible is set at RMB 3,000 and the compensation is 50%~66%, without a ceiling.[56] Once the Taicang Model began to be put in effect, coverage reached 99% of the population. The financial burden of healthcare was clearly reduced for policy holders and the level of fairness was somewhat improved. Through the regressive compensation and periodic settlement of individual's self-paid expenses, medical resources are now more inclined to flow toward patients with major disease. The Taicang Model alleviates the phenomenon of being 'driven into poverty or back into poverty as a result of illness.' In a public-benefiting system, namely the basic medical insurance system, it allows for more or 'special' benefits on top of the fundamentals.

4.4.4.3.1.2 FRONT END: SUSTAINABLE FINANCING

The Taicang Model is essentially a way for social insurance to purchase reinsurance from commercial insurance, for the purpose of insuring major illness. The social insurance entity uses funds in the medical insurance fund to pay the premiums. The per capita amount of funding is set at RMB 50 per year per individual account in the urban basic medical insurance, and RMB 20 per year per account in the urban and rural residents' medical insurance account (people insured under this include non-formally employed residents as well as rural residents).[57] The prerequisite for this program to work involves a fairly high level of funds consolidation and a substantial balance of funds available in the medical insurance fund. This also provides an important guarantee for ongoing funding. The Taicang Model adheres to the fundamental principles of insurance. The incidence of major disease is small but losses can be huge. Because of this, the per capita premiums can be small yet the total funding is still enough to cover spending on catastrophic medical events. This is a manifestation of the mutual-aid nature of insurance. Generally speaking, spending on compensation for major disease takes up only 3% to 4% of the balance of medical insurance funds, a figure which is fully affordable by the Taicang municipal social insurance department. The program also satisfies the requirement that the social insurance fund increase in value, and it satisfies the need for funding to be sustainable.

4.4.4.3.1.3 MIDDLE: CONTROL OF COSTS

In the Taicang Model, the insurance company is inserted into the tripartite system of social insurance entity, hospital, and insured person. This builds a way to control costs into the system due to the supervisory function of the insurance company, which oversees spending on medical services. The social insurance entity delegates its authority to review medical costs to the commercial insurance company. The company uses its professional expertise to inspect hospitalization practices, supervise expenses, and do sample checks on cases. It then reports to the social insurance authorities on the results. Based on these results, the authorities impose penalties for any violations of regulations. At the same time, the social insurance authorities exercise regulatory control over the insurance company, including control over profits. Each of the two parties, social and commercial insurance, carries out their respective roles, one as the judge or 'umpire' and the other as the 'player.' This prevents medical costs from growing too quickly and it also allows for government to transition from being actively engaged in business to becoming a regulator of business.

4.4.4.3.1.4 REAR END: RISK-SHARING MECHANISMS

The Taicang Model adheres to the idea of 'conserving principal while allowing for a modest profit while sharing risk.' Once the profit-loss ratio exceeds 5%, the rule is that both parties take an equal share in the amount over that figure. This establishes a risk-sharing mechanism for insuring major illness, on the basis of an actuarial balance. It ensures the stability and sustainability of operations. 'Conserving principal while allowing for a modest profit while sharing risk' is fully in line with the desire of the insurance company to make a profit, while it also shares risk in a reasonable way. This is conducive to ensuring the stability of the whole system. The funding for insuring major illness, and the compensation standards, are determined on the basis of an actuarial balance. They take into consideration the deductible amount, the list of reimbursable items that are covered, and so on, but they are also subject to dynamic adjustment according to actual expenditure items. Systemic adjustments that allow the insurance company to reimburse for items not on the national list, and that allow for removing the ceiling on compensation, enable the insurer to create accurate estimates of spending on major disease, and to avoid running through the funds in the social insurance account. Effective integration with the basic medical insurance system is a vital precondition for the model to work, for people to feel that taking out insurance for major illness is getting them something in return. A whole series of mechanisms provide powerful support for the sustainability of the Taicang Model, including risk sharing, return of surpluses to both parties, adjustment of funding depending on aggregate risk, and so on.

4.4.4.3.2 The Zhanjiang Model: new-type reinsurance that features commercial insurer's participation in value-added businesses of social security funds

The Zhanjiang Model is a prime example of insuring major illness through the practice of buying reinsurance (see Figure 4.45). It alleviates the problem of 'being driven into poverty as a result of illness,' since it raises the ceiling on the maximum amount of compensation. It uses premiums that are already being paid into the medical insurance fund and thereby does not increase the financial burden on policy holders. A reasonable amount of risk sharing and disclosure of public finances allows for the ongoing ability to insure for major illness, and means the practice of 'maintaining the principal and making a small profit' can be continued. This motivates the insurance company to participate and it guarantees steady operations of the insurance for major illness.

4.4.4.3.2.1 MAIN COMPONENTS OF THE ZHANJIANG MODEL AND RESULTS IN ACTUAL PRACTICE

The Zhanjiang Model is a prime example of cooperation between social and commercial insurance in economically backward regions. Prior to introducing

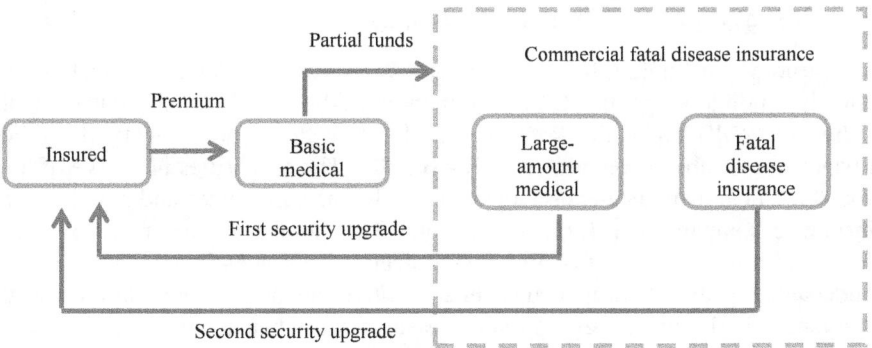

Figure 4.45 Zhanjiang model.

the system of reinsurance for major illness, in 2009, the Zhanjiang municipal government combined the two 'tracks' or systems of insurance that previously had been called the new rural cooperative insurance and the urban residents' medical insurance. It set up a universal medical insurance system that unified the insuring of both urban and rural residents. This raised coverage for basic medical insurance from 85% of the population in 2009 to 92.8% in 2015.[58] It dealt with urban and countryside as one unit and it pooled funding at the municipal level. In 2012, Zhanjiang set up a system for insuring major illness in order to improve the degree of safeguards provided under this basic insurance. The municipal government authorized the Zhanjiang Branch of PICC to handle its basic medical insurance at no cost to the government, but at the same time the government purchased insurance coverage for major illness from PICC through a standard insurance contract. The account of the city's insurance fund was divided into two parts, one for 'spending for compensation of insurance claims' and the other for 'purchase of insurance for major illness.' The fiscal spending of the government did not change, nor did the payments of individuals. Thirty percent of the insurance fund was now used to buy large-sum supplementary medical insurance from the insurance company.

Within the scope of what is insured by the insurance, individual's self-paid expenses are reimbursed at two different levels depending on amount paid out. The percentages are 50% and 80%, with the higher percentage reimbursed for greater self-paid amounts. The two ceilings for compensated amounts are RMB 300,000 and RMB 500,000.[59] To a certain degree, this substantial increase in the amount that can be reimbursed has alleviated the problem of people being driven into poverty as a result of major illness. In terms of getting reimbursed for treatment, the residents of Zhanjiang can opt to undergo medical treatment in any of the city's 182 designated hospitals. They can be referred to non-local hospitals or vice versa, and can receive immediate reimbursement. This not only reduces the amount of time a resident spends on insurance issues, but it resolves the problem of uneven geographic distribution of medical resources and the resulting difficulty some people have in accessing medical care.

4.4.4.3.2.2 FRONT END: SUSTAINABLE FUNDING

The structure of funding for the Zhanjiang urban-rural residents' medical insurance is: 'individual payments + government subsidies.' Individuals contribute at either the RMB 50 or the RMB 80 level, while the various levels of public finance pay a subsidy per person of RMB 320.[60] The authorities in charge of the social medical insurance excise a portion of the insurance fund and pay it to the insurance company as a form of premium. This purchases insurance coverage for major illness on behalf of all policy holders. The system is predicated on the understanding that there is a substantial positive balance of funds in the social insurance fund and that appropriate measures are taken to mitigate risk. The Zhanjiang Model has improved the efficiency of health insurance as well as level of safeguards, but has done so without increasing spending on the part of the government or increasing payments on the part of Zhanjiang residents. It is therefore highly sustainable.

4.4.4.3.2.3 MIDDLE: COST CONTROL

The commercial insurance company and social insurance authorities have combined forces and jointly carry out a number of tasks, including inspection rounds of medical services, auditing of compensation cases, settlement of expenses, management of files containing policy holders' information, performance evaluations of designated hospitals, and review of qualifications for opening an outpatient clinic. As authorized by the social insurance authorities, the commercial insurance company has assembled a team for making rounds to check on medical services. It has personnel stationed at each of the high-volume top-class (Grade Three) hospitals, as well as travelling teams that check on other hospitals. It conducts strict audits of the costs of major illness insurance and investigates such fraudulent behavior as false claims and fake registration at hospitals, in order to reduce improper spending.

The system of payments made to hospitals operates on an advance-payment basis. At the beginning of each month, the administrative authority governing the social insurance fund disperses 80% of the average monthly amount for the previous year to a designated hospital. It waits to disperse another 10% until the end of that month, after the audit by the administration has cleared, and it settles up the remaining 10% at the end of the year, depending on whether or not the hospital meets its targets. If medical costs for policy holders at a hospital exceed the total allocation for the hospital in that same year, then the hospital must bear the cost of the extra spending. This effectively controls the increase in improper medical spending at the source.

4.4.4.3.2.4 REAR END: RISK SHARING MECHANISMS

When the social insurance fund operates at a loss, the ultimate responsibility for paying bills rests with the public-finance department of the local government. This ensures that the social insurance fund does not run out of money. At the same time, the commercial insurance company and social insurance entities agree in advance on a flexible way to deal with profit and loss in the fund. That is, if either profits or losses are within 3% of the total that year, the People's Insurance Company of China handles the profit or loss on its own. If premium income exceeds 3% of the total amount that year, PICC extracts 50% of the amount that is over and deposits it into the urban-rural residents' medical insurance fund. If losses are more than 3% of the total in that year, the company shares 50% of the extra cost with the medical insurance fund.[61] If, however, catastrophic losses occur in the plan for insuring major illness, then supplementary clauses in the agreement are brought into effect by which the public finance authorities in the local government step in to increase public funds. This is to make sure that the major illness insurance is able to maintain principal while allowing for modest profit. Appropriate risk-sharing helps the insurance company control risks and ensures the sustainability of Zhanjiang Model.

4.4.5 Summary of China's experience

The above ways in which commercial and social insurance cooperate can be divided into three general types, depending on the relationship between the commercial insurance company and China's publicly-funded basic medical insurance. Those three are defined as 'handling (or undertaking),' 'cooperative,' and 'supplementary.' Irrespective of whether commercial insurance is authorized to handle basic medical insurance, or whether it simply provides secondary compensation for major illness insurance, all forms of cooperation inevitably require close integration with the basic medical insurance system and they require the insertion of commercial insurance into that system. That is how they are able to build a healthcare system that provides universal coverage and strong safeguards. The following conclusions come from summarizing the experience of various places.

First, cooperative models between commercial and social insurance must be informed by local conditions. China's small and dispersed style of agriculture determines the fact that any attempt to improve rural medical safeguards has to suit local conditions. The degree of economic development, extent of public finance, cultural and ethnic features of each part of China are different. The way in which medical insurance is administered has to be different, as well as the list of things that are covered under insurance. Forms of cooperation must respect the realities of different places and must try to devise the optimum model for each place.

Second, forms of cooperation should be based on county-level public finance. Since China's agriculture is small-scale and dispersed, at the most granular level this mode of agriculture determines the fact that the funding for rural medicine is also dispersed. The fundamental point about the funding of China's rural medicine is that it depends on the finances of the county. Because of this, it is hard for China to adopt one optimum development model that applies universally when it looks at financing rural healthcare. China can only adopt models that may be second-best overall but are actually best when it comes to a specific place. Such models must match the level of economic development, condition of public finance, and cultural and ethnic features of the place.

Third, mandatory supplementary health insurance can be developed by embedding new policies in the system. In the Jiangyin Model, to get supplementary commercial health insurance people voluntarily pay fees, and those who do can enjoy remote medical services. For a relatively low premium, such insertion of value-added services can actually result in universal coverage of supplementary health insurance. This shows that developing the new public-benefiting insurance through systems design can bring about supplementary health insurance that is invisibly mandatory. On the basis of this now-universal coverage, the degree of safeguards can gradually be improved.

Fourth, the key to realizing powerful safeguards lies in breaking through the confines of the reimbursement list in a sustainable way. Since the start of the new medical reform, China has basically put in place universal coverage. In order to go further now and reach the goal of stronger safeguards, it is crucial to increase the percentage of claims that can be reimbursed, to lower self-paid fees, and to break through the restrictions of the list of drugs and medical services that can be reimbursed under basic medical insurance. One of the key objectives of the cooperation between social and commercial insurance must be to break through this list in a sustainable way.

Fifth, the insertion of commercial insurance into the system is of ultimate important in pulling together a healthcare industrial chain. Commercial insurance has professional expertise in many areas including information management, statistical analysis, and policy consulting. Inserting companies into the funding and payment process of medical insurance can improve the unequal status of commercial insurance with respect to hospitals, and can enable companies to play an important role in overseeing how patients are being treated in hospitals. On that basis, by making use of the force of capital, commercial health insurance can help build an entire system that has preventive medicine and health management at the front end, reasonable levels of treatment in the middle, and rehabilitation and long-term nursing care at the end.

Sixth, risk-balancing mechanisms that are based on actuarial laws are the key to sustainable development of the industry. It is crucial to make accurate use of insurance, to allow insurance for major illness to play a supplementary role, and to establish risk-sharing mechanisms that are reasonable. We can only control risk at the rear end effectively through accurate understanding of the 'insurance' attributes of major illness insurance, and by setting prices scientifically through relying on the laws of big data and actuarial rules. Only then can we realize a situation in which insurance funds are being put to use in a stable and sustainable way.

4.5 COMMERCIAL HEALTH INSURANCE IN CHINA FROM A NEW, PUBLIC-BENEFITING PERSPECTIVE: PRINCIPLES, APPROACHES, AND POLICY RECOMMENDATIONS

4.5.1 Principles: maintaining a balanced approach

4.5.1.1 Give equal weight to fairness and efficiency

Indicators about fairness look at the coverage rate of the basic medical insurance system as well as degree of security. Indicators about efficiency stress such things as controlling medical costs and improving the quality of services. Given that we must have social insurance achieve broad coverage, we should take advantage of the market mechanisms of commercial insurance to raise operating efficiencies. We use it to realize sustainability in the front-end process of pooling funds, to achieve real results in the middle processes in terms of holding down expenses, and to achieve a rebalancing of risk at the rear end. Ultimately, the goal is to establish a new public-benefiting health insurance system that has powerful safeguards and is stable and sustainable.

4.5.1.2 *Give equal weight to government and market*

The 'benefits' attribute of the new public-benefiting insurance requires that China's medical reform take advantage of both government and the market. The reform should use the government's administrative power and ability to concentrate and deploy resources. Government can achieve very broad coverage through mandatory-like methods of requiring insurance. It can set up risk-adjusting mechanisms and resolve issues of adverse selection, while realizing rebalancing of risk and sustainable development. The medical reform should also, however, make use of the market's regulating mechanisms. It should introduce competition and incentives into the business, and should allow commercial health insurance companies to participate in establishing a managed style of medicine.

4.5.1.3 *Give equal weight to risk and rewards*

Mandatory insurance and prices that are set by the public raise the level of risk for insurance companies. This is one side of the equation. Dealing with this requires using risk-adjusting mechanisms and reinsurance mechanisms in order to dissolve the possible systemic risk. On the other side of the equation, the system must satisfy the desire on the part of commercial health insurance companies to make a reasonable profit. It therefore should allow insurance companies to offer options that carry a certain degree of risk when providing supplemental health insurance. Companies should be allowed to offer expanded-type and additional-type health insurance for customers with special needs, in order to strengthen their ability to make a profit.

4.5.1.4 *Give equal weight to regions themselves and the disparities among regions*

Given China's vast territory and uneven economic development, there are obvious disparities between cities and rural areas and between the basic medical insurance systems of each. Models for growth are different as well as the degree to which these models work. In developing the new public-benefiting style of health insurance, we must respect these differences and seek to apply appropriate solutions and development models. Given that, however, we must also make every effort to reduce the difference in medical insurance treatment among regions and the disparity in quality of services. The aim is to achieve a high level of fairness and public benefit.

4.5.2 Approaches to take in developing commercial health insurance

4.5.2.1 Adapt solutions to local conditions. Segment China's market for commercial health insurance by region. Encourage different places to adopt models that suit the local conditions and encourage medical insurance systems to experiment with innovative approaches

Since China's agriculture is small-scale and dispersed, at the most granular level this mode of agriculture determines the fact that the funding for rural medicine is also dispersed. The fundamental point about the funding of China's rural medicine is that it depends on the finances of the county. To develop the new public-benefiting insurance, we should bear in the mind the actual conditions of county finances. We should give full consideration to regional characteristics. We should aim for appropriate solutions to local conditions while also attempting to achieve synergy across regions. In addition, we need overall systemic support from the Central Government.

1   Development models should suit local needs. With respect to how to improve their health insurance systems, different regions should use a unified approach that is within the framework of the new public-benefiting insurance, but they also should segment the market and encourage the use of models that are appropriate for local conditions.
2   Maintain synergies between regions. Being defined by region does not mean being closed off. The insurance markets of each region should have open competition with one another. Using the health exchanges as a platform, they should allow consumers to make their own choices and allow capital and manpower to flow freely. The aim is to strengthen synergy and mutual assistance.
3   Set up a national laboratory for exploring innovative approaches to medical insurance. We should establish a national laboratory to support systemic innovations in medical insurance and to support reforms. It should provide models for such things as new payment methods and medical services that have been tested and proven effective, for use throughout the country.

4.5.2.2 Synergistic efforts from both the demand and supply sides

4.5.2.2.1 Innovations on the supply side

The emphasis of product research and development should be on improving and extending the industrial chain as well as segmenting it into different tiers. In terms of improving the industrial chain, insurance companies should use their expertise in actuarial science and risk management to improve safeguards and also the actual percentage of reimbursement of claims for major illness and chronic disease. In terms of extending the chain, insurance companies should gradually shift their focus from post-event compensation to pre-event preventive medicine and disease management. In terms of segmenting the chain, insurers may target special-needs groups and high-end customers for individualized products.

Product pricing should be allowed to segment the market by regions, and mandatory and voluntary health insurance products should be regulated separately. With respect to mandatory health insurance products, the public itself should set pricing by regions. Insurance companies are forbidden to refuse insurance to people or select the levels of risk they choose to insure. With respect to expanded-type and additional-type insurance products, however, insurance companies may make their own decisions on acceptable levels of risk and may also set pricing based on actuarial principles.

With respect to claims settlement, we should incorporate mechanisms that relate to managed medicine, with the aim being to control costs and make reimbursement more convenient for the patient. First, that means constantly trying to simplify the payment process—ultimately, the insurance entity should settle with the hospital directly and in real time. Second, it means creating new methods for figuring payment. The insurance company may use a variety of methods to calculate reimbursements to hospitals, including by type of disease, by person, by a lump sum, and so on. Meanwhile, insurance companies must strengthen routine audits as well as targeted audits and they should be proactive in monitoring medical practices.

With respect to regulation, health insurance should be regulated as a separate industry given its unique nature and given its risks.[62] This will require improving China's statistical and actuarial systems and the systems that apply to financial accounting. We should establish tables on incidence of disease and incidence of losses.[63] We should push forward regulatory systems that address health insurance compensation rates and set limits on medical compensation rates.[64]

With respect to taxation, we should establish preferential tax policies on health insurance earnings as a way to stimulate the growth of the health insurance industry. In levying the value-added tax, this means policies that lower the tax rate on premium income or exempting the tax altogether. In levying the income tax on company earnings, this means learning from the experience of developed countries and adopting a floating rate in order to lower corporate income taxes.[65]

With respect to administrative permits, we should explicitly define market-entry requirements and should also loosen requirements to the appropriate degree. We should make every effort to reform the system of certification that applies to health insurance entities. That includes setting up defined standards for market entry, standardizing the process of market entry, and encouraging social (private) capital to invest in the health insurance industry.

With respect to technology, we should apply big data and Internet-based smart technologies as well as refined management techniques to the research and development of products, healthcare services, and managed medicine. We should use advanced information technologies to make full use of data mining of customer demand and to guide customers in the direction of healthy behavior, and we should realize a situation in which data collection, analysis, and monitoring link directly to hospital systems.

4.5.2.2.2 Innovations on the demand side

We should go further in granting preferential tax treatment to buyers of health insurance. For individual buyers, this means raising the amount that can be deducted from individual income as a result of paying premiums, and it also means tilting the policy incentive in the direction of low- and middle-income people. For group buyers of insurance, including corporations and employees, we should lower or exempt taxes and increase the percentage of allowable pre-tax expenses.

With respect to organizational initiatives, we should make every attempt to have more forms of group insurance that are available to consumers. We should encourage corporations, institutions, community organizations, and groups of people suffering from specific diseases, such as diabetes, to take the initiative in purchasing group insurance. In that regard, we should set up third-party exchange platforms, and allow individual consumers to purchase health insurance as part of a group plan so as to get a discount on premiums.

We should set up pilot programs in super-large organizations that experiment with self-insuring employees' health, as an example of encouraging all kinds of demand-side systemic innovations. As test sites, we can relax regulatory restrictions on such super-large entities as institutes of higher education and allow them to self-insure their employees. In such instances, they would in turn grant insurance companies the authority to provide third-party management services and be responsible for underwriting policies, carrying out claims settlement, setting up case files, managing data, and controlling medical costs.

With respect to 'smart' medical technologies, such things as Internet-based technologies and Internet-of-Things technologies can be applied to managing the health of policy holders. That would include the whole process from diagnosis to post-illness nursing, and it would allow for integrating preventive medicine, treatment, and rehabilitation. Through the O2O (online-to-online) model of health insurance, it is possible to set up a closed medical services cycle that integrates health management, online consultation, offline first diagnosis, online re-diagnosis, online drug purchase and delivery, real-time health information monitoring, and nursing care after medical treatment.[66]

4.5.2.2.3 Synergistic efforts

The path taken by the new public-benefiting insurance is a third route that combines the efforts of government and the market. Its core concept is to turn social medical insurance into a marketable commodity and thereby enable it to be provided by a third party, namely insurance agencies. As intermediaries, they manage the entire process from evaluation to budgeting to quotas, payment, and supervision.

4.5.2.3 *Improving security in a progressive manner*

The new public-benefiting insurance system consists of three layers of security: quasi-compulsory supplementary health insurance, expanded-type health insurance and additional-type health insurance to meet special demands (see Figure 4.46).

The outer layer is the most crucial in terms of realizing public benefits. It involves providing a standardized package of supplementary health insurance provisions which include the following: reimbursement of self-paid expenses that fall within the medical insurance list, reimbursement of drugs and treatment services that are outside the list, management of chronic illnesses, long-term care, and so on. This supplementary insurance is aimed at everyone and is to make up for inadequacies of the basic medical insurance, particularly those people suffering from chronic disease, the elderly, and the disabled.

Health insurance at this layer should rely on public pricing and should abide by the principle of mutual assistance within society. While this is a quasi-mandatory form of insurance, at the same time it should be paid for by everyone's sharing the burden, with limited subsidies. Each provincial government can determine what the level of disposable income should be for receiving subsidies—if disposable income is below a certain level, the government may provide an appropriate amount of public-finance subsidies in order to pay premiums. For people whose disposable income is above the threshold, the mandatory nature of supplementary health insurance means they should be granted tax relief.

The second and third layers are market-oriented commercial health insurance. The public-benefiting nature of the insurance and market profitability can be harmonized by having an appropriate degree of sharing but also by segmenting the high end of the market. The primary audience for expanded-type insurance is middle- and high-income groups of people. This offers insurance for such things as preventive medicine and disease interventions, fitness and rehabilitation, psychological issues, dental and vision assistance, and so on. Additional-type insurance mainly targets the special needs of high-end customers by offering them high-end services. It offers channels for going abroad for medical care and precision medical services. The insurance company itself conducts a risk analysis and sets prices according to the incidence of diseases.

In terms of the spectrum of products, single disease insurance, as represented by critical illness insurance, plays a certain role but should not occupy too great a percentage of the totality of products. Moreover, as the spectrum of diseases changes in China, the safeguards provided under a critical illness policy should be expanded to the appropriate degree. Priority should be given to developing advance-payment types of products.[67]

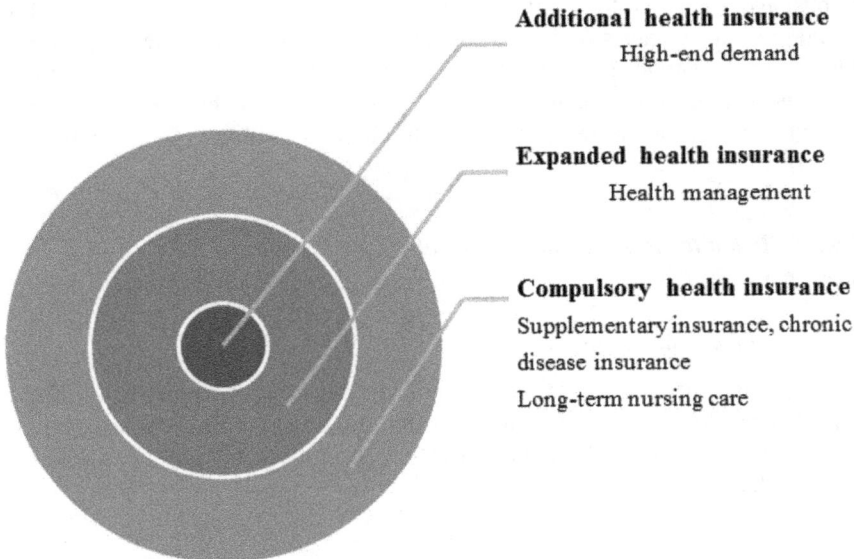

Additional health insurance
High-end demand

Expanded health insurance
Health management

Compulsory health insurance
Supplementary insurance, chronic
disease insurance
Long-term nursing care

Figure 4.46 Three-layer progressive structure of China's public-benefiting commercial
health insurance.

4.5.2.4 Complete integration: integrate social insurance and commercial insurance resources by using 'Pharmacy Benefit Managers.' Link up technology, organization, information, and resources

'Cooperation, sharing, and co-existing' is fundamentally a matter of making sure that insurance data, information, and resources are interconnected between the two kinds of insurance. We recommend that the starting point for this kind of integration be the model called 'Pharmacy Benefit Managers' (PBM). Pharmacy Benefit Managers tie together resources related to medicine, social insurance, and commercial insurance. These entities sign contracts with pharmaceutical companies, medical services organizations, and insurance companies. The core purpose of this is to lower overall spending on medical costs, with the understanding that the quality of medical services will not be compromised, and to increase the utility of pharmaceuticals. The experience in the United States can serve as a reference for specific forms of cooperation. One form is that the insurance company either sets up a PBM company directly or it acquires one. The prime example is OptumRX under United Health, which is the largest health insurance company in the U.S. OptumRX is a pharmacy benefit management company. A second acquisition is that of Aetna by CVS Health, which owns the second-largest PBM in America. The situation in China at the present is that 'medicine' and 'pharmaceuticals' have not yet separated into two different lines of business. Meanwhile, pharmacies are prohibited from selling drugs online. Certain policy obstacles prevent insurance companies from cooperating directly with pharmaceutical companies. As policies gradually remove constraints, however, insurance companies will move deeply into this business, particularly if the next step is to remove the prohibition on selling prescription drugs online.[68]

4.5.2.5 Risk allocation: create a risk balancing fund and a reinsurance system

4.5.2.5.1 Risk balancing mechanisms

We have investigated the ways in which developed countries handle risk overall. With respect to risk balancing mechanisms, this report has also designed two models that might apply to China's situation, the American Model and the European Model.

4.5.2.5.1.1 AMERICAN MODEL

In the American Model, the risk-balancing mechanisms of the new public-benefiting insurance are divided into two parts. One is the risk allocation program, and the other is the transitional risk corridor. The risk allocation program is a permanent (government-funded) program. Its main purpose is to balance the cost differences among insurance companies. The risk corridor is a transitional type of program, an institutional arrangement. It is used to deal with mistakes in evaluating risk during the early period, when technologies are not yet mature.

4.5.2.5.1.1(a) Risk allocation program

Institutional framework: The province is the unit of administration. Under this program, provincial authorities set up risk adjustment plans for the new public-benefiting insurance. All insurance companies that offer mandatory supplementary health insurance policies must participate, by regulatory fiat. The program sets up a risk fund at the provincial level of administration, which is a funding (or funds pooling) organization (see Figure 4.47). Funds are assembled from within the risk balancing system. Transfer payments are made between insurance companies with high and low risk. The net payments of the entire system come to zero.

Methods of evaluating risk: Based on risk factors,[69] the objective is to calculate the risk score of each insurance company that provides mandatory supplementary health insurance. Once that is done, then the average risk score for all companies within the province is calculated. Companies who score higher than the average must pay out into the fund. Those who score lower are able to receive risk compensation. Risk allocation is mainly a

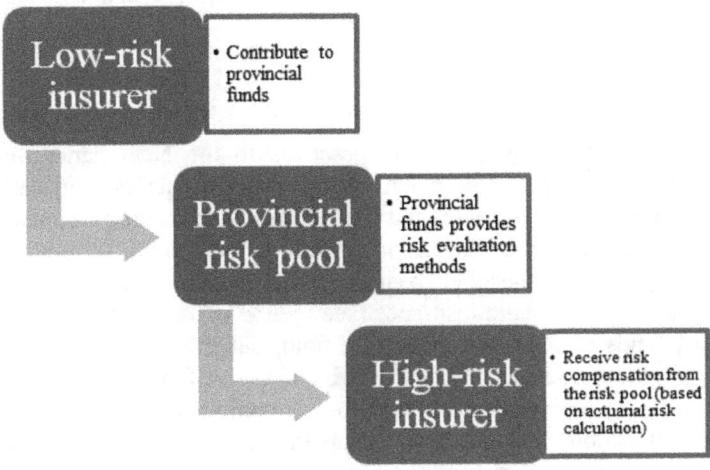

Figure 4.47 Risk balance of new public-benefiting insurance.

matter of cross-subsidies among insurance companies and of transfer payments. It does not involve the insertion of public finance in any way. It is meant to achieve a balance between premium income and expected medical expenses.

Design of the risk-evaluation model: Risk evaluation models mainly include three types, prospective type, consistent type, and retrospective type. In the early period of setting up the system (the first one to three years), the consistent model will be applied which uses information on demographics from that same year and estimated cost of diagnoses for that same year. Once the risk allocation program is more mature, the database on health statistics will be set up and information from hospitals and insurance will be interconnected. Given that foundation of data, it will be possible to introduce the prospective model and make risk compensation arrangements in advance. If advance compensation turns out to be inadequate, then the system can introduce the retrospective model to accomplish post-event compensation. Post-event compensation should not, however, exceed 20% of risk compensation costs.

4.5.2.5.1.1(b) Transitional risk corridor

The risk corridor program is a transitional program (three years), with a risk fund operated at the provincial level. At the outset, the funds will be injected into the program from public finance. The risk corridor program is mainly set up to alleviate mistakes made in the course of evaluating the cost of risk and therefore to supplement the actual costs of insurance companies. If actual costs diverge from the target value by more than 3%, then the provincial level risk fund is responsible for making up the difference. Companies with an excess in their balance of funds must pay into the fund; companies that overspent on costs can receive supplementary compensation.

4.5.2.5.1.2 EUROPEAN MODEL

The European model is mainly based on practices in the Netherlands and Germany. This plan sets up a risk balancing mechanism that is constantly updated, based on incidence of disease, and uses the province as the administrative unit. It involves setting up a risk-balancing fund in each province. Sources of funds include government subsidies, basic medical insurance premiums, and the mandatory supplemental health insurance (see Figure 4.48). The government directly allocates funds into the risk balancing fund, but it also provides subsidies in the form of tax revenues. The latter two sources of funds are collected from local social insurance departments and from commercial insurance companies. The risk-allocation funds are divvied up in a uniform way within the province, and are for pre-event risk adjustment and post-event risk compensation. Pre-event risk allocation funds are based on the forecasted estimate of what insurance companies will have to reimburse to policy holders for spending on medical costs in a given year, under the mandatory supplemental health insurance policies. (See reference to the Netherlands, section 4.4.1.1.3.)[70] Since pre-event adjustment mechanisms may not be completely accurate, it is necessary to make further adjustments by using post-event compensation mechanisms at the end of a given year. Post-event compensation mechanisms include limits on costs and outlier risk sharing.

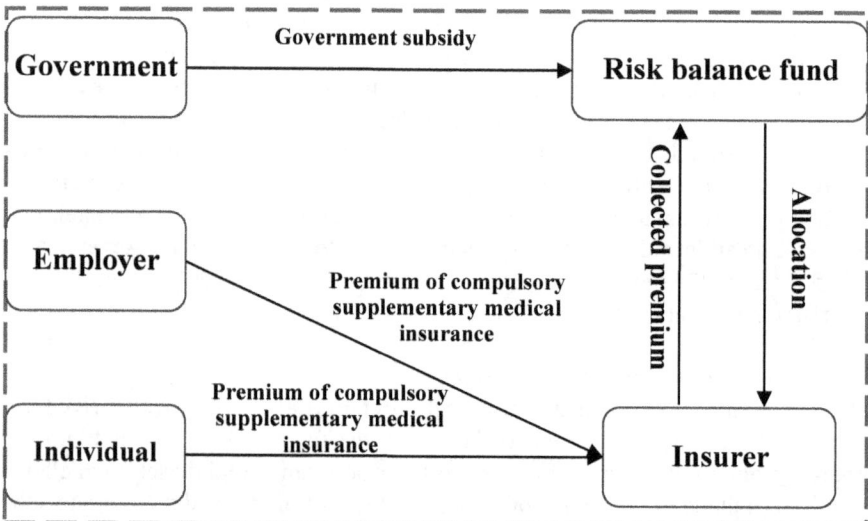

Figure 4.48 Provincial risk balance mechanism.

4.5.2.5.2 Reinsurance mechanisms

To mitigate the large-sum risk of excessive spending on medical costs, we should set up reinsurance companies at two administrative levels, regional and national. The regional reinsurance companies mainly have three functions. First, they reinsure the policies of the social insurance (government) departments. Second, they reinsure the policies of insurance companies who insure for mandatory supplemental health insurance. Third, they reinsure the policies of insurance companies who insure for voluntary-type policies. The national reinsurance companies take the dispersal of risk a step further by covering risk across all jurisdictions.

4.5.3 Policy proposals

After summing up the situation of commercial health insurance in China, including its positioning, principles for its development, and paths by which it can develop, we present the following nine main recommendations. The first three relate to top-level design. The middle three are policy recommendations regarding the industry. The last three take a micro perspective in making specific policy recommendations.

4.5.3.1 Strengthen systemic design at the top-tier level of government

4.5.3.1.1 We recommend establishing a national laboratory for innovations in medical insurance

In terms of technology, setting up such a laboratory will provide powerful support for China's reform of medical insurance and for implementation of the Healthy China strategic plan. It will provide a storehouse of technology that can be used to raise the efficiency of China's social insurance and medical insurance systems. It will mainly have the following responsibilities.

1   Based on systemic innovations in the payment of medical insurance which are value enhancing, this laboratory should lead the way to fundamental reform of controls over medical costs. It should use the American Center for Medicare and Medicaid Innovation as a model in how to operate. The primary task of China's equivalent will be to develop, research, test, and take charge of implementing a new form of payment system. The current traditional method of payment will move toward an improved method that is based on medical results. Controlling medical costs is an immediate goal for the present, but the ultimate goal of innovations in medical insurance must be to raise the value of medical services, so that patients have the sense they are getting something in return for their medical expenditures.

2   The laboratory should set up systems for evaluating China's medical services and its medical insurance system, including appraisal standards. It

should also conduct an in-depth evaluation of China's experience and lessons that have been learned. It should speed up the process of improving standards by which to evaluate the quality of China's medicine and its system of providing services. In this regard, it may take the system used in the United States as a point of reference. This system evaluates from a number of perspectives, including a ranking of medical institutions, evaluation of medical quality, degree of satisfaction on the part of patients, and so on.[71] In addition, the lab should set up evaluation standards for appraising the effectiveness of cooperation between social and commercial insurance. China must set up a system of standards for evaluating basic medical insurance that can converse in the same language with global standards in this field. On the one hand, the lab should summarize the experiences of the past and lessons learned, but on the other it should serve as a compass for guiding China's future health insurance system.

3   The lab should set up actuarial balancing standards and basic norms for tenders for underwriting major illness insurance. We recommend that the Taicang Model be publicized and promoted, that is, the 'actuarial balance' method. Only after basic standards have been formulated and basic rules for major-illness actuarial balancing have been set up can we take the next step to competitive bidding.

4   The lab should provide support for other key technologies. This refers particularly to standards for building China's medical insurance high-speed information highway. It should push forward the interconnectedness of medical insurance information, and should avoid the current situation in which the Ministry of Health, Ministry of Human Resources and Social Security, and China Insurance Regulatory Commission have all set up different standards for transactions. This should be an entity that is led by government but independent and that works out the national standards for medical insurance transactions. It should be the entity to establish China's medical information highway.

4.5.3.1.2 We recommend establishing China Health Insurance Exchanges

The establishment of health insurance exchanges in China will form a new platform for balancing supply and demand. The products traded on the exchanges, 'basic medical safeguards packages,' should comply with standardized regulations in terms of coverage of safeguards, setting of fees, sharing of costs, actuarial values, and so on. Only when consumers buy policies through the exchange can they enjoy subsidies from public finance and preferential tax treatment. Policies offered outside of the exchanges do not need to comply with standards or requirements, but they are still subject to the same degree of regulatory oversight.

4.5.3.1.3 We recommend setting up risk balancing mechanisms for China's health insurance

China's risk balancing mechanisms for health insurance are essentially non-existent. Despite that, whether you take the United States or Europe, risk-balancing mechanisms are a core systemic requirement for the development of health insurance. We recommend:

1 With funding at the provincial level of government administration, set up a risk-balancing mechanism that is based on incidence of disease. Use the risk evaluation model and risk factors to calculate the risk scores and expected medical costs of each insurance company within the system so as to allocate risk between high- and low-cost companies.
2 Risk factors should take into consideration the age, gender, region, cost group of pharmaceuticals, and cost group of diagnosis, among other factors. As the risk-balancing mechanism is applied, factors should be added or deleted. Risk adjustment should primarily be pre-event, with post-event compensation done as a supplementary measure to minimize moral hazard.
3 In the early period of applying the risk-balancing mechanism, the risk corridor can be used as a transitional systemic arrangement in order to make up for losses of insurers as a result of inaccurate risk evaluations.

4.5.3.2 Take a firm middle-road perspective with regard to industry policy

4.5.3.2.1 Managing the demand side

Encourage organizational innovations that take a variety of forms, allow organizations to operate on both a for-profit and not-for-profit basis in order to enrich the forms by which consumers can purchase insurance. Encourage all kinds of demand-side systemic innovations. First: encourage the purchase of group health insurance through such things as third-party exchange platforms, enterprises, institutions, community organizations, and self-organized groups of people with particular diseases such as diabetes. Second: set up pilot programs that test the use of self-insurance by employees in super-large organizations. For example, employees of universities could experiment with allowing a self-insurance component on top of the government reimbursement program with the self-insured premiums receiving preferential income tax treatment.

4.5.3.2.2 Taking a sequential approach

Take a staged and planned-out approach to gradually setting up managed care in China. Make use of the role of commercial health insurance companies to restructure the value chain of China's medical services.

Create the conditions, both institutional and policy-wise, that enable commercial health insurance companies to enter into the process of paying medical insurance payments, as a first step, and then into the entire process of controlling medical expenses. Use market forces to restructure the value chain of China's medical services. In order to set up an effective form of managed care in China, we must do the following.

1　Shift the priority away from just payment of medical expenses to things like improving the quality of medical services and health education. After insurance companies take on the role of handling basic medical insurance, they must be proactive in evaluating and supervising the quality of hospitals. They should participate in the pricing of medical services and the reform of payment methods, among other activities.

2　Make full use of the leverage and guiding role that the medical payments system can have on medical services, as well as the support it can provide for setting up a tiered medical care system. Through models such as HMO (Health Maintenance Organization) and PPO (Preferred Provider Organization), and through economic leverage, mandatory referrals, and other methods, stimulate the formation of a tiered medical care system that consists of 'first diagnosis at the grassroots level, two-way referrals, separate kinds of treatment for emergency and chronic cases, and top-to-bottom synergies.'

3　Set up a managed-care form of medicine in China, by taking advantage of the reform that will eliminate the institutional system that governs public hospitals (reform of the *bianzhi* system). Encourage social forces (private forces) to manage medical facilities and work to establish a diversified pattern of ownership of medical organizations. Encourage insurance companies to become involved in medical care through audits of medical services and supervision of medical quality.[72] By using general practitioners as gatekeepers, guide patients in the direction of reasonable treatment. Promote the practice of payments according to type of illness or by headcount. Look into using DRGs (diagnosis-related groups), payment depending on performance, payment methods that fall under a compound form of total budget management.[73] Reduce the risk of illness by allowing insurance to cover preventive medicine and health education, so as to reach the goal of treating people before they get sick.

4.5.3.2.3　Establish a regulatory system that is specific to the health insurance industry

Departments that deal with regulating insurance in China should strengthen the power of an entity that focuses specifically on health insurance. First, this means regulating health insurance separately, internally setting up a 'department' that solely handles this kind of regulation (the current administrative level of 'division' is too low). Second, it means setting up a regulatory system that is specifically aimed at health insurance, which includes an independent accounting system and rules on reimbursement procedures and risk controls. Third, it means setting up professional techniques that are specific to the industry, such as a health insurance actuarial system, reserve funds that are tailored to the unique aspects of health insurance, standards for compensation capacity and solvency, minimum levels of compensation, and so on.

4.5.3.4 More specific policies

4.5.3.3.1 Reform of health insurance products: we recommend having a system that includes mandatory basic medical insurance and quasi-mandatory supplementary medical insurance

4.5.3.3.1.1 ESTABLISH A COMPLETE SUPPLY SYSTEM THAT CONSISTS OF MEDICAL INSURANCE EXCHANGES AND COMMERCIAL INSURERS

First, the exchanges should provide compulsory 'basic medical insurance packages' that include basic medical insurance and critical illness insurance as well as preventive healthcare and health services. Second, insurers may launch quasi-compulsory supplementary products that meet customer demand and that allow for differences in the obligations of the insurance. Third, on the basis of expanding preferential tax treatment for health insurance products, define a more complete spectrum of health insurance products that includes medical insurance, disease insurance, disability insurance, long-term nursing insurance, and insurance for management of chronic diseases.

4.5.3.3.1.2 SPECIFIC PRODUCTS WOULD INCLUDE BUT SHOULD NOT BE LIMITED TO PUBLIC-BENEFITING NURSING INSURANCE, SUPPLEMENTARY MEDICAL INSURANCE FOR THE RETIRED, SPECIAL INSURANCE FOR VULNERABLE GROUPS, AND MEDICAL LIABILITY INSURANCE

First, individual insurance accounts of urban workers should be activated to develop public-benefiting nursing-care insurance. In essence, these accounts are a form of compulsory savings, which have functions that include both payment and savings. Individuals should be allowed to use funds in their accounts to purchase public-benefiting type nursing insurance, so as to make better use of the money.

Second, we should develop public-benefiting supplementary medical insurance for the retired by referring to the Medigap program of the United States. The U.S. Medicare program has certain limitations such as non-reimbursibles, mutually insured amounts, and excluded liabilities, so that some elderly and disabled people purchase private insurance when coverage is inadequate—that is, they use Medigap as a supplement. In taking a lesson from this American example, China may also think of developing a form of public-benefiting supplementary medical insurance for retired people that is offered by commercial insurance companies and that lowers the out-of-pocket amounts that specific groups of people need to pay while still improving the degree of coverage.

Third, we should design products that target the demand of vulnerable groups of people in order to improve the public-benefiting aspect of health insurance. Specifically, while creating more nursing homes that provide in-house medical care for the elderly, we should also provide health management products that include long-term nursing care. A suite of services could be offered as a package that includes everything from hospital stays during treatment, nursing care during rehabilitation, assistance with daily living during the stabilization period, to terminal care.[74] With respect to disabled people, we should develop insurance products for nursing care. This strengthens China's ability to finance facilities for rehabilitation as well as long-term care giving. Insurance for loss of income due to disability should be provided as a way to help all people mitigate losses due to disability over the course of an entire life.[75]

Fourth, through the use of mutual-insurance institutions, we should develop a new public-benefiting form of medical liability insurance. By drawing on the experience of the 'medical occupation liability insurance' of the Japan Medical Association (JMA) and the mutual-assistance medical liability insurance of the UK's National Health System (NHS), we should have mutual-insurance institutions underwrite new public-benefiting medical liability insurance to protect the lawful rights and interests of both physicians and patients.

4.5.3.3.1.3 IN ITS EARLY STAGE, SUPPLEMENTARY MEDICAL INSURANCE SHOULD BE FUNDED PRIMARILY BY THE MODEL 'GOVERNMENT SUBSIDIES + VOLUNTARY PARTICIPATION,' IN ORDER TO PROVIDE AN INCENTIVE FOR PEOPLE TO PURCHASE THIS FORM OF INSURANCE

By a combination of government subsidies and preferential tax policies, the idea is to stimulate purchase on a voluntary basis with self-determined choices. As products gradually become more mature and people's disposable income rises in China, participation in supplementary health insurance can transition from being voluntary to being mandatory.

4.5.3.3.2 We recommend expanding measures that encourage the insurance industry to 'handle' China's basic medical insurance

4.5.3.3.2.1 WE SHOULD FORMULATE MANAGEMENT PROCESSES THAT DEFINE HOW TO HANDLE BASIC MEDICAL INSURANCE

A number of government departments are involved in basic medical insurance, which leads to institutional overlap and unclear authority. Those include the Ministry of Human Resources and Social Security and the National Health and Family Planning Commission, among others. As a result, the national level of government must lead the way in formulating management procedures for basic medical insurance and must straighten out and streamline the current situation. It should unify the functions involved in administering basic medical insurance and should explicitly define the scope of authorities and responsibilities of participants.

4.5.3.3.2.2 IN A STAGED MANNER, WE SHOULD PUBLISH EXPLICIT PLANS THAT ELEVATE THE DEGREE OF PARTICIPATION IN BASIC MEDICAL INSURANCE BY COMMERCIAL INSURANCE COMPANIES

In provinces where basic medical insurance is already being handled quite well, such as in Henan and Jiangsu, we should expand the number of pilot programs to cover the entire province. We should place specific limits on the numbers of how many insurance companies can be involved in handling basic medical insurance, or the percentage of business each handles. Through design of systems, we should encourage commercial insurance companies to promote supplementary health insurance to policy holders of basic medical insurance, which would provide additional services at relatively low premium rates. The aim is to raise the degree of safeguards on top of the existing foundation of universal coverage, in a form that is invisibly mandatory.

4.5.3.3.2.3 WE SHOULD DECIDE THAT MANAGEMENT FEES FOR HANDLING BASIC MEDICAL INSURANCE SHOULD BE DRAWN FROM THE MEDICAL INSURANCE FUND

Right now, it is hard to have basic medical insurance buy services since local governments are reluctant to raise further funds for management fees. We recommend issuing regulations on how to deal with management fees for handling basic medical insurance. Taking a lesson from the experience in Germany and other countries, these regulations should require that management fees be withdrawn directly from the basic medical insurance fund. The regulations would place a ceiling on use of funds for this purpose, and they would strengthen regulatory supervision and audits of the funds.

4.5.3.3.3 *We should vigorously promote connectivity between commercial health insurers and China's basic medical insurance systems*

4.5.3.3.3.1 WE SHOULD SET UP A PLATFORM THAT ALLOWS FOR COOPERATIVE USE OF INFORMATION AMONG MEDICAL INSURANCE, HOSPITALS, AND COMMERCIAL HEALTH INSURANCE

Information relating to medicine should be standardized. We should establish standards that define how to collect and transmit information so that information shared by medical insurance, hospitals, and commercial health insurance is organically consistent. Using the information platform, we should ensure statistical connectivity between commercial health insurance and hospitals, and go further in supporting instant settlement of regular commercial health insurance claims.

4.5.3.3.3.2 THE GOVERNMENT SHOULD INTEGRATE THE MEDICAL DATA
OF RELEVANT INDUSTRIES IN ORDER TO CONSTRUCT DATABASES
THAT CONTAIN INCIDENCE OF DISEASE DATA AND MEDICAL
COST DATA

That data should be a shared resource, such that commercial health insurers can use their actuarial abilities to set prices for health insurance in a more scientific way and can improve their capacity to estimate risk.

4.5.3.3.3.3 WE SHOULD ENABLE COMMERCIAL HEALTH INSURANCE TO
PLAY A ROLE IN HOLDING DOWN THE COSTS OF MEDICAL SERVICES
AND DRUGS

The United States and other countries use the medical resources network that links hospital—doctor—insurance company, which can serve as a reference in this regard. That allows commercial insurance to serve as a third-party payer for medical services and drugs. Not only does this help hold down costs, but it breaks down the unequal status of insurance companies with respect to hospitals.

4.5.3.3.3.4 WE SHOULD MAKE USE OF THE VERTICAL MANAGEMENT OF
INSURANCE COMPANIES, THEIR NATIONWIDE INSTITUTIONAL
NETWORKS AND INFORMATION SYSTEMS, AND GET THEM TO
PARTICIPATE IN BASIC MEDICAL INSURANCE AT A NATIONAL LEVEL

They also should be working in health insurance at the provincial level, building a platform for referrals within a province, and allowing for non-local hospital visits as well as instant settlement services.

4.5.4 Outlook: the positive role that commercial health insurance can play in China's medical reform

The Healthy China strategic plan was set forth in 2016 in a document called *Healthy China 2030 Planning Outline*. This made the following five points with respect to China's medical reform and the deployment of health industries in the country. Looking forward, commercial insurance organizations have much to do in the medical reform work of the future.

4.5.4.1 Instituting a situation in which physicians have freedom of movement

Reforms are taking initial steps to do away with the *bianzhi* system in public hospitals, and initial steps to do away with bureaucratization of hospitals. As they do this, and as a system of allowing doctors to be employed in multiple places takes hold, insurance companies can help establish new human-resource systems and more reasonable levels of compensation. This includes providing annual bonuses and incentive mechanisms in order to attract medical personnel. Companies can also organize physicians' groups under the banner of the company in order to break through the monopoly situation that has a hold on the best doctors. They can help push along a more reasonable distribution of doctors.

4.5.4.2 Contributing to a tiered medical treatment system

The current system requires that hospitals receive approval to be designated as an institution that can reimburse insurance claims. As this system of being a 'designated provider of medical insurance' is eliminated, and as doctors are allowed to work in multiple locations, commercial insurance companies should be able to enter into the system of providing basic medical and healthcare services at the grassroots level. In doing so, they can raise the quality of 'initial-visit' services at grassroots entities, which will be able to retain those patients who have only moderate health problems. That should relieve the pressure on major hospitals, where all patients now try to get treatment. Meanwhile, insurance companies can join the process of building up the medical chain. Through managed care, they can cultivate family doctors who serve as gatekeepers and who determine whether or not a patient needs to be referred on to specialists. Depending on the level of medical institution, companies can set different mutual payment rates, thereby forming a tiered system of healthcare that includes 'initial visits at the grassroots level, two-way referrals, different handling for emergency and chronic problems, and synergy between top and bottom.'

4.5.4.3 Pushing forward appropriate pricing for medical care and drugs

Hospitals currently subsidize their medical services with overly expensive drug prescriptions. To end this situation, it is necessary to break the monopoly that public hospitals have when it comes to retailing pharmaceuticals. This requires lifting controls on who can fill prescriptions at the retail level. This will in turn force medical services to set more reasonable prices.[76] Under the system of Pharmacy Benefit Managers, companies (that serve as PBM) represent insurance companies in negotiations with pharmaceutical companies and receive discounts on drugs. (They help decide which medications are covered by health insurance plans, and are thereby able to set reimbursement rates to pharmacies.) These companies also represent patients in carrying out audits of prescribed drugs and they make sure that patients are using drugs correctly.[77] By setting up ties with pharmaceutical companies and retail drug outlets, commercial insurance companies break down the way in which 'hospitals use high-priced drugs to cover their costs.' This leads to more reasonable pricing and more reasonable use of medical services.

4.5.4.4 Achieving a diversity of entities that handle medical care

The *Healthy China 2030 Planning Outline* includes language that gives social forces (private as opposed to government) priority in setting up non-profit medical institutions, and that says non-profit private hospitals are to be treated on an equal basis with public hospitals. The *Outline* points out that 'efforts should be made to gradually create a fair-competition market environment for public and private medical institutions.' It goes on to say that the government supports the idea of allowing insurance entities to invest in and set up medical institutions. It supports redeploying the medical industry, taking away the monopoly position of public hospitals in the medical system, and forming a more diversified pattern of medical care.

4.5.4.5 Providing quality health services

Insurance companies have a number of advantages including platforms, excellent human resources, and technologies. They can make use of big data, the Internet, and 'smart' medical practices to construct health-management platforms, formulate individualized health management plans, and guide health resources away from treatment of disease toward pre-event prevention and whole-process health management. In doing this, they create a health industry chain that incorporates health management into health products, managed care, supply of pharmaceuticals, and physical examinations.[78]

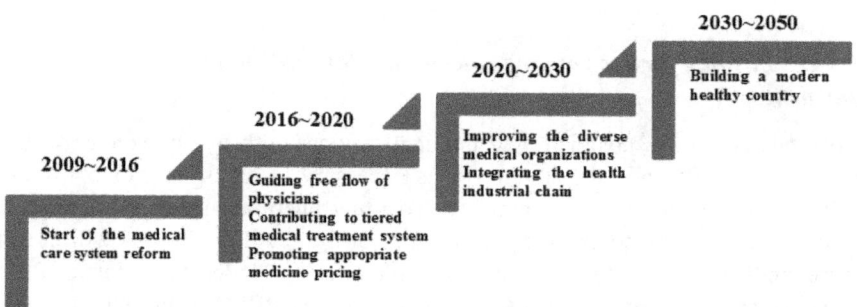

Figure 4.49 Role of commercial health insurance in China's medical reform.

Notes

1 Li Haoyue, Yanzhu and Liang Yunxi of the School of Finance, Renmin University of China (in no particular order) also contributed to the Report. Special thanks go to Zhang Jing.

2 Source: *China Healthcare and Family Planning Yearbook*.

3 Source: *China Healthcare and Family Planning Yearbook*.

4 people.com.cn; The Average Life Expectancy of Chinese Residents Grows by One Year over 2010. www.3news.cn/2015/1222/59539.html.

5 people.com.cn; The Average Life Expectancy of Chinese Residents Grows by One Year over 2010. www.3news.cn/2015/1222/59539.html.

6 Source: *China Statistics Yearbook*.

7 The State Council Information Office Hosts Press Conference on the Innovative Development of Fatal Disease Insurance for Urban-rural Residents. Website of Central Government of the People's Republic of China, www.gov.cn/xinwen/2016-10/19/content_5121874.htm.

8 CIRC. *2015 Annual Report on the Insurance Market of China*. China Finance Publishing House, Beijing, June 2015.

9 Source: *China Statistics Yearbook*.

10 Source: website of National Bureau of Statistics.

11 Source: *China Statistics Yearbook*.

12 Report of Market Prospective Investment Strategy Planning on China Medical Information Industry (2013–2017).

13 BOC International's Special Report on Medical Informatization in China (2016).

14 BOC International's Special Report on Medical Informatization in China (2016).

15 BOC International's Special Report on Medical Informatization in China (2016).

16 BOC International's Special Report on Medical Informatization in China (2016).

17 BOC International's Special Report on Medical Informatization in China (2016).

18 BOC International's Special Report on Medical Informatization in China (2016).

19 Dong Haisong. A Study on the Development of Commercial Medical Insurance from the Perspective of the Ten New Rules of the State Council [J]. *Journal of Finance and Economics*, 2015 (11).

20 K.J. Arrow. The Welfare Economics of Medical Care. *American Economic Review*, 1963, 53(5): 941–973; G. Arkerlof. The Market for Lemons: Quality Uncertainty and the Market Mechanism. *Quarterly Journal of Economics*, 1970, 84(3): 488–500.

21 M. Rothschild and J. Stiglitz. Equilibrium in Competitive Insurance Markets: An Essay on the Economics of Imperfect Information. *Quarterly Journal of Economics*, 1976, 90, 629–650.

22 Wang Jun, Gao Feng. A Study on the Co-existence of Adverse Selection and Positive Selection at China's Health Insurance Market [J]. *Journal of Financial Research*, 2008 (11): 160–170.

23 K. Arrow. The Welfare Economics of Medical Care. *American Economic Review*, 1963, 53(5): 941–973; M. Pauly. The Economics of Moral Hazard: Comment, Part 1. *American Economic Review*, 1968, 58(3): 531–537.

24 Wang Jun, Gao Feng, Leng Huiqing. Examining the Moral Hazard in the Market for Health Insurance [J]. *Management World*, 2010 (6): 50–55.

25 Li Tao. A Study on the Development Strategy for China's Commercial Health Insurance. *Finance and Economy*, 2015.

26 Wang Yincheng. Transaction Cost at the Insurance Market and Control Measures [J]. *Insurance Studies*, 2003 (5): 11–16.

27 Gong Yisheng. *A Study on the Development Strategy of China's Commercial Health Insurance* [D]. Nankai University, May 2012.

28 P.H. Schurr, J.L. Ozanne. Influences on Exchange Processes: Buyers' Preconceptions of a Seller's Trustworthiness. *Journal of Research*, 1985, 11(7): 939–953.

29 Wang Guojun. IT Application and Establishment of Reliance Mechanism in the Insurance Industry [J]. *Finance World*, 2013 (5): 112–113.

30 David Dranove, translated by Huang Cheng, Xu Yongguo. *The Economic Evolution of American Health Care: From Marcus Welby to Managed Care* [M]. Shanghai SDX Joint Publishing Company, December 2015.

31 Ma Shuai. A Sociological View of the Impact of Public Reliance on the Growth of Insurance Industry [J]. *Journal of Insurance Professional College*, 2012 (10): 40–43.

32 Zhu Hengpeng. Defects of the Medical System and Distorted Drug Pricing [J]. *Social Sciences in China*, 2007 (4): 89–103.

33 Zhu Hengpeng. Establishing the Level-by-Level Medical System to Mitigate Hospital-patient Disputes [N]. *China Pharmaceutical News*, March 24, 2014.

34 Zhou Qin, Tian Sen, Pan Jie. Inequality behind the Impartiality: Theoretical and Empirical Study on the Benefit Accessibility of Urban Resident Basic Medical Insurance [J]. *Economic Research Journal*, 2016 (6): 172–185.

35 Xu Ling, Jian Weiyan., An Empirical Study on the Benefit Accessibility of China's Basic Medical Insurance System [J]. *Mediscience and Society*, 2010 (11).

36 Social security authorities retain the power to collect and supervise basic medical insurance funds.

37 Xiang Junbo. Developing Commercial Health Insurance to Serve the Reform of Medical System Reform [J]. *Insurance Studies*, 2014 (12): 3–13.

38 R.A. Musgrave. *The Theory of Public Finance*. New York and London: McGraw-Hill, 1959.

39 R.W. Boadway, D. Wildasin. *Public Sector Economics*. China Renmin University Press, 2000.

40 J.G. Head. Merit Goods Revisited [J]. *Finanzarchiv*, 1969, 28 (2).

41 Zhang Ying. *A Study on the Integration Mechanism for Commercial Health Insurance and Social Medical Insurance System* [D]. Wuhan University, 2012.

42 Huang Jian. Social Failure: Intension, Expression and Inspiration [J]. *Party and Government Forum*, 2015 (2): 23–26.

43 Yang Guangli. *A Study on Risk Management of China's Commercial Health Insurance* [D]. Shandong University, November 30, 2015.

44 Implement Separate Regulation of Health Insurance. *Shanghai Financial News*, May 24, 2011.

45 Source: *Ten-year Exploration and Successful Experiences of Jiangyin Mode of New Rural Cooperative Medical System*.

46 Source: Jiangyin statistics, http://tjj.jiangyin.gov.cn.

47 *Actively Participating in and Building a Uniform Platform for Policy-oriented Medical Insurance Services*.

48 *Actively Participating in and Building a Uniform Platform for Policy-oriented Medical Insurance Services*.

49 Zhang Chunsheng. Luoyang Model Helps Farmers Afford Medical Services. *China Insurance News*, June 5, 2009.

50 Liu Yong. A Pioneer of Administration-Handling Separation: Luoyang Model of New Rural Cooperative Medical Scheme. *21st Century Business Herald*, April 23, 2012.

51 *Actively Participating in and Building a Uniform Platform for Policy Medical Insurance Services*.

52 Hao Jun. *A Study on the Feasibility and Strategy of Introducing Commercial Insurance to the Basic Medical Insurance of Beijing* [D]. Academy of Military Sciences PLA China, 2013.

53 Piloting Coinsurance Piloted in Pinggu. *Medicine Economic Reporter*, September 3, 2014.

54 Source: *Regulations on Reinsurance of Fatal Disease and Hospitalization Insurance Supplementing Social Medical Insurance (Trial)*, T.R.S.Z., 2011, No. 5.

55 Source: *Regulations on Reinsurance of Fatal Disease and Hospitalization Insurance Supplementing Social Medical Insurance (Trial)*, T.R.S.Z., 2011, No. 5; *Notice on Revising the Rules on the Reimbursement List of Fatal Disease and Hospitalization Insurance of Taicang City*, T.R.S.Y., 2014, No. 2.

56 *Rules on 2015 Subsidy Standards for Outpatient Fatal Disease Insurance*, T.R.S.G.Z., 2016, No. 4.

57 Source: *Regulations on Reinsurance of Fatal Disease and Hospitalization Insurance Supplementing Social Medical Insurance (Trial)*, T.R.S.Z., 2011, No. 5.

58 Source: Zhanjiang social security funds administration, www.gdzjsi.gov.cn/outside.

59 Source: *Zhanjiang: Improve Zhanjiang Model, Explore New Form of Medical Insurance*, www.mof.gov.cn/xinwenlianbo/guangdongcaizhengxinxilianbo/201603/t20160307_1896967.html.

60 Source: *2015 Policy on Zhanjiang Urban-Rural Resident Basic Medical Insurance.*

61 Source: *Zhanjiang: Improve Zhanjiang Model, Explore New Form of Medical Insurance*, www.mof.gov.cn/xinwenlianbo/guangdongcaizhengxinxilianbo/201603/t20160307_1896967.html.

62 Li Yuquan. A Study on Separated Regulation over Health Insurance [J]. *Insurance Studies*, 2011 (9).

63 Health Insurance should be Subject to Separate Regulation. *Shanghai Financial News*, May 24, 2011.

64 Zhu Minglai, Cui Jingjing. Experiences of USA in Compensation Rate Regulation over Commercial Medical Insurance [J]. *Commercial Insurance*, 2015 (8): 64–67.

65 Shen Hong. *A Study on China's Tax Policy on Commercial Health Insurance* [D]. Guangxi University, June 2014.

66 Qiu Hui. A Study on the Innovation in the O2O Mode of Health Insurance in the Internet Era [J]. *Reformation and Strategy*, 2016 (2): 29–32.

67 Caihui, Wu Haibo. Severe Disease Insurance and Fatal Disease Insurance: Policy Comparison and Integrative Development [J]. *Health Economics Research*, 2015 (12): 44–47.

68 Some insurers are making plans in this regard (China Life and Cachet cooperate in medical expense control; Pingan acquired Anhui Hefei Kuaiyijie E-commerce Co. Ltd. which has medical B2B license).

69 Risk factors are determined as per time and regional factors. In the early stage of the program (1–3 years), the evaluation is made on the basis of age, gender, region, and diagnosis. According to their diagnosis information, individuals are put into corresponding disease groups and scored according to their age, gender, and region. If an individual suffers from more than one disease, each disease is counted in. If an individual suffers from more than one syndrome, the interactions between the diseases are counted in. In the stable stage of the program (3–5 years), new risk factors would be introduced, e.g. use of prescription drugs, use of treatment devices, and annual changes of the insured. In the mature stage (5 years later), more risk factors, e.g. preventive services (physical examination, early intervention) and orientation factors (specific remedy, new treatment technology) may be brought in and the evaluation models will be regularly calibrated according to historical data.

70 The information about income includes income source and income level and region includes average morbidity risk and average income level of the region; medicine cost group concerns the chronic disease identification condition based on the province's prescription drugs for chronic diseases; diagnosis cost group is the identification condition for fatal diseases necessitating huge follow-up expenditure, and is based on the International Classification Code of Diseases. The fund management should set up a dedicated participants' information system to collect the individuals' information from insurers, social security authorities, and medical service suppliers of the province. Because of the possibility of new disease emergence and diagnosis improvement, the fund management should conduct annual discussions on the addition,

deletion, or modification, as well as the weight of existing risk adjustment factors, so as to ensure the mechanism is forward-looking and updated.

71 Comprehensive ranking of medical institutions as reflected in the 'Best Hospitals' of US News and World Report; evaluation of medical service quality in the 'Hospital Comparison' of US Center for Medicare and Medicaid Services (government authority) and '5-star Medical Evaluation' of Healthgrades Company (the third party); patient satisfaction evaluation in the 'Hospitals' Consumer Medical System Evaluation' of the Center for Medicare and Medicaid Services and the 'Patient Satisfaction Survey' of Press Ganey Company (third-party).

72 Huang Hai. US Managerial Medical Services Shed Light on China's Medical Expense Control: A Game between Medical Quality and Medical Expenses [J]. *Hospital Directors' Forum. Journal of Capital Medical University (Social Sciences)*, 2014 (2): 58–63.

73 *Healthy China 2030 Planning Outline*, paragraph 2, Chapter 11, Section IV.

74 *Healthy China 2030 Planning Outline*, paragraph 2, Chapter 10.

75 *Healthy China 2030 Planning Outline*, paragraph 3, Chapter 10.

76 Zhu Hengpeng. Defects of the Medical System and Distorted Drug Pricing [J]. *Social Sciences in China*, 2007 (4): 89–103.

77 Zhao Wen. *Application of Drug Benefit Management to Medical Insurance and Commercial Health Insurance in China* [D]. Southwestern University of Finance and Economics, 2014.

78 Li Jie. *The Advantages of the Insurance Industry in Promoting Health Management* [N]. China Insurance News, August 19, 2015.

Bibliography

A Pioneer of Administration-handling Separation: Luoyang Mode of New Rural Cooperative Medical Scheme. *21st Century Business Herald*, April 23, 2012.

Akerlof, G. The Market for Lemons: Quality Uncertainty and the Market Mechanism. *Quarterly Journal of Economics*, 1970, 84(3): 488–500.

Arrow, K.J. The Welfare Economics of Medical Care. *American Economic Review*, 1963, 53(5): 941–973.

Boadway, R.W., Wildasin, D. *Public Sector Economics*. Beijing: China Renmin University Press, 2000.

Cai Hui, Wu Haibo. Severe Disease Insurance and Fatal Disease Insurance: Policy Comparison and Integrative Development [J]. *Health Economics Research*, 2015 (12): 44–47.

Dranove, David (translated by Huang Cheng, Xu Yongguo). *The Economic Evolution of American Health Care: From Marcus Welby to Managed Care* [M]. Shanghai: SDX Joint Publishing Company, 2015.

Dong Haisong. A Study on the Development of Commercial Medical Insurance from the Perspective of the Ten New Rules of the State Council [J]. *Journal of Finance and Economics*, 2015.

Gong Yisheng. *A Study on the Development Strategy of China's Commercial Health Insurance* [D]. Tianjin: Nankai University, 2012.

Hao Jun. *A Study on the Feasibility and Strategy of Introducing Commercial Insurance to the Basic Medical Insurance of Beijing* [D]. Academy of Military Sciences PLA, China, 2013.

Head, J.G. Merit goods revisited. [J]. *Finanzarchiv*, 1969, 28 (2).

Health Insurance should be Subject to Separated Regulation. *Shanghai Financial News*, May 24, 2011.

Huang Hai. US Managerial Medical Services Shed Light on China's Medical Expense Control: A Game between Medical Quality and Medical Expenses [J]. *Hospital Directors' Forum. Journal of Capital Medical University (Social Sciences)*, 2014 (2): 58–63.

Huang Jian. Social Failure: Intension, Expression and Inspiration [J]. *Party and Government Forum*, 2015 (2): 23–26.

Li Jie. The Advantages of the Insurance Industry in Promoting Health Management [N]. *China Insurance News*, August 19, 2015.

Li Tao. A Study on the Development Strategy for China's Commercial Health Insurance, *Finance and Economy*, 2015.

Li Yuquan. A Study on Separated Regulation over Health Insurance. *Insurance Studies*, 2011 (9).

Liu Yong. A Pioneer of Administration-Handling Separation: Luoyang Mode of New Rural Cooperative Medical Scheme. *21st Century Business Herald*, April 23, 2012.

Ma Shuai. A Sociological View of the Impact of Public Reliance on the Growth of Insurance Industry. *Journal of Insurance Professional College*, 2012 (10): 40–43.

Qiu Hui. A Study on the Innovation in the O2O Mode of Health Insurance in the Internet Era [J]. *Reformation and Strategy*, 2016 (2): 29–32.

Qiu Jionghua. Coinsurance Piloted in Pinggu. *Medicine Economic Reporter*, September 3, 2014.

Rothschild, M., Stiglitz, J. Equilibrium in Competitive Insurance Market: The Economics of Markets with Imperfect Information. *Quarterly Journal of Economics*, 1976 (90): 629–650.

Schurr, P.H., Ozanne, J.L. Influences on Exchange Processes: Buyers' Preconceptions of a Seller's Trustworthiness. *Journal of Research*, 1985, 11 (7): 939–953.

Shen Hong. *A Study on China's Tax Policy on Commercial Health Insurance* [D]. Guangxi University, 2014.

Wang Guojun. IT Application and Establishment of Reliance Mechanism in the Insurance Industry [J]. *Finance World*, 2013 (5): 112–113.

Wang Jun, Gao Feng. A Study on the Co-existence of Adverse Selection and Positive Selection at China's Health Insurance Market [J]. *Journal of Financial Research*, 2008 (11): 160–170.

Wang Jun, Gao Feng, Leng Huiqing. Examining the Moral Risk at the Market of Health Insurance [J]. *Management World*, 2010 (6): 50–55.

Wang Yincheng. Transaction Cost at the Insurance Market and Control Measures [J]. *Insurance Studies*, 2003 (5): 11–16.

Xiang Junbo. Developing Commercial Health Insurance to Serve the National Medical Care System Reform [J]. *Insurance Studies*, 2014 (12): 3–13.

Xu Ling, Jian Weiyan. An Empirical Study on the Benefit Accessibility of China' Basic Medical Insurance System [J]. *Mediscience and Society*, 2010 (11).

Yang Guangli. *A Study on Risk Management of China's Commercial Health Insurance* [D]. Shandong University, 2015.

Zhang Chunsheng. Luoyang Model Helps Farmers Afford Medical Services. *China Insurance News*, June 5, 2009.

Zhang Ying. *A Study on the Integration Mechanism for Commercial Health Insurance and Social Medical Insurance* [D]. Wuhan University, 2012.

Zhao Wen. *Application of Drug Benefit Management to China's Medical Insurance and Commercial Health Insurance*. Southwestern University of Finance and Economics, 2014.

Zhou Qin, Tian Sen, Pan Jie. Inequality behind the Impartiality: Theoretical and Empirical Study on the Benefit Accessibility of Urban Resident Basic Medical Insurance [J]. *Economic Research Journal*, 2016 (6): 172–185.

Zhu Hengpeng. Defects of the Medical System and Distorted Drug Pricing [J]. *Social Sciences in China*, 2007 (4): 89–103.

Zhu Hengpeng. Establishing the Tiered Medical Care System to Defuse Hospital-Patient Disputes [N]. *China Pharmaceutical News*, March 24, 2014.

Zhu Minglai, Cui Jingjing. Experiences of USA in Compensation Rate Regulation over Commercial Medical Insurance [J]. *Commercial Insurance*, 2015 (8): 64–67.

5   Research Topic 4

Policies and regulations relating to commercial health insurance

Zhu Minglai

5.1 INSURANCE REGULATORY SYSTEM

5.1.1 Overview

5.1.1.1 Objectives and principles of regulation of insurance

The unique functions of the insurance industry, and the way it operates, determine the objectives of regulating the industry. The ultimate goal of insurance regulation is to ensure that these functions are fulfilled. The particularity of the insurance industry can be seen mainly in the nature of its liability obligations, security, and breadth of operations and in the complexity of its products. Meanwhile, market failure and the uniqueness of the industry itself may cause chaos in the allocation of resources and a waste of resources that pose a serious threat to the legitimate rights and interests of the insured, as well as to the normal operations of the insurance industry. It is necessary, therefore, for the government to intervene in the insurance market, keep the market in order through regulatory means, and thus promote its healthy, efficient, and fair development.

The operations of the insurance industry must conform to the operating laws of the economy as a whole. Under the market economy, insurance companies must be subject to regulation according to law. For the sake of the insurance industry and the insured, insurance regulation should be authoritative and in earnest, mandatory, and consistent, to ensure that the regulation is effective. According to Article 134 of the *Insurance Law of the People's Republic of China,*

> insurance regulatory entities shall, under the principles of legality, openness and fairness, supervise and administer the insurance sector according to this Law as well as duties prescribed by the State Council, so as to maintain the order of the insurance market and protect the legitimate rights and interests of insurance applicants, insurants and beneficiaries.

5.1.1.1.1 Principle of legality

The principle of operating according to law requires that an insurance regulatory body must supervise and administer the insurance industry in accordance with law, and must carry out administrative functions according to legally stipulated objectives, measures, procedures, and conditions. It must not overstep its authority. Regulatory entities should not only be legitimate entities but must perform procedures according to law. At the same time, they should establish mechanisms that handle violations in a timely manner by carrying out supervision and determining accountability.

Another manifestation of the principle of operating according to law requires that regulation be adequate and appropriate. This means that the government should not directly intervene in the normal internal operations of insurance entities. Insurance companies are corporate legal persons that operate independently and assume full responsibility for their profits or losses; they have the right to determine their own operating policies and measures independently within the confines allowed by laws and regulations. In particular, under a market economy, insurance regulators shall not intervene in the operations of insurance companies so long as companies do not violate relevant laws, regulations, and policies, harm public interests, or run counter to public ethics. Interfering in the normal and legal operations of insurance companies is in fact an overstepping of authority and is in itself illegal. In addition, overly strict regulation often backfires, resulting in new types of market failure and undermining the original state of normal competition. Such regulation is counter-productive. Not only is it unable to protect consumer rights and interests effectively but, in the long run, it leads to damaging consumers' interests.

5.1.1.1.2 Principle of openness and fairness

The principle of openness requires that insurance regulators disclose the processes or results of relevant administrative actions according to law. For example, they should hold hearings regarding legislation or law enforcement, and make the relevant documents and information available to the public in accordance with law. As required by the *Regulation of the People's Republic of China on the Disclosure of Government Information*, insurance regulators must voluntarily take the initiative to make known to the public all regulations and regulatory policies that have been formulated in accordance with law. They must make public all administrative approvals (permits or licenses), administrative penalties, and so on. They shall also carry out procedures relating to information disclosure requests from citizens, legal persons, and other entities according to legally prescribed procedures. When information is required to be made public, it will be done so within the legally required timeframe and manner and within the full scope of what is required.

The principle of fairness requires that insurance regulators treat those being administered equally. They must make the same administrative decisions under the same circumstances; under different conditions they must arrive at different conclusions. They shall exercise discretionary powers impartially, within the scope of legally defined objectives, and they must listen to the opinions of those subject to administrative action before making decisions against them.

5.1.1.1.3 Principle of organic unity

The principle of organic unity has three levels of meaning. First, regulators at different levels shall have unified regulatory standards. They shall not take the law unto themselves, administer as they wish, or regulate in a way that is redundant or in a way that allows for loopholes. Second, macro regulation and micro regulation should be unified. Micro policies, measures, and methods should conform to the general policies on macro-economic and financial development and stay relatively stable and consistent. Third, domestic regulatory requirements and international requirements should be unified. Domestic regulatory laws and regulations should gradually be brought in line with international rules.

5.1.1.2 Evolution of the insurance regulatory system

In the early period after New China was established, the insurance industry was under the aegis of the Finance Ministry. It was, moreover, an independent accounting unit within the national public finance system. Starting in 1959, the domestic insurance business basically came to a halt. Only foreign-related insurance businesses continued to operate. The insurance industry was then put under the administrative leadership of the People's Bank of China and became a Division under that bank's Foreign Business Department.

In 1979, the State Council approved the *Minutes of the meeting of branch presidents of the People's Bank of China*, and made the major policy decision to 'gradually restore domestic insurance operations.' Once domestic business resumed, the insurance industry continued to be administered and supervised by the People's Bank of China. The People's Insurance Company was a bureau-level subsidiary directly under the People's Bank of China. In 1983, the People's Insurance Company was separated from the People's Bank of China and became an economic entity directly under the administration of the State Council. The purpose of this was to make the People's Bank of China function solely as the central bank of the country, and to reinforce the financial regulation functions of the bank. It weakened the direct leadership functions of the bank over the insurance industry and strengthened its functions as regulator. In March 1985, the State Council issued the *Interim Regulations on the administration of the insurance industry*. Article 4 of this explicitly states that 'the national administrative body for the insurance industry is the People's Bank of China.' To put the *Interim Regulations on the administration of the insurance industry* into full effect, the People's Bank of China gradually established and then strengthened its internal bodies charged with regulating the insurance industry. The initial regulatory body was the Insurance Credit Cooperation Division under the Financial

Management Department of the bank. In May 1994, this was turned into the Insurance Division under the Non-Bank Financial Institutions Management Department. With the enactment of the *Insurance Law*, in July 1995 the People's Bank of China set up an Insurance Department to oversee China-invested insurance companies, in order to strengthen regulatory controls over insurance. During this period, foreign-invested insurance companies and the representative offices of foreign insurance companies in China were under the regulatory control of the insurance division of the Foreign-Funded Financial Institutions Management Department. Auditing of insurance companies was the responsibility of the Inspections Bureau of the People's Bank of China. The People's Bank of China also increased efforts to build up regulatory entities within its system. It required branches to set up insurance sections, and for branches below the provincial level, it required that certain staff be assigned to work specifically on insurance regulation.

As the operating models of separate industries evolved for banking, securities, and insurance, the State Council approved the establishment of a China Insurance Regulatory Commission (CIRC) on November 18, 1998. This body was then specifically responsible for regulating the insurance industry. Starting from the end of 1999, the CIRC set up agencies in provinces, autonomous regions, municipalities directly under the administration of the Central Government, and certain cities specifically designated in the national plan. This went a step further in improving the nationwide insurance regulatory system. In 2003, the CIRC was formally upgraded to become a ministerial-level unit directly under the State Council. Its quota for the number of functional departments, agencies, and personnel headcount was increased accordingly. At present, the CIRC consists of 16 functional departments and has 36 agencies (insurance regulatory bureaus) spread throughout the country. In 2010, it extended its network of agencies to local regions on a pilot-program basis by setting up regulatory sub-bureaus in Tangshan, Suzhou, Wenzhou, Shantou, and Yantai.

5.1.2 Main components of insurance regulation

Insurance regulation is targeted at insurance operations. Those operations mainly are expressed as business activities, although they also relate to the organizations themselves. The business activities that insurance companies engage in are not 'normal' in the sense of producing material goods or trading goods. Instead, they are a unique kind of activity that supplies society with insurance safeguards, that is, insurance products. The core concept behind insurance products is insured security—the various types of insurance that such security takes are the products of the industry. By function, such products can be defined as producing safeguards and producing the ability to shift or transfer risk. As the insurance industry has grown, the implications of its products and the functions of those products have expanded. Modern insurance companies produce products that manifest themselves at three different functional levels: first, core products that insure for security; second, insurance products that provide direct services on behalf of handling business; and third, other services that are provided in response to customers' requirements, or what could be called 'functional insurance.' The business of insurance companies can be divided into three types that correspond to these three levels, namely risk-type, savings-type, and service-type business. Among these three, however, the core of the industry is risk-type business. That is, the industry produces products that insure for security. With today's integrated economy and integrated forms of finance, the business of insurance companies can no longer be limited to traditional underwriting of policies or provision of security against risks. Nevertheless, with respect to regulating the industry, all of the above activities or businesses of insurance still fall within the purview of 'insurance regulation.' One key difference is that some activities (such as the use of insurance funds) require harmonized regulation among different regulatory bodies (such as the China Securities Regulatory Commission.) In more specific terms, the tasks of regulating insurance include the following.

5.1.2.1 Regulatory supervision over institutions

Regulatory supervision of insurance entities mainly takes the form of industry-specific legislation in various countries. This provides rules and regulations on the organizational form that insurance companies can take. For example, in China, the *Insurance Law* provides that the organizational form of insurance companies can only be either state-owned enterprises or joint-stock (shareholding liability-type) companies. Generally, an insurance company is composed of the headquarters and branches. Some specific rules regarding insurance companies are a supplement to laws and comprise the legal system for regulatory management of insurance institutions, together with relevant laws. Almost all countries have specific rules of various kinds that require insurance companies to apply for permission to operate within the scope of a given jurisdiction. Licensed applicants must meet local government's requirements with respect to organizational form, financial affairs, operations, and commitments, before they can be qualified to operate.

5.1.2.2 Regulatory supervision over business

This kind of supervision mainly has to do with restrictions on business scope, operations, contracts, the formulation of rates, reinsurance policy, and so on. Business supervision enforces constraints mainly in the form of contract law. Business supervision varies from country to country. Generally, business supervision is comparatively more relaxed in mature markets, the reason being that companies in such markets have more incentive to carry out self-restraint by disciplining themselves. In contrast, in markets like China, which are still in the initial stages, tightening up regulatory supervision over business helps lead the market into a virtuous cycle as early as possible.

5.1.2.3 Regulatory supervision over finance

An important part of financial supervision is supervision over the assets and liabilities of insurance companies, especially liabilities. Strict asset supervision requires a prudent attitude toward the asset structure and asset risks of insurance companies to ensure their safety and stability and thus protect the interests of consumers. Supervision over liabilities is primarily about regulating insurance reserves. Such reserves are intended to pay off future debts or contracted liabilities. Drawing from them has a bearing on the insurance company's future capacity to settle claims with due compensation. Therefore, insurance regulators of various countries generally take regulating reserve funds to be a core part of regulatory supervision of the liabilities of insurance companies.

5.1.2.4 Regulatory supervision over capital operations

China's *Insurance Law* stipulates that the areas in which an insurance company's funds can be invested are limited to deposits in banks, the purchase of government bonds and financial bonds, and such other forms of utilizing capital as the State Council agrees upon. For these things, moreover, the percentage of the reserve fund that is invested must also be determined by the insurance regulators. The purpose of doing things this way is to require insurance companies to adopt a cautious approach to investing as they choose channels of investment. It is also to prevent any negative results that arise from radical assumptions made in the course of designing products and setting rates.

5.1.2.5 Regulatory supervision over solvency

Regulatory supervision over solvency, or the insurance companies' ability to pay out compensation, is a core part of insurance regulation. It relates to the question of whether or not an insurance company has the capacity to carry on normal operations and to safeguard the financial assets of the people (whose money they are entrusted to manage). In order to ensure that insurance companies have the capacity to make reimbursements, insurance laws of different countries have formulated specific measures that relate to such things as capital requirements, drawing on earnest money, setting up safeguarded money, and determination of minimum requirements for capacity to pay out reimbursements, i.e. solvency as defined in insurance company terms. Insurance regulators generally use specific indicators as ways to regulate the solvency of insurance companies. They monitor minimum capital adequacy ratios and the amount of capital at risk. They monitor insurance and information indicator systems, and they carry out on-site inspections. Meanwhile, they also set up an insurance guarantee fund in order to provide certain supplementary support to insurance companies in the event those companies have insufficient funds to cover their obligations. This avoids the possibility that bankruptcy of a company will damage society at large.

5.2 COMMERCIAL HEALTH INSURANCE REGULATION

5.2.1 Overview of China's commercial health insurance regulatory system

5.2.1.1 Evolution of the regulatory system

China's insurance regulation began in 1985 when the State Council released the *Interim Regulations on the management of insurance companies*. In 1989, the General Office of the State Council issued the *Notice on strengthening management of the insurance industry*, which proposed a series of measures and methods to rectify the insurance market and addressed important issues such as the allocation of tax revenue from insurance companies and the establishment of new companies. At that time, the People's Bank of China was the government entity with authority over the insurance sector. To emphasize the importance that authorities placed on rectifying the insurance market and to deal with the problems found in different regions during the implementation of the *Notice on strengthening management of the insurance industry*, in 1991 the People's Bank of China issued the *Notice on further regulating and strengthening management of the insurance business and insurance institutions*. Prior to the *Insurance Law* taking effect, this *Notice* served as the key basis on which insurance regulators in the various levels of the Bank supervised insurance business and insurance institutions. During this period, regulation of the entire insurance industry in China was in its infancy. There was no specialized regulatory approach. In addition, no laws or regulations related specifically to commercial health insurance had been set up.

The *Insurance Law* came into effect on October 1, 1995. To assist in implementing it, on July 5, 1996, the People's Bank of China issued the *Interim Regulations on managing insurance*. While the regulatory system governing insurance gradually took shape, there was still no specialized regulation aimed at commercial health insurance, and so efforts in that direction were still conducted under the framework of the *Insurance Law*.

In 1998, the State Council established the China Insurance Regulatory Commission [CIRC]. This was in order to put a specific policy directive into actual practice, that is, the policy of separating out banking, insurance, and securities industries from one another in terms of their own operations and also administering them as separate industries. This was done in order to strengthen regulatory controls over insurance. On December 16, 2002, the CIRC released the *Guiding Opinions on accelerating the development of the insurance industry*. With respect to regulatory management of commercial health insurance, this proposed operating and administering the industry in a more specialized and professional way. It recommended that the industry be proactive in exploring new models for risk management, that it increase efforts to cultivate health insurance professionals, that it expand international exchanges and cooperation while also bolstering exchanges and cooperation within the industry. The unique risk features of health insurance place higher demands on specialized operations and require the formulation of specialized laws and regulations. At the same time, methods by which regulatory controls are applied to the industry must be uniform—since the operations of health insurance companies are different, this may lead to inconsistencies in how they are regulated, which in turn affects the results of regulation. Therefore, in order to stimulate the development of the health insurance industry but also standardize its operating behavior, and in order to protect the legitimate rights and interests of relevant parties, on August 7, 2006, the CIRC issued the *Measures on administering the health insurance industry* (Bao Jian Hui Ling [2006] No. 8). This was the first set of departmental rules aimed specifically at the commercial health insurance industry. It includes stipulations about health insurance operations, products, sales, actuarial science, and reinsurance, among other things. It explicitly defines the legal responsibility that insurance companies are liable for if they violate laws and regulations. It mainly covers the following topics: the basic types of health insurance; the business scope of and requirements for health insurance operators; regulations on the cooperation between insurance companies and medical institutions; product management systems for short-term, long-term, and group health insurance; obligations and forbidden behavior when insurance companies undertake the sale of health insurance products; the reporting system that applies to health insurance actuarial practices and various requirements on reserve funds; regulations on reinsurance; and punishments for violating regulations on business management, product management, protection of the insured, and so on. In a word, the *Measures on administering the health insurance industry* have now set forth the basic system for health insurance operations. They also have led to greater standardization of health insurance and a greater ability of the industry to operate within the bounds of rules and regulations.

In 2008, the CIRC drew up standardizing documents concerning the statistical systems used by health insurance companies with respect to the business they were authorized to handle for China's basic medical insurance programs. In order to meet the requirements that the *Opinion on medical reform* set forth for the insurance industry, in June, 2009, the CIRC issued *Opinion on having the insurance industry fully comply with carrying out the Opinion on medical reform, and having it participate in the building of a multi-tiered medical safeguards system.* This clarified the pathway toward building such a system, and specified concrete tasks. To promote the development of commercial health insurance in order to meet people's needs for healthcare, on November 17, 2014, the General Office of the State Council released the *Opinions on accelerating the development of commercial health insurance* (Guo Ban Fa [2014] No. 50). This described the need to improve regulatory cooperation among the various departments. It recommended a division of labor according to responsibilities in order to strengthen regulatory supervision over commercial health insurance entities and investigations of those entities. It brought forth the need to improve laws and the regulatory system pertaining to health insurance operations, and to refine the specialized nature of regulation of this sector. It called for strengthening regulation over the various components of the business, including sales, under-writing, reimbursements, services, and so on. It called for strict investigation into and punishment for such behavior as misleading people when making sales and engaging in irrational competition. It called for standardizing and regulating market order. It called for improving market entry and exit provisions with respect to the business of handling urban and rural resident's major illness insur-ance, as well as business that 'handles' other kinds of medical safeguards. It called for improving the systems that govern tenders for that business, as well as the systems that govern reimbursement, services, and so on. At present, the various regulations and systems adopted by the China Insurance Regulatory Commission constitute the basic framework for regulating health insurance as a specialized and distinct industry. These things create a beneficial environment in which health insurance can operate and grow.

5.2.1.2 Constructing the regulatory system that governs commercial health insurance

5.2.1.1.1 Rules on how to regulate the 'handling' of social insurance by commercial health insurance

In recent years, the insurance industry has actively participated in the handling of the urban employees' and urban residents' basic medical insurance, as well as the new rural cooperative medical insurance program in certain regions. To do this, they have used their experience in actuarial science, their professional ser-vices and risk management technologies, and they have built up experience and achieved a measure of success. The Jiangyin, Xinxiang, Luoyang, Zhengzhou, and Pinggu models have emerged from this process. In order to take full advantage of this social management function of insurance, and to encourage it and standardize the ways it is being done, in July 2008, the China Insurance Regulatory Commission issued the *Notice on certain issues to do with the work of the insurance industry in participating in the handling of social medical insur-ance* (Bao Jian Fa [2008] No. 60). This mainly presented detailed regulations on various considerations, including mode of cooperation, required qualifications, risk management, business demands, and so on. Specifically, in terms of mode of cooperation, in principle the industry should adopt the 'entrusted manage-ment' model in providing operating services. In addition, as per relevant regula-tions pertaining to 'entrusted management,' health insurance companies should sign authorization contracts with government and provide the corresponding management services. The insurance company takes in management service fees for this 'entrusted management,' but it is not required to take a measure of investment risk in the medical insurance fund, or be responsible for the fund's profits and losses. Insurance companies under contract to participate in the hand-ling of basic medical insurance must abide by relevant provisions of the *Meas-ures on administering the health insurance industry*. When conditions are ripe, they should gradually shift to the authorized management mode by providing appropriate local solutions for the local situation. With respect to operating conditions, in principle, insurance companies should meet the following requirements: first, they should meet all conditions as outlined in Article 8 of the *Measures on administering the health insurance industry*. Second, they should get approval and support from their headquarters to carry on this handling business. Third, they should have a sound organizational structure and strict internal controls, a good service network with subsidiaries in the corresponding regions. Fourth, they should assign dedicated staff for handling the basic medical insurance business. Fifth, they should have a sound medical services network and a sound information management system. With regard to risk management and control, they should set up a system dedicated to managing this specific fund for purposes of doing the basic medical insurance handling business, and they should conduct strict financial management to ensure the safety of social insurance funds. They should strengthen their ability to do statistical analysis, and be able to conduct real-time monitoring of business operations. They should keep a close eye on changes in national policies with regard to basic medical insurance, and guard against policy risks and moral hazard. They should strictly abide by relevant national laws and regulations, and conduct their authorized handling accordingly. In addition, insurance companies should take effective measures to improve the management of basic medical services. They should develop a smooth and efficient business process that complies with the characteristics of basic medical services. They should streamline medical expense reviews and reimbursement procedures, and shorten the time needed for reimbursement. They should build a relatively independent IT system for handling the basic medical insurance business that has sound functions and can operate safely and smoothly, and they should cooperate with relevant government departments to build a medical services network that features a reasonable structure and standardized management, provides high quality and convenient services for the insured, and is conducive to risk control.

5.2.1.1.2 Regulatory rules on policy-type health insurance business

At present, China's policy-type health insurance business mainly consists of products that enjoy individual preferential-tax treatment. Through a number of policy notices and measures, detailed regulations have been put out regarding such products and their market-entry provisions, product design, protection of consumers' rights and interests, and so on. Those include the following: the *Interim Measures for administration of health insurance business involving preferential individual tax treatment* (Bao Jian Fa [2015] No. 82), the *Notice on the pilot program of individual income tax policies for commercial health insurance* (Cai Shui [2015] No. 126), the *Insurance Law*, and various other documents.

5.2.1.1.2.1 MARKET ACCESS

According to the *Interim Measures for administration of health insurance business involving preferential individual tax treatment* (Bao Jian Fa [2015] No. 82), insurance companies that provide such products shall meet the following conditions. Their solvency ratio at the end of the previous year and the end of the most recent quarter shall not be less than 150%; they should have suffered no serious administrative punishments over the last three years; if they are a life insurance company, they should have a health insurance division that is focusing on just health insurance; they should have a relatively independent health insurance information management system that is connected to the commercial health insurance information platform; and they should have a professional team, in which no less than 50% of staff have work experience in health insurance and no less than 30% have medical backgrounds.

5.2.1.1.2.2 PRODUCT DESIGN

The *Notice on implementing the pilot program of individual income tax policies for commercial health insurance* (Cai Shui [2015] No. 126) stipulates that products should be developed based on the *Framework guidelines and template for health insurance business involving preferential individual tax treatment*. At the same time, they must be an all-purpose type of insurance that not only has the function of providing safeguards but also offers accounts with minimum guaranteed yields. That is, they must meet the two different obligations of medical insurance and personal savings accounts. If the insured person is a taxpayer over the age of 16 and below the statutory retirement age, insurance companies cannot refuse to insure him due to past medical history and they must guarantee continued insurance. In addition, there are also stipulations on the insured amounts, operating principles, and coverage of insurance policies.

5.2.1.1.2.3 PROTECTION OF CONSUMERS' RIGHTS AND INTERESTS

The *Interim Measures for administering health insurance business involving preferential individual tax treatment* (Bao Jian Fa [2015] No. 82) describes the standardized operating behavior of insurance companies. They are required to operate health insurance business that involves preferential individual tax treatment in line with the requirements for long-term health insurance. The companies may not reject insurance applicants because of their past medical history and they must guarantee continued insurance.

5.2.1.1.2.4 MARKET EXIT

When insurance companies are dissolved, have their license revoked, or go bankrupt, the liquidation of health insurance business that involves preferential individual tax treatment shall be conducted according to the *Insurance Law* and other applicable laws.

5.2.1.1.3 *Regulatory rules on the protection of consumers' rights and interests*

Protecting the rights and interests of consumers is the whole premise of and foundation for the survival and development of the insurance industry. At the core of all regulatory policies is the protection of consumers' rights and interests. This is reflected in many aspects, but is particularly notable with respect to market entry and exit and how sales are conducted.

First, regulations highlight insurance companies' obligation of disclosure. Due to the particularity of health insurance, the sales personnel of insurance companies are usually obliged to disclose a certain amount of information. According to Article 17 of the *Insurance Law*, when the insurer provides an insurance contract that has standard clauses in it, those clauses shall be explained in an attachment and the insurer will explain the clauses to the person being insured. Upon executing the contract, the insurer will clearly indicate any clause under the contract that exempts the liability of the insurer on any of the documents that serves as proof of insurance, including the insurance slip, insurance policy, or other insurance certificates. The insurer will explain such clauses in either written form or by telling the person being insured—if this is not done in explicit fashion, the relevant clause does not come into force.

Second, regulations strengthen management over those who sell insurance products. As stipulated in the *Opinions on strengthening protection of the rights and interest of insurance consumers* (Bao Jian Fa [2014] No. 89) issued by the CIRC in November 2014, insurance companies shall adopt a sales system that segments potential consumers into different groups according to their ability to tolerate risk and the specific features of a given product. Companies are not allowed to promote products with misleading sales pitches regarding the quality of services or the coverage of insurance clauses. In the course of selling products, they are not allowed to prevent consumers from performing the obligation of truthful disclosure or dissuade them from performing the obligation; they cannot falsify or alter insurance contracts without authorization, or provide false certificates to consumers; they must not exaggerate the benefits of insurance products, conceal important details of insurance contracts, or provide false information about the products. They may not sign insurance contracts on behalf of consumers without their written authorization or approval of recognition, or carry on other behavior that violates laws and administrative regulations and the CIRC's stipulations. Where insurance products are sold via telephone or the Internet, phone records and online evidence concerning the rights and obligations of both parties shall be kept. The insurance companies shall bear the responsibility for any illegal sales behavior undertaken by intermediaries on its behalf, and shall therefore also be responsible for improving and standardizing the contracts that it has with those intermediaries.

Third, the regulations standardize regulatory supervision over health insurance products. The *Measures on administering the health insurance industry* include comprehensive and systematic regulatory provisions on the management of health insurance products. It establishes China's 'basic system' for health insurance products and covers such aspects as insurance clauses, insurance rates, the permitting process for products (review and approval process) and their registration, and responsibilities regarding insurance. Since China has several kinds of medical safeguard systems, the medical insurance products provided by commercial health insurance, which are of a type that reimburses expenses, are to a certain degree an alternative to China's other forms of insurance including publicly funded medical insurance and the social basic medical insurance. Because of this, the *Measures on administering the health insurance industry* point out that, when designing medical insurance products which reimburse expenses, insurance companies should attempt to differentiate these from other kinds of insurance the insured person may have, through the use of different clauses, rates, and compensation amounts. In addition, health insurance products are often closely connected to forms of medical treatment. To protect the interests of the insured, the *Measures on administering the health insurance industry* prescribe that insurance companies shall respect the rights of the insured to access suitable medical services and may not include in the terms and clauses of insurance products any compensation requirements that are unreasonable or go against general medical criteria.

Fourth, the regulations standardize market entry requirements. Given the particularity of health insurance, the *Measures on administering the health insurance industry* detail the specific provisions that insurance companies must meet in order to operate a health insurance business. These cover such aspects as an independent accounting system, actuarial system, risk management system, underwriting and compensation system, data management system, information management system, and human resource requirements.

Fifth, the regulations strengthen the management responsibilities of insurance companies. Insurance companies are required to upgrade the management and training of their marketing personnel and intensify supervision over their insurance agents. In addition, insurance companies should be extremely concerned about protecting the privacy of the insured person and should establish a system that protects customers' information and ensures confidentiality.

5.2.1.3 Core regulatory requirements relating to commercial health insurance

At the present time, a fairly large number of problems still need to be addressed with regard to the operations and behavior of the health insurance business. For example, critical illness insurance products are designed in a flawed manner in that the responsibility for safeguards is not made explicit and the products are more like 'quasi-life insurance' than health insurance. This has led to a considerable number of controversies and complaints. To a degree, it has affected the image of the insurance industry and consumer confidence. Fee-based medical insurance cannot effectively carry through on the principle that losses should be compensated, and does not accurately reflect the degree of risk in sufficiently differentiated levels of pricing. Under the pressure of intense market competition, a number of irregular operating practices have emerged, such as inducing policy holders to purchase redundant forms of medical insurance that reimburse expenses. There is vicious competition among companies, including the lowering of health insurance premium rates in a 'blind' fashion, which increases risk to the industry as a whole. The health insurance industry has followed the practice of the life insurance industry by operating in an 'extensive' mode. This means that operations often disregard customer service, the necessary disclosures are not made to customers, explanations about medical terminology are unclear, and so on, all of which has led to considerable numbers of consumer complaints. These things have a negative impact on developing the market for health insurance and on the image of the insurance industry. Strict regulatory supervision of the health insurance market is therefore necessary, including controls over such aspects as operations and management, insurance products, sales behavior, and actuarial reports. Specifics are listed below.

5.2.1.3.1 Regulatory supervision relating to operations and management

Legally, every insurance company in China may enter the field of health insurance. According to Article 7 of the *Measures on administering the health insurance industry*, life insurance companies and health insurance companies that are established according to legal procedures can, after being approved by the CIRC, operate a health insurance business. Insurance companies that fall outside the scope of life or health insurance companies can, once approved by the CIRC, engage in a health insurance business if it is short-term. It can be seen that insurance companies must obtain approval from the CIRC before they carry on any health insurance business. In this regard, the CIRC can either approve the qualifications of a company or reject them, depending on such things as true extent of capital, technical strength, operating conditions, capacity to make reimbursements (solvency), and market behavior. This is to preserve market order and to protect the interests of consumers,

The health insurance market in China is still at an initial stage of development. Multiple forms of entities are currently operating in the business. Life insurance companies have secured a chunk of the market, while specialized health insurance companies only occupy a small share. However, for the health insurance industry to grow it must take the path of specialization—this is already the consensus of the industry as a whole. The key to specialized operations is to put in place an operations and a management mode that is suited to the risk features of health insurance. This does not necessarily signify the need to set up dedicated institutions or monopolistic operations. Instead, as per the unique nature of health insurance, it means laying a firm foundation for specialized operations by putting strict requirements on each link of the business and requiring long-term investment.

In addition, given the characteristics of health insurance, cooperation between insurance companies that provide health insurance and medical institutions is the universal practice among countries around the world. The cooperation between insurance institutions and healthcare institutions breaks down the traditional tripod relationship among the insurance company, the insured person, and the medical services institution, however. The insurance company and the medical services institution may then team up to form an alliance of interests, or a linked entity, which turns the relationship with the insured person into a binary relationship. If the relationship between the insurance company and the medical services institution is not adequately regulated and standardized, it is easy for the insured person to be harmed, for example by receiving inadequate medical care. For this reason, the tenth clause of the *Measures on administering the health insurance industry* stipulates that 'the cooperation among insurance companies, medical institutions, and health management service entities cannot be used to harm the legitimate rights and interests of those who are insured.'

5.2.1.3.2 *Regulatory supervision relating to products*

Regulatory supervision relating to products mainly includes the review and approval process, confirmation of insurance liabilities, and premium rate adjustments for short-term insurance products. The headquarters of an insurance company must apply for approval or registration of insurance products in ways that are strictly in accordance with the provisions of the CIRC. The *Measures on administering the health insurance industry* stipulate that insurance companies must submit their drafts of health insurance clauses and premium rates to the CIRC according to relevant requirements, for approval and then for filing once they have been approved.

Regulating the obligations of insurance, that is, insurance liability, lies at the heart of regulating insurance in general. It involves the interests of both parties. Depending on whether the safeguards are long-term or short-term, commercial health insurance provides long-term and short-term types of policies. The main products of long-term health insurance are specific-term insurance and life-long major disease insurance. Given the need to control risk, long-term disease insurance usually involves protecting the insured person in the eventuality of death, the liability for death, so as to indemnify the person against medical expenses caused by certain diseases whether or not that person dies. Other than that, medical insurance, nursing care insurance, and income loss insurance do not include the liability for death, except death from the diseases covered in the clauses.

Short-term health insurance products have floating rates, meaning that when insurance companies are selling products, they can price those products within a certain reasonable range for different groups or regions after determining a benchmark rate. The purpose of this is to meet diverse needs—it is a necessary part of a market-based insurance rate system. Determining the benchmark rate is the core element of product pricing, and should follow two principles. First, it should be fair and adequate. 'Fair' means that insurance companies should set reasonable prices, and the net risk premium should be equal to the sum of estimated compensation costs plus an additional risk coefficient. Reasonable prices should not compromise the interests of the insured. 'Adequate' means keeping back a certain risk coefficient, still under the premise of ensuring fairness, that is used to make up for the costs incurred by the insurance company (including taxes) as well as to make the insurance company a reasonable profit. The second principle is that the benchmark rate should be reasonable. The benchmark rate for short-term personal health insurance products with floating rates should be a binding reference for the range of floating rates. Insurance companies should be cautious about determining insurance rates and should not change them frequently. Because of this, the determination of the benchmark rate requires support from data accumulated by insurance companies over a number of years.

5.2.1.3.3 Regulatory supervision relating to sales

Regulatory supervision relating to insurance company sales includes two components, supervision over products and supervision over sales staff. Supervision over insurance products focuses on insurance premium rates. When selling insurance products, insurance companies should strictly follow the already-approved insurance terms and rates or those that have been registered and are pending approval. It is forbidden to change terms or rates at will. This is to avoid undermining the interests of policy holders, to avoid destroying market competition, and to avoid endangering the company's ability to pay compensation.

The behavior of sales staff should be regulated. Insurance operations call for a high degree of specialization and professionalism. They are highly technical and the demands on staff are considerable. Training and education of insurance staff is an important part of the government's role in administering the insurance industry. When selling the kind of medical insurance that reimburses expenses, salespeople should first ask people about their social medical insurance, and may not tempt them into buying products that duplicate the same or similar functions. At the same time, they may not exaggerate the health safeguards that their products are offering, hide any exemptions from liability that the insurance company may have, or mislead insurance applicants or policy holders in any other way.

5.2.1.3.4 Regulatory supervision over actuarial procedures

Health insurance companies, life insurance companies, and other insurance companies operating a health insurance business must submit actuarial reports that comply with the requirements of the CIRC. An actuarial report is a document that contains the conclusions and recommendations of actuaries on certain areas of work. The purpose, contents, and accountability requirements of an actuarial report are related to the specific regulatory requirements and the development level of actuarial science. Actuarial reports should contain the methods and procedures that support the actuaries' conclusions and proposals, to such an extent that the relevant parties and departments can understand the conclusions and proposals and can communicate on the basis of them. In particular, the report on the liability reserve fund lies at the heart of actuarial reports. The accuracy of the assessment of liability reserves is crucial to the financial accounting, objective disclosure of operating results, and solvency of insurance companies. Therefore, Article 121 of the *Insurance Law* stipulates that 'an insurance company shall engage actuaries who are certified by the insurance regulatory authority of the State Council to establish the actuary reporting system.' According to Article 35 of the *Measures on administering the health insurance industry*, insurance companies that undertake the business of health insurance shall submit the actuarial report or assessment of reserves report for the previous year according to relevant requirements of CIRC. In detailed fashion, these reports will cover the basis, method, and results of the calculation of reserves, as well as how the capacity to pay compensation (solvency) influences the company. The reports must be signed by the actuary who is responsible, and that person must confirm that the report abides by prudent principles.

5.2.1.4 Influence of regulatory policies on developing the health insurance market

As noted above, commercial health insurance in China is at a preliminary stage of development. Effective supply is insufficient, the overall size of the market is too small, the level of specialization is low, products are far too homogeneous, and the ability of health insurance to control risk is very fragile. The external environment for the industry is also in need of improvement. At the same time, the unique risks of health insurance place a high demand on companies to have specialized operations. It is highly significant therefore to have regulatory policies in place that optimize the environment in which the industry can operate and grow. Policies must be consistent and reasonable as well as incentivizing. Regulatory policies are significant as well in defining the legitimate rights and interests of those who are in the health insurance industry.

In more specific terms, the following regulatory policies have been published. Several *Notices* pushed forward the realization of health insurance products that allow for preferential individual tax treatment: CIRC and the Ministry of Finance and the State Administration of Taxation (SAT) jointly issued the *Notice on launching work on the pilot program of individual income tax policies for commercial health insurance, Notice on implementing the pilot program of individual income tax policies for commercial health insurance*, and *Framework Guidelines and template for administering health insurance business involving preferential treatment for individual income taxes*. With regard to statistics, the *Statistical System for Critical Illness Insurance* strengthened the statistical foundations of the business. It provided the statistical support for policies and measures to be formulated in a scientific way, which thereby enables health insurers for major illness to operate in accordance with laws and regulations according to defined rules. In August 2015, the General Office of the State Council released the *Opinions on the comprehensive implementation of critical illness insurance for urban and rural residents*. This aims to have all urban and rural residents with basic medical insurance also be covered by critical illness insurance by the end of 2015, and it aims to establish a comprehensive critical illness insurance system by 2017. Recently, the CIRC formulated and released five documents that have to do with bidding on tenders, standards for services, financial accounting, risk adjustments, and market exit terms and conditions. Those were: *Interim Measures for the administration of insurance company bidding for critical illness insurance for urban and rural residents*, *Regulations on the services of insurance companies for critical illness insurance for urban and rural residents (trial)*, *Interim Measures for financial management of insurance companies that handle critical illness insurance for urban and rural residents*, *Interim Measures for risk adjustment of insurance companies that handle critical illness insurance for urban and rural residents*, and *Interim Measures for exit of insurance companies from the critical illness insurance market for urban and rural residents*. As explicit regulations and requirements, these five linked documents go a step further in improving the systemic framework for critical illness health insurance. They are a concrete expression of how administering the industry has been brought into line with national policy. This further consolidates understanding of the industry and social consensus about how it functions, and it upgrades the way in which government administers insurance company operations. These policies help ensure that the business of critical illness insurance can proceed on a sustainable basis.

5.2.2 Main problems with the regulatory system that applies to commercial health insurance

5.2.2.1 Inadequate laws

Laws govern and standardize the behavior of government, the public, legal entities, and other forms of organization and they must be respected and followed. In the sphere of commercial health insurance, business must also be conducted according to law, while specialized regulation of the commercial health insurance industry must be carried out along the lines laid down by law. The industry can develop and grow only if the country has set up a complete and sound set of laws, regulations, and rules, yet at present this is lacking in China. No law related to the commercial health insurance industry has been put in place. The *Measures on administering the health insurance industry* is the only relevant guidance, but this belongs to the category of a 'departmental rule.' It has less binding force than either 'law' or 'administrative regulation.' At the same time, however, China's health insurance industry is de facto continuing to grow, and reforms relating to the country's medical system are continuing to move more deeply into institutional structures. As a result, a number of new circumstances and problems have arisen. The *Measures on administering the health insurance industry* came out in 2006. Quite some time has passed since then so it is unavoidable that the *Measures* should be outdated to a certain extent. What's more, commercial health insurance impacts the physical wellbeing of people, and deals with such issues as indemnifying them for financial loss. In recent years, the industry has moved into a stage of high-speed growth, and in the coming period it will be ever more necessary to have it proceed according to standardized and regulated processes as defined by laws and regulations. The specialized work of regulating commercial health insurance can only use law as an effective and powerful weapon if that work is done within a sound legal system. Only if there actually is law can the industry operate according to law. Only then can regulation proceed smoothly along the tracks laid down by law.

5.2.2.2 Low level of specialization

As one form of insurance, health insurance does insure an individual person, yet it is quite different from life insurance. It differs in actuarial principles, risk management and controls, operating models, and in many other respects. Specifically, the basis for setting prices is different, the per capita premium is lower, and it is a quasi-public good in terms of its business nature. In addition, it touches upon a broad sphere of interests, has a long service chain, a wide range of participants, and complicated risk factors. Claims are frequent and operating costs are high. Enormous inputs are needed at the early stage and it takes companies a long time to break even or make a profit. All of these characteristics determine the fact that health insurance must be separated out from life insurance and property insurance. The original model of having all three mixed together and developing in an 'extensive' kind of growth pattern is already unworkable. Health insurance must begin to comply with its own internal laws of development and must operate according to its unique features. It must follow the path of being a specialized profession unto itself. This is, moreover, the way health insurance operates internationally and it is also the way the CIRC has consistently felt it should operate. In contrast, however, if you look back on the path the industry has actually taken, it is hard to be optimistic. Over the past ten years, insurance companies have indeed made efforts to carry on health insurance as a specialized business. Strictly speaking, however, few companies are well equipped to conduct specialized operations. The market at one point had high hopes for several companies, including PICC Health Insurance Co. Ltd., Ping An Health, Kunlun Health Insurance Co. Ltd., Hexie Health Insurance and CPIC Allianz Health Insurance Co. Ltd. These have, however, developed only slowly and remain small and relatively weak in terms of profitability. They are still in a formative stage.

In 2006, the CIRC issued the *Measures on administering the health insurance industry* which were quite explicit with regard to the qualifications and business management systems required for operating a health insurance business. They included things like the market entry system and setting up independent accounting, actuarial and risk management systems. In practice, however, these provisions have not been implemented effectively. The result has been that the threshold for market entry has remained low and life insurance companies dominate the health insurance market while specialized health insurance companies only occupy a relatively small market share. The 'quasi-life insurance' nature of health insurance products on the market is pronounced. Currently, almost all property insurance companies and life insurance companies are allowed to engage in the health insurance business. Since they are accustomed to operating this business as they do property and life insurance, rather than taking its unique features into account, they do not fare well. Some insurance companies even regard health insurance as a lost leader, a way to crack open the door to other business, and they use it to wage a price war. They then make up for losses from health insurance with profits from other business. This not only puts customers' interests at risk but it also abuses the resources of the health insurance market and affects the image of the industry.

5.2.2.3 Lack of supporting policies

Since health insurance plays such an important role in safeguarding people's livelihoods, and since the development of health insurance is inseparable from a favorable environment for the industry, including the support of government policies, many countries around the world have adopted special policies to foster its development. In China, however, looking at the realities as they stand today, the environment is not ideal and supportive policies are ineffective. The first indication of this was when policies in support of commercial health insurance came out in the early period of the industry but were never implemented effectively. Examples would be exempting insurance companies that engage in health insurance from the business tax and income tax, allowing units to include a certain amount of commercial health insurance expenses in pre-tax costs, and deducting a designated amount of commercial health insurance premiums paid by individuals before calculating personal income tax. Since the policies themselves were not forceful enough, they were not able to speed up the development of a market for commercial health insurance and so did not play the guiding role that was intended. Policies not only need to be improved upon but they need truly to be put into effect. Second, commercial health insurance has long been regarded merely as a supplement to the basic medical insurance of the social security system. It has never become an organic component of the national medical security system. Social security departments in some regions have even mandated the use of large-sum supplementary corporate medical insurance that they themselves provide. This business should by all rights belong to commercial insurance. Such practices have put pressure on the multi-tiered medical insurance safeguards of commercial health insurance by reducing the space in which it can play a role in the system. They have severely curtailed the growth of commercial health insurance. Finally, centralized government purchase of services from commercial insurance institutions is still in a trial stage. Government attitudes have not fully turned around yet, plus there is no uniform set of laws and regulations to deal with the situation. We lack the corresponding laws, regulations, and rules, and an effective regulatory system.

5.2.2.4 Lack of laws and regulations that relate to the healthcare industry

With the ongoing deepening of industry reforms in general as well as changes in insurance business models and the legal environment, the insurance industry should take advantage of the possibilities and should strengthen itself. Right now, financial capital is yet again in pursuit of health insurance. Fosun United Health Insurance Co. Ltd. received approval to incorporate in 2017; Alibaba Health announced a partnership with the Alibaba Group, China Taiping, and Taiping Life Insurance in 2016 to set up Alibaba Health Insurance Co. Ltd., which will be specializing in online health insurance. Among companies vigorously applying to get a license to carry on a health insurance business, the brightest highlight is the emergence of cross-sector alliances. Examples are the alliance of Ling Kang Pharmaceutical Group and Bsoft Limited, and that of Sunshine Insurance Group and Neusoft. This, industry analysts believe, will give birth to insurance giants like UnitedHealth Group Inc. of the United States. This kind of feverish activity reminds people of the evolution of America's own health insurance markets, when all kinds of capital were angling to get a share. In China's own cross-sector alliances, people are thinking they see the embryonic form of United Health Group. The alliance of Ling Kang Pharmaceutical Group and Bsoft Limited will merge the advantages inherent in healthcare and big data industries, thus getting a head start in the insurance market. In a situation in which public hospitals have an absolute advantage, insurance companies lack the ability to insist on negotiated pricing. They also are finding it impossible to have effective digital communications with hospitals, or to track and intervene in medical processes. All they can do is sit back and pay reimbursements in a passive way. Not only are losses unavoidable in such a scenario but it is impossible to get to any kind of scale. Because of this, it may very well be that China's health insurance market will move in the direction of an integrated mega-insurance industry. The Alibaba Group, Ping An, and Fosun have all mapped out plans for the entire healthcare industry. This will require massive amounts of capital and a long time, however, as well as the inclination of policy to support the effort as well as to guide it.

5.2.2.5 Legal grey zone of overseas health insurance: 'overseas health insurance is swimming outside the bounds of regulation'

With respect to overseas health insurance, at present there are two different forms of regulatory vacuum. The first relates to 'underground policies,' referring to insurance policies that overseas insurance companies, mainly based in Hong Kong and Macau, sell to residents on the Chinese mainland. These have not been through the approval process of the China Insurance Regulatory Commission. Overseas insurance companies send salespeople to the mainland or employ local people to promote their insurance products. The salespeople of these overseas insurance companies come into China to publicize their goods and introduce products of the overseas company, or they educate residents inside China on how to invest in policies that are outside China, and so on. As the degree to which China opens to the outside world increases daily, the number of residents inside China who are purchasing foreign insurance is increasing at a rapid pace. Overseas insurance companies have gone to great lengths to attract customers, even at the expense of violating laws and regulations. In 2015, Chinese mainlanders paid premiums of HKD 31.6 billion to buy insurance in Hong Kong. China's enormous insurance market has had the effect of fostering a massive grey zone when it comes to regulation. The second form of regulatory vacuum is one that is quite commonly seen, namely a model of cooperation between domestic and overseas insurance companies. The foreign insurance company provides products and services while the domestic insurance company is responsible for issuing policies. The products are mainly high-end medical insurance products. Domestic insurance companies that are in the business of high-end medical insurance can basically adopt one of two business models. Either they can borrow the products, services, and medical-network resources of an overseas company, or they can do their own R&D of products, and set up their own medical network. The main purpose of engaging in high-end medical insurance, however, is to have access to better overseas medical resources. This means the insurance company has to provide managed care services, and that the demands on it in terms of specialization and network are higher than those for normal medical insurance. Because of this, when domestic insurance companies sell the high-end kind of product, in most cases they take advantage of cooperating with a foreign company to use its products and network. The result is that in reality, in the course of doing business, some domestic insurance companies are selling products in name only. In reality, they have not provided any services—sometimes all they provide is a sales platform. The foreign insurance company sends in salespeople to do the selling. This is equivalent to bringing 'underground policies' into the light of day. Not only is it more complex than having a domestic insurance company write the policies, but it is very difficult to regulate.

The fact that overseas insurance companies enter the high-end insurance market of China in disguised forms leads to chaos in the market, which is difficult to deal with since a 'vacuum zone' still exists in regulation. Once these companies withdraw their business, the follow-on services that customers may require are no longer covered, and customers' interests may well be harmed. The only relevant regulation is the *Measures on administering the health insurance industry*. In this, Paragraph 2 of Article 10 stipulates that 'cooperation between insurance companies and medical service institutions and health management service institutes shall not harm the legitimate rights and interests of the insured.' However, there is still no official regulatory policy in this regard.

5.2.2.6 Inadequate experience in how to regulate online short-term health insurance business

The wave of the Internet has already swept up all economic and social activities in China. In 2016, the online business of insurance grew rapidly as more and more users became used to searching for insurance products online. Young people make up a majority of online insurance consumers. A health insurance product of Zhong An Online P&C Insurance even became an online hit. Compared with traditional insurance products, marketing of online products has an advantage since it allows for easy access to product information and premium rates, but the subsequent links of purchase, services, and claims are still at a preliminary stage. The user experience also needs to be improved. In regulatory terms, there is no substantive difference between online health insurance products and traditional health insurance—both must follow the regulations that apply to traditional insurance. Nonetheless, in the context of such rapid development of online insurance, the traditional regulatory mode is unable to meet the regulatory needs, and there now is a need to formulate more specific rules.

5.2.3   International experience of regulating commercial health insurance, using healthcare reform in the United States as an example

5.2.3.1 Background of the healthcare reform

The United States has the most advanced commercial health insurance market in the world. It is mainly composed of two main categories, employer-sponsored group health insurance and individual health insurance. High medical expenses and astronomical insurance premiums have, however, forced many American people to give up health insurance. According to the Current Population Survey (CPS) conducted by the U.S. Census Bureau in 2009, the number of uninsured Americans reached 46.34 million at the end of 2008, which was 15.4% of the total population. Other statistics show that, in 2007, 79 million American people had trouble paying medical bills, and 80 million could not afford medical treatment. With the economic downturn and rise in medical costs, American families face a serious medical security crisis. The Congressional Budget Office predicts that if reform does not take place, 54 million non-elderly persons will have no medical insurance by 2019. Compared to people who do have medical insurance, these people have lower incomes, less education, and few of them work full time. A majority are black or Latino; they are younger but in poorer health.

The medical insurance crisis not only puts a heavy burden on American families, but is an important factor behind the way America's healthcare system is operating at a sub-optimum level. America's medical services show a tremendous disparity with other countries in terms of accessibility, quality, and efficiency. According to research of the U.S. Institute of Medicine, the penetration of medical insurance is the most important factor in determining the accessibility of medical services. Since many Americans have no health insurance or inadequate insurance, the accessibility of medical services is extremely inequitable. Poor accessibility and low quality of medicine are closely related. The uninsured have little access to routine diagnoses, preventive health examinations, and reasonable control of chronic diseases. They are in poorer health than those with insurance and have a shorter life expectancy. People without insurance also contribute to ineffective disease monitoring and ineffective medical delivery. Their medical history is hard to retrieve and examine, and the varied nature of their medical needs makes it hard to control medical costs. These things also make for low efficiencies when it comes to funding medical care for this segment of the population.

In 2008, people with no insurance, in the group described above, paid only one-third of their medical expenses. That left about USD 56 billion in unpaid bills. The government covered 75% of the otherwise unpaid bills, and the remaining roughly USD 14 billion was transferred in invisible form to commercial health insurance companies. People without health insurance not only often forego medical treatment due to inability to pay but, even more likely, go bankrupt as a result of inability to pay.

5.2.3.2 Basic components of America's healthcare reform bill

To ensure the rights and interests of consumers, this round of the healthcare reform placed higher demands on commercial insurance companies with respect to such aspects as eligibility for insurance, product pricing, benefits, and insurance exchanges.

5.2.3.2.1 Eligibility for being insured

To achieve the ideal of universal coverage, the healthcare reform made it mandatory for all eligible people (except special groups) to participate in health insurance. Not doing so would incur a fine. In 2014, the fine was set at the greater of USD 95 per person or 1% of household income. It was raised to USD 325 per person or 2% of household income in 2015, and to USD 695 per person or 2.5% of household income in 2016. The fine was halved for children, and the total fine paid by each household was not to exceed USD 2,085. There were exceptions for special groups: if the lowest level of premiums exceeded 8% of income, these people were exempted from fines; if income was below the Federal Poverty Level (FPL), insurance was not mandatory, as it also was not for some other specific groups. If income was below the minimum taxable income level (which is USD 9,350 for individuals and USD 18,700 for households under the 2009 *Tax Law*), then these people were also not required to buy insurance.

The government was to provide premium subsidies for low-income households, to encourage them to participate in insurance plans through the insurance exchange mechanism. The range of subsidies was set at between 100% and 400% of the Federal Poverty Level of income (for a family of four, the income standard for 2009 was between USD 29,327 and USD 88,200). The subsidies were determined based on the percentage of household income taken up by premiums (see Table 5.1). Meanwhile, limits were set on the percentage of medical expenses that individuals or households had to pay if they had government-subsidized insurance policies. From the perspective of insurance product-pricing principles, rules governing the level of the actuarial value of essential benefits were set forth in order to make sure that the insurance did truly function as a form of safeguards. At the same time, these rules were a form of price-control measure for insurance products in the market.

According to the Congressional Budget Office forecast, if the policy proceeds according to the bill proposed by the House of Representatives, the federal government will provide total subsidies of USD 602 billion from 2010 to 2019 to insurance exchanges. It will provide around USD 436 billion according to the Senate's proposal. Meanwhile, according to the latest actuarial report of the Centers for Medicare and Medicaid Services under the Department of Health and Human Services, the subsidies will come to USD 506.5 billion based on the 2010 *Budget Reconciliation Bill*.

The Health Care Reform Bill also strengthened the requirements on employers to provide insurance for employees. This round of proposals required any employer with more than 50 full-time employees to buy group insurance for their employees, or they would be fined USD 2,000 per employee (fines for the first 30 employees could be exempted). If employees paid premiums that were over 8%–9.8% of their income, then the employer providing group insurance had to provide 'free choice vouchers' to anyone whose income was lower than 400% of the Federal Poverty Level. That person could then choose whether or not to give up group insurance and instead buy personal insurance through insurance exchanges. The value of vouchers was to be equal to the employers' cost of group insurance. Free choice vouchers are tax-exempt, but their recipients cannot then also enjoy a tax credit.

Tax relief was provided to small businesses to encourage them to buy group insurance for employees. For tax years 2010 through 2013, companies with less than 25 full-time employees whose annual wages averaged less than USD 50,000 were entitled to tax credits of up to 35% of employer premiums, and employers with less than 10 employees whose annual wage averaged less than USD 25,000 were entitled to tax exemptions. After 2014, the maximum credit increased to 50% of the premiums paid by small business employers that have fewer than 25 full-time employees and pay average wages of less than USD 50,000 a year for at least two consecutive years, and employers with less than 10 employees whose annual wages average less than USD 26,000 were then exempt from paying tax on premiums.

Ultimately, supplements to the *Budget Reconciliation Bill* determined that companies with more than 50 full-time employees, if unable to pay group insurance (premiums exceed 9.5% of their income) and provide a standard level of safeguards, could also be exempt from the fines of USD 2,000 per employee provided they paid subsidies of USD 3,000 per employee through the insurance exchange mechanism.

Table 5.1 Premium subsidies and security levels in three U.S. healthcare reform proposals

Premium subsidy capping

Proposal by Senate		Proposal by House of Representatives		Budget Reconciliation Bill (Final)	
Income levels	Premium as % of income (%)	Income levels	Premium as % of income (%)	Income levels	Premium as % of income (%)
100~133% FPL	2.0	100~133% FPL	1.50	100~133% FPL	2.00
133~150% FPL	4.0~4.6	133~150% FPL	1.5~3.0	133~150% FPL	2.0~4.0
150~200% FPL	4.6~6.3	150~200% FPL	3.0~5.5	150~200% FPL	4.0~6.3
200~250% FPL	6.3~8.1	200~250% FPL	5.5~8.0	200~250% FPL	6.3~8.05
250~300% FPL	8.1~9.8	250~300% FPL	8.0~10.0	250~300% FPL	8.05~9.5
300~350% FPL	9.80	300~350% FPL	10.0~11	300~400% FPL	9.50
350~400% FPL	9.80	350~400% FPL	11~12		

Actuarial value of essential benefits

Proposal by Senate		Proposal by House of Representatives		Budget Reconciliation Bill (Final)	
Income levels	Actuarial value (%)	Income levels	Actuarial value (%)	Income levels	Actuarial value (%)
100~150% FPL	90	133~150% FPL	97	100~150% FPL	94
150~200% FPL	80	150~200% FPL	93	150~200% FPL	87
–	–	200~250% FPL	85	200~250% FPL	73
–	–	250~300% FPL	78	–	–
–	–	300~350% FPL	72	–	–

5.2.3.2.2 Product pricing

Insurance companies are prohibited from differential pricing based on health status. Limits are set on the extent to which prices can be based on age (the ratio can be no more than three to one), as well as on health habits (the maximum ratio of premiums for smokers to premiums for non-smokers is 1.5 to 1). Differential pricing is allowed based on whether the insured's family is covered by insurance and whether or not the insured participates in a health promotion program; pricing can also vary by geographic locations and other factors. Insurance companies may not exclude people from group insurance coverage or from child insurance due to prior conditions. They may not add unreasonable limits to single-year or whole-life compensation amounts, unreasonably extend the length of the waiting period for insurance, or terminate contracts for false disclosure, except for fraud. Group insurance policies must cover employees' children until they are 26 years old if those children are still financially dependent on their parents. This helps to cover the gap in insurance for newly graduated young people.

It should be pointed out that, due to information asymmetry, insurance companies rely on accurate disclosure by insurance applicants to decide whether or not to provide insurance and to determine the level of premiums. Generally speaking, since the cost of doing so is high, insurance companies will not verify in great detail the physical conditions and medical records of the insured when reviewing applications. They do check some policies more carefully after signing the contracts. If high medical expenses were already incurred, insurance companies generally do not take responsibility for those. Compared with meticulous prior investigations, this approach can reduce the underwriting costs and premiums, but may also give rise to contract disputes. Traditionally, state laws allow the insurer to terminate insurance contracts based on material non-disclosure that affects the insurer's decision on underwriting or the level of premiums. Some states restrict the insurer's right to terminate contracts more than others. They rule that the insurer can only exercise the right to rescind a contract when false or inaccurate statements directly result in insurance events.

For a long time, the right to rescind contracts has sparked controversy and been a focus of regulatory attention. According to a special study conducted by the National Association of Insurance Commission (NAIC) in 2009, the right of rescission was exercised in 27,246 cases, or 3.7% of the 6.7 million medical expense insurance policies sold by the surveyed 52 insurance companies between 2004 and 2008.

In June 2009, the Committee on Energy and Commerce of the House of Representatives held a special hearing on the right of rescission. By investigating up to 11.6 million pages of documents from the three largest health insurers in the U.S., it was found that 19,776 policies were terminated based on false disclosure between 2003 and 2007, and the right of rescission was mostly exercised after the insured had already become ill. This allowed the three companies to save up to USD 3 billion.

Investigators also conducted a detailed study on 13 cases where the insurers were accused of abuse of rights. They found that, in at least five cases, insurance companies finally restored coverage over the insured; in five cases, insurance companies terminated the contracts based on inadequate disclosure irrelevant to insurance accidents; in two cases, insurance companies terminated coverage of the whole family based on false statements; and in another two cases, the false disclosure was caused by the insurance agents.

In order to fully protect the rights and interests of consumers, the proposals put forward by the Senate and the House of Representatives both stipulate that the insurer may not exercise the right of rescission unless an insurance fraud by the insurant is proved. Meanwhile, to prevent insurance companies from evading the restrictions on rescission or offsetting the cost by increasing premium rates or rejection rates, the proposals also specify such things as premium rates and pricing factors, the percentage of medical expenses to be paid by the insured, and exclusion of prior condition. This brings the proposals in line with the rules on the right to rescind contracts.

5.2.3.2.3 Benefits

The new standardized insurance benefits would prevent adverse selection in the insurance market, provide more transparent price information for customers, promote fair competition, and ensure that the federal government's premium subsidies remain the same for different healthcare plans. The benefits of the new general insurance (personal and small business insurance) are almost the same as those provided by large groups. To this end, the Secretary of the Labor Department conducted investigations on group insurance in 2010 to determine the basic coverage. The criteria of the new health insurance plan were determined by the Department of Health and Human Services. The basic safeguards must include ambulance services, emergency services, hospitalization, maternity services and neonatal care, mental health and behavioral health, prescription drugs, rehabilitation services and equipment, nursing care, preventive services (including services recommended by the Preventive Services Task Force and vaccinations recommended by the Centers for Disease Control and Prevention), chronic disease management, and pediatric services (including vision and dental care).

To prevent families from going bankrupt because of medical bills, the healthcare reform established four levels of cost-sharing standards and capped annual self-paid expenses. For small business health insurance policies, the deductibles may not exceed USD 2,000 per person or USD 4,000 per household. For personal health insurance, deductibles may not exceed USD 5,950 per person or USD 11,900 per household. For preventive services, there is no sharing component or deductible—this is to encourage the growth of preventive medicine and better health management.

5.2.3.2.4 *Insurance exchanges*

One highlight of this round of healthcare reform was the creation of the insurance exchange mechanism. This is an alternative or supplement to the existing personal insurance and small business insurance markets and it is to conform to the same market rules (such as rules on underwriting and premium rates). For products sold through the insurance exchange mechanism, the actuarial value, deductibles, and so on are subject to the approval of insurance regulators. Governments at the state level or below are to complete the establishment of the insurance exchange mechanism by 2014. In the future, the government will only subsidize premiums and shared costs of individuals and families insured through the insurance exchange mechanism. In 2010, the Secretary of the Department of Health and Human Services, as well as state governments, established an annual review process for premium increases. This was part of determining the eligibility of insurance companies to participate in insurance exchange mechanism.

There has been a relatively large schism between the Senate and the House of Representatives on the issue of whether or not to establish a national insurance exchange mechanism. The House of Representatives proposed national insurance exchanges as a way to replace the existing personal insurance market. Although states can have their own insurance exchange systems, they must comply with very strict rules. The Senate called for the coexistence of an interstate or regional insurance exchange mechanism and the existing insurance market, urging the federal government to provide grants for insurance exchange mechanisms at the state level. Individuals and groups with less than 100 members could purchase insurance through insurance exchanges. The states could impose restrictions on groups with less than 50 people before 2016, and allow groups with more than 100 members to choose insurance plans on their own from 2017. Ultimately, the Senate's proposal was adopted.

Although the Senate bill passed, in reality the insurance exchange mechanism proposed by the House of Representatives' bill has three considerations that are more likely to reduce premiums and increase the market share of the insurance exchanges. They are: (1) the exchange mechanism must completely replace the existing personal insurance market; (2) the insurance exchange mechanism must be directly administered by the federal government; (3) by establishing public insurance institutions, the Secretary of the Department of Health and Human Services may directly participate in the development of insurance plans and increase the ability to have negotiated premiums.

The proposal of the House of Representatives emphasizes the federal government's direct control of the insurance exchange mechanism on two grounds. First, the insurance regulatory systems of state governments are weak, and the state insurance market and regulatory policies are often controlled by large insurance companies. Second, a unified national insurance exchange mechanism (or trading system) may save on administrative costs, while 50 state-based systems may lead to redundant administrative procedures and a waste of resources. Research indicates that some state-based exchanges may eventually be closed because of the small number of participants. This is especially true if the personal and small group insurance markets are allowed to operate outside the exchanges. Experts believe that, for a pooling arrangement to be stable, it should cover at least 100,000 people, which is a size too large for some less populated states. Meanwhile, an exchange should hold at least 25% of the private market share. Otherwise, it is unable to reduce adverse selection and attract insurance companies to join in the pooling arrangement. However, state-based exchanges also have advantages. Since Medicare is still a partnership of the federal and state governments and operated by state governments, state-based insurance exchanges would help to effectively link the program to subsidized private insurance.

In addition, the proposal of the House of Representatives emphasizes the control of the entire non-group insurance market through the insurance exchange mechanism, that is, the replacement of the existing personal insurance market with the exchange mechanism. In the Senate plan, small group and personal insurance markets can continue to operate outside the exchange mechanism, but without government subsidies. This is somewhat like the 2006 healthcare reform of Massachusetts. In the Massachusetts reform, people with high income who are not eligible for subsidies are allowed to purchase insurance products from outside the state insurance system, that is, outside the reach of people who at the time were called 'Connectors.' As a result, this reduced the Connectors' potential market share of the personal insurance market, but it also reduced their ability to manipulate prices.

According to estimates of the Congressional Budget Office, about 30 million people will be insured through the insurance exchange mechanism by 2019.

5.2.3.3 Key lessons to be drawn from the U.S. health reform process when it comes to China's own commercial health insurance regulation

The Chinese government should make full use of its 'guidance role' in healthcare reform. As a highly developed market economy, the U.S. has begun to place ever greater emphasis on strengthening the government's role in the healthcare system. Not only is the U.S. requiring the government to increase regulatory controls over the market for medical services, but it is requiring the government to take more responsibility for funding health insurance. This suggests that, under a market economy, giving full play to the guiding and regulatory role of the government is essential to ensuring sustainable development of the medical insurance system and fair access to health resources.

Dealing with health reform through legislation, and approaching the funding of healthcare through a budgeting process, are things that provide health reform with strong legislative safeguards and funding support. In the U.S., the healthcare reform plan was drawn up by the legislature and is to a degree legally binding after being adopted by the legislature. This provides its implementation with a basis in law. At the same time, the U.S. healthcare reform plan has involved substantial budget planning. Inputs are put into a budget, projects are defined as funding items, enforcement is assigned to specific organizations. This too helps in setting up reliable funding guarantees. It allows for strong budgetary constraints and also enforceability. These things are worthy of our attention as they have valuable implications for China.

The U.S. example shows that it is important to improve health insurance products and strengthen supervisory regulation of premium rates in order to serve the entire system and protect the interests of consumers. In terms of regulatory controls over products, attention should be given to the extent to which commercial health insurance products are complementary to social medical insurance, and also to the adverse effects that unreasonable design of commercial health insurance products may have on the operations of social medical insurance. Right now in China, increasingly fierce market competition is leading to a situation in which some insurance companies are racing to lower deductibles and the percentage of self-paid expenses. They are doing this to the extent of cancelling cost-sharing altogether. Cost sharing, however, is one of the main mechanisms by which to avoid moral hazard in social medical insurance. As for price supervision, close attention should be paid to the impact that changes in the healthcare system have on the way commercial health insurance prices risk factors.

5.3 REGULATORY POLICIES RELATING TO THE HANDLING OF SOCIAL INSURANCE BY COMMERCIAL INSURANCE COMPANIES: CRITICAL ILLNESS INSURANCE AS A CASE IN POINT

5.3.1 Regulatory policies of the China Insurance Regulatory Commission on critical illness insurance

The China Insurance Regulatory Commission regulates critical illness insurance in several key ways: top-level design, institution building, daily supervision, and capacity building. With respect to top-level design and institution building, the CIRC played an active role in the design of the critical illness insurance system. When the system was first implemented on a pilot basis, it set forth regulatory measures to supervise the business. The CIRC conducts monthly checks, does quarterly analysis, and generates a six-month summary of results. It organizes inspections on a regular basis, and deals with any violations in a timely manner. Since commercial health institutions started to engage in critical illness insurance, the CIRC has punished the subsidiaries of companies such as China Continent Insurance and PICC, issued nearly 50 regulatory letters to more than ten insurance companies, and held talks on regulatory issues with more than 200 people.

Most recently, the CIRC has formulated five administrative policy documents: *Interim Measures on how to administer the process of having insurance* companies bid on critical illness insurance for urban and rural residents, *Regulations on the services of insurance companies that are handling critical illness insurance for urban and rural residents (Trial)*, *Interim Measures for financial management of insurance companies that handle critical illness insurance for urban and rural residents*, *Interim Measures for risk adjustment of insurance companies that handle critical illness insurance for urban and rural residents*, and *Interim Measures for market exit of insurance companies that are handling critical illness insurance for urban and rural residents*. These five policy documents specify the provisions and requirements on how to conduct bidding, on the service standards, financial accounting, risk management, and market exit terms of insurance companies, and on how to improve the critical illness insurance system. The five documents are a concrete expression of policy involvement in regulatory management of critical illness insurance. They will further consolidate the consensus of the industry and society on how to improve regulatory supervision over the way insurance companies handle social insurance operations. Each is described in more detail below.

5.3.1.1 Regulations pertaining to bidding

The *Interim Measures on how to administer the process of having insurance companies bid on critical illness insurance for urban and rural residents* explicitly set forth the processes involved in bidding: pre-bid, bidding, bid winning, and contract signing process. They require that documents to do with bidding conform to the historical statistics on basic medical insurance of the government entity that is extending the tender as well as the management service requirements for which the insurance company is bidding. Bidders are required to evaluate underwriting risks according to that data as well as management service costs. They are to determine the premiums, amount of insurance, threshold amounts, and payment ratios, and include in their bid documents the target groups of critical illness insurance, term of insurance, scope of responsibility, exclusions, models of payment, profit-loss adjusting mechanisms, dynamic changes to the terms of contract, how they intend to handle managed care, the standards of their services, and measures by which to achieve results. Insurance companies may not participate in bidding for projects that provide no empirical data or inadequate data. They may not offer prices that incur obvious losses, or bid for projects that have no risk adjusting mechanism, require service fees, commissions, or consulting fees of the insurance company after it has won a the bid.

5.3.1.2 Management services

The *Regulations on the services of insurance companies handling critical illness insurance for urban and rural residents (Trial)* set forth specific requirements for insurance companies that are handling critical illness insurance. It covers such aspects as capacity building, insurance plan design, claim verification, payment, customer service, supervision of medical behavior, and management of case files. With respect to building capacity to provide services, it makes recommendations of a guidance nature about creating a network of service outlets, deployment of personnel, and information systems. With respect to data management for critical illness insurance, it recommends adopting an actuarial management system, using the data of the basic medical insurance to a reasonable degree, and setting up a critical illness insurance database. With respect to payment, it recommends a 'one-stop mode' of settlement services. It also recommends looking into setting up a system for getting feedback on claims settlement. With respect to customer services, it notes that insurance companies should put in place an effective mechanism for handling complaints that relate to critical illness insurance. In terms of controlling medical risk, it notes that insurance companies should strengthen communications with and coordination with the relevant local government departments. With support from the local healthcare administrative body and the department handling basic medical insurance, they should establish a medical review system for critical illness insurance. They should also assist in formulating standards for testing and evaluating medical services as provided by the insurance company and they should set up a system whereby the designated medical institution gets reviewed and evaluated. They should work smoothly with the regulatory bodies that govern medical behavior. In terms of managing files, insurance companies should use a combination of hard-copy (paper) and digital files on reimbursements. They should implement a method of saving files that provides for 'one case—one document,' (i.e. each case has a traceable document associated with it). They should facilitate retrieval through case numbering as well as indexing by the insured person's information. They should, moreover, strengthen their work relating to file confidentiality.

5.3.1.3 Financial management

The *Interim Measures for financial management of insurance companies handling critical illness insurance for urban and rural residents* stipulate that the cardinal principle of financial management when it comes to insurance companies that handle critical illness insurance is 'separation of income and expenses, safety and efficiency.' These *Measures* also include detailed provisions on such things as the accounting rules to use when contracting for 'entrusted management' of insurance funds, how to handle expenses, reporting requirements and how to submit reports, as well as information on regulatory supervision and inspections.

5.3.1.4 Risk adjustment

Insurance companies should establish a dynamic risk adjustment mechanism through negotiations with relevant departments of the local government. They should adopt proper risk-adjusting methods to deal with any surplus balances during the insurance term and any losses that are of a 'policy nature,' i.e.

incurred on behalf of government requirements. The aim is to guarantee the sustainable development of the critical illness insurance business. Risk-adjusting mechanisms to do with critical illness insurance should adhere to the principle of balancing income and expenses, as well as the principle of conserving principal while allowing for a modest profit. The *Interim Measures for risk adjustment of insurance companies operating critical illness insurance for urban and rural residents* points to situations in which policy-type losses might occur and suggests countermeasures to deal with these in terms of risk adjustment. So-called 'policy-related losses' can refer to losses caused by inaccurate pricing, or to governmental changes in basic medical insurance policies, or to other policy-related factors. Insurance companies should ask relevant departments of local government for local basic medical insurance data and relevant variables, including diagnosis and treatment data, participation rate in basic medical insurance, hospitalization rates, and increase in per capita medical expenses over the past three years. They should design risk-adjusting measures accordingly.

5.3.1.5 Market exit management

Improving the market exit mechanism is highly significant for protecting the interests of consumers and for ensuring that the critical illness insurance system continues to operate in a steady manner. The *Interim Measures for market exit of insurance companies that are handling critical illness insurance for urban and rural residents* set forth clear rules on things that are not included in the required qualifications for handling critical illness insurance. They specify how much registered capital must be held by the headquarters company and what its solvency requirements are. If either the headquarters or the subsidiaries of a company have violated rules and regulations in the course of handling critical illness insurance, and received 'administrative punishment,' then the *Measures* provide that they must ensure a smooth transition of their accounts according to regulations and withdraw from the business. Such violations can include but are not limited to using documents in the course of bidding that violate regulations, and fraudulent behavior and ill-will types of competition in the course of bidding.

These five new policies focus on regulatory controls over how to actually implement critical illness insurance and they put forward specific requirements on the capacity building of commercial insurance companies. The refinement of regulatory procedures in the practice of critical illness insurance represents an enormous advance at the regulatory level. The most notable highlights of this round of reform are as follows.

First, they contain detailed regulations on the specific services provided by insurance companies. The *Regulations on the services of insurance companies that are handling critical illness insurance for urban and rural residents (Trial)* require insurance companies to provide the insured with 'one-stop' settlement services by using their own institutional and information networks. They also require companies to provide long-distance settlement services for an insured person who has to be treated in a different jurisdiction and who cannot settle bills immediately when leaving the hospital.

Second, they set forth actuarial requirements. The *Interim Measures on how to administer the process of having insurance companies bid on critical illness insurance for urban and rural residents* stipulate that insurance companies may not participate in bidding for projects if they do not provide empirical data or if their data is inadequate, if they tender a bid that will obviously incur losses, if they have no risk adjusting mechanism, or if they pay service fees, commissions, or consulting fees after winning the bid. The *Regulations on the services of insurance companies that are handling critical illness insurance for urban and rural residents (Trial)* require insurance companies to design critical illness insurance plans that are based on data provided by local basic medical insurance authorities that either span the past three years or meet actuarial requirements.

Third, they set forth regulations on the financial management of insurance companies, and specifically require them to operate at the provincial or municipal level of administrative jurisdiction. This puts the administrative level at which funds for critical illness insurance are pooled at a higher level.

Fourth, in terms of risk adjustment, they emphasize the principle of balancing income and outflow and preserving principal while allowing a modest profit. In this regard, they put forth the specific implications of 'policy-type losses.' Policy-type losses are losses in critical illness insurance that result from inaccurate setting of prices by administrative bodies, from changes in basic medical insurance policies, or from other policy-related factors. In order to ensure the sustainable development of the critical illness insurance business that is handled by insurance companies, it is necessary to adjust the circumstances that cause such policy-type losses.

5.3.2 Case study: Taicang model

5.3.2.1 Institutional design of the Taicang model

The Taicang model is a form of 'critical illness reinsurance' that uses a partnership between social insurance and commercial insurance. Under the Taicang model, local departments of human resources and social security invite tenders from commercial insurance institutions thereby incorporating commercial methods of handling insurance. The mechanism uses the surplus in the pooled funds of Taicang's basic medical insurance. If, on the basis of already receiving basic medical insurance, an insured person's self-paid expenses come to more than RMB 10,000 in total, then commercial insurance companies provide a degree of compensation for the extra amount. The self-paid expenses can consist of items both inside and outside the government-designated medical catalogue for basic medical insurance.

5.3.2.1.1 Compensation standards

In 2011, the compensation standards of critical illness reinsurance were determined through bidding: the reimbursement rate was 53% for self-paid medical expenses of RMB 10,000 to RMB 20,000; it increased by 2.5% per RMB 10,000 for self-paid medical expenses of RMB 20,000 to RMB 100,000; and the rate was 75%, 81%, and 82% for self-paid medical expenses of RMB 100,000 to RMB 150,000, RMB 200,000 to RMB 500,000 and above RMB 500,000, respectively. No ceiling was set on the amount of compensation. To prevent a loss in the basic medical insurance fund, commercial insurance institutions can draw no more than 5% of the total critical illness insurance fund if there is a surplus at the end of the year, while the rest of the surplus must be returned to the government's special account for critical illness insurance as the risk adjustment fund. If a risk event occurs in the critical illness insurance fund at the end of the year, risk adjustment funds are to be used; if those are insufficient, the cost of risk-adjustment funds is to be shared equally by the two parties.

5.3.2.1.2 Funding

Using the standard amounts that participants in the urban employees' basic medical insurance program and urban and rural residents' basic medical insurance program must pay per year, which are RMB 50 and RMB 30 respectively, Taicang collected RMB 21.68 million for critical illness insurance in 2011. This was roughly 3% of the surplus in the medical insurance fund. With this, it provided critical illness insurance compensation to 2,604 patients in Taicang. Among these, 207 had hospitalization expenses that exceeded RMB 150,000, and the actual reimbursement rate increased from 50% to 80%. In 2011, the critical illness insurance fund operated in a sound manner with a total amount in funding of RMB 21.68 million. Of this, compensation paid out came to RMB 18.4 million, while commercial insurance institutions took in RMB 980,000 as service fees, leaving a surplus of RMB 2.3 million.

5.3.2.1.3 Insurance participants

Among participants in critical illness insurance, urban employees accounted for 67.5% and urban and rural residents for 32.5%. Urban employees paid 84% of the total premiums, while urban and rural residents paid 16%. These two groups of people paid differentiated rates of premiums but received equalized benefits. This form of 'secondary distribution' reflected the policy inclination in favor of disadvantaged groups and rural areas and was in line with the goal of having urban areas 'pay back' their debt to rural areas and achieve a more equal situation.

5.3.2.1.4 Insurance company's engagement in medical treatment processes

The Jiangsu Branch of PICC Jiangsu Branch partnered with the Taicang Human Resources and Social Security Bureau in setting up a 20-member team to manage and oversee the medical treatment being provided at hospitals. The team was authorized by the Bureau to do this and it operated under Bureau guidance. The expenses for this mechanism were drawn from the critical illness insurance fund, according to a specific percentage of the total. In 2011, the percentage was 4.5%. The total drawn from the fund was RMB 980,000, while the insurance company's actual operating cost in the first half of the year was RMB 650,000.

5.3.2.2 Main regulatory measures

5.3.2.2.1 Establishing a profit margin for insurance companies

To strengthen regulation over critical illness insurance operations of insurance companies, in March 2014 the Jiangsu Bureau of CIRC released the *Interim Measures for regulating the critical illness insurance business of insurance companies* (Su Bao Jian Fa (2014) No. 28). This was a 'standardizing document,' which provided detailed rules on such aspects as qualifications, management of the bidding process, business statistics, operations management, information exchange, and regulatory supervision.

5.3.2.2.2 Regulatory supervision over bidding for critical illness insurance

The Jiangsu Bureau of CIRC established a whole-process regulatory system that dealt with preliminary aspects of insuring critical illness, the actual process of insuring, and post-insuring oversight. First, it pushed forward the process of calling for tenders in a sound and reasonable way. It authorized the insurance associations of the various localities to organize the participation of corporate members in developing the plans for making bids for critical illness insurance. The emphasis was put on funding, risk-sharing mechanisms, period of cooperation, the risk fund, and data calculation. Second, it strengthened supervision over the bidding process, established a database containing the insurance industry's operating costs for critical illness insurance, and collected basic data on costs in 93 regions involving the subsidiaries of 18 eligible insurance companies. Those costs included human resources, vehicle and electronic equipment expenses, and daily operating costs. Third, with respect to post-insurance processes, it established a regular ongoing mechanism for supervision and inspections. Companies that are handling critical illness insurance are subject to on-site inspections every half year to encourage them to carry out orderly operations that are in line with regulations.

5.3.2.2.3 Standardizing the regulations that govern the basic services of subsidiaries of insurance companies

To improve the critical illness insurance services of insurance companies, the Jiangsu Bureau of CIRC issued the *Basic Regulations on critical illness insurance services provided by subsidiaries of insurance companies (Trial)*. This was based on in-depth research and surveys. It provided standardized approaches to such things as capacity building, claims settlement, customer service, medical behavior supervision, and file management of insurance companies. It set basic standards for staffing, vehicles, and service outlets according to the characteristics of the groups and regions served. It called for interconnectedness of the information systems that underlie critical illness insurance. It confirmed that a 'one-stop' payment process and long-distance payment option should be realized, and it confirmed the need to set up a system for getting feedback on critical illness insurance reimbursements.

5.3.3 Main problems and recommendations on improvements

5.3.3.1 Standardize the request for tenders and the bidding process, and develop proper methods by which to evaluate bids

In the testing stage of the critical illness insurance system, a strange phenomenon has appeared as pilot programs are implemented in various places. In the process of asking for tenders, some social insurance departments have been overly domineering and have set basic prices that are too low (the per capita level of funding). In addition, companies themselves have competed by lowering prices in order to capture the business. This kind of price war leads to even greater losses and makes the whole concept of making a modest profit while conserving capital unworkable. In looking for the cause of this problem, it turns out that the authorities in many places base the winning of tenders solely on price, rather than on such things as quality. The lower the price, the higher the score of the bidder, which concentrates the attention of bidders on price alone. To deal with this problem, we need to standardize the way in which bidding is conducted and also standardize management controls over contracts. These should be explicit about what services are offered and what the cost-control indexes should be. Prices should be established at a reasonable level so as to prevent vicious price competition. We should speed up the process of evaluating bids in a comprehensive way and we should carry out comprehensive evaluations of insurance entities that participate in tenders with respect to such things as capacity to do the business, per capita funding amounts, profitability rates (that is, costs and expenses), and so on. Among these things, the weighting of the per capita funding amount should be lowered in evaluating bids, whereas that for the capacity to provide services should be raised. The idea is to guide insurance entities to focus on quality of service. Given comprehensive evaluations of a company's capacity, a company with sufficient capacity will also have sufficient margin to negotiate on prices. This then will curb unreasonable price wars and allow for a pattern of competition that is standardized and orderly.

In addition, as to the funding standards (per capita contribution) in tendering documents, we should gradually bring in third-party teams of experts to establish a 'lowest' or base price using historical data for calculations. These teams should participate in the process of bidding. They should also establish a price-finding model for critical illness insurance that takes into account a number of factors—overall consideration of the level of economic development, incidence of major illness leading to high-priced medical costs, level of safeguards for critical illness insurance, and so on. This should be done based on the advantage that experts hold in actuarial sciences and it should be done using historical data. This kind of effort should gradually become a required condition for participating in a tender.

5.3.3.2 Explicitly define methods for handling (underwriting) the business, and be clear about the responsibilities on both sides

The ways in which insurance companies can handle critical illness insurance fall into two categories: authorized operations and contracted purchase of their insurance. The responsibilities of the two sides are different for these two categories. Under the existing modes of cooperation, the division of labor is fairly clear for both categories, but the division of risk is not. That is, the mechanisms that apply to risk-sharing are unclear.

With respect to having commercial insurance companies handle critical illness insurance, we believe we should adhere to three principles in thinking about how to define operating costs and profits in a reasonable and scientifically calculated way.

First, a scientifically determined distinction should be made between the profits and losses that accrue to 'policy-type' insurance and 'management-type' insurance. The profits and losses due to compensation for so-called 'policy-type' insurance are caused by changes and improvements in medical insurance policies. Examples would be when the authorized list of medicines for medical insurance is changed, or the level of funding is adjusted, or when there is a sudden public-health crisis. In such cases, social insurance departments can calculate the expected compensation rate (loss ratio) based on historical data of the basic medical insurance. In contrast, the profits and losses due to compensation of the management-type insurance are caused by the operating activities of the company itself and the insurance company should take its portion of either profits or losses. That is, its portion is the difference between the expected loss ratio (policy profit or loss) and the actual loss ratio.

Second, the handling cost for critical illness insurance should be determined through 'scientifically derived estimates, market competition [public bidding], and substitution.' Where insurance companies are willing and able to undertake critical illness insurance business at reasonable costs, the government can determine the operators through public bidding. If insurance companies cannot accept the pricing, social insurance departments can substitute themselves in doing the business.

Third, the expected profit of insurance companies should not be included in the management cost as a fixed charge; instead, an effective incentive mechanism should be formed through the risk-sharing model. The professional advantage of insurance companies is reflected in their operational efficiency. Their profitability should depend on their putting in quality resources in order to strengthen their operating and management capability.

5.3.3.3 *Leverage the advantages of insurance companies to expand value-added services in critical illness insurance*

Commercial insurance companies should increase investment in R&D systems related to critical illness insurance business. They should connect their information systems with the basic medical insurance information system to achieve the ability to do comprehensive reviews of medical expenses, to distinguish substandard, normal, and suspicious cases through systematic screening, and to manage and control medical expenses in accordance with expert opinions and local policies. The development of the medical expense 'smart' review system should be strengthened and the model 'smart review+medical expert review' should be adopted to enhance medical risk management control and reduce fraud, waste, and unreasonable expenses. At the same time, relying on their extensive network of subsidiaries, insurance companies should establish a way to coordinate medical services over a long distance. They should experiment with setting up a bank of medical experts in various places to ensure that the reviews of medical costs are fair and reasonable.

One important indicator that can be used in assessing the performance of insurance companies who handle critical illness insurance should be the following: such companies should make full use of very granular data on medical insurance to leverage their actuarial expertise, to set reasonable overall fee rates, to manage in a more meticulous way, to strengthen controls over medical risk, and to prevent medical costs from rising too quickly. At the same time, they should strengthen their controls over information security. The *Opinions of the General Office of the State Council on accelerating the development of commercial health insurance*, published in November 2014 (Guo Ban Fa [2014] No. 50), points out that 'relevant government departments and commercial insurance institutions should strengthen the security of the personal information of the insured to prevent leakage and abuse of such information.' To prevent any losses to social security departments and the insured caused by the exit of insurance companies and the possibility they take data with them, it is necessary to formulate information security and confidentiality agreements that are uniform, to establish an independent operating platform, to develop relevant software, and to build an interface-based firewall between that platform and the social security database. We should also improve a joint operating mechanism that involves multiple insurance companies, and put in place an information security evaluation system targeting insurance companies that have withdrawn from the market.

Insurance companies should also specify in tender contracts that the following items are to be included in how their services are evaluated: the establishment of medical records on critical illness for the insured, follow-up investigation of people who were reduced to poverty because of critical illness, patient satisfaction surveys, and the blacklists of both medical institutions and individuals who violate regulations pertaining to critical illness insurance.

5.3.3.4 Elevate the level at which funding for critical illness insurance is pooled and managed, and formulate templates for standardized contracts

Elevating the level of pooling includes looking into funding critical illness insurance at the provincial level. On the one hand, this allows commercial health insurance companies to make better use of their more qualified personnel at provincial-level organizations. This is particularly true with respect to the R&D and design of products. On the other hand, this can prevent overly fragmented management of critical illness insurance while also allowing for greater dispersal of risk, since this would enable flexible allocation of funds at the municipal level. At present, among the 29 provincial regions that have launched critical illness insurance plans, Anhui, Shaanxi, Zhejiang, Jiangsu, Henan, Jiangxi, and Hainan explicitly proposed to develop provincial contract templates. As critical illness insurance moves forward on a nationwide basis, all provinces and municipalities should take steps to develop provincial contract templates and elevate the administrative level at which pooled funding takes place.

Inviting tenders at the provincial level also allows insurance regulators to select qualified insurance companies at a higher level and according to stricter standards. It allows them to evaluate and upgrade products that can serve as models to emulate on a regular basis, and it allows them to improve the statistical systems that apply to critical illness insurance companies, as well as the unique accounting regulations that apply to their finances. By going through the provincial critical illness insurance information platform, insurance associations in different areas can set up ways to share core data. They can deal strictly with any price wars or other unfair methods of competition on the part of insurance companies. They can more easily maintain market order and ensure that critical illness risk operations have long-term stability.

5.3.3.5 Improve regulatory management services and establish a performance evaluation system

The *Statistical System for critical illness insurance (Trial)* (Bao Jian Fa [2013] No. 77) requires regulatory bureaus and insurance companies to submit statistical statements on critical illness insurance every quarter. We recommend that the

CIRC release national reports on critical illness insurance on an annual basis to disclose in detail the progress, achievements, and problems in how it is being implemented. At the same time, we recommend that insurance companies be required to disclose special financial reports on critical illness insurance on a regular basis every year. They should use as reference the financial disclosure system that is required of compulsory automobile liability insurance. These reports should be reviewed by eligible auditing institutions, so as to ensure the adequacy and transparency of critical illness insurance operations.

Since critical illness insurance is being passed to commercial insurance companies for handling, we should develop indicators that evaluate both the operational efficiency of insurance companies and the regulatory efficiency of regulators. These indicators should include method of selection of operators and bid success rate of operators, relevant financial and business experience, staffing, structure, and capacity, the soundness and coverage of relevant information systems, rate of violations, complaints, and service satisfaction. We should establish an investigation and evaluation system for pilot programs of critical illness insurance in order to identify problems and causes of problems. The process should be objective, comprehensive, fair, and accurate. It should also summarize lessons learned and seek patterns, in order to provide policy advice for the formulation of more scientific policy. Through both quantitative and qualitative analysis, we want to achieve more fine-grained management of critical illness insurance systems.

5.3.3.6 Adhere to administration that operates by the rule of law and encourage institutional innovation

Article 64 of the *Social Insurance Law* stipulates that China's social insurance funds 'are earmarked for specific purposes and no organization or individual is allowed to embezzle or misappropriate them.' The *Interpretations of the Social Insurance Law* was drafted by the Legislative Affairs Commission of the Standing Committee of the National People's Congress, the Legislative Affairs Office of the State Council and the Ministry of Human Resources and the Social Security Department. These *Interpretations* of the law state that 'earmarked for specific purposes' means that social insurance funds are mainly used for social insurance benefits and may not be disbursed unless otherwise stipulated by the state. The *Guiding Opinions on the work of critical illness insurance for urban and rural residents*, the *Notice on cost management measures for the purchase of critical illness insurance from insurance companies with basic medical insurance funds* (Cai She (2013) No. 36), and other documents also point out that critical illness insurance funds are used to pay social insurance benefits. Having commercial insurance companies handle them for the purpose of critical illness insurance, therefore, does not qualify as 'embezzling' or 'misappropriating funds.'

Article 72 of the *Social Insurance Law* stipulates that 'Staff expenses and basic operating costs of social insurance-handling entities, as well as management fees, are to be safeguarded at the same level of public finance as per State [national] regulations.' The question remains, and awaits legal clarification, as to whether or not commercial insurance companies who handle critical illness insurance for urban and rural residents can use the stipulations of Article 72 and get paid for their handling expenses by public finance allocations, instead of drawing the expenses from the pooled fund itself. This still needs to be clarified by laws and regulations.

Currently, critical illness insurance is operated in ways that are overly uniform. That is, social security agencies are responsible for organizational guidance, regulatory supervision, and policy formulation while insurance companies conduct specific operations. From a practical standpoint and long-term perspective, we recommend that local solutions be devised by localities themselves. Innovations should be encouraged, as well as pilot programs that turn entities handling medical insurance into legal persons that are professional and that provide occupations for people. These legal-person entities should be allowed to bid for critical illness insurance business in competition with commercial insurance companies. This is in the interests of upholding the principle of fair competition.

5.4 PREFERENTIAL TAX TREATMENT FOR COMMERCIAL HEALTH INSURANCE, AND ANALYSIS OF REGULATORY POLICY

5.4.1 Comparisons of international tax incentive policies for health insurance

5.4.1.1 Health insurance preferential tax policies of the United States

5.4.1.1.1 Overview of health insurance tax incentive policies

Modern commercial health insurance in the United States originated from such non-profit organizations as Blue Cross and Blue Shield in the 1930s (also known as the Blue Plans.) These provided plans for insuring hospital costs and the cost of doctors' services. For-profit insurance companies then started to enter the market, driving its rapid development. In the early days, Blue Plans and insurance companies only provided health insurance for groups, since group health insurance had distinct advantages for them—lower risk of adverse selection and lower management costs, and group plans met the government's requirement for labor protection. In 1942, the *Stabilization Act* was passed in the context of World War II. It allowed employers to provide health and security plan benefits to employees as a way to retain them, given the strict controls during the war on prices and workers' wages. It therefore raised salaries for people in a camouflaged way. In 1943, an administrative tax court ruling specified that the group medical and hospitalization insurance premiums that employers paid to insurance companies could be considered employee income and therefore exempt from tax. This further strengthened the connection between health insurance and employment. This policy was a prelude to tax incentive clauses of the *Internal Revenue Code* (IRC) of 1954. Those landmark clauses removed uncertainty about tax incentives available to employers and motivated them to buy group health insurance for employees.[1]

The tax incentive policies of health insurance in the United States mainly include three aspects.

First, group health insurance: group health insurance premiums paid by employers for employees can be itemized as pre-tax operating expenses, and not be regarded as taxable income of employees, so they are tax-free for both employers and employees. Where employers do not purchase group health insurance for employees but instead pay the same amount to employees as wages, then taxes shall be collected by the federal government, state government, and even local government. For example, the federal income tax rate of a worker in the District of Columbia is 25%, the social security tax rate is 15.3% (including that of employers and employees), and the state income tax rate is 9.5%, so tax subsidies for group health insurance reach up to 50% of the expenditures. According to Section 125 of the IRC, under certain conditions, group health insurance premiums paid by employers and employees can be deducted from pre-tax profit and income and there is no limit to such deductions, so the purchasers will get a very low 'tax price.' Where the employer does not buy employees group health insurance but pays that amount of money to employees in cash, then it shall be included in the taxable income of employees, who will get far less tax benefit from personal health insurance than from group health insurance.

Table 5.2 provides an illustrative example. Two workers, A and B, earn almost the same amount of salary. B participates in group health insurance with premiums of USD 10,000, all of which is paid by the employer. Since the premiums can be deducted before calculating income tax and the Federal Insurance Contribution Act tax (FICA tax), the amount of money saved on not paying tax comes to USD 3,030. If the employee himself adds, say, USD 1,500 to the premium, this part is fully tax-deductible under Section 125 of the IRC, saving an additional USD 450.

Second, personal health insurance: according to law, if the deductibles (medical expenses paid by individuals) of a personal commercial health insurance product are no less than USD 1,050 per person or USD 2,100 per family, the purchaser is entitled to tax subsidies through a personal health savings account (HSA). Contributions to this account are eligible for pre-tax itemized deductions, but the upper limit is the greater of the value of individual deductibles or USD 2,700. The total deductibles per family that can be itemized as pre-tax expenses cannot exceed USD 5,450. In addition, if a person does not have a group health insurance plan and the sum of personal health insurance premiums and other medical expenses exceeds 7.5% of adjusted gross income (AGI), the amount in excess can be itemized as a pre-tax expense. According to the *Affordable Care Act* (ACA), the

Table 5.2 Case: Influence of group insurance tax incentives on insurance purchase costs

(a) Compensation and tax liabilities of two workers: with and without health insurance, 2006

	Person A (without health insurance)	Person B (with health insurance)	Difference (A–B)
Total compensation	**$50,000**	**$50,000**	**$0**
Taxable wages	$50,000	$40,000	$10,000
Employer contributions to health insurance premiums	$0	$10,000	–$10,000
Taxes	**$10,810**	**$7,780**	**$3,030**
Federal income taxes	$3,160	$1,660	$1,500
Employer FICA	$3,825	$3,060	$765
Employee FICA	$3,825	$3,060	$765

(b) Compensation and tax liabilities of two workers offered health insurance: with and without a section 125 plan, 2006

	Person B1 (without 125 plan)	Person B2 (with 125 plan)	Difference (B1–B2)
Total compensation	**$50,000**	**$50,000**	**$0**
Taxable wages	$40,000	$38,500	$1,500
Employer contributions to health insurance premiums	$10,000	$10,000	$0
Taxes	**$7,780**	**$7,331**	**$450**
Federal income taxes	$1,660	$1,440	$220
Employer FICA	$3,060	$2,945	$115
Employee FICA	$3,060	$2,945	$115

Source: Kaiser Family Foundation, 2008.

Note
Amounts may not sum to totals due to rounding effects.

threshold for claiming an itemized deduction on medical expenses would rise from 7.5% (effective in 2013) to 10% of AGI for those under age 65; for those 65 or older, the 10% threshold would be effective after 2016 (Sec. 9013 of the Patient Protection and Affordable Care Act).

Third, health insurance for the self-employed: there was no clear tax preference policy on health insurance for the self-employed until the *Tax Reform Act of 1986*, which said that 25% of the premiums paid by a self-employed person could be deducted from income when calculating tax. This percentage was then increased to 30% and then 40% with the implementation of new acts, before the *Taxpayer Relief Act of 1997* decided to gradually increase it to 100%. It went up from 45% in 1998 and 1999 to 50% in 2000 and 2001, 60% in 2002, 80% from 2003 to 2005, and 90% in 2006, and then to 100% after 2007. In general, sole proprietors, partners, and people who hold 2% or more of a small corporation can all benefit. In some cases, self-employed people are eligible for group health insurance; if the insurance is provided by the employer of a spouse, however, the self-employed person is no longer entitled to tax exemptions.

Tax benefits for the self-employed are subject to the following restrictions. First, tax benefits are not available if either the self-employed worker or his or her spouse has subsidized coverage provided by the employer; second, the amount of tax benefit may not exceed net profit and other business income; and third, the benefits are only applicable to income tax—that is, the premium amounts can only be itemized as expenses against income tax. When calculating self-employment tax based on net earnings from self-employment, they cannot be deducted.

5.4.1.1.2 Updates on tax credit policies under Obamacare

The ACA, which was fully enacted in 2014, places particular emphasis on support for the new state health insurance marketplaces (exchanges). The government took the lead in establishing these exchanges, which use tax credit policies to encourage individuals and small groups to participate in health insurance plans. For states that have already extended the traditional Medicaid income standard to 133% of the Federal Poverty Level, the federal government will provide tax credits on premiums paid for households with incomes between 133% FPL and 250% FPL in addition to subsidies for self-paid medical expenses. It also provides such tax credits for households with incomes between 250% FPL and 400% FPL, but not the subsidies for self-paid medical expenses.

5.4.1.1.3 Fiscal cost of preferential tax policies

Tax-type spending refers to intentional deviations from the normal tax structure in order to achieve certain policy objectives. The aim of such deviation is to give certain designated groups of taxpayers preferential tax treatment in order to provide either tax relief or tax incentives. The reduction in national tax revenue that results from this deviation from a base line of normal tax revenue is 'tax-type spending.' In essence, tax-type spending is a kind of subsidy. It is done to achieve specified policy objectives and to strengthen certain economic behavior as a form of macro-adjustment of the economy. In return for this, the government pays the price of less tax income.

The U.S. government's financial support for healthcare is mainly reflected in three programs. The first is Medicare, a federal health insurance program for the elderly, on which fiscal spending in 2006 was USD 380 billion. The second is Medicaid, a relief program for poor people, on which fiscal spending in 2006 was USD 190 billion. These two programs are under the jurisdiction of the Department of Health and Human Services. The third program is administered by the Internal Revenue Service of the United States, and relates to the tax-type spending that preferential tax policies de facto create. In 2006, total tax-type fiscal spending by the federal government on health insurance or other health-related services was estimated at USD 143 billion.[2]

Employee-sponsored group health insurance policies enjoy stronger benefits from tax-revenue subsidies than non-group insurance policies. A certain amount of the premium that employees pay on behalf of employers can be deducted by the employee from his pre-tax income. In 2006, this amount of deducted expense came to USD 132.7 billion. To date, this is the largest tax-type subsidy for expenditures on health in the country. Moreover, Section 125 of the Internal Revenue Code allows employees to pay premiums with pre-tax money, so all of an employee's contributions are tax-free. These two subsidies account for about 95% of all health-related tax-type spending in the United States.[3]

5.4.1.2 Commercial health insurance preferential tax policies of Australia

5.4.1.2.1 Incentive policies to do with commercial health insurance

Australia has used a multi-barreled approach of both incentives and constraints in order to get people to purchase commercial health insurance. The aim has been to go further in dispersing the risk of medical costs and to encourage wealthier people to be treated at private hospitals so as to relieve congestion at public hospitals. To accomplish these objectives, the government has mainly adopted the following measures.

First, it has increased medical care options. If patients who are covered by the publicly funded system go to a public hospital, they only need to pay for such things as the bed fees, dental expenses, and ophthalmology expenses but they have no choice over what doctor to see or which ward they are put in. In order to increase options for its residents, Australia has allowed self-paying patients, defined as those who participate in commercial health insurance, and patients who are in private hospitals to select their doctor as well as room. In these cases, however, the government will only pay 75% of the given standard rates for treatments and services. The rest must be paid by others, whether that is the individual or his insurance company.

Second, the Australian government provides subsidies for health insurance premiums and also levies fines for not being insured. On July 1, 1997, the *1996 Private Health Insurance Incentives Bill* was formally put into effect. This is considered to be Australia's first major policy adjustment in private health insurance. The Bill states that the government must provide premium subsidies to customers who purchase commercial health insurance. The government provides between AUD 25 and AUD 125 per year in premium subsidies for those whose annual income is less than AUD 35,000 for an individual and AUD 70,000 for a family (the amounts differ depending on the type of product). People with an annual income of between AUD 35,000 to AUD 50,000 and families with an annual income of more than AUD 70,000 are not entitled to subsidies. At the same time, individuals with an annual income of more than AUD 50,000 or families with an annual income of more than AUD 100,000 who are not covered by private health insurance must pay a 1% punitive medical care surtax. The *1998 Private Health Insurance Incentives Bill*, effective on January 1, 1999, increased these subsidies. It ruled that all Australians eligible for the universal healthcare system, regardless of their income level, would now be entitled to 30% of premium subsidies for private health insurance. Starting on April 1, 2005, the Australian government further raised premium subsidies to people aged 65 and above, granting a subsidy amounting to 30% of the premium to those aged between 65 and 69 and up to 40% to those above 70. Private health insurance premiums are subsidized in two ways. In the first, the individual pays the premium to the insurance company with the deduction already taken out. The government pays the deducted portion to the insurance company. In the second, the individual pays the entire amount to the insurance company and either is reimbursed for that amount in a tax rebate, or he fills in a form applying for the reimbursement and takes it to any one of many healthcare agencies to get reimbursed. Most Australians opt for the first method.

Third, the government encourages people to participate in health insurance plans when they are still young. In Australia, private health insurance products are priced by communities, and the premiums are the same for people within the same area, regardless of age. Health insurance companies are not allowed to reject insurance applications, but they have the right to adjust a product's premiums for an entire group of people. Any adjustment to premiums requires approval from regulatory authorities, and customers must be informed of such adjustment in advance. Because of this, the percentage of young people purchasing private health insurance is not high. In July 2000, the Australian government launched the Lifetime Health Coverage (LHC) initiative. On the first July 1 after a person has reached the age of 30, if a person has not taken out commercial health insurance then they have to pay an additional 2% for every year that they delay. The highest loading of this bill on top of premiums is 70%. Once a resident has paid continuously for ten years, the additional fee is eliminated. To bridge short time periods when a person may not be insured, such as when he is switching insurance companies or going to work abroad, Australia has determined that a person can go without hospital coverage for a maximum of 1,094 days in a lifetime (that is, three years less one day), without having it bring into play the additional load on their premiums.

Starting in July 2012, Australia made adjustments to premium subsidies and the medical care surtax. Premium subsidies remain unchanged for low- and middle-income groups. For high-income groups, not only are subsidies no longer offered on premiums but the medical care surtax rate is increased (up to a maximum of 1.5%). By adopting the above measures, in 2013, Australia was able to have 47% of its population covered by commercial health insurance.

5.4.1.2.2 Results of policies

Australia's 'commercial health insurance incentives policy' and the 'Lifetime Health Coverage loading initiative' are complementary to each other. The former provides government subsidies whereas before an individual had to pay the entire amount of premium themselves. The sharing of the cost of premiums has motivated people to buy insurance and also made insurance more affordable. Meanwhile, for high-income people who have not bought health insurance, the punitive surtax also increased the percentage of policy holders. The Lifetime Coverage Health initiative has expanded the coverage of private health insurance, and to some extent promoted stable participation among young groups. The two combined have played a key role in boosting people's enthusiasm for private health insurance and increasing their participation. In 1999, fewer than 6 million Australians were covered by private health insurance. In 2013, the number exceeded 10 million, accounting for more than 47% of the total population.

5.4.2 Analysis of China's commercial health insurance tax policies

5.4.2.1 Policy background

Commercial health insurance has developed rapidly in China in recent years. In 2014, premium income from original (or direct) health insurance policies reached RMB 158.718 billion, an increase of 41.27% over the previous year. Among the different types of life insurance, premiums for health insurance grew fastest. Health insurance reimbursements and grants amounted to RMB 57.116 billion, an increase of 38.92% over the previous year. The share that commercial health insurance held in life insurance as a whole rose from 6.95% in 2009 to 12.18% in 2014. From January to October 2015, premium income from direct health insurance reached RMB 202.725 billion, which represented a 48.35% increase over the previous year. From these figures it can be seen that the commercial health insurance market enjoys robust demand and huge development potential.

To further promote the development of commercial health insurance, on May 6, 2015, the Standing Committee of the State Council decided to draw on international experience and launch preferential tax policies for individuals on a pilot-program basis. The aim was to encourage people to buy comprehensive-type commercial health insurance policies that were aimed at the general public. Given the cost of premiums, each person was permitted to deduct an average of RMB 2,400 from income before figuring taxes. According to our projections, commercial health insurance premiums will exceed RMB 800 billion by 2020 if calculated based on an average annual growth rate of 25%. Taking into account the 'releasing' effect of the preferential tax policies, the premiums may actually reach more than RMB 1 trillion, and commercial health insurance will become one of the three main insurance businesses, the other two being property insurance and life insurance.

5.4.2.2 Analysis of relevant regulatory policies

Following the *Opinions on accelerating the development of commercial health insurance*, released by the State Council in 2014, in order to further advance the growth of the industry, the State introduced and improved upon a set of preferential tax policies on commercial health insurance.

In May 2015, the Ministry of Finance, the State Tax Administration, and the China Insurance Regulatory Commission jointly issued the *Notice on the work of launching the pilot program of individual income tax policies for commercial health insurance* (Cai Shui [2015] No. 56) as a way to vigorously promote the related pilot-program work. According to this *Notice*, individual purchasers of commercial health insurance are entitled to a pre-tax deduction of up to RMB 2,400 per year from their premium cost. The *Notice* designated Beijing, Shanghai, Tianjin, and Chongqing as pilot areas for testing the program.

Following that, in November 2015, the Ministry of Finance, the State Tax Administration, and the China Insurance Regulatory Commission jointly issued the *Notice on implementing the pilot program of individual income tax policies for commercial health insurance* (Cai Shui [2015] No. 126). This included more detailed provisions on the preferential tax policies for commercial health insurance. According to these guidelines, meant to serve as a framework for product design, commercial health insurance products involving preferential taxes should take the form of all-purpose insurance. At the same time, they carry two kinds of obligations, namely medical insurance and also personal savings accounts. People being insured should be taxpayers over the age of 16, and below the statutory retirement age. In terms of the obligation to provide medical safeguards, reimbursements should cover self-paid medical expenses within the scope of the benefits of the local basic medical insurance funds, as well as a portion of the expenses outside the scope of these benefits.

On July 27, 2016, the China Insurance Regulatory Commission made public the list of commercial insurance companies that have already received permission to engage in the business of preferential-tax type commercial health insurance products. They include PICC Health Insurance Co. Ltd., Sunshine Life Insurance Corporation Ltd., Taikang Life Insurance Co. Ltd., China Life Insurance (Group) Company, China Pacific Life Insurance Co. Ltd., Ping An Life Insurance Company of China, New China Life Insurance Co. Ltd., Taiping Life Insurance Co. Ltd., CCB Life Insurance Co. Ltd., General China Life Insurance Co. Ltd., Taiping Pension Co. Ltd., Soochow Life Insurance Co. Ltd., Union Life Insurance Co. Ltd., PICC Life Insurance Co. Ltd., Lian Life Insurance Co. Ltd., and Shanghai Life Insurance Co. Ltd.

This round of formulating policies to do with preferential tax treatment of commercial health insurance illustrated the important role and functions that this kind of insurance plays in supplementing China's basic medical insurance system. On the one hand, its coverage and its targeted group of customers point to its unique ability to provide high-level medical safeguards. On the other hand, the government has imposed constraints on this kind of insurance through regulating how insurance companies operate, which shows that preferential tax-type health insurance also bears a certain social responsibility.

Specifically, commercial health insurance enjoying preferential tax policies for individuals mainly targets people who have participated in basic medical insurance and want compensation for self-paid expenses on top of the benefits of basic medical insurance. It also targets those who want to be insured against high medical expenses that result from critical illness. The purpose of such insurance is to compensate for high-end medicine costs.

Commercial health insurance involving preferential taxes provides comprehensive protection. Within the scope of compensation liability are hospitalization costs, outpatient expenditures before and after hospitalization, certain outpatient treatment expenses, and outpatient treatment expenses for chronic diseases. The benefits of each item are shown in Table 5.3.

Commercial health insurance products involving tax preferences are available to both healthy people and those with prior conditions. In other words, insurance companies may not reject insurance applicants based on their medical history. Moreover, there is no requisite waiting period.

As to the term of policies, regulations state that insurance companies must guarantee continuous coverage until a policy holder's statutory retirement age. They may not refuse to continue coverage due to a change in the person's health status during this period.

In addition, with respect to the overall loss ratio, health insurance products are to follow the concept of conserving principal while allowing for a modest profit. When the simple loss ratio of the medical insurance part of a policy is lower than the prescribed ratio as according to regulations, the insurance company must return the difference in ratios to the individual policy holder's

Table 5.3 Benefits of commercial health insurance products involving tax preferences (RMB)

The insured Medical insurance liability	With anamnesis when first covered	Without anamnesis when first covered
I Annual medical expenses of a single policy	200,000	40,000
i Hospitalization costs and outpatient expenditures before and after hospitalization	200,000	40,000
Of which: single material cost	30,000	5,000
ii Certain outpatient treatment expenses	20,000	5,000
iii Outpatient treatment expenses for chronic diseases	3,000	1,000
II Ceiling on accumulated compensations within period of guaranteed continuous coverage	800,000	150,000

Source: CIRC. *Notice on circulating the guidelines and template for health insurance products involving tax preferences* (Bao Jian Fa (2015) No. 118), December 16, 2015.

account. If the actual reimbursements that a company makes to a policy holder are less than 90% of the medical expenses of the insured within the agreed-upon range in the contract, the insurance company must automatically make up that amount to the policy holder. These stipulations go to show that insurance with preferential tax treatment is different from normal commercial health insurance and bears a certain social responsibility.

5.4.2.3 Influence of preferential tax policies on the health insurance market

On May 12, 2015, the China Insurance Regulatory Commission, the Ministry of Finance, and the State Tax Administration jointly issued the *Notice on the work of launching the pilot program of implementing individual income tax policies for commercial health insurance.* To ensure the smooth implementation of the pilot programs, this *Notice* selected a core city in each of China's main regions in which to launch the pilot program initiative. Of these cities, four are under the direct jurisdiction of the Central Government, namely Beijing, Shanghai, Tianjin, and Chongqing. In the provinces and autonomous regions, cities were chosen on the basis of having a large population as well as having fairly high comprehensive management ability.

We expect that the preferential tax policies will provide incentives to people to purchase commercial health insurance—the policies will stimulate an increase in actual demand and will have a positive influence on expanding the market. We also feel that this positive influence, namely the stimulus effect on demand of the preferential tax policies, will be expressed in the following two ways.

The first way relates to the tax-avoidance result of the preferential tax policies. Premiums for health insurance can be itemized as expenses against pre-tax income, which allows the policy holder to gain some tax benefits and which indirectly lowers the price of the commercial health insurance. As a result, given the role of price elasticity, this increases the demand for commercial health insurance. If an urban employee who purchases commercial health insurance enjoys the highest tax-avoidance benefit as allowed for in the *Notice*, which is to say they purchase RMB 200 per month of commercial health insurance, then we can use this figure to calculate the actual benefits of the preferential policy to employees who are at different levels of income.

The second way preferential tax policies have a stimulus effect relates to the demonstration effect. Publicity about the policy as well as government behavior can raise people's awareness and understanding of commercial health insurance. Strict regulatory control by government over this kind of insurance sets up a beneficial image in people's minds, and an attitude of public confidence. This in turn draws others in the category of 'potential demand' into buying the insurance even if they are not motivated by the tax avoidance feature.

Our research used the fitted employee income distribution in China and integrated that with data from questionnaire surveys conducted in the Binhai New Area of Tianjin. It used a two-part model of demand and income. By using the estimated probability of purchasing preferential-tax type commercial health insurance and the percentage of people at different income levels to the total number of employees, we could then predict the number of people willing to purchase preferential-tax type commercial health insurance as well as the amount of premiums they would be willing to pay. As a result, we predicted the size of the commercial health insurance market given the incentive of preferential tax policies.

The results of the quantitative model show that the incentive effect of preferential tax policies is massive. The premium income from preferential-tax type commercial health insurance is expected to reach RMB 35.633 billion per month, and the corresponding tax preferences will amount to RMB 1.481 billion per month. According to our calculations, the ongoing annual increase in premiums will then be roughly RMB 427.596 billion if potential demand is fully released. What's more, the model reckons that the annual total amount of foregone taxes due to the preferential policy will be roughly RMB 17.016 billion. China's actual revenues from individual income taxes in 2014 were RMB 737.7 billion. As compared to that figure, the foregone tax revenue is only about 2.3%. The influence of the policy on China's overall tax revenue structure is not large.

In 2014, China's tax revenue from individual income taxes totaled RMB 737.7 billion, which represented an increase of 12.9% over the previous year. Large cities that are in relatively more developed parts of the country represent a substantial percentage of that amount. In 2014, for example, China's tax revenues from individual income taxes in the top 16 cities came to RMB 411.4 billion or 55.77% of the national total. Those 16 included such cities as Shanghai, Beijing, and Shenzhen. It is particularly important, therefore, to calculate the effect of preferential tax policies on potential demand for insurance in the largest cities. This research estimated the potential market for commercial health insurance in cities based on the percentage of actual income tax revenue in those cities in 2014 as a percentage of the national total.

We can see from our projected results that preferential tax policies will have a very considerable incentive effect on potential demand for health insurance in cities with the highest level of individual income taxes. For example, the market for commercial health insurance is estimated to increase by more than five times in such cities as Shanghai, Ningbo, Shenzhen, Suzhou, and Nantong. Meanwhile, the additional market value is estimated at more than RMB 10 billion in just the five cities of Shanghai, Beijing, Shenzhen, Guangzhou, and Suzhou.

5.4.3 Health insurance with preferential tax treatment for individuals: current situation and problems

Pilot programs were launched nationwide on January 1, 2016. Since that time, the China Insurance Regulatory Commission has successively issued five lists of names of companies licensed to operate health insurance with preferential tax treatment. In all, 26 companies are now qualified to do this business, which represent roughly 32% of all insurance companies in the country.

The *Notice on the pilot program of individual income tax policies for commercial health insurance* stipulates that such products shall be in the form of all-purpose insurance that provides insurance safeguards but also sets up accounts for policy holders that have a minimum guaranteed income. The products are therefore to incorporate two kinds of obligations, namely health insurance and personal savings accounts. At present, the value-added services and scope of safeguards differ for the various companies, but they all have added targeted therapy for malignant tumors to their coverage and they reimburse 100% of costs under the social insurance program and 80% of costs outside that program or a composite figure of no less than 90%. It should be said that such products greatly increase the level of safeguards for insured groups of people. Moreover, insurance companies also provide health management and other value-added services outside the scope of the basic medical insurance, which means they are playing their proper role in establishing a multi-tiered system of medical insurance safeguards in China.

However, at present the main problems with these products are their limited size of business and the inadequate range of people they cover. According to publicly available data, by March 31, 2017, there were a total of 67,272 policies in the 31 cities conducting pilot programs. These policies represented 1% of the number of people eligible to be covered by this kind of preferential-tax health insurance policy in these cities. Roughly 58,000 were participating in the program, and the total value of their premiums came to around RMB 118.4 million, which is a very small figure. The per capita premium amount was RMB 1,760 a year, which was RMB 640 less than the RMB 2,400 ceiling on itemized deductions. Obviously, the development of commercial health insurance that includes tax preferences is not ideal. The incentive effect of tax policies on demand for insurance has not come up to expectations. The main reasons are as follows.

First, consumers are not highly motivated by the relatively low tax benefits—the incentive effect is not at all obvious. Policy holders can write off up to RMB 2,400 in premium expenses against income, but this is actually a relatively low figure. It is insufficient to stimulate demand. For example, based on the RMB 2,400 ceiling, an employee with a take-home pay of RMB 6,000 per month will pay RMB 240 less a year in income taxes. If that RMB 240 is put to buying commercial health insurance involving tax preferences, however, that employee still needs to pay out RMB 2,160 a year. Table 5.4 shows the maximum degree of preferential tax treatment, by level of wages. It also shows the necessary amount of premium payments after the total amount of the tax-preferenced income is spent on premiums.

Second, the preferential personal tax policies benefit a small group of people. Commercial health insurance is a supplement to basic medical insurance in China. It provides a higher level of protection so it caters to a higher-income group. But high-income groups of people, or those in large corporations, generally already have supplementary insurance and there is considerable overlap of the coverage that different policies provide. Moreover, the number of people

Table 5.4 Premium expenditure on top of preferences (RMB)

Level	Take-home pay per month	Maximum tax reductions per year	Premium expenditure on top of preferences	Income tax preferences as % of annual income
1	3,500~5,000	72	2,328	0.12
2	5,000~8,000	240	2,160	0.25
3	8,000~12,500	480	1,920	0.32
4	12,500~38,500	600	1,800	0.13
5	38,500~58,500	720	1,680	0.10
6	58,500~83,500	840	1,560	0.08
7	Above 83,500	1,080	1,320	–

Note
The income tax preferences as % of the annual income is the ratio of the annual maximum tax preferences to the highest annual income at the corresponding income level.

who pay personal income tax in China is relatively small. In 2015, there were 28 million people with a monthly income of over RMB 3,500, which is the threshold for paying tax. That figure represents 2.07% of the total population. The number of people with incomes of more than RMB 120,000 who actually self-declared their taxes was around 5 million. This figures accounts for 0.37% of the total population. China has been granting subsidies for preferential tax policies but the scope of coverage is quite small and demand for the policies is inadequate. The result, this year, is that while we can applaud the attempt we cannot say that there is much of an audience doing the same.

Third, inadequate product promotion has led to a lack of understanding among consumers. From the perspective of companies and their profitability, the *Interim Measures* place considerable pressure on operations and operating risk. The *Measures* stipulate that commercial health insurance that has preferential tax treatment shall have no deductibles, the amount insured shall not be less than RMB 200,000, applicants with pre-existing illness cannot be turned down, and the compensation ratio shall not be less than 80%. Companies are therefore cautious about taking on this business. Meanwhile, the relatively low extent of marketing has led to insufficient understanding by consumers and indeed ignorance that such products even exist. As a result, the market has not developed as well as people had hoped it would.

Fourth, the actual process of handling the tax-related business has not yet been smoothed out. Tax refunds are a key link in commercial health insurance involving preferential tax treatment. Refunds require close collaboration among insurance companies, employers, and tax authorities. However, most regions have not yet issued operating procedures on refunds. At the same time, this type of product has to do with individuals signing up for policies, but individuals actually report their taxes through the entity for which they work. For insurance companies that received permits to undertake the tax-preferential type of insurance, this has led to an overlap between the group insurance for those entities and people's individual insurance. Not only has this influenced management efficiency in insurance companies but it has dampened the enthusiasm of taxpayers to sign up for policies.

Fifth, models by which social insurance can cooperate with commercial insurance are not yet in existence, which means that it is impossible to take advantage of leveraging the scale of social insurance. Commercial health insurance that involves preferential tax treatment should be tied in to China's basic medical insurance in effective ways if it is to be an effective supplementary form of insurance. In terms of the safeguards that commercial policies offer, however, each company is different when it comes to coverage that falls outside the scope of the government-designated list of items covered under social insurance. There is no unified standard. Moreover, in most places, large-sum supplementary insurance has been added to the basic medical insurance for urban employees, but there is no comprehensive plan for how to link it with commercial health insurance.

5.4.4 Lessons and recommendations

First, raise the tax benefits to encourage participation among taxpayers. The current ceiling of RMB 2,400 that can be deducted from pre-tax income is relatively low. Table 5.5 lists maximum amounts of itemized deductions and their percentage of per capita income in some developed countries. This international experience indicates that the amount of tax deductions under similar policies of developed countries accounts for about 10% of average income. Statistics released by the National Bureau of Statistics show that, in 2015, the annual average income of urban workers in the non-private sector was RMB 62,029. It therefore would be advisable to increase the amount of allowable tax deductions to RMB 6,000 per year.

On a superficial level, the increase in deductible tax amounts would appear to reduce government tax revenue. In reality, however, due to the resulting expansion of the commercial health insurance market, it would have a positive effect on the fiscal balance between revenue and spending. The basic medical insurance funds are facing pressure in all parts of the country, due to the rigid nature of welfare benefits and the natural rise in medical expenses. A large part of the deficit in these funds will have to be covered by public finance at the national level. If commercial health insurance can become an effective supplement or substitute for basic medical insurance, effective leveraging of the preferential tax policies will help moderate pressures on national finance.

Second, integrate the policies that deal with 'supplementary medical insurance for corporate employees' and 'health insurance with preferential tax treatment for individuals,' and establish unified standards for tax deductions and models of coordination. The *Pilot Program for improving the urban social security system*, released by the State Council in 2000, stipulates that 'eligible enterprises may provide their employees with supplementary medical insurance, if the amounts deducted from wages for this purpose are less than 4% of total

Table 5.5 Income tax deductions in some developed countries

Country	Pretax itemized reduction limit (Home currency)	Pretax itemized reduction limit (USD)	Per capital income (USD)	Pretax itemized reduction limit as % of per capita income	Monthly limit (RMB)	Annual limit (RMB)
Italy	EUR 3,615.20	4,988.61	29,340	17.00	730	8,750
Germany	EUR 2,800	3,863.72	32,640	11.84	508	6,094
Austria	EUR 2,920	4,029.31	41,244	9.77	420	5,029
U.S.	USD 3,250	3,250	39,156	8.30	356	4,272
Greece	EUR 1,200	1,650.48	22,313	7.40	317	3,809
Republic of Korea	KRW 1 million	951.6	34,836	2.73	117	1,405

Source: Insurance Association of China. *Private Health Insurance: An International Perspective.* Beijing: China Financial Publishing House, 2015.

wages. The amount so deducted can be itemized as part of operating costs.' From January 1, 2008, the percentage was increased to 5%. In practice, however, to enjoy the 5% policy, enterprises that purchase supplementary medical insurance from insurance companies must have such insurance designated as supplementary medical insurance by social security authorities, and they must submit applications to local State Tax Administration offices. This process takes a long time, and only a miniscule number of enterprises have actually benefited from the policy.

Since commercial health insurance that provides preferential tax treatment is obliged to cover taxpayers with pre-existing illness, as well as to guarantee continuous coverage, insurance companies face a high risk of adverse selection. In contrast with individual policies, employer-sponsored supplementary medical insurance is group insurance that covers employees regardless of their pre-existing conditions. (This also applies to the supplementary employment insurance of non-corporate types of units.) Having everyone in the group purchase the insurance helps to spread settlement risks and strengthen the scale effect. Because of this, we recommend that tax authorities refer to the way of doing things put forth in the 2013 *Notice on issues concerning personal income taxes on enterprise annuities and occupational annuities.* This would put both kinds of insurance under integrated management, namely the supplementary medical insurance and the individual insurance with preferential tax treatment. The supplementary medical insurance premiums paid by enterprises should be a part of operating costs before business income tax, but they should also be deducted from the taxable income of employees before personal income tax. We recommend gradually raising the percentage allowed for deductions from 5% to between 8 and 10%, and simplifying the application procedures for getting supplementary medical insurance designated and getting tax exemption. At the same time, the supplementary medical insurance should be tied in to commercial health insurance for which employees pay fees, so as to encourage more enterprises and individuals to enroll and so as to improve the multi-tiered medical insurance system.

Third, make full use of the opportunity provided by the individual-account reform in the basic medical insurance for employees. Use the social insurance platform effectively, and invigorate the link between the funds in social security accounts and tax-preferential commercial health insurance in order to increase participation in that form of insurance. For a long time, the ways in which money in personal accounts could be spent were strictly controlled. This led to a massive amount of idle funds in such accounts, which were used very inefficiently. During the 13th Five-Year Plan period, various provinces and municipalities rolled out policies to relax restrictions on the use of funds in personal accounts and to allow account holders to purchase commercial health insurance with them. However, at this point there are a multitude of commercial health insurance products on the market and their quality is highly uneven. In contrast, health insurance products that offer preferential tax treatment enjoy preferential policy treatment from the government, and their premium rates, terms, and levels of profit are strictly controlled by regulatory departments. They are quasi-public goods and therefore they also have the most reasonable pricing of all products on the market. Their safeguards are the most complete. In general, they are the products most worth buying.

We recommend that insurance regulators and social security departments jointly formulate policies to redefine the use of funds in social security accounts to allow them to be funds that can buy commercial health insurance products involving preferential tax treatment. We recommend that they guide and encourage people to use their social security account funds for such purchase. Not only can this increase the efficiency with which the funds are being used, but it can expand the number of people who hold tax-preferential-type insurance policies. In bringing into play the principle of large numbers, this will also reduce the adverse selection and settlement risks of insurance companies. By having whole families participate in insurance plans, the group of insured can be expanded to include direct relatives of employees. This can be effective in resolving the problem of catastrophic medical spending when a family runs into a crisis. It can therefore help alleviate the risk of being forced into poverty or returned to poverty as a result of illness.

Fourth, further refine and standardize regulatory policies on commercial health insurance that offers preferential tax treatment. As per the rule of 'conserving principal while allowing for a modest profit,' the *Interim Measures for the administration of health insurance operations that provide preferential tax treatment for individuals* stipulate that where the simple loss ratio is lower than 80%, the difference in amounts is to be returned to the personal account of the insured. However, the *Framework of guidelines for health insurance products with preferential tax treatment for individuals,* as issued by the China Insurance Regulatory Commission, explicitly defines the simple loss ratio as all losses and extra expenses (used to provide value-added services to the insured) as a percentage of all premiums in a fiscal year. At the same time, this *Framework of guidelines* does not specify how the difference can be refunded nor does it give any unified rules on this, leaving the matter up to the decision of insurance companies.

We recommend that regulators further clarify whether the difference shall be refunded in cash or deducted from the premium for the next year, and that they specify the scope of 'extra expenses,' including what categories of health management expenses should be included and whether expenses for such value-added services as physical examinations and immune system tests are included in cost expenditures or not. Regulators need to define all of these things and constantly refine the standards of compliance. They need to be explicit about what costs belong to whom, so as to leave insurance companies with a certain profit margin. This is to elevate the enthusiasm of insurance companies towards carrying on the preferential tax-type business and to increase their confidence in making it profitable. It is to improve the way these products develop in the market.

Fifth, further the building of the information platform used by tax authorities. Upgrade the convenience of actually operating the system, strengthen the force of policy publicity and product promotion, and enable people to understand more about commercial health insurance with preferential tax treatment so as to make them more enthusiastic about participating in the insurance. On the one hand, insurance regulatory departments should go further in coordinating their work with tax authorities. As fast as possible, they should set up and perfect a tax management platform and information sharing mechanism. They should clarify the rights and obligations of those who are insured, formulate complete, convenient, and efficient operating procedures by which taxes are refunded. They should improve the experience of the individual in enrolling in these insurance products and truly bring policy benefits to the great mass of people who pay taxes. On the other hand, insurance regulatory bodies, insurance associations, and insurance companies should put more force behind their promotion of the policies and products, in order to increase people's understanding and generate more enthusiasm for enrolling.

5.5 MEASURES FOR IMPROVING THE REGULATION OF COMMERCIAL HEALTH INSURANCE

5.5.1 Place higher demands on the regulatory management of specialized operations of health insurance

Regulatory bodies should establish regulatory departments that are solely responsible for overseeing health insurance. In order to achieve more specialized operations of health insurance and create a policy environment that is conducive to the growth of health insurance, we must take advantage of the regulatory forces of insurance regulatory bodies. One important part of this will be to set up a dedicated regulatory body for health insurance under the China Insurance Regulatory Commission. First, through independent regulation, regulators can strengthen research and guidance on health insurance, draw up regulations that are specifically directed at health insurance, and improve the overall regulatory system that governs health insurance. They can strictly regulate market access by standardizing entry provisions, and gradually realize a situation in which health insurance is handled by companies that only do health insurance. In that way, they can push for making the field more professional. Second, setting up a body within CIRC that is dedicated to regulating health insurance will be beneficial to establish better communications and coordination with relevant departments at a higher level, including social security, medical, and health departments. The aim is to achieve a more beneficial policy environment.

5.5.2 Promote legislation at a higher level of government and foster a good external policy environment

Commercial health insurance involves a wide range of activities, many management links, a large amount of work, and complex and miscellaneous services. Its operations involve not only the insurer and the insured but also medical institutions and social security agencies. Given the number of participating entities, regulating the business requires a coordinated approach by many different government departments. Commercial health insurance plays a supplementary role in China's medical safeguards system, and as such it is subject to not only social insurance policies and medical policies but also the considerable influence of the institutional structures within which it operates. Because of this, regulatory departments must actively communicate with social insurance and health departments in addition to increasing regulatory controls over insurance companies and guiding them toward standard operations. Moreover, regulatory departments should seek to have support from legislation and policies that are established at a higher level of government. This includes improving upon such things as the *Social Insurance Law* and the *Healthcare Law*. The status of different components of health insurance should be defined in a more specific way, including medical insurance, medical services, commercial health insurance, and medicine vis-à-vis pharmaceuticals. The rights and obligations of these things should be clarified in the course of their interaction. Management of the greater health industry of the future must proceed on the basis of law.

5.5.3 Strengthen the protection of consumers' rights and interests

Insurance regulators should speed up completion of the amendment to the *Measures on Administration of Health Insurance*. They should pay particular attention to the protection of consumers' rights and interests, and strengthen regulation over behavior harming the rights and interests of consumers. In particular, dedicated plans should be developed to regulate online insurance companies and insurance products sold by overseas insurance companies through informal channels.

5.5.4 Improve industry standards and build information and data exchange platforms

Given that the pricing basis of health insurance is different from that of life insurance and property insurance, it is necessary to establish an independent actuarial system based on the incidence of disease data and medical expenses to accurately identify and evaluate business risks and provide effective support for product pricing and risk control. The information system should make a point of enhancing information exchange with the systems of insurance companies, social security agencies, health authorities, and medical institutions to achieve real-time sharing of data.

5.5.5 Improve and implement health insurance tax policies

Insurance regulators need to integrate the supplementary medical insurance and preferential personal tax policies, establish unified standards for tax deductions and modes of coordination, streamline the designation and tax exemption application procedures, and align supplementary medical insurance with commercial health insurance involving tax preferences, so as to encourage participation from enterprises and individuals and improve the multi-tiered medical insurance system.

We recommend that insurance regulators and social security departments jointly formulate policies that facilitate the use of funds in social security accounts for purchase of commercial health insurance involving tax preferences. At the same time, they should adopt a form of 'family insurance.' This can be a way to extend the target group to immediate family members of employees, in order to cover catastrophic medical bills and prevent poverty brought on by illness.

5.5.6 Maintain strict regulation over critical illness insurance

Insurance regulators should attempt to control the quality of insurance companies 'at the source' by strengthening procedures that govern market entry. They should increase reviews and investigations into such things as qualifications required for the industry, ability to pay reimbursement compensation, and so on. They can experiment with establishing a market-entry blacklist to screen out offenders. They should strengthen regulatory management over market behavior and put high pressure on any improper forms of competition or illegal activity—these should be dealt with severely, as per laws and regulations, in order to maintain market order. Regulators should strengthen their supervision over the quality of services. They should push for open information, and should require periodic and timely reports on the status of major illness insurance operations as well as regulatory conditions. They should themselves be willing to accept the regulatory oversight of the public.

5.5.7 Seek to establish non-profit commercial insurance institutions

Efforts can be made to reform social insurance agencies, transform their functions, and establish non-profit commercial insurance institutions, which have no shareholders and offer no dividends. 'Non-profit' does not mean that these entities are required to suffer losses. Instead, their profits, if any, should mainly be used to employ more professional personnel to provide better services for consumers. At the present time, social insurance entities have control over substantial amounts of information. The process of reform called 'de-administration' should help to allow for better coordination among departments such that information can be shared in real time. This too will contribute to improving the operating models of commercial insurance companies.

Notes

1 M.A. Thomasson. The Importance of Group Coverage: How Tax Policy Shaped U.S. Health Insurance. *American Economic Review*, 2003, 93(4): 1373–1384. doi:10.1257/000282803769206359.
2 Joseph Antos. Is There a Right Way to Promote Health Insurance through the Tax System? *National Tax Journal*, 2006 (59). doi:10.17310/ntj.2006.3.05.
3 Paul Fronstin. Savings Needed to Fund Health Insurance and Health Care Expenses in Retirement. *EBRI Issue Brief* (Employee Benefit Research Institute), 2006 (1): 4–31.

6 Research Topic 5

Impact of comprehensive medical reform on commercial health insurance

Zhu Hengpeng, Zan Xin, and Sun Mengting

Counting from the 1980s, commercial insurance has been functioning in China for more than 30 years. Commercial *health* insurance, dealing more specifically with healthcare, appeared in the early 1990s and is by now becoming ever more important in the eyes of the government and society at large. Commercial health insurance had its inception before China's 'basic medical insurance system' began, and then had to become 'supplementary' to that system as time went on. By now, however, primarily in the past two years, China's Central Government documents are noting that commercial insurance should become a 'main pillar' in China's system of social safeguards. Changes in China's healthcare and medical systems have consistently impacted the growth of commercial health insurance, and this situation is likely to continue in the future.

Factors that affect changes in China's healthcare and medical systems come primarily from two aspects. One is public policy as it relates to the medical reform process, specifically the stream of policy documents that have come out since the new medical reform was launched in 2009. The other is the social and economic transformation caused by China's ongoing process of transforming its mode of development. This is seen specifically in such things as higher standards of living, an increase in consumer demand, the release of demand for medical care, changes in the spectrum of disease, and technological advancements.

It is obvious that both of these aspects will have an extremely pronounced effect on the development of commercial health insurance. The effect of the former can be seen in the 'policy intent' of the government to put major effort behind support of commercial health insurance. On a nationwide basis, 'room to implement this policy effort' is gradually increasing, as China's central policy-makers work behind the scenes to use commercial insurance (that is, market mechanisms) to take China's medical reform into deeper waters. The effect of the latter reflects changes in the national awareness of insurance, the increase in demand for insurance products that are multi-tiered and diversified, and the opportunities for innovation brought on by the advance of Internet technologies.

This report will focus on the impact of 'comprehensive medical reform' on the development of commercial health insurance. It will include an analysis of relevant policies, a forecast of the development of China's medical and healthcare systems, and a specific analysis of the space into which commercial health insurance can develop.

6.1 REFORM OF CHINA'S MEDICAL AND HEALTHCARE INSTITUTIONS: STAGES IN THE EVOLUTION OF THE REFORM AND THE EARLIER INFLUENCE ON COMMERCIAL INSURANCE

The earliest stage of China's healthcare system reform can be traced back to the 1980s, so reform has been going on for some time. Due to changes of those in power, among other things, the context for reforms has kept changing and it is hard to describe each round of reform in a logical or consistent way. Each round had its own emphasis and its own policy adjustments. From all of the documentary material we have sifted through, the start of commercial health insurance began at very nearly the same time as the launch of the earliest health reform. At least one could say it came immediately following on that. After that, however, the patterns of reform and patterns of institutional structures again began to influence the development of commercial health insurance in different ways.

6.1.1　From the 1980s to 1998: initial marketization of the supply of medical services and the embryonic development of commercial health insurance

In 1985, the State Council approved and passed on for implementation the *Report by the Ministry of Health on a number of policy issues to do with the work of healthcare reform.* This is generally regarded as the start of China's healthcare system reform. This *Report* pointed to the need to 'loosen policies, streamline administration and devolve authority to lower levels of government, raise funds from multiple sources, open up a broader path to developing healthcare careers, and invigorate [resuscitate] the work of providing healthcare.' All the way up until 1998, this concept of 'invigorating' (or resuscitating) continued to influence the development of the systems that provide medical services in China.

The Ministry of Health, Ministry of Finance, and other Central Government departments then issued a whole series of reform policies. By giving greater autonomy to medical institutions at lower levels, by allowing medical institutions to increase the amount of income that they could distribute on their own, by allowing doctors in medical institutions to have income that was derived from moonlighting medical services, and so on, these stimulated medical institutions to provide more medical services. At the same time, these policies encouraged social forces (private or non-governmental) to participate in providing medical care. This expanded the supply of services and improved their quality as well as their efficiency.[1] The supply of medical services began to be market-oriented to an initial degree. That is, via the actions of different market entities, including medical institutions, doctors, and patients, resources began to be allocated independently as opposed to being allocated solely by administrative directives, as had been the situation before. (For example, in the past, patients of different social status or rank could only get medical care at medical institutions that were administratively designated for them.)

Total healthcare costs increased rapidly during this period. Between 1985 and 1991, total expenditures on healthcare nationwide went from RMB 27.9 billion to RMB 89.3 billion, roughly a three-fold increase. By 1997, they reached RMB 319.7 billion, or 11.5 times the figure in 1985. However, the core element in the ability to supply medical services, namely professional medical personnel, did not in fact show a correspondingly ferocious increase during this period. The supply side of resource allocation did not change that much (see Figure 6.1.) The main reason for this is that the training of doctors relied to a large extent on medical institutions, but those same medical institutions were almost completely 'public' institutions with all that the public system implied. The number of people that institutions could cultivate as professionals was subject to severe restrictions. Meanwhile, medical institutions that were managed outside the public system, by 'society,' found it hard to attract the outstanding doctors away from public institutions. Their failure to grow effectively limited any increase in the number of physicians overall.

With little increase in supply but a sharp increase in costs, it can well be imagined that residents felt the increase in costs in a visceral way (we do not even take into account the influence of changing prices on this situation.) What this

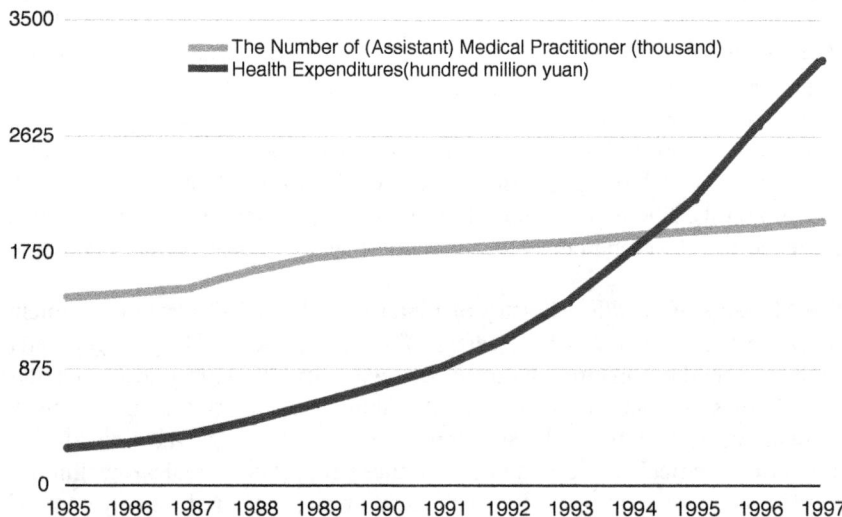

Figure 6.1 National health expenditure and changes in physician resources between 1985 and 1997.

Source of data: *China Health Statistical Yearbook.*

did, however, was to provide room in which commercial health insurance could develop. As the very first company to deal in the health insurance business, the People's Insurance Company of China (PICC) had already begun offering personal insurance products to the market in the early 1980s. The number of participants at the time was roughly 2 million. By the end of 1992, the cumulative balance of insurance funds in PICC had reached RMB 23.69 million.[2] Around 1993, the China Pacific Insurance Company (CPIC) and Ping An Insurance (Group) Company of China (Ping An) also launched their first group and individual health insurance products.

Given the passage of time, we were not able to obtain data on the growth of commercial health insurance during that period, but documentary materials do indicate that this period could, at the very least, be defined as the 'embryonic stage' of commercial health insurance in China. Back then, people necessarily had only the most rudimentary awareness of their own risk, given that the government intervened in every aspect of people's lives. People's level of income was also low, so that purchasing power was not enough to support buying health insurance. Urban residents had somewhat higher spending capacity, but they also had a much greater reliance on publicly funded medicine and the labor insurance program run by the government. Awareness of commercial health insurance was therefore miniscule, whether it stemmed from the public or the private sector. Not only were there essentially no policy documents on the subject, but commercial insurance entities were themselves only beginning to test the water.

6.1.2 From 1998 to 2009: gradual improvement of China's basic medical insurance system and the growth of commercial health insurance

In 1998, in order to meet the needs of transforming China's model for social and economic development, and in order to reduce the pressures brought on by reform of China's State-Owned Enterprises, which was adding fuel to the flames at the time, the Central Government issued a policy document setting up a system called the *Medical insurance system for urban employees*. The Central Government also laid down a path for 'having China become a country with a social security system.' Meanwhile, the State Council formally abolished the old system of publicly funded 'labor insurance medical safeguards.' This was done by the *Decision on the establishment of a basic medical insurance system for urban employees* (issued by the State Council [1998] No. 44). This called for vigorous exploration into establishing a system of social medical insurance that would provide low levels of security to a broad number of people. The funding model for this medical insurance would combine pooled funding from the public with individual accounts. This *Decision* also mentioned the role of commercial insurance for the first time: '... medical expenses that exceed the allowed limit of compensation can be resolved by such means as coverage from commercial health insurance.'

In terms of reforming supply-side systems, this period no longer emphasized such things as expanding the autonomy of medical institutions or turning them into corporations. Instead, relative to the previous period, government not only did not reduce interference in the affairs of public medical institutions but it increased interference. Doctors were no longer encouraged to use their spare time to provide medical services. Salaries were adjusted somewhat but this came mainly from fine-tuning personnel salary systems within public hospitals and was not related to any institutional or structural reforms. With regard to having society (private entities) manage hospitals, for the first time the Central Government issued a document that explicitly called for managing hospitals in different categories and it included clear mention of for-profit medical institutions and non-profit medical institutions. However, there was no clear policy support during this period of having 'society managing hospitals,' or 'releasing the vitality of social forces in managing hospitals.'

This may have been related to the very tight situation in public finance at the time. Policymakers who were involved may have worried that an overly fast rise in medical costs would jeopardize the urban employees' basic medical insurance fund that had just been set up. They were worried it might not hold up under excessive spending pressure. In fact, when this fund was just set up, a great portion of the funding came from 'a one-time lump sum transfer' meant for the employees who had been let go from State Enterprises as a result of State-Owned Enterprise reform. These lump-sum transfers came from public finance at different levels of government administration. The Enterprises themselves paid some into the fund, and individuals paid in premiums, but the majority came from public finance. The first appearance of the idea of commercial insurance in Central Government documents may have been related to this. That is, there was a hope that the power of commerce could help play more of a role in payment links, which would reduce the burden on the basic medical insurance fund. At the time, the hope was that this would maintain social stability.

In order to support the development of commercial insurance, the Ministry of Finance then issued a document regarding establishing 'supplementary medical insurance' for employees. This noted that the insurance fees for the supplementary insurance could be drawn from employee wages, to a maximum of 4% of total wages. These funds could be itemized as dealing with welfare benefits. This was a clear sign of support for the development of commercial health insurance. Beijing, Xiamen, and other economically developed parts of the country took the lead in exploring how to set up commercial supplementary insurance that would be appropriate to their own local level of economic development and that could tie in to their local system for urban employees' medical insurance. In addition to this, various comprehensive medical insurance products began to appear in quantity with coverage for both outpatient visits and inpatient hospital stays. A richer diversity of commercial health insurance products became more available.

During this stage, the number of entities handling commercial health insurance business increased significantly. The PICC monopoly had dominated the business but now a number of domestic companies came into the market, including Ping An, CPIC, Taikang, Xinhua Life Insurance, among others, and also including foreign-funded commercial insurance companies. The health insurance market expanded rapidly, going from RMB 3.65 billion in 1999 to RMB 24.19 billion in 2003. The average annual growth rate reached as high as 60.4%. In 1999, commercial health insurance accounted for only 0.9% of total health expenditures, while the figure rose to 3.7% in 2003.

In 2003, the 'new rural cooperative medical system' was established, followed by the 'basic medical insurance system for urban residents' in 2007. With these, a basic medical safeguards system began to provide universal coverage in China. In objective terms, this could be seen as a kind of squeezing out of commercial health insurance. At this stage in China's growth, the country and its people regarded the reimbursement of expenses as their primary need when it came to medical safeguards. With the government providing more and more safeguards directly, the scope of commercial insurance coverage and the people to whom this coverage could be sold were naturally diminished. To take commercial health insurance coverage of young people as an example: before the urban residents' basic medical insurance system was set up in 2007, many parts of China had already put out commercial insurance products that were targeted at young people and children. After the basic medical system incorporated this group of people into its coverage, however, these products could either take on another form, as supplementary to the basic medical insurance, or they could simply cease to exist.

Statistics reflect the fact that once commercial health insurance reached 3.7% of total healthcare spending in China, which was in 2003, it stopped growing. Between 2003 and 2009, the percentage hovered around 3.5%, reaching 4% only in 2008.

Even though the market share of commercial insurance slowed down, however, during this period the government began issuing more policies with respect to the industry—these both encouraged it, and regulated and standardized it. In 2003, the China Insurance Regulatory Commission issued *Guiding Opinions on accelerating the development of health insurance*. This document explicitly ruled that health insurance had to be specialized as a distinct and separate part of insurance as a whole, and it required insurance companies to set up specialized operations for health insurance. This thereby guided the industry in the direction of fast and sound growth. In 2004, the China Insurance Regulatory Commission approved the establishment of five specialized health insurance companies (PICC Health, Ping An Health, Zhenghua Health, Kunlun Health, and Sunshine Health Insurance.) In 2006, the China Insurance Regulatory Commission promulgated the *Measures on [administrative] management of health insurance*. This went a step further in clarifying regulatory rules to do with the health insurance industry.

With the aim of propelling further reforms to develop the insurance industry, in 2006 the State Council issued *Various Opinions of the State Council on reforming and developing the insurance industry*. The text within this document that referred to commercial health insurance specifically noted:

[We] encourage and guide the people of the country to participate in insurance, including such forms as commercially offered old-age insurance and health insurance. This has tremendous practical meaning when it comes to improving China's social safeguards system, and raising the level of safeguards for all people.

This was the first time commercial health insurance had been elevated in a Central Government document to the strategic level of 'improving the social safeguards system.' Nevertheless, specific policies in support of this declaration have not yet been issued.

During this period, reform of supply-side systems stagnated, which greatly hindered the development of commercial insurance. In 2009, commercial health insurance claims accounted for only 2% of the business income of medical institutions nationwide. Spending by the basic medical insurance program, however, was also only 37.7% of total business income. That is to say, close to 60% of medical expenses was paid for out-of-pocket by patients themselves. (This does not rule out the possibility that a very small amount was paid by charitable institutions, civil relief organizations, and so on.) The fact that China's general income level is relatively low may have to do with the reluctance to spend money on commercial health insurance products. Second, it may have to do with the short period of time in which commercial health insurance has developed and the relatively low level of the industry as a whole. Third, however, it may have even more to do with the monopoly system of the institutions within public hospitals, a system that still pertains to the supply side. Medical institutions are under the absolute control of rigidified public institutions, so it is very hard for commercial medical insurance to find room to begin to use market mechanisms to optimize the allocation of medical resources. This makes it impossible to improve the quality of products and also impossible to cultivate a large-scale customer base for commercial health insurance.

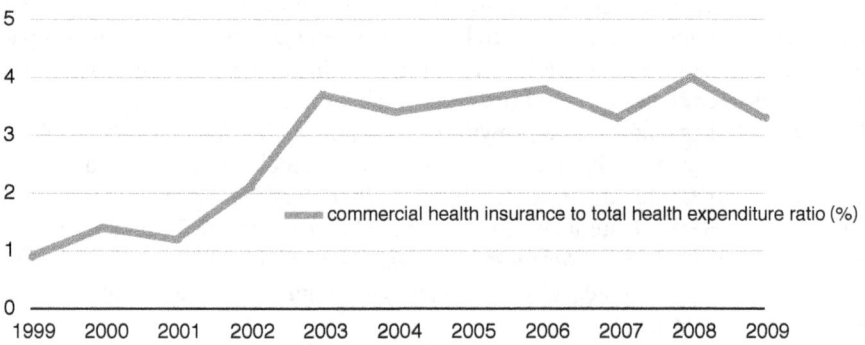

Figure 6.2 Commercial health insurance to total health expenditures ratio between 1999 and 2009.

Source of data: *China Health Statistical Yearbook*; *China Insurance Yearbook*.

6.1.3 From 2009 till now: launch of a new round of medical reform, and transforming the way commercial health insurance is positioned in policy terms

In 2009, the Central Government issued *Opinions on deepening reform of the institutional structures that govern medicine, pharmaceuticals, and healthcare.* This officially launched a new round of reform of the institutional structures that govern the medical and healthcare systems. The focus of the reform was the question of how to resolve problems encapsulated by the phrase 'it is difficult and expensive to see a doctor.' It addressed all-round reform of the institutional structures that govern medicine, pharmaceuticals, and health insurance in China. The overall mindset of the reform turned up even more contradictions and stalemates at the beginning, such as on the one hand trying to strengthen government intervention in supply-side systems—examples would be implementing an essential-drugs system at the grassroots level and carrying out price reform of drugs in public hospitals. On the other hand, the reform also required the basic medical insurance system to play a bigger role as the medium by which market mechanisms were to be put into place. It sought to adjust the allocation of medical resources through reform of payment methods.

No substantive reform has ever really touched upon doctors, however, the core production factor in the whole medical field. As a result, 80% of doctors are still monopolized by public medical institutions. It has been impossible to create a competitive market for human resources, one that allows the flow of professionals who are able to enter the market as well as to leave it. As a result, from 2009 right up to the present, this reform has not made any substantive breakthroughs. Meanwhile, the idea of trying to strengthen government intervention in supply-side systems has not in fact changed the way diagnosis and treatment have been distorted for a long time—one example would be the way hospital costs are covered by pushing drugs. Doctors have long complained about the way the government sets their salaries through the 'compensation system.' With respect to demand-side systems, reform of the methods of payment for basic medical insurance remains a formality with no substance behind it. Medical insurance attempts to control costs have stirred up general opposition on the part of both hospitals and doctors. The majority of medical institutions prefer to transfer the pressure on controlling costs on down to the patient. This includes such things as refusing to treat patients with basic medical insurance, encouraging patients with basic medical insurance to take their complaints to the administrative bodies that manage insurance, and so on.

It is against this backdrop that commercial health insurance has experienced a great transformation in how policy initiatives define its position in China. As Figure 6.3 shows, commercial health insurance did not in fact show any breakthrough growth in the years between 2009 and 2013. Premium revenue as a percentage of total healthcare costs dropped from 3.3% in 2009 to 2.8% in 2011, then rose to 3.6% in 2013, but its performance has still not reached the stable level of around 3.5% between 2003 and 2009. Nevertheless, the terminology

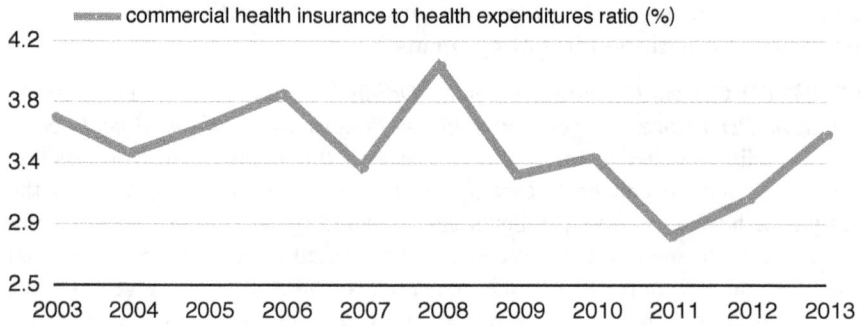

Figure 6.3 Changes of commercial health insurance to health expenditures ratio between 2003 and 2013.

Source of data: *China Health Statistical Yearbook; China Insurance Yearbook.*

used by Central Government documents to describe commercial health insurance has changed. At the outset of reform in 2009, government language simply emphasized things like making sure commercial insurance became 'professional,' and 'used its industry-specific advantages to provide handling services for basic medical insurance.' By 2014, when the State Council issued the *Various Opinions on accelerating the development of a modern insurance services industry*, this document explicitly mentioned that commercial health insurance 'should become a major pillar of China's social safeguards system,' that it should become the 'primary handler' of individual and family commercial health insurance plans, an 'important provider' of healthcare plans for old age, 'an active participant in the marketized operations of social insurance.' With these statements, the policy orientation of commercial insurance realized a 'qualitative leap forward.' (See Table 6.1.)

As more and more problems began to erupt in China's healthcare system, and as social contradictions intensified by the day, and as it was increasingly clear that the role State-owned units and government departments could play in changing this was minimal (as represented by the organizations that manage basic medical insurance), Central Government policymakers turned their hopes in the direction of commercial health insurance entities. Those hopes had been placed on prying the medical reform into action by using the government-run health insurance entities. The very least that can be said about all this is that policymakers now realized that market mechanisms ultimately must go through entities that are genuinely market-oriented (and not State-owned administrative units still dominated by government administration) if they are to be effective. Policymakers now placed high hopes on a combination of released demand for health services, as a result of social and economic development, and encouraging the strong growth of commercial health insurance. In the newest round of health reform, this became the goal and the breakthrough point for reform.

Table 6.1 Portion of Central Government documents relating to commercial health insurance between 2009–2015

Document title	Issued by	Time	Core statement	Development goal
Opinions on deepening the reform of medical and health system from the State Council	State Council	March 2009	(1) Actively develop commercial health insurance (2) Actively promote the government to purchase medical security services, explore entrusting qualified commercial insurance institutions to run various types of medical security management services	To accelerate establishment and improvement of multi-level medical security system with basic medical security as the main body, and other forms of complementary medical insurance and commercial health insurance as the supplement, covering both urban and rural residents
Views on the insurance industry's deep implementation of health care reform and its active participation in the construction of multi-level medical security system	China Insurance Regulatory Commission	May 2009	Meet the diverse needs of healthcare, actively participate in basic medical security management services, and improve the operation mode that is separated from administration; actively explore and participate in the construction of medical service system; strengthen management; put forward conditions that commercial insurance organizations should have in management of basic medical security	To continuously improve the health insurance service capacity of the industry, to establish and improve the multi-level medical security system, to meet diversified needs of health support, and to promote good and fast development of the industry

continued

Table 6.1 Continued

Document title	Issued by	Time	Core statement	Development goal
Outline of the social security development plan for the '12th Five-Year' period	Ministry of Human Resources and Social Security, National Development and Reform Commission; Ministry of Civil Affairs; Ministry of Finance; Ministry of Health; Social Security Foundation	2012	Gradually establish complementary medical insurance system suitable for different groups and grades, implement and perfect the tax support policy, and encourage the complementary role of commercial insurance; encourage the government to purchase the service, and entrust qualified commercial insurance organizations to handle medical security services	To actively and steadily develop a multi-level social security system, to speed up urban and rural social security, and to steadily promote the integration of the protection system and administrative services
Guidance on the participation of commercial insurance institutions in the handling of new-type rural cooperative medical services	Ministry of Health; China Insurance Regulatory Commission; Ministry of Finance; Office of Deepening the Reform of Medical and Health System of the State Council	April 2012	Establish the basic principles for commercial insurance organizations to participate in the handling of the new-type rural cooperative medical service, strictly control the admission of commercial insurance organizations to new-type rural cooperative medical service, request to standardize the management of handling service, perfect the operation mechanism, and guarantee sustainable development; put forward	To introduce the competition mechanism, to reform the government public service delivery mode, to reform the management of social undertakings, to strengthen the handling service consciousness of the new-type rural cooperative medical service, to improve the service quality, to upgrade the service level, to improve the ability of the commercial insurance organization to develop the non-basic medical insurance products, satisfying the rural residents' differentiated medical security demand, and to promote the multi-level medical security system construction

the conditions that commercial insurance organizations should meet to participate in the handling of new-type rural cooperative medical service

| *Guidance on the development of urban and rural residents' critical illness insurance* | National Development and Reform Commission; Ministry of Health; Ministry of Finance; Ministry of Human Resources and Social Security; Ministry of Civil Affairs; China Insurance Regulatory Commission | August 2012 | (1) Take the manner in which critical illness insurance is purchased from commercial insurance institutions
(2) Encourage commercial insurance institutions to provide diversified health insurance products
(3) Put forward the conditions that commercial insurance institutions must have to provide critical illness insurance | To reduce the burden of medical expenses on people with critical diseases, to solve the problem of disease-caused poverty, to establish and perfect the multi-level medical security system, to promote the construction of universal health insurance system, to promote the interaction between health insurance, medical services, and medicine systems, and to promote the combination of the leading role of the government and market mechanism, to improve the level and quality of basic medical security |

continued

Table 6.1 Continued

Document title	Issued by	Time	Core statement	Development goal
State Council's views on promoting the development of health services	State Council	September 2013	(1) Encourage commercial insurance institutions to invest in the medical service industry in various forms, such as building new medical institutions, participating in the restructuring of existing medical institutions, trusteeship, and running public medical institutions, etc. (2) Encourage commercial insurers to provide diversified, multi-level and standardized products and services (3) Encourage government-purchased services to entrust qualified commercial insurance agencies to handle various medical insurance services (4) Establish the mechanism of cooperation between commercial insurance companies and medical, physical examination, and nursing institutions	To further improve health insurance services, diversify commercial health insurance products, greatly increase the number of insured persons, increase the proportion of commercial health insurance expenditure in the total health cost, and form a better health insurance mechanism

State Council's views on speeding up the development of modern insurance services	State Council	August 2014	(1) Develop diversified health insurance services; encourage insurance companies to vigorously develop various types of commercial health insurance products, and link with basic medical insurance (2) Support insurance institutions to participate in the integration of the health service industrial chain, to explore the use of equity investment, strategic cooperation to establish medical institutions and participate in public hospital restructuring (3) The government, through the purchase of services from commercial insurance companies, actively explores the promotion of qualified commercial insurance institutions to handle various types of old age, medical insurance services (4) Improve the health insurance related tax policy	(1) To make commercial insurance the key pillar of the social security system (2) To make insurance the basic means of risk management and wealth management for the government, enterprises, residents, and an important channel to improve the level and quality of security, and an effective tool for the government to improve public services and strengthen social management; allow insurance to play an effective role as the social 'stabilizer' and the economic 'booster'

continued

Table 6.1 Continued

Document title	Issued by	Time	Core statement	Development goal
Opinions of General Office of State Council on speeding up the development of commercial health insurance	General Office of State Council	October 2014	(1) Expand the supply of commercial health insurance (2) Promote the improvement of healthcare service system, comprehensively promote and standardize commercial insurance institutions to provide for urban and rural residents critical illness insurance, and steadily promote the participation of commercial insurance institutions in various types of medical insurance management services, improve the cooperation mechanism between commercial insurance institutions and medical and health institutions (3) Improve the management and service level (4) Improve the development of commercial health insurance support policy	(1) Make commercial health insurance play a 'fresh force' role in deepening the reform of medical and health system, developing health service industry and promoting economic quality and efficiency upgrading (2) By 2020, establish a complete market system, product-form rich, operating integrity norms of modern commercial health insurance services

Notice on the pilot work of personal income tax policy on commercial health insurance	Ministry of Finance; State Administration of Taxation; China Insurance Regulatory Commission	May 2015	(1) Grant personal income tax benefits to individuals in the pilot area for expenses on designated commercial health medical insurance (2) Propose the scope of taxpayer's tax preferential policy applicable to commercial health insurance, and the definition of commercial health insurance products in accordance with the provisions (3) In order to ensure the smooth implementation of the commercial health insurance personal income tax policy, select a central city in every region as the pilot city	To implement *State Council's views on promoting the development of health services* (No. 40, 2013)
Views of the General Office of State Council on the comprehensive implementation of the insurance for urban and rural residents	General Office of State Council	July 2015	(1) Strengthen the connection of medical insurance systems (2) Support commercial insurance institutions to provide critical illness insurance (3) Strengthen the supervision of the operation of critical illness insurance	(1) Before the end of 2015, critical illness insurance should cover all urban residents covered by the basic medical insurance for urban residents, the new-type rural cooperative medical system (referred to collectively as urban and rural residents' basic medical insurance) (2) By 2017, to establish a relatively perfect insurance system for critical diseases

Source: Compiled by the research group based on public documents. Documents released by the Central Government with basically repeated contents are not listed here.

6.2 MAIN WAYS IN WHICH COMMERCIAL INSURANCE HAS PARTICIPATED IN THE MEDICAL REFORM UP TO NOW, AND ANALYSIS

Before 2014, when the Central Government upgraded the position of commercial insurance to being a 'key pillar,' official government documents expressed ways that commercial insurance could participate in the medical reform in two main regards. First, qualified insurance entities could be commissioned to handle the management of the basic medical insurance program, with services being purchased by government. In this regard, government theoretically returned to its fundamental roles: formulating policy, organizing and coordinating, and regulating and inspecting. This was to realize the principle of 'separating out administrative oversight from actual handling of the business,' with specific regard to the management structure that oversaw basic medical insurance. Second, social forces, including commercial insurance, could be encouraged to set up medical institutions, provide healthcare services as a business, as a way to optimize the allocation of medical resources. (Since commercial insurance companies develop all kinds of insurance products that are not within the scope of medical reform policies and regulations and are therefore not very subject to the influence of medical reform, this study does deal with them. Such products are mainly developed through the companies' own R&D capabilities.)

This approach, however, basically limited the scope within which commercial insurance could participate in the medical reform. That is, commercial insurance entities were allowed to provide handling services for basic medical insurance and to provide capital for establishing medical institutions. The problems that most concerned the public, however, were not addressed by this arrangement. Those problems were structural or institutional in nature, and related to such things as distorted pricing of drugs and the administrative monopoly over allocation of doctors. Commercial insurance entities had no say about these things. That is, through two-way transactions they could indeed handle basic medical insurance and they could negotiate with providers of medical services (mainly public hospitals), and they could carry out settlement of claims, but they had no ability to explore other kinds of price-forming mechanisms within the context of a market. Other issues were similarly outside their range. Commercial insurance companies could set up hospitals themselves, but they were incapable of resolving the problem of a scarcity of doctors on their own, just as other social forces had been incapable of this.

In recent years, the emerging Internet-based medical care has provided a new opportunity for commercial insurance companies to further participate in and promote medical reform. Ultimately, this technology is also pushed forward by the reform. However, use of such technologies is limited by the way other institutional or structural reforms have not gone forward. At the current time, Internet technologies cannot provide genuinely leapfrogging development to commercial insurance.

In what follows, we comb through several mainstream models that various parts of China are using to enable commercial insurance to participate in the medical reform. We analyze each briefly. Finally, in the third part of this study, we elaborate on why we think commercial insurance has not yet made any clear progress in affecting the medical reform.

6.2.1 Role of commercial insurance in improving and reforming demand-side systems

6.2.1.1 Handling of basic medical insurance

Over the past ten or more years, the main way in which commercial insurance has sought to participate in the medical reform and to propel its own development in the process has been to provide handling services to local governments for their basic medical insurance programs.

First, Central Government documents have long since expressed clear support for this approach. The hope is that it will allow the system to be managed more professionally. Second, the workload on government departments that manage health insurance has become an extremely heavy burden, as the insurance system expands coverage, funds increase, and people's demand for medical care is released. This has led to the twin problems of 'unending work' and 'work that is done poorly.' As a result, some local governments have expressed the hope that public finance funds can provide support for having commercial insurance come in and help share the load, as well as improve the efficiency of services. On their side, commercial insurance entities have their own motivations. By taking on the handling of services for basic medical insurance, they can gather management experience, train up their human resources and teams, and gain greater public acceptance. At the same time, given the information resources they can obtain in the course of providing handling services (such as statistics on medical insurance), they can develop products of their own that are outside the scope of basic medical insurance. With multi-tiered, diverse products, they can take market share.

Zhanjiang city in Guangdong province was one of the first to have commercial insurance companies participate in handling their basic medical insurance program. The model of that participation has become known as the Zhanjiang Model. In the early period, it was regarded by insurance companies as the model that should be promoted nationwide. It works as follows. The Zhanjiang Social Security Bureau (the Bureau) signed an agreement with an insurance company, namely the Chinese People's Health Insurance Co. Ltd. (PICC Health). PICC Health provides the Bureau with a portion of the handling services for the basic medical insurance fund, at no charge. In return, the Bureau purchases large-sum supplementary medical insurance from PICC using 15% of the individual contributions paid into the basic medical insurance fund. The two parties have agreed on a certain level of hospital costs for individual hospitalization. If reimbursable costs come in below that, the basic medical fund carries out settlement of claims by itself. If the costs come in above that level, PICC Health handles settlement.

This model is described in shorthand as 'one system, two grades (tiers), pooled funding of both urban and rural areas, and voluntary options.' That is, the basic medical insurance of urban and rural residents of Zhanjiang is divided into two tiers. Individuals pay different rates for each tier, and the amount of reimbursement they get is different. All of those enrolled in the insurance, no matter what their *hukou* (residence permit) status, whether urban or rural, may voluntarily choose one or the other tier depending on need for level of medical care and depending on income. Premiums are paid on an annual basis. The first tier costs RMB 30 in premiums per year, and the second costs RMB 60. The maximum reimbursable amount for hospital stays in a year under the basic medical insurance program is RMB 160,000 for the first tier. For the second tier, it is RMB 180,000. Once the reimbursable costs of an insured person go over RMB 50,000 but are under RMB 160,000 (RMB 180,000 for the second tier), 50% of out-of-pocket costs will be covered by critical illness supplementary insurance. Once costs go over RMB 160,000 (RMB 180,000 for the second tier), the amount that is reimbursable goes to 70% if those costs are within the prescribed scope of things covered by medical insurance policies.

In theory, this way of doing things is very beneficial for the commercial insurance company. The company gets itself inserted into the entire chain of managing basic medical insurance funds. The difficulty of controlling costs in the medical insurance fund makes more hospitalized patients come within the scope of the insurance company's large-sum supplementary insurance, which only increases the company's need to pay more reimbursements for reinsurance products. The insurance company can dodge this by adopting the Zhanjiang model. In addition, it can gather in the experience of handling insurance that the basic medical insurance system has already accumulated. It can get more in-depth understanding of the behavior patterns and cost characteristics of medical institutions and develop more mature handling models which it can later promote to the rest of the country.

Jiangyin city in Jiangsu province operates in a similar way. This place brought in commercial insurance fairly early in the course of handling the new rural cooperative program. In fact, since the new rural cooperative system was set up in 2001, it has been handled by the China Pacific Insurance Company, and that continues to be the case today. Jiangyin set up a new rural cooperative management committee. The municipal leader serves as chairman of the committee and the head of the Healthcare Department serves as vice-chairman. The office, under this committee, is responsible for day-to-day affairs and for the work of cooperating with commercial insurance. In corresponding fashion, the China Pacific Insurance Company established a business management center just for this business. The center employs 57 people. These people manage the medical insurance services counter, they provide medical treatment, they oversee and investigate costs, and so on. In 2009, on the basis of years of insurance handling experience, China Pacific Insurance Company developed a supplementary commercial health insurance product for voluntary enrollment by local people.

6.2.1.2 Handling of supplementary health insurance

According to the *Social Security Law*, mandatory participation in insurance should by all rights be only through the basic medical insurance system. In many areas, however, local governments feel that the people in their jurisdiction need a higher level of medical safeguards so they have added a layer of mandatory supplementary insurance on top of the basic medical insurance. This lightens the load on people when they develop critical illness and it lowers the risk of falling into poverty or back into poverty as a result of illness. In economically developed areas where the pressure of an aging society on the medical insurance fund is somewhat less intense, the premiums for this kind of supplementary insurance can come from the surplus balance in the basic medical insurance fund. In less developed areas, the participants in the insurance must raise funds from elsewhere to pay premiums. This kind of supplementary insurance, set up as an additional safeguard by government, is handled by commercial insurance companies in many places.

Xiamen city in Fujian province is among those that have chosen to have a commercial insurance company handle the business. Xiamen has a high level of income and funding of its insurance program is correspondingly high. At the same time, the great majority of insured people are young people, a group that spends very little on medical care. This means that in regular years the medical insurance fund has a tremendous surplus. In 2010, Xiamen purchased supplementary insurance handling services from a commercial insurance company using funds from its basic medical insurance (urban employees' medical insurance and urban and rural residents' medical insurance). The applicant for the policy was the Xiamen City Social Security Center. The two parties signed an agreement whereby medical spending above a certain level of costs would be compensated by the 'large-sum supplementary medical insurance,' with coverage that included all critical illness. Both the employees' and urban and rural residents' insurance for critical illness was implemented at the municipal level, using unified systems, so that even if a person's residence status changed, he would still receive uninterrupted coverage under the insurance. Any surplus in the supplementary insurance fund was allowed to go to the commercial insurance company as recognition of the principle of conserving capital while allowing for a modest profit. Risk, on the other hand, was borne by both parties as per their agreement.

At present, the annual premium for Xiamen's critical illness insurance for employees is RMB 84 per person. Of this, the pooled basic medical insurance fund pays RMB 48 and the individual pays RMB 36. The annual premium for the urban and rural residents' critical illness insurance is RMB 10.3 per person, all of which is paid out of the pooled funds of the urban and rural residents' fund. The cooperative agreement stipulates that these premiums may not be adjusted due to any 'policy-type' factors or any changes in medical fees. (Policy-type factors would include such things as [the] drugs and medical treatment items [on the official list of covered items], changes in the way of settling medical costs, or limits to the maximum paid by basic medical insurance.) When medical expenses of the insured person exceed the figure of RMB 100,000, as the maximum allowed under basic medical insurance, the employees' critical illness insurance compensates 95%, with a maximum compensation total of RMB 400,000. The urban and rural residents' critical illness insurance compensates 80% with a maximum total of RMB 350,000. These figures are vastly higher than the nationally prescribed 50%.

Zigong city in Sichuan province has adopted a different method of raising funds for its insurance program. In 2016, people in Zigong paid RMB 150 per person per year into the urban employees' medical insurance fund as a premium for supplementary insurance. This was a compulsory deduction from wages, along with the premium for basic medical insurance. The social security bureau of Zigong then purchased supplementary insurance handling services from the China Life Insurance Company (China Life). If at some point the insurance company becomes unable to participate in the handling of basic medical insurance, however, the increase in compensation is likely to 'release' an excessive amount of demand for medical treatment. A 'conspiracy' among medical institutions, doctors, and patients pushes medical fees up, creating a situation in which too many patients meet the requirements for the supplementary insurance, as a result of which the commercial insurance company faces losses year after year.

In addition, since such supplementary insurance is established and organized completely by government, such things as the catalogue of approved items and methods of payment are also decided upon by government. For example, government may limit compensation to only things either on or off the catalog, or may dictate that medical insurance payments must be done by the same method as that for basic medical insurance, and so on.

6.2.1.3 'Taking on and handling' critical illness insurance

In 2012, the National Development and Reform Commission and other five ministries and commissions issued the policy document called *Guiding Opinion on launching procedures for critical illness insurance for urban and rural residents*. This required local governments to purchase critical illness insurance from commercial insurance companies on behalf of people with relatively low levels of safeguards in the two insurance programs called urban residents' medical insurance and new rural cooperative medical insurance. Local governments were to use a portion of the surplus balance in their funds for this purpose. At the time, this was seen as a golden opportunity for commercial insurance entities, as a way to participate in the Medical Reform.

By the end of 2013, 28 provinces nationwide had issued plans for implementing the critical illness insurance. Eleven insurance companies had started handling this critical illness insurance business in 144 'fund-pooling jurisdictions' of 25 provinces. Coverage extended to 360 million urban and rural residents.[3] In 2015, the General Office of the State Council issued *Opinion on full implementation of the urban and rural residents' critical illness insurance*, which explicitly described methods by which commercial insurance entities were to take on and handle the business of critical illness insurance. It called on them to implement the program accordingly. Local governments and commercial insurance companies together agreed upon the level of premium income that the company could derive from this business (this generally was within 5% of the total amount of pooled funds). At year-end, any balance that exceeded the agreed upon income would be returned to the local government and put into the insurance fund to be used the following year. If, on the other hand, there was a loss, then the local government and commercial insurance company would both bear the risk.

Specific arrangements are up to localities. Some areas, such as Taicang city in Jiangsu province, use the balance to set up critical illness insurance. Some, as in Shenzhen, Guangdong province, have residents pay out their own fees in order to enroll in the insurance, either on a voluntary or mandatory basis.

Taicang city in Jiangsu province was one of the earliest places to have a system for critical illness insurance. Before the six ministries and commissions issued the policy document on this subject in 2012, Taicang was also one of the key places for doing research and conducting surveys. The basic medical fund in Taicang has a fairly large surplus balance but it also has a large risk of 'being forced into poverty as a result of illness,' since the compensation rate under its basic medical insurance system is low and patients bear a heavy spending load. As a result, the local government decided to use the surplus in the basic medical fund to ask commercial insurance companies to bid on a tender for critical illness insurance, in order to lighten this load. PICC Health (Jiangsu Branch) won the bid for providing handling services for critical illness insurance, but in addition it then has been able to access statistical data on basic medical insurance expenses as it helps the local social security bureau carry out supervision and inspections.

At the current time, a designated amount per person per year is drawn from the basic medical health insurance pooled fund for paying for critical illness insurance. For employees it is RMB 84 per year. For urban and rural residents it is RMB 20. The insurance itself, however, does not differentiate between employees and urban and rural residents in terms of coverage. It provides insurance coverage at a progressive rate of compensation for claims (53% to 82%) for every insured person, with the rate of compensation getting higher as the range of expenses goes up. The compensation starts after medical costs exceed RMB 10,000, and there is no ceiling on the total amount.

Shenzhen city in Guangdong province only began implementing a critical illness insurance program in 2015. In this case, however, residents are able to decide whether or not they wish to pay into the insurance. Initially, the Shenzhen government set a fairly low payment threshold of RMB 20 per person per year. It bolstered its case for this insurance by using official propaganda channels, encouraging all holders of basic medical insurance to enroll in the new insurance and pay premiums. In order to make better use of the accumulated surplus balance in individual accounts, the social security bureau deducts the cost of premiums directly from personal accounts if their balance exceeds 5% of average wages in Shenzhen in the previous year. In addition, some people have their premiums paid for them by the civil welfare fund and the disability protection fund—specifically, those people with Shenzhen residence permits (*hukou*) who are living on subsistence allowances or are orphans, people in need of special attention and care, severely disabled people, and so on, that is, those who are not able to pay for the insurance but have relatively high needs.

One major feature of the Shenzhen model is its high level of safeguards. This is a characteristic common to all developed areas in China. The insurer covers 70% of medical expenses over a deductible of RMB 10,000, which must be paid by the individual. If the insured person suffers from illness, 70% of the medical drug expenditures within the list of medical drugs for critically serious diseases of Shenzhen can be covered by the insurer, with the maximum limit of RMB 150,000.

6.2.1.4 Case study: Qingdao city

Commercial insurance companies participate in handling basic medical insurance or supplementary/critical illness insurance in different ways throughout the country, but most places adhere to the three core characteristics as described above. Qingdao city in Shandong province is an exception, however. It is an exception in the degree to which government allows commercial insurance to participate in reform, and the role that commercial insurance plays in reform. The relationship between the two parties, departments in charge of social security and the commercial insurance company, has gone from simple provision of services by the company to full partnership in pushing forward reform of the structural institutions that govern medicine and healthcare in China.

6.2.1.4.1 Design of the basic framework of the Qingdao model

In 2013, the Qingdao municipal social security bureau proposed the idea of comprehensive cooperation with commercial insurance companies. That is, on the basis of having the social security retain the authority to formulate policy and the functions of regulator, through an open tender the municipality would authorize several commercial insurance companies, concurrently, to handle the basic medical insurance and supplementary medical insurance of the city in its entirety. This extended to the entire chain of social medical safeguards. The people of Qingdao could make their own decisions about which company to select, based on quality, which established market competition among the handlers of insurance.[4]

In February 2014, three commercial insurance companies won the bidding, namely PICC Health, Ping An Endowment Insurance, and Taiping Life Insurance. These three began to provide whole-chain social health insurance services for the insured in Huangdao District, Chengyang District, and Laoshan District. Given that they had the support of information technology and network platforms, their services focused on health management for minor problems and paid safeguards for major diseases. Both sides synchronized their approach to reform, namely the regulator and those being regulated. Taking advantage of the commercial company's nationwide network, they provided insured people with the ability to undertake medical treatment in non-local places, and they strengthened systemic-type examinations of funds payment, and so on.

Under this model of cooperation, social security departments are responsible for formulating policies on local health insurance, for the budgeting of the health insurance fund, for managing the agreements between designated medical institutions and commercial insurance companies and doing performance assessments of their services, as well as integrating related medical and healthcare resources, and for ensuring the reasonable allocation of medical and healthcare resources. The commercial insurance company is responsible for providing services to those who enroll in the insurance. They are responsible for managing designated medical institutions, participating in the joint construction of a 'smart' medical insurance Internet platform that includes the diagnostic service center, and they are responsible for exploring diversified payment mechanisms and cooperation mechanisms with medical institutions. Data that they obtain during this process can be used to develop other supplementary insurance products.

Part of design work for the medical insurance system also incorporated the participation of commercial insurance companies. Three commercial insurance companies have participated in the research and basic data analysis of Qingdao urban and rural residents' health insurance policy, the formulation of policies and creating more detailed rules for the implementation of critical illness medical aid, long-term care insurance, and accident insurance, and so on. The idea is to make sure that insurance companies are familiar with the thinking behind policy regulations before they undertake specific tasks. They therefore can be more prepared to work effectively and more able to deepen cooperation between the two sides.

The core of the entire cooperative project is the framework design of the Internet platform for 'smart medical insurance.' 'Smart medical insurance' is meant to guide the reform of the entire healthcare system, starting from the handling services for social health insurance, including payment services, and extending to all medical services. It is aimed at ensuring higher quality medical services, reducing medical costs, and ultimately achieving a transformation of the entire healthcare system—from a focus on diagnosis and treatment of disease to a focus on health management. Diagnosis centers, third-party testing centers, surgery centers, doctors' groups, and other new organization models for medical services can all be integrated through this platform. Not only can supplementary insurance products other than the basic medical safeguards make convenient use of this platform to development, display, provide insurance through this platform, but non-basic medical insurance can also register to be on the platform. This provides more options to the potential insurer. All kinds of information and statistics are pulled together through this process. The convenience and effectiveness of regulatory oversight are therefore greatly increased, for both the medical service entities themselves and the entities handling medical insurance.

Three pilot areas cooperated in being frontline experiments of the cooperation between social and commercial insurance. Those carried out three projects related to wellness and management of chronic diseases—one on diabetes, one on controlling the dependence on tobacco, and one on high blood pressure. That is, these projects adopted new ways by which several parties could work together, including medical insurance, government departments, and commercial insurance, with commercial insurance providing the manpower and technical support. To take the project on controlling tobacco dependency as an example, the Taishan Insurance Company worked with the Laushan district to set up an online information platform that policy holders and doctors working to control tobacco could access once they were registered. Doctors would upload relevant data onto the platform each time they had performed services, so as to 'keep online records of offline operations.' This established a real-time monitoring system by which project managers could keep informed of the doctors' treatments and the behavior of smoking patients. Since treatment of tobacco dependency is fairly standardized, this kind of real-time monitoring system can fully track the behavior of both doctors and patients being treated for that problem. The experiment has provided valuable empirical experience for the entire community with respect to building out the healthcare system and specifically controlling chronic disease. The project was recognized by the World Health Organization (WHO) which awarded it a 'Best Practices of Healthy Cities award' in 2014.

The primary significance of the Qingdao tobacco project lies not in controlling the use of tobacco but rather in exploring effective models by which China's medical services system can transition from a 'treatment of illness' model to a 'management of health' model. In the tobacco case, the parties explored ways to bring such government entities as the basic medical insurance program and healthcare departments together with all kinds of social forces, especially community medical institutions, in an effective collaborative effort to control chronic disease and improve wellness. Ultimately, the idea was to establish an effective tiered, classified, diagnosis and treatment system with clear division of labor that would achieve the transition from treating illness to managing health. This transition is one of the chief goals of the entire institutional reform of healthcare and medical structures in the country.

6.2.1.4.2 *Ways social security is collaborating with commercial insurance in Qingdao*

The Qingdao model of cooperation is different from others in that it is comprehensive whereas others simply authorize a commercial insurance company to handle tasks for social medical insurance. The main features of the Qingdao model are as follows.

First, it provides an incentive for the commercial insurance company as a result of intensifying market competition and allowing for comprehensive cooperation. The simpler form of just 'purchasing services' means that a government insurance entity is simply outsourcing certain handling tasks to the commercial insurance company while at the same time paying that company a management fee. Under such a model the commercial insurance company has no authority over managing the medical insurance funds and is unable therefore to earn the profits that might derive from effective use of the funds. As a result, the company is not motivated to contribute to controlling the costs of the medical insurance institutional structure. In contrast, under a model of comprehensive cooperation, the commercial insurance company directly handles business, directly settles accounts with designated medical institutions, and directly serves patients. Based on the actual situation of each insured person, the insurance company can also develop personalized supplementary insurance policies and provide a full suite of insurance services. This opens up tremendous space into which the company can develop its business. In addition, the design of mechanisms aimed at market competition also stimulates the insurance company to provide better and more diversified services, in order to draw in potential customers.

Second, the Qingdao model strengthens information systems and uses an Internet platform for integrating resources. It forms a cooperative mechanism whereby social medical insurance and commercial health insurance can benefit one another and join forces to create a effective tiered, classified (divided into categories), diagnosis and treatment system with clear division of labor. The 'smart medical insurance' Internet platform is a joint effort that is headed by social health medical insurance (government) departments with the commercial health insurance company investing manpower, capital, and technology. It is not limited to the traditional simple business of paying compensation out of the medical insurance fund but instead extends to the full range of health safeguarding services. The services that the platform provides include diagnostic support services, patient guidance, remote consultation services, return visits after treatment, rehabilitation consultations, two-way referral assistance, and so on, so as to achieve a seamless connection among the various parties including the insured, medical institutions, and entities handling medical insurance. The medical institutions, third-party testing agencies, and other related institutions participating in various services are organized and coordinated by the social health insurance departments. As compared to having government set up the platform by itself, this way of doing things obviously saves on costs and allows the system to be more relevant to the needs of the person who is insured. The insured person can have easier access to health management and healthcare through the platform. Health insurance departments in this process can more easily guide the allocation of medical resources in order to improve service quality and efficiency and save on medical costs. On their side, the commercial insurance companies can take advantage of the accumulated information on the platform as well as the policy holders it attracts, to extend their product line to more diversified forms of insurance policies and healthcare services.

Third, the Qingdao model strengthens the checks and balances between stakeholders. The 'smart health insurance' platform takes its strength from information technology and sets up four 'assessment systems.' These are: the assessment by the insured person of the way the commercial insurance company is handling services as well as the way the designated medical and pharmaceutical entities are handling their services; the assessment by the designated medical and pharmaceutical institutions of the commercial health insurance company; the assessment by the commercial health insurance company of the designated medical and pharmaceutical institutions; and the assessment by the social insurance departments of the commercial insurance company. This provides a way to have checks and balances on all four sides. It helps incentivize and also constrain the social insurance departments. At the same time it highlights the right of the insured person to have a say in the process and it gives that person the ability to carry out regulatory oversight. It is therefore beneficial to the rights and interests of the insured.

6.2.2 The participation of commercial insurance companies in the supply-side reform

International experience shows that many commercial health insurance companies have directly funded their own medical institutions. Having an insurance company run a medical institution allows it to have more systematic control over medical processes and over the structure of medical costs. Some foreign commercial insurance companies even mainly operate in this manner, by providing medical services for the insured through their own medical institutions. In 2013, the policy document called *Various Opinions of the State Council on promoting the development of the health services industry* explicitly encouraged the same practice in China. The policy document 'encourages enterprises, charities, foundations and commercial insurance institutions to invest in medical services by funding new hospitals, participating in the restructuring of existing ones, serving as trustees, and by operating public medical institutions.'

In fact, before this document came out, in 2011 the Ping An Trust Co. Ltd. had already co-established the Hospital of Traditional Chinese Medicine with the Longgang District Government in Shenzhen. This was the first local case of a commercial insurance institution participating in the establishment of hospitals since the new Medical Reform began. In 2012, however, due to various coordination issues, Ping An announced it was withdrawing and the cooperation failed. In 2012, Xinhua Insurance Company tried to build a network of health management agencies. By 2013, it had invested a total of RMB 180 million in Qingdao, Yantai, Wuhan, Xi'an, Baoji, Chongqing, Changsha, Chengdu, and Zhengzhou. This was to set up clinics mainly offering health management and to promote the industry chain known in shorthand as 'health management+medical services+nursing services,' but the results were mediocre.

In the process of building a new Grade Three (top) hospital, Weifang city in Shandong province found that funding was tight and finally decided to bring in a commercial insurance institution to be a shareholder, together with the government and the local medical school. In July 2012, Sunshine Insurance signed a cooperation agreement with Weifang called the 'Cooperation Agreement on market-based operating of a public health center,' to jointly build the Sunshine Union Hospital. The municipal government approved the use of a piece of land measuring 5,000 *mu* [roughly equivalent to 823 acres], and it provided RMB 300 million in funding support. This was to be used on building the hospital as well as a restaurant and apartment building, for organic farming, and for other services. Sunshine Insurance invested RMB 800 million and was responsible for building the hospital. On May 8, 2016, the hospital officially opened in Weifang. Sunshine Insurance, the Weifang Municipal Government, and Weifang Medical College are shareholders, with Sunshine Life holding a 55% share. The hospital is a designated Grade Three hospital under the basic medical insurance system. It offers comprehensive services and has 2,000 beds that are open to the public. With Sunshine Insurance as its co-investor, patients can choose to buy from the hospital health insurance products developed by the company, and get real-time reimbursement of claims.

However, public documentation has not yet clarified a number of things about the hospital. As a hospital in which the government is also a shareholder, it is unclear what kind of management mechanisms the organization uses. Is the structure run under the rule of law with independent operations, or not? Does the institution enjoy direct subsidies from public finance, or not? Are hospital staff still under the *bianzhi* personnel system, as normally applies to public institutions? Does it use the performance-evaluation system by which wages are determined, on a nationwide standardized basis, by governmental human resources and social security departments? Are drugs for the hospital procured through province-wide unified bidding procedures? It is also unclear whether or not Sunshine Insurance, as the largest shareholder in the hospital, carries out claims settlement with the hospital in accordance with drug prices as stipulated by national regulations. Can it, instead, explore new health insurance payment methods that are more in line with the characteristics of the 'new type' of health insurance. All of this remains to be clarified. At this point, it is uncertain how much of a role this hospital will play in pushing forward the reform of China's medical and healthcare institutional structures.

6.2.3 The participation of commercial health insurance companies in Internet-based medical services

As the economy has grown and technology has developed, Internet-based medical care has emerged rapidly in China over recent years, particularly in the field of mobile medical care. In 2011, the website called HaoDF ['good doctor,' *hao* 'good,' DF: *daifu* 'doctor'] developed the first mobile app, which marked the start of mobile medical care in China. Subsequently, other 'light consultation' online products such as Spring Rain Doctor were launched, through which patients can consult doctors online through the apps. According to the CICC Report, the online medical service market in 2013 was RMB 2 billion, and is expected to maintain an annual growth rate of 50% to 80% in the next three years. The market for wearable devices in 2017 is expected to exceed RMB 5 billion.

The emergence of Internet-based medical services has created an opening in the traditional medical services system through which market-oriented forces, including commercial insurance entities, can enter. Online consultation products like Spring Rain Doctor have begun to provide private doctor's services. They are exploring how to customize both service items and prices, which in essence is the start of price formation by a market for medical services.

In 2014, Ping An Health Insurance Co. Ltd., a subsidiary of China Ping An Insurance Company, launched the 'Ping An Health Cloud' mobile app. This does business in online consulting, online-to-online drug services, electronic health records, chronic disease management, and so on, by providing online medical services by family doctors and specialists and by the use of big data mining and the construction of an online drug exchange network. At present, this includes the services of more than 50,000 physicians who rank above the title of 'attending doctor.' Among these are 5,000 doctors from Grade Three hospitals, of whom more than 300 are self-employed specialists and more than 500 are experienced contracted doctors from Grade Three hospitals. The platform also extends its services to offline business. It has contracted with more than 3,000 hospitals, clinics, and medical centers, and 1,200 pharmacies, and plans to build its own offline diagnosis and treatment platform to provide users with health services that combine online health consulting and offline healthcare, as well as drugs, medical devices, electronic health files, health insurance and commercial insurance payment and other services. The aim is to integrate the medical network, drug network, and information network, and to form a closed loop of 'medical services + insurance.'

By June 2016, 'Ping An Health Cloud' had over 80 million registered users, with 250,000 daily online inquiries, and was ahead of the vast majority of mobile medical consultation products. However, the business is similarly constrained by the slow pace of reform in the personnel system of public hospitals. It still must rely on doctors from Grade Three hospitals and is unable to form its own team or train up its own long-term resource. This remains its largest constraint.

6.3 DIFFICULTIES AND BOTTLENECKS THAT COMMERCIAL INSURANCE COMPANIES FACE IN PARTICIPATING IN CHINA'S MEDICAL REFORM

The most immediate goal of the medical reform is to resolve the problem of difficult and expensive access to medical care. At a more profound level, however, the significance of the reform lies in setting up positive functioning of the entire system, with a high-quality and highly efficient medical services and safeguards system so as to improve people's wellbeing. The most obvious problems in the medical system lie in such things as using revenue from drug sales to support hospitals and doctors. The root cause of this is that the core resource of medicine, namely doctors, are trapped in the institutional structure that governs public institutions. They cannot move freely, and when factors of production cannot move freely it is impossible to form well functioning markets. The monopoly of public medical institutions has distorted behavior in a whole series of ways.

If commercial insurance is to join into the process of reforming China's medical system, therefore, indeed to the extent of leading it, we must find a way to 'liberate doctors.' Only then can there be market-driven price-forming mechanisms and only then is there the possibility of supply and demand both having a say in business consultation. The current situation, however, is that commercial insurance is faced with a number of both internal and external restrictions in its attempt to lead the 'liberation of productive forces.' These include the binding constraints of the external environment in which commercial insurance companies operate, but they also include the bottleneck of improving their own capacities.

6.3.1 External constraints on commercial insurance companies that keep them from entering into medical reform

6.3.1.1 Policy environment constraints that derive from the institutional structures of the medical and healthcare system

First, for the past seven years of medical reform, the reform of public hospitals has been mired in a deadlocked situation, yet public hospitals represent the most important entities with which commercial insurance does business. Reform of hospitals can be summed up in the following three categories. None of these, however, has touched upon the fundamental problem of institutional structure. Indeed, it could be said that all three try to evade real reform.

The first category involves reforming the relationship between government and public hospitals. This includes such things as separating out administration (officials) from operations (professionals), and exploring the setting up of governance structures that operate by a rule of law. In 2010, the former Ministry of Public Health issued an *Opinion* called *Guidance Opinion on pilot-program reform of public hospitals*. This called for setting up entities specifically for managing public hospitals that could substitute for and replace the functions of government in managing hospitals, and at the same time it called for establishing legal-person governance structures in public hospitals. Beijing, Chengdu, and Shenzhen have carried out initiatives in this direction, but in practice all they have achieved is to shift the functions of what had been the governmental health division in hospitals to a different government department. The transfer of power has been within government. The boundaries of government functions have not been adjusted to allow for 'release' of decision making authority down to hospitals themselves, not to mention setting up independent and autonomous governance structures that operate under rule of law (legal-person governance structures).

The second category involves strengthening intervention by government in certain aspects of the micromanagement of public hospitals. Specifically, this refers to separating out the business of medicine from the business of drugs, that

is, eliminating the mark-ups on drugs and increasing the prices of medical services. The intent of the policy of eliminating mark-ups on drugs is to take away
the incentive that hospitals have to push drugs, particularly expensive drugs.
However, eliminating the 15% mark-up does not in fact touch upon the roughly
20% income that hospitals receive in the form of rebates on drugs, nor does it
touch upon the roughly 30% income that doctors receive in the form of kickbacks on the sale of drugs. The reason hospitals and doctors have the ability to
demand rebates and kickbacks is that they have a market monopoly under the
system of public hospitals. So long as their monopoly continues, they will continue to have the ability to take in monopolistic earnings.

The third category involves changing the behavior of public hospitals by
reforming the method of payment under the basic medical insurance system. The
most commonly practiced method of handling payment right now is the 'total
amount controlled method.' Departments of medical insurance set quotas for the
total amount of spending that is allowed in a given pooled-fund jurisdiction. The
quotas are in accord with the budget of the basic medical fund of that district.
This total amount is divvied up by designated medical institutions. The division
is done according to the principle of 'setting expenditures based on income, and
maintaining a balance between income and expenditures.' The implied incentive
and restraint mechanism, to control costs, is described as 'allowing the balance
to remain with the institution for its own use, while sharing the burden of overspending with others.' That is, the hospital may keep any excess of funds, while
any overspending is shared between the designated hospital itself and the
medical insurance fund. The retention and sharing ratios vary from place to
place. Other payment methods are similar to the 'package payment' method of
the 'total amount controlled method,' but they are ineffective due to the fact that
the institutional structure of public hospitals has not yet been reformed and the
monopoly position of hospitals has not yet changed. (Such other methods include
payment of basic medical insurance according to individual kinds of illness or
according to number of bed-days.) The public-institution structure of public hospitals dictates that hospitals cannot use any excess of funds to increase salaries
of staff. At the same time, hospitals have neither the ability nor the motivation to
control the grey income of doctors. Under the constraints of the 'total amount'
system, hospitals frequently reject patients who are covered by basic medical
insurance. This stirs up problems between patients and the entities that handle
medical insurance who then try to coerce the medical insurance departments to
increase quota.

The fact is, however, that even these new methods of payment, these so-
called 'package payment' methods, have not changed the way in which the
National Development and Reform Commission sets planned-type pricing. At
the end of the year, when the hospital and medical insurance calculate whether
or not there is an excess of spending over the 'total amount,' the calculations are
still done by prices set by the National Development and Reform Commission.
That is, the prices of drugs and medical care are not determined by negotiations
between the health insurance department and the hospital as equal parties to the

transaction. This situation pertains even to government-run healthcare handling entities, not to mention commercial insurance companies. In the face of strong, government-backed public hospitals, commercial insurance companies as a passive 'payer' can do nothing but foot the bill issued by the hospital. They have no room for negotiation and no power of regulation.

Meanwhile, with respect to the even more critical personnel system, the past seven years have not seen the slightest breakthrough in reforms. Despite the many policies that the Central Government has issued that allow doctors to practice medicine in more than one place, the essential personnel status of doctors as being part of a 'unit' has not changed. In 2011, the Beijing municipal government passed a document called *Beijing administrative methods for allowing doctors in the Beijing municipality to practice in more than one location (Trial)*. This attempted to push forward the development of private medical institutions. By May of 2015, however, the number of doctors actually registered to work in more than one location came to just 5,122. This was not even 5% of the total number of doctors in the city. In 2015, a survey of the situation was carried out by the Beijing Committee of the Chinese Peasants and Workers Party. It showed that 76% of the doctors surveyed were willing to practice in multiple medical institutions, but as many as 38% of the respondents said that their hospitals prohibited or hindered them from doing so due to a variety of unwritten rules and restraints.

There is an essential difference between multipoint practice and freelance practice. The essence of freelance practice is that the market allocates the resource of medical professionals. Doctors are free to choose where they want to work—they make their own determinations about market conditions and then decide on where to practice or how many different places to practice in. The decision is not subject to the constraints of administrative approvals. As a member of society (as opposed to a member of a unit), determinations regarding compensation, method of employment, method of cooperation, and so on are the result of negotiations by both sides. In contrast, with multipoint practice, the doctor remains a member of a unit. His former status as a member of a unit does not change. He has absolutely no room for negotiation with the hospital in which he is working and no freedom. If the hospital forbids him to practice elsewhere then he cannot openly provide services in another place—all he can do in that case is violate rules by moonlighting. The places in which he might want to work and number of places are all subject to administrative controls. The healthcare administrative departments do not change the assigned place of work of the 'checked and ratified' doctor, no matter whether he is practicing in one place or two or three. Practicing in multiple locations does not change the essential nature of the controls exercised over that doctor.

Without market-oriented mobility of doctors, it is impossible to have market-determined pricing of doctor's salaries and even less possible to have market-determined pricing of doctor's services. At the same time, so long as doctors are imprisoned in the institutional structure of public hospitals, non-public medical forces will find it hard to grow. The entities that pay the funds to commercial health insurance will remain public institutions that hold over 80% of medical resources (doctors). Meanwhile, if insurance companies themselves set up hospitals, as 'social [private] forces,' they will lack sources of human talent.

Second, the original intent of Central Government policies that encouraged commercial insurance companies to 'handle' basic medical insurance was to achieve a breakthrough in the existing system. However, given that the human resources departments were unwilling to let go of power, and that 'administration' and 'operations' were not in fact separated out from one another, commercial insurance companies were used simply as cashiers. They did not become cooperative partners, which put massive constraints on their further growth.

Suppose that human resources departments and the social security system were indeed willing to cooperate to a deeper extent with commercial insurance. Suppose they even delegated authority to commercial insurance companies— this would give commercial insurance a certain room to grow under a situation in which government still formulates funding standards and calculates a minimum level of security. It would give them permission to develop multiple levels of insurance products, among which basic medical insurance would be included. Patients could choose the most basic insurance, provided by government, or they could select that plus supplementary insurance. Both Medicare in the U.S. and Germany's social medical insurance operate in this way. The United States allows all kinds of supplementary insurance on top of Medicare, and it also allows commercial insurance to supply products that substitute for traditional Medicare. The managers of Medicare pay a per-head fee to commercial insurance (with the standards for the fees mainly being determined by government tenders). In contrast, Germany allows critical illness funds as managed by social medical insurance to have a certain degree of authority to adjust rates, for differentiated competition.

China's situation, however, is that commercial insurance has no power at all to make adjustments to medical insurance policies. On the contrary, funding and compensation are unilaterally determined by government. Commercial insurance companies that handle basic medical insurance are not even allowed to participate at all in the government's decision making process. All they can do is sit and wait for the government to 'notify them of results.' Two examples are described above of places that adopted a cooperative model fairly early on between commercial insurance and social security departments (the Jiangyin and Taicang cases). Despite having cooperated for many years, there has been no obvious break-through in the work of administering medical insurance, not even with the development of supplementary commercial health insurance on top of basic medical insurance.

In theory, commercial insurance companies and government should enjoy equal standing as market entities. That includes companies whether they handle basic medical insurance, or are authorized by government to undertake supplementary or critical illness insurance. As the purchaser of services, the government should be on equal footing with the supplier of services. What we have discovered in our research, however, is that the posture of government is far 'stronger' than that of commercial insurance companies. In the handling of medical insurance services, the government dominates nearly every aspect of the transaction, while the commercial insurance company is more like an entity that executes administrative orders and simply serves as 'cashier' for disbursing money out of the medical insurance fund. The commercial insurance company's ability to negotiate is highly limited when it comes to managing medical insurance, handling services, or even developing supplementary insurance products. It is forced into a passive position.

Jiangyin can serve as example. In 2009, on the basis of managing the basic medical insurance program, CPIC (China Pacific Insurance Company) also developed a supplementary commercial health insurance product in which residents could voluntarily participate, but the financing and compensation estimates of the product had to go through local government approval before they could be implemented. This ensured standards of safeguards which local government felt should 'not be too high.' Ultimately, the financing level of the supplementary insurance was set at RMB 90 per person per year and has not been adjusted so far. When it comes to residents' health safeguards, the government's functions extend outwards in boundless fashion. Commercial insurance companies find it difficult to gain any room for independent development.

Since it had been through the bidding process, in its negotiations with the government regarding division of rights and responsibilities and distribution of fund balances, at least PICC went through 'discussions' by which local social security bureau officials allowed it to handle the critical illness insurance and even allowed it to have a 'modest profit.' Nevertheless, the Taicang model was very hard to replicate in other parts of Jiangsu province. In 2012, the State Council's Medical Reform Office issued a document that pushed for nationwide implementation of critical illness insurance. Jiangsu responded to the requirements of this document by setting up critical illness insurance systems across the province and bringing commercial insurance into the process. Since PICC had been handling this insurance earlier, and had the experience, it participated in the bidding in all parts of the province. According to the explanation of a senior person in the Jiangsu branch of PICC, however, some cities asserted that the basic medical insurance fund was intended to enable common people to have medical care—it was not for enabling insurance companies to make money, and if one of them did want to handle the critical illness insurance in that place, then they had better be ready to lose money. Anyone who did not want to lose money might as well not participate in the bidding.

Since local governments were mostly averse to having commercial insurance companies make any profit off 'handling' or 'taking on' the business, very few companies have actually carried out these operations. Since 2012, the Insurance Regulatory Bureau of Jiangsu province has given approval to 23 companies to participate in bidding on tenders for critical illness business, but as of 2016 only 6 companies were engaged in the business. Other than PICC, the others are either showing losses or having trouble growing.

Third, in the past seven years, in response to the requirements of the New Medical Reform, public finance has increased spending on China's medical and healthcare systems. This includes not only an increase in funding of public medical institutions (subsidies for daily operations, spending on projects, and so on), but also public-finance subsidies for the urban and rural residents medical insurance and the new rural cooperative insurance. To a certain degree, this has further solidified the distortions of the monopoly pattern and only increased the difficulties of commercial health insurance.

Public medical institutions can serve as an example. China's public-finance structure is hierarchical, as described by the phrase 'management at each tier of administration and each eating at its own hearth' (i.e. separate budgets for each). This has meant that the higher the level of public medical institution, the greater the degree of public-finance support over these past seven years. In such cities as Beijing and Shenzhen, first-line cities with powerful financial resources, for every RMB 100 of income in municipal public hospitals, as much as around RMB 20 can come from public-finance subsidies.

Grade Three hospitals have expanded very rapidly. Between 2010 and 2014, the number of doctors in such hospitals went from being 32% of the national total to 42%. The number of beds went from being 31% to 38%. The number of patients choosing to see a doctor in a Grade Three hospital went from being 37% to 47%. The number of patients choosing to actually be hospitalized in a Grade Three hospital went from being 33% to 41%. For every two patients getting medical care at a hospital, that is to say, there was a third choosing to go to a Grade Three hospital.

Throughout China, the increase in public-finance support for the building of hospitals and purchase of equipment has been quite apparent. This too has been a consequence of the demands of the New Medical Reform. However, building buildings, adding beds, renovating equipment has also simply strengthened the monopoly force of Grade Three hospitals and added further to the medical fees of patients.

In the face of the tyrannical-type power of Grade Three hospitals, which have the government at their back, commercial insurance companies naturally cannot be equal partners to any transaction in a market situation. At the same time, the more private hospitals grow in power, the more reluctant doctors are to leave them—they don't dare go out on their own.

Meanwhile, public-finance subsidies have increased year after year with respect to the financing of the urban residents' health insurance and the new rural cooperative medical insurance. Given the increase in the total amounts of the funds, government departments have even begun to fight among themselves over power to manage them—specifically, the social security departments and the health departments. It goes without saying that they are not willing to grant the right to manage the basic medical insurance funds to commercial insurance companies.

6.3.1.2   Constraints due to China's stage of social development

Quite apart from the various policy constraints, the growth of commercial health insurance in China is also affected by the country's stage of social development. In 2016, the State Statistical Bureau made public the following data: China's GDP in 2015 was RMB 67.67 trillion, which ranked second in the world. But GDP per capita was just RMB 52,000 or around USD 8,016. This was still a certain distance from levels in such developed countries as the United States, Japan, Germany, and the UK, where the figure was over USD 37,000.

Looking more specifically at economic structure, we can see that China is still a country in transition and 'in the midst of developing' as opposed to being developed. The percentage of tertiary industries in a country is one important indicator of that country's level of development. In recent years, although the share of primary and secondary industries have both fallen in China's economic structure, and the share of tertiary industries has risen, that share just went over 50% in 2015. Meanwhile, structural problems within industries are pronounced. Modern service industries are still extremely weak, including the insurance industry. This economic context for the growth of the insurance industry is something that cannot be ignored—the extent to which commercial (health) insurance is retarded is consistent with this overall kind of environment.

The tradition of 'strong government' in China is another thing that has been holding back commercial insurance from developing. Beijing, Shenzhen, and other top cities are already among the ranks of developed economic bodies, but the people in those cities are far more conscious of government-provided welfare benefits than they are of the advantages of sharing risk through buying commercial insurance. Moreover, the public-finance resources of these places are generally excellent since basic medical funds are flush with money—people tend to be younger and the funds are not faced with the problem of sustainability due to the aging of society. As a result, governments in these places frequently provide greater insurance compensation for a broader range of safeguards out of 'generosity.' Seen objectively, this too squeezes out commercial insurance to a certain extent.

The same holds true for people with higher incomes. Under the tradition of 'strong government,' people within the institutional structure of government generally have higher incomes than those who are outside of it. Incomes of the type earned in government departments, public institutions (units), and State-Owned Enterprises are fairly high, and purchasing power is quite strong. Medical demand among these people is at a higher level and demands on commercial insurance are also high. However, these people have no risk of having to pay high costs, since 'government,' 'units,' and 'State-Owned Enterprises' already provide quite substantial supplementary safeguards. In some State-Owned Enterprises in which welfare benefits are quite good, such as the Industrial and Commercial Bank of China, employees essentially incur no spending costs at all when they get sick. In addition to the basic medical insurance and the supplementary medical insurance of the unit, they also have welfare supplements such as the unit's 'comfort subsidies.' What these people see as important is whether or not commercial insurance can provide higher quality and more convenient service. For example, can it help them reduce waiting times, get through the 'green channel' to see a specialist, and so on. These services, however, are precisely what commercial health insurance is unable to provide under the existing institutional structure.

6.3.2 Bottlenecks within commercial insurance that affect its participation in the medical reform

It cannot be denied that a number of external factors have led to the slow development of commercial health insurance—unassailable forces that have held it back. This does not mean, however, that the commercial insurance industries does not have internal problems all its own. When the planned economy was just beginning to loosen up the system of 'control by officials,' in the 1980s, newly emerging market forces were subject to restrictions but there still were plenty of industries that weathered hardship to grow up in the cracks. If commercial insurance is to play a larger role, it needs to make changes in a number of regards, including its own industry environment, policies, and management concepts.

Nevertheless, the core reason for the weak development of insurance relates to the powerful way government officials control the insurance market. Since it is hard for private enterprises to enter the field of insurance, most insurance companies are State-Owned Enterprises. Only a very small number are shareholding companies, such as Ping An Insurance (which still does not change the very powerful government 'background' [connections] of such companies). Insurance companies lack any motivation to improve management, raise efficiency, or improve product quality, since they are not competing in a beneficial way among themselves. Meanwhile, State-Owned Enterprises are generally aiming to be largest, not to have the most beneficial results. This contributes to the problem of vicious competition among State-Owned insurance companies.

The Jiangsu area, where we conducted our research, is an example. In the course of bidding for government tenders to handle basic medical insurance, some companies were interested only in 'snatching and occupying' market share, whatever the cost might be. In one city of Jiangsu, the requirement for bidding was that an insurance company agreed its profits would be limited to 20% of the surplus balance of the fund every year. The Jiangsu branch of People Insurance Company of China calculated that there were 400,000 insurants in that city, each contributing RMB 20 to the pooled funding every year so that the total amount in the fund was roughly RMB 8 million. The cost of handling the fund would come to at least RMB 400,000 (20% of an estimated RMB 2 million balance). If a commercial insurance company took on the business and intended at the very least to not make a loss, then all it could pay out in compensation every year was RMB 6 million. The remainder of the RMB 2 million would be drawn on for other expenses. Ultimately, the winning bid came from a different insurance company. Its winning proposal was that it would return 100% of the surplus back to the local government. In addition, the insurance company assigned 20 people at its own cost to do the handling work and provided two cars for government use, without taking in a penny. According to the explanation of the person at the Jiangsu branch of PICC, this way of competing to get bids is common and exists to this day.

In order for there to be a healthy competition among commercial insurance companies who handle basic medical insurance, two conditions should be present at the very least. First, the insured person, that is, the ultimate consumer of insurance, should have the right to assess the services being provided and to provide direct feedback to the provider of the services—this ability to provide feedback should be built into the system, so as to improve services. Our understanding of the actual situation from doing our research, however, was that insurance companies mainly were responsible only to government. They did accept performance evaluations by government, but the results of these were not made public. Even though the insured person was the one paying the fees for insurance, all they could do was passively accept whatever service they received. The insured person does indeed have the right to express an opinion either to a commercial insurance company or to the government departments managing medical insurance, but there are no institutional safeguards to guarantee that the ensured person's rights are actually realized.

Second, commercial insurance companies should be able to make comparisons among themselves quickly and effectively. Pros and cons are only apparent once there is a comparison. In the places we researched, however, the inclination was to stick with a given company once it had been settled upon at the beginning. Other companies were then not allowed to participate in handling medical insurance services. This made it impossible for there to be sustained, long-term competition among companies. As a result, not only did the winning bidder have no incentive to improve, but it had no yardstick by which to measure itself against others. This might look as though government was 'protecting' the commercial insurance company as it provided handling services to government. Instead, however, the practice held down beneficial competition among commercial insurance companies and prevented their sound growth.

Without pressure from competition, commercial insurance companies will also not fully release their potential 'productivity of services.' Between 2001 and 2016, CPIC provided handling services for Jiangyin's new rural cooperative insurance program—15 years of handling services. During this time, it was allowed to share in accessing data on the people who were insured in medical insurance, in order to help oversee the behavior of hospitals. To this day, however, CPIC has not even considered using this accumulation of data to carry out big-data R&D, not to mention developing supplementary insurance products that are multi-tiered and diversified and targeted at different types of illness and different groups of people. Instead, the company's energies have been focused on how to expand the Jiangyin 'handling model' to more parts of the country. They have not focused on building up stronger and more refined service capabilities.

Naturally, commercial insurance companies have confronted a variety of problems, including the short time-span for growth, the long-term suppression of their room for growth, and the severely inadequate supply of human resources and experience. This has led to an inability break open markets, develop products, and improve service capabilities. These limitations do exist. The systems, organizations, and technology that relate to gathering information on critical illness risk need to be improved. This includes setting up databases that would support the industry in general (including data on the medical history of insured people and their non-medical behavior), setting up companies that do surveys (surveys of information on patients), and granting legal rights to disclose information on patients' medical history. However, how to collect accurate information and data still depends, ultimately, on deepening reform of medical institutions. Right now, the value and usefulness of data coming out of medical institutions is extremely limited, due to the long-term distortions of cost structures and medical behavior.

6.4 FUTURE TRENDS IN THE OVERALL DEEPENING OF MEDICAL REFORM, AND ROOM INTO WHICH COMMERCIAL INSURANCE CAN DEVELOP

The impetus for deepening China's medical reform comes not only from the will of policymakers. Objectively speaking, it is also being pushed by the way society is developing. Take the current situation: even though the interests of various departments and the benefits of the industry have led to reform being mired in stalemate, which has weakened the ability of Central policymakers to push forward commercial insurance as well as such private forces as non-public medical institutions, when you look at that in combination with the way the economy and society are developing, in fact commercial insurance has quite a promising future.

The various factors that obstruct policies intended to develop commercial insurance, as described above, should gradually become less important. This is due to the downturn in the economic situation and the way fiscal revenues are increasing at a slower pace. In 2015, the rate at which public-finance revenues increased slowed to 8.4%. This was the lowest rate of increase since 1992. Between 1992 and 2013, public-finance revenues consistently grew at a double-digit pace. The very substantial power of public finances is what enabled the government to allocate resources during this period, which in turn provided key support for interventions. By 2014, however, after the rate dropped to 8.6%, it continued to decline in 2015. (See Figure 6.4.)

This decline in the pace at which public-finance revenue has been increasing is now confronting rigid spending requirements on such things as pensions. Such required spending has served to increase financial pressures. Within the next few years, more of government's diminished public-finance income will have to go toward filling in the system's previously created 'hole.' This includes dealing

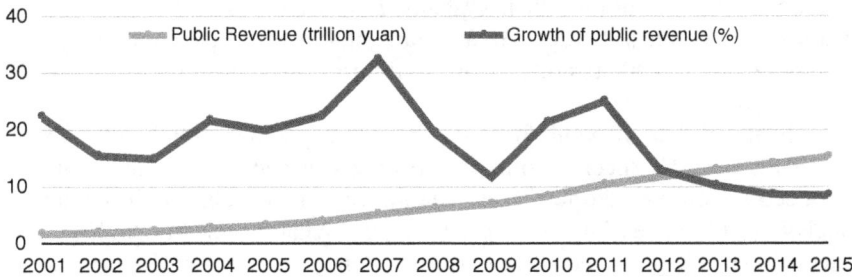

Figure 6.4 China's public revenue and changes in its growth rate between 2001 and 2015.

Source of data: *China Statistical Yearbook 2001–2015.*

with the pressure of running out of money for pensions. Public finance can no longer use surplus funds to continue to finance the high-cost and high-safeguard requirements of public medical institutions. The same holds for the urban residents' medical insurance and new rural cooperative insurance programs. The entire country is currently engaged in integrating two types of medical insurance systems. In order to reduce the social conflicts this involves, most areas are adopting methods that pull together and equalize the level of benefits offered by the two systems. Benefits under the new rural cooperative system are being increased. In the next few years, subsidy funds from public finance will focus more on smooth integration of the two systems than they will on simply raising benefits under one system. Local governments will be adopting a more conservative posture when it comes to continuing to have high pooling requirements for medical insurance funds—this is to avoid financial pressures when systems are consolidated.

As the ability of government to make adjustments grows weaker, we believe that at the very least the following four things will change in quite obvious ways as wholesale reform of China's medical and healthcare systems moves into deeper levels.

First, public hospitals will face significant financial pressure. The economic downturn will inevitably affect the ability of people to consume. Since the start of the new medical reform, the improvement in basic medical insurance benefits has already released demand to its maximum level, whether that demand was already potential or was further induced. What's more, the basic medical insurance funds are already running dry. Hospitals may well hope to continue to increase revenues at a fast pace, but they are losing the source of those revenues. In addition, since public hospitals are 'public-institution units,' their spending is often of a rigid nature (the salaries of personnel in such units can only increase, they cannot decline.) Low income and high outflow must necessarily lead to a large group of public hospitals facing extremely high financial risk. Meanwhile, government no longer has the surplus financial clout to reach into its pocket for hospitals. This may well force some local governments to push public hospitals in the direction of reforming their systems, in order to lessen their own (local governments') financial burden. As a result, some medical personnel may also be pushed toward 'marketization,' which will bring changes to the entire supply side of the medical system.

The financial data of public hospitals has already shown trends of this kind since 2013. In 2013, income noticeably declined in contrast to many years of high-speed growth prior to that year. The increase in spending on hospital personnel was still increasing by 2015, however. What's more, after 2011, the increase in spending on personnel was consistently higher than the increase in total business revenue. The inability of hospitals to balance revenues and expenses must inevitably become a critical problem within the near future. (See Figure 6.5.)

Second, the pressures on the basic medical insurance funds continue to intensify. Factors that mean the funds may run dry include the way private hospitals have intensified their monopoly position in these past few years, the rapid development of high-grade hospitals, and excessive and hard-to-control medical treatments, but they also include the way the basic medical system is combining two systems into one and also pushing forward critical illness insurance.

Areas with an older population will be the first to face the collapse of medical insurance. Over the past few years, due to the way economic development in different areas has become more strongly unbalanced, large quantities of young labor have flowed toward more developed regions. This has contributed to the pooling of medical insurance funds in those regions (young people pay more but cost less money) while the 'old and sick' have remained in the less developed areas. The policy for China's urban employees' medical insurance says that

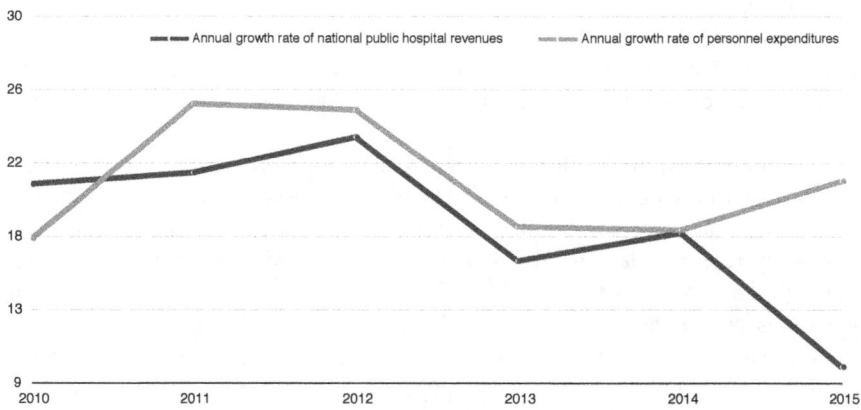

Figure 6.5 Annual growth rate of national public hospital revenues and personnel expenditures between 2010 and 2015 (%).

Source of data: National Health Financial Statement.

employees no longer need to pay contributions once they have retired. This brings into sharp relief the pressures on employees' insurance funds in lesser developed regions. These areas are constantly calling on the State to raise the administrative level at which fund-pooling takes place in order to merge the funds of lesser developed regions with those of more developed regions. The hope is that this will relax the pressure on the former.

However, developed regions are already at the point where they do not have that much 'surplus grain' to contribute to pooling. Given the contributions that so many young people have made who have come in from other areas, more developed regions have generally improved the benefits of their medical insurance and they have greatly increased the safeguards that they provide to retired people. Meanwhile, those people were originally in a good position to pay into the fund and the medical institutions near them have fairly high standards and charge high fees. Although developed regions pool more money, they also spend more and their surplus balance is limited.

From data published by the Ministry of Human Resources and Social Security, we can see that between the years 2001 and 2013 the disparity in amount of systemic support for employees under the employee insurance system was widening, that is, the coefficient of variation which represents the extent of statistical scattering. It increased from 0.26 in 2001 to 0.44 in 2013. In contrast, the per capita spending out of the fund and per capita cumulative balance had a coefficient of variation that kept declining. While medical costs were rising rapidly in developed regions, medical costs in underdeveloped regions were also quickly 'catching up,' due to the aging population and loss of control over public medical institutions. (The more underdeveloped a region, the more public institutions can become monopolies, since such areas are more conservative in terms of allowing private forces to run hospitals.) These trends reduced the gap between developed and underdeveloped regions. In terms of surplus balances, developed regions have up to now enjoyed a 'demographic dividend' and therefore the advantage of high surplus balances. This too is being lost in recent years. Underdeveloped regions are the same—all are facing the crisis of running out of money.

This will bring opportunities to commercial medical insurance in two ways. First, the pressures on funding in the underdeveloped areas will force policy-makers to consider raising the administrative level at which pooling of funds takes place. However, the administrative level at which pooling takes place in developed regions is already fairly high, while it is the opposite in less developed regions and the difficulties in achieving coordinated pooling are substantial. At the same time, there is the unavoidable risk of moral hazard (both sides have an incentive to pay less into the system while spending more.) Reforming the funding mechanism of the employees' insurance nevertheless becomes possible because of this. That is, first adjust the funding level of the two types of areas to the same level (that is, reduce the funding of the developed area); then reduce the scope of basic medical insurance to limit the difficulties of managing the fund once the administrative level of pooling is raised in underdeveloped areas.

Developed regions will therefore pay less in contributions—their excess can be used to purchase commercial insurance, which ensures that the actual benefits of insured people in developed areas do not decline. The second way the situation can benefit commercial medical insurance is as follows. Without even taking into consideration any adjusting of the level at which funds are pooled, all areas are already feeling pressure on their medical insurance funds. They have already begun to shift that pressure from the departments that manage medical insurance to medical institutions. Hospitals, faced with the 'total amount control system' of medical insurance departments and their refusal to provide supplementary funds for excess spending (overrun costs), are increasing the number of 'self-pay' items required of patients in order to maintain salaries and reduce pressure from medical insurance to control costs. This is happening particularly in areas where funds have already run dry. The actual percentage of compensation coming from the basic medical insurance is declining. Patients' 'self-pay' portion of bills is increasing. This too opens up room into which commercial health insurance can grow.

Third, as China's economy develops and people's incomes increase, as demographic structures change and the spectrum of disease shifts, changes in demand for medical care are becoming obvious. Demand is becoming stratified and also diversified.

First of all, over the past dozen years, the ongoing rise in national income and significant widening of the income gap have made people's demand for medical care change—it has gone from 'trying to see a doctor' to 'wanting to see a good doctor' and 'wanting not to get sick at all.' On the one hand, patients not only

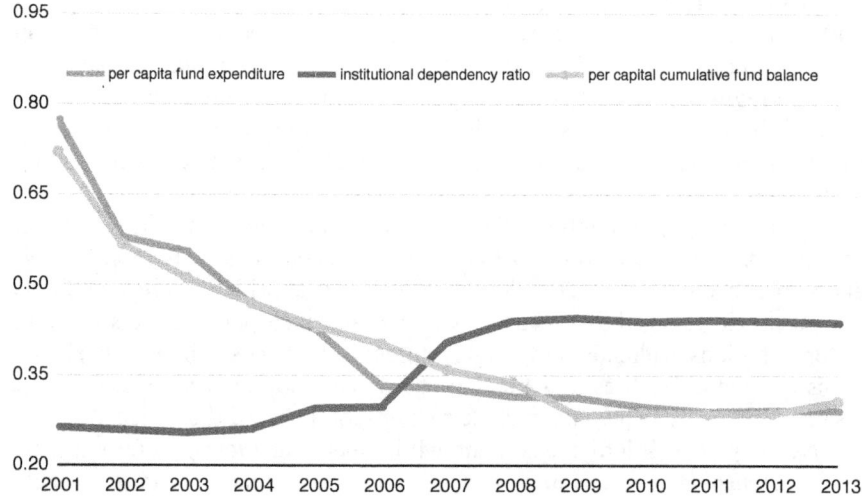

Figure 6.6 Variation coefficient of indicators related to urban staff medical insurance of 30 provinces and cities between 2001 and 2013.

Source of data: *China Labor Statistical Yearbook.*

want to receive a higher level of professional care and better hospitals as well as better doctors, but they want a better medical experience overall—that is, they require a better attitude and efficiency of service. On the other hand, the disparity in ability to pay has created a differentiation in demand for medical services. There is now a market for higher levels of medical service and more detailed categories of medical care.

Second, changes in the spectrum of diseases have had an extremely large influence on the categorization of medical services. In addition to that, life-threatening diseases prior to the 1950s mainly included such things as acute infectious diseases, parasitic diseases, and malnutrition that were treated by targeted biomedical means. As society progressed, by the period between 1990 and 2012 the primary cause of death had changed to chronic diseases and included such things as chronic infectious diseases, malignant tumors, cardiovascular disease, and endocrine and metabolic system diseases. The biggest different between chronic disease and acute disease is that acute disease generally requires drastic 'cliff-hanging-type' treatment which is prescribed as a result of actual symptoms. Chronic disease, on the other hand, calls for proactive prevention of disease prior to its active stage while post-onset of disease requires continuous health management—that is, ongoing, diversified kinds of health management services. Obviously, China's existing public medical institutions are not set up to deal with the new kinds of demand. They primarily offer a non-continuous style of medical service that focuses mainly on acute disease. In addition, the quality and efficiency of services is determined by doctors whose status is 'national

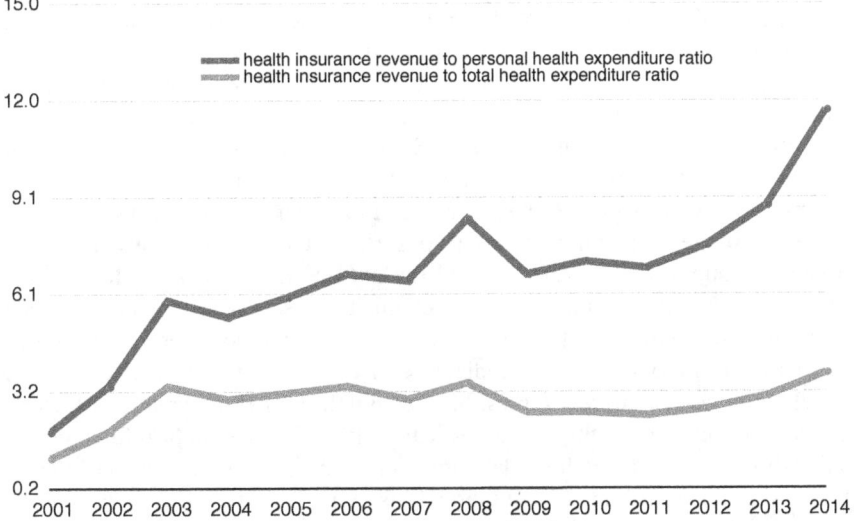

Figure 6.7 National health insurance revenue to personal health expenditure and total health expenditure ratio between 2001 and 2014 (%).

Source of data: *China Health Statistical Yearbook; China Insurance Yearbook.*

cadre' under the existing personnel system. This again provides space in which commercial health insurance can explore new models of providing healthcare services.

The new spectrum of diseases has created a demand for new kinds of safeguards. It is very hard, however, for such things as health services, management of chronic disease, and nursing care during the period of rehabilitation, things that are now available from privately run medical institutions, to get entered into the designated scope of basic medical insurance items. This vacuum in safeguards is therefore also providing room for commercial insurance to grow in a sustainable way—in terms of both expanded coverage and development of new kinds of policies.

Fourth, as resources within the institutional structure of medicine contract, that is, as public-sector resources pull back in an overall way, the attractiveness of public institutions to doctors will decline. Meanwhile, the appearance of new models of providing medical care, including Internet services and doctors' groups, will provide a golden opportunity to rejuvenate medical personnel resources. Spring Rain Doctor can serve as an example. By 2016, the Spring Rain Doctor platform had attracted more than 500,000 doctors. This means that about one in six of the country's 3.03 million doctors were practitioners on the platform, and this is only one corner of the Internet-based medical services. According to incomplete statistics online, there are now more than 2,000 mobile medical apps in China, and a growing number of doctor platforms are being established on the Internet.

This has opened up a channel by which doctors can interact directly with insurance companies. In the past, the root cause of many of the constraints on policies put forth in the Medical Reform was that doctors were tied into being 'members of units' in the public institution system. There were no market-set prices for medical services, since market prices could not be set by a mobile pool of medical professionals. Meanwhile, commercial insurance could not step across public medical institutions to reach doctors directly and negotiate with them on reimbursement standards and methods of cooperation. This is now changing, however, as doctors begin to face a broader group of patients, given the support of new technologies. (The basic medical insurance system is not motivated to support these doctors, and the entities that handle medical insurance under government control are often unable to do so.) This provides a golden opportunity for commercial insurance. Not only can commercial insurance become the 'primary payer' of medical services, and explore how to allocate medical resources via market forces, but it can help propel the creation of price-formation mechanisms in the entire medical system. This can in turn force public hospitals to reform. Meanwhile, data amassed from information on the Internet will also provide assistance to commercial insurance companies as they improve their actuarial capacities and develop more products.

In fact, statistics from commercial insurance after 2013 are already reflecting this trend to a certain degree. After many years of being 'squeezed' by basic medical insurance, and experiencing sluggish growth, commercial insurance is beginning to show an increase in its percentage of premium income overall as well as its percentage in the spending made by individuals on healthcare. The increase in the share of commercial health insurance in personal healthcare spending has been particularly notable, rising from 6.7% in 2009 to 11.7% in 2014. In absolute value terms, per capita health-insurance income rose from RMB 33 in 2009 to RMB 96.3 in 2014. The increase between 2013 and 2014 alone was 38.6%, or RMB 69.5 in absolute terms. (See Figure 6.8.)

However, any resolution of the internal problems of the commercial insurance industry is going to be determined by adjustments in national financial policy. This relates particularly to the very powerful 'rule by officials' or control over the industry. Even if financial policies cannot be loosened over the short term, the various positive factors as described above can still bring a degree of prosperity to commercial insurance markets. They can address such problems as low internal efficiency and vicious competition practices. There is some hope of an easing in the situation, therefore, as the overall environment moves in a more market-oriented direction every day.

6.5 POLICY RECOMMENDATIONS

To sum up what has been said above, the development of China's commercial health insurance will depend primarily on several things: the quantity of medical resources that are available to it, the extent to which government entities have occupied the insurance market, and the extent to which resources are allocated by administrative methods. The motivation for growing commercial health insurance will primarily come from the will of policies and measures, their actual experience when put into practice, and changes in the social and economic environment. It may be that the development of commercial insurance, and indeed its ability to 'break the ice' in reforming the entire institutional structure of medicine in China, will have to wait for the ongoing decline of public institutions. It may also be, however, that the determination of policymakers will be

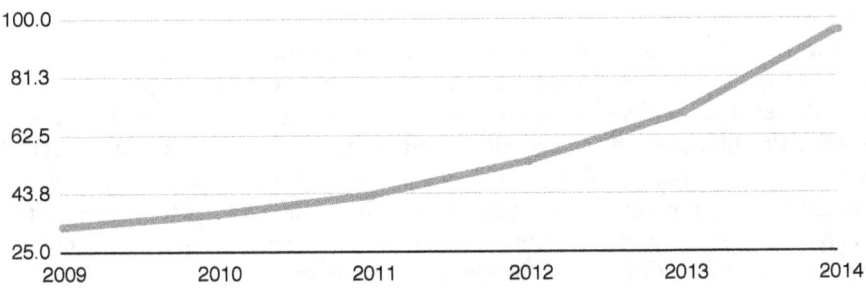

Figure 6.8 National per capita health insurance revenue between 2001 and 2014.

Source of data: *China Health Statistical Yearbook; China Insurance Yearbook.*

able to reform the situation, before the absolute end of the road is reached in the current way in which resources are allocated administratively. Through the use of more force, policymakers may be able to bring about real implementation of policy documents that, prior to this time, have not been implemented. That would allow commercial insurance to be injected into reform at an earlier time and help to turn around a dire situation.

Our policy recommendations are as follows.

6.5.1 Using reform of the personnel salary mechanism as the breakthrough, push supply-side reform of medicine into the deeper structures of institutions

Liberating medical personnel is the key to developing commercial insurance, and indeed to the entire undertaking of Medical Reform. Without marketizing the human resource of medicine, there can be no market price for medical services. Resource allocation will remain severely distorted and commercial insurance will be unable to become a professional 'third party' in the system. China's medical reform will remain mired in a deadlocked situation. Specific recommendations are as follows.

First, cancel the *bianzhi* system in public hospitals, that is, the staffing quota that applies to public institutions and that is registered as a quota in the government budget. For employees who are already registered on the personnel rolls under this system, we might adopt the principle of 'applying the old rules to older people and new methods to newer people.' Employees who have a public-institution status (or identity) under the *bianzhi* system could maintain that status (identity) without having their benefits changed. This would include having them continue to enjoy old-age pensions from their public-institution 'unit.' After 2016, when reform is initiated with respect to the old-age pensions of public-institution units, we can refer to relevant documents that applied to the reform of State-Owned Enterprises. That is, we can provide 'status (identity) changeover' subsidies as we cancel the *bianzhi* registrations in the government budget. New employees in the future will no longer be registered on public-institution personnel rolls. Instead they will, in a unified way, participate in China's social pension (old-age) insurance.

Second, explore ways in which hospitals and doctors can cooperate on more equal terms. This would include having doctors rent hospital equipment as they provide services, and allowing them to work part-time in hospitals. Encourage hospitals to find their own methods of compensating doctors that are in accord with the unique nature of the healthcare industry. Stop having administrative officials dictate the number of places in which a doctor can practice medicine. Encourage doctors to participate in Internet-based medicine and to strengthen the 'radiating' effect of outstanding medical resources.

Third, encourage hospitals to look at new ways to evaluate doctors (performance evaluations), either on their own or in alliance with doctors themselves, so as to weaken the importance of the job-designation (title) system. Encourage third parties, such as industry associations, to help raise the standards of professional management in the medical industry. Ensure that all relevant parties have a role in evaluations, including peers in the industry, employers, and the public at large.

6.5.2 Promote reform that turns public medical institutions into institutions run by society at large. At the same time, push forward the process of having non-public forces (private forces) manage hospitals

In developed countries and regions throughout the world, there is no such thing as a public medical institution that does not have an independent legal-person governance structure. There is also no such thing as a public medical institution that has become a 'tiger in the road' blocking development of non-public forces that manage medical institutions. Our specific recommendations are as follows.

First, abolish the administrative grading system of public medical institutions. Explore modern legal-person governance structures for medical institutions that use a board of directors as the core governing body. Move toward having the head of the hospital be a professional manager.

Second, abolish direct payments into medical institutions from public finance. Set up a system of public-finance 'rewards and subsidies' that is based on performance reviews, or directly change the system to 'subsidizing those in need.'

Third, with respect to pricing, refer to the 2014 document issued by the National Development and Reform Commission (NDRC). That is, move in the direction of having market-oriented public medical institutions no longer implement the pricing of medical services that was earlier prescribed by the NDRC. Instead, have benchmark pricing be determined through negotiations between hospitals and entities that handle medical insurance.

Fourth, allow medical institutions to adjust the scope of their business depending on their own circumstances. That includes having hospitals determine their own operating costs and make their own purchases, such as drugs, materials, and so on.

Fifth, with respect to privately run medical institutions, no longer limit the forms or mediums by which medical services are provided, and no longer limit the scope of services to the specific grade of the medical institution. Encourage all medical institutions with legitimate qualifications to determine the scope of their services in a flexible way, depending on their own capabilities and the needs of the market. Encourage the establishment of health-examination centers, surgery centers, and rehabilitation centers with nursing care, and support the development of new models for providing medical care in order to enable the entire healthcare industry to flourish.

6.5.3 Be explicit about the differences between basic medical insurance and commercial health insurance and how they are positioned in China's system; push forward reform of health insurance handling and payment mechanisms

Commercial insurance must be allowed to retain its autonomy, whether or not it is handling basic medical insurance, or just carrying on its own business. Otherwise, it will be impossible for market mechanisms to play their necessary role. Our specific recommendations are as follows.

First, pull in the 'pooled funding' boundaries of basic medical insurance and grant commercial insurance more space in which to develop. At the same time, set up a unified system of universal social medical insurance that has a low level of benefits but broad coverage. Use this to change the current situation of doubtful sustainability of funds, and the way lesser developed regions are subsidizing (paying back) more developed regions.

Second, reform the existing system by which government entities are handling medical insurance and move towards having the handling done by private entities and legal-person entities. For specifics, refer to the above discussion of public medical institutions. Introduce competitive mechanisms. Allow insured people to decide for themselves who they want to handle their medical insurance—this could well be commercial insurance entities or it could be privatized government entities.

Third, separate out management (administration) from operations in the process of managing medical insurance. Departments that manage medical insurance should no longer be allowed to intervene in micro-management of medical insurance funds. This includes intervention in such things as payment methods. Instead, these things should be determined by medical institutions themselves in consultation with handling entities depending on the conditions of the fund and supply-side considerations. Departments that manage medical insurance should focus exclusively on regulatory oversight of the industry, on maintaining its proper functioning and healthy operations.

Fourth, establish a medical insurance physician's system. Guide and constrain improper behavior of individual doctors in terms of diagnosis and treatment, and use this as an important measure by which to support doctors' ability to practice independently.

Fifth, open up greater market access for specialized health insurance companies. Encourage the development of private commercial insurance companies that are at the small and medium-sized level, as well as non-profit, non-governmental, insurance organizations. Set up a health information-sharing platform. Improve the laws and regulations that apply to these things.

6.5.4 Implement a regulatory system that calls for openly available information, mandatory information disclosure, and participation by all sides including individuals, society at large, and government.

Push for including the participation of third-party entities, industry associations, and social organizations. Guide the industry in the direction of self-discipline, with all parties involved in consultations.

Note

1 S. Hillier, J. Shen. Health Care Systems in Transition: People's Republic of China. Part I: An Overview of China's Health Care System. *Public Health*, 1996, 18 (3): 258–265.
2 Duan Jiaxi. Historical Opportunities for China's Commercial Health Insurance Development. *China Insurance*, 2008, 8: 14–21.
3 Li Hang, Sun Dongya, Zhang Lei, Zhang Junxing. Research in China's Commercial Health Insurance Development. *China Medical Insurance*, 2014, 9: 22–24.
4 This idea is not put into practice. Instead, it's decided that different insurers shall handle the basic medical insurance in different administrative regions to pave way for the free choice of the insured in the future.

7 Survey report on demand for commercial health insurance in China

Qiu Yue and Guo Pei

7.1 BACKGROUND AND PURPOSE

Commercial health insurance is not only an important part of China's multi-tiered medical safeguards system, but it is inherently necessary if we are to achieve the strategy of a 'Healthy China.' As economic and social progress continue in China, as the 'aging population' trend accelerates and patterns of the prevalence of diseases change, people are placing ever greater demands on health services and healthcare safeguards. At the same time, China's economy has entered a 'new normal' stage of development. The rate at which fiscal revenues increase is slowing down. Pressures on the country's medical insurance system are enormous. The government, faced with the fundamental reality of fast-paced increases in the demand for healthcare, but inability to cover that demand through the basic medical insurance system, has been highly concerned about developing the commercial health insurance industry. It has issued a host of important documents aimed at spurring on that development.

Attempts to develop commercial health insurance in China fall within the general scope of 'supply-side structural reforms.' Not only do such reforms require firm adherence to policies that introduce new ways of doing things, but they require adherence to the principle of being guided by demand. In recent years, China has conducted a number of national surveys and investigations in the realm of healthcare. Surveys that had to do with the demand for commercial health insurance, however, mainly focused on insurance companies as the primary entities involved. They rarely, moreover, covered the subject on a nationwide basis. In order to understand and truly grasp the demand for commercial health insurance in China, in June and July 2017, we conducted a nationwide telephone survey on 'the demand for health insurance among urban and rural people' in the country. This report offers a statistical analysis of the data that resulted from that survey. We hope that it will provide statistics and reliable information to support the formulation of relevant policies and plans in China.

7.2 SURVEY DESIGN

The actual work of conducting the survey on the 'demand for health insurance among urban and rural populations in China' was entrusted to the Opinion Polling Center of the National Bureau of Statistics of China. The questionnaire covered basic information on those being surveyed, including participation in social insurance and assessments of that program, purchase of commercial health insurance and evaluations of that insurance, future demand, and so on. Respondents were between the ages of 18 and 75 who lived in the area being surveyed for more than six months of each year. Sampling decisions used a nationwide grid of designated administrative districts above the level of sub-district (streets or local communities) and townships. The 'unit' of sampling was the telephone number. A total of 20,000 samples were chosen from the framework (grid) using multi-level, multi-stage, proportional, and simple random sampling techniques.

For purposes of the sampling process, the country was divided into five levels. China's three directly administered provincial-level cities were defined as a single level (Beijing, Shanghai, and Tianjin). The other four were China's four large economic zones (east, central, west, and northeast China), each divided separately into sampling areas. A sample of 1,000 respondents was drawn from each of the three municipalities. The remaining respondents were drawn from the four major economic zones in proportion to their population: 6,000 were drawn from east China, 4,800 from central China, 4,800 from west China, and 1,400 from northeast China. Samples in directly administered cities were drawn directly. In each of the four economic zones, a PPS (probability proportional to size) sampling method was used to draw samples from each prefecture-level city (the sampling unit) according to population in the city and ranked by per capita GDP. Between 350 and 400 samples were drawn from each sampling unit. At the same time, in each unit we maintained the proportion of urban and rural sampling areas as in the total, to ensure that the samples were representative. The survey covered three municipalities directly under the Central Government and 43 prefectural-level cities, as shown in Figure 7.1. We collected a total of 19,999 samples. The distribution of sample quantities is shown in Table 7.1.

7.3 BASIC INFORMATION ON RESPONDENTS TO THE SURVEY

7.3.1 Socio-demographic characteristics of the target population

7.3.1.1 Urban/rural, regional, gender, and age distribution of respondents

The number of statistically valid samples of this survey was 19,999, of which 60.7% were drawn from urban areas and 39.3% from rural areas. In terms of

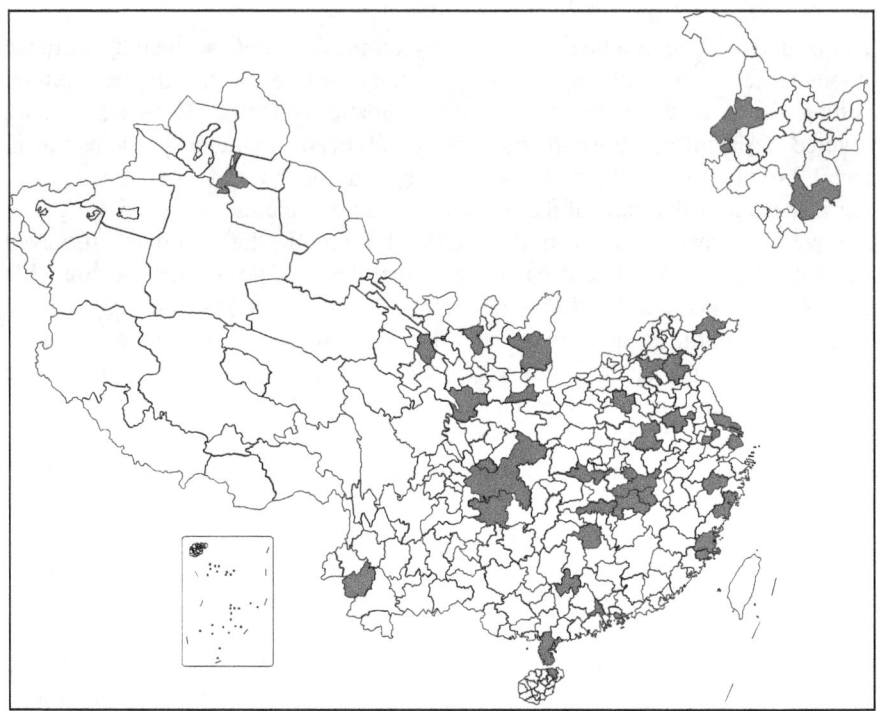

Figure 7.1 Forty-six cities from which samples were drawn.

distribution by region, 15.0% of the total samples were drawn from provincial-level municipalities, 30.0% from east China, 24.0% from central China, 24.0% from west China, and 7.0% from northeast China. In terms of distribution by gender, men accounted for 56.3% of the total samples and women for 43.7%. In terms of distribution by age group, the two largest age groups were 18–29 years old and 30–39 years old. These two groups accounted for 25.8% and 25.7% of the total samples, respectively. They were followed by the age group 40–49, which accounted for 19.7%; the smallest age group was 70–75, accounting for 4.4%. For details, see Table 7.2.

7.3.1.2 Distribution of respondents by education and occupation

Samples with senior high/secondary vocational/technical school education accounted for the largest percentage of the total valid samples (24.2%), followed by samples with a bachelor's degree and those with a junior high school diploma, accounting for 23.6% and 20.3%, respectively. The number of samples with a master's or higher degree was the smallest, accounting for 2.9%. For details, see Table 7.3.

Table 7.1 Number of effective samples by province/city and urban or rural area

Province	Prefectural-level city	Number of samples	Number of samples drawn in urban areas	Number of samples drawn in rural areas
Beijing	–	1000	852	148
Tianjin	–	1000	709	291
Shanghai	–	1000	851	149
Hebei	Qinhuangdao	400	240	160
	Baoding	400	184	216
Jiangsu	Wuxi	400	225	175
	Nantong	400	207	193
Zhejiang	Wenzhou	400	200	200
	Jinhua	400	166	234
Fujian	Fuzhou	400	275	125
	Putian	400	184	216
Shandong	Yantai	400	200	200
	Jining	400	200	200
	Linyi	400	200	200
Guangdong	Shenzhen	400	360	40
	Foshan	400	362	38
	Zhanjiang	400	164	236
Hainan	Haikou	400	286	114
Shanxi	Taiyuan	400	336	64
	Luliang	400	183	217
Anhui	Chuzhou	400	196	204
	Lu'an	400	172	228
Jiangxi	Nanchang	400	211	189
	Jiujiang	400	208	192
	Yichun	400	180	220
Henan	Zhoukou	400	152	248
Hubei	Huangshi	400	243	157
	Jingzhou	400	202	198
Hunan	Changsha	400	297	103
	Hengyang	400	285	115
Inner Mongolia	Wulanchabu	400	238	162
	Hezhou	400	231	169
Chongqing	Yongchuan District	400	301	99
Sichuan	Guang'an	400	144	256
Guizhou	Zunyi	400	245	155
Yunnan	Lincang	400	142	258
Shaanxi	Xi'an	400	203	197
	Yan'an	400	221	179
Gansu	Longnan	400	155	245
Qinghai	Haidong	400	226	174
Ningxia	Zhongwei	400	245	155
Xinjiang	Urumqi	400	350	50
Liaoning	Shenyang	350	224	126
Jilin	Jilin	349	283	66
	Yanbian Korean Autonomous Prefecture	350	248	102
Heilongjiang	Qiqihar	350	161	189
Total		19,999	12,147	7,852

Table 7.2 Urban/rural, regional, gender and age distribution of respondents

	Type	Percentage
Urban/rural distribution	Urban	60.7
	Rural	39.3
Regional distribution	Province-level municipalities	15.0
	East	30.0
	Central	24.0
	West	24.0
	Northeast	7.0
Gender	Male	56.3
	Female	43.7
Age (years)	18–29	25.8
	30–39	25.7
	40–49	19.7
	50–59	14.5
	60–69	9.9
	70–75	4.4

Table 7.3 Distribution of respondents by education (%)

Primary and lower education	Junior high education	Senior high/ secondary vocational/ technical school education	Vocational college education	Bachelor's degree	Master's and higher degree
10.0	20.3	24.2	18.9	23.6	2.9

Among the samples drawn from urban areas, employees of state-owned units, including Party and government organs and public institutions, accounted for the largest percentage (24.5% of the total). This was followed by employees of private enterprises (12.1%), and private business owners (10.4%). The percentage of self-employed people and those working in other forms of urban employment was the smallest (0.7%). Among the rural samples, the number of farmers was the largest, accounting for 13.1%, followed by migrant workers (including those working for fixed terms and non-fixed terms) and unemployed individuals, accounting for 6.9% and 5.5%; individuals in other forms of employment in rural areas accounted for only 1.0%. For details, see Table 7.4.

7.3.1.3 Distribution of respondents by marital status

Of those surveyed, 75.8% of the respondents were married, 20.4% unmarried, 2.4% divorced and 1.4% widowed.

Table 7.4 Distribution of respondents by occupation (%)

Basis for distribution	Occupation	Percentage
Urban samples	Employees of state-owned units	24.5
	Employees of collectively owned enterprises	5.2
	Private business owners	10.4
	Employees of private enterprises	12.1
	Freelancers	0.7
	Other forms of employment in urban areas	0.7
	Unemployed	7.2
Rural samples	Farmers	13.1
	Migrant workers	6.9
	Owners of township collectively owned or private business	3.7
	Employees of township collectively owned or private business	4.7
	Employees of government agencies or public institutions	4.4
	Other forms of employment in rural areas	1.0
	Unemployed	5.5
Total		100

7.3.2 Family income

The largest number of respondents had an annual family income of RMB 50,000–100,000 (20.6%), followed by respondents whose annual family income was RMB 100,000–300,000 (18.7%) and then RMB 300,000–500,000 (17.1%). The number of respondents whose annual family income was more than RMB 500,000 was the smallest, accounting for only 2.0%. Another 8.0% of the respondents' annual family income was either unclear or unanswered. For details, see Table 7.5.

Table 7.5 Distribution of respondents by annual family income (%)

Basis for distribution	Income (RMB)	Percentage
Annual family income	Less than 10,000	11.1
	10,000–30,000	18.7
	30,000–50,000	17.1
	50,000–100,000	20.6
	100,000–150,000	11.5
	150,000–250,000	7.3
	250,000–500,000	3.7
	More than 500,000	2.0
	Unclear/unanswered	8.0

7.3.3 Health status and health-monitoring behavior

Most of the respondents were in fairly good health, but 11.4% suffered from long-term illnesses or critical illnesses, including such things as heart disease and diabetes. With respect to physical examinations, about half of the respondents took a physical exam once every year; about one-fifth of the respondents had had no physical exam within five years. For details, see Table 7.6.

7.4 ENROLLMENT IN CHINA'S BASIC MEDICAL INSURANCE PROGRAM AND EVALUATION OF THAT PROGRAM

7.4.1 Social basic medical insurance

7.4.1.1 Distribution of respondents by enrollment in the basic medical insurance program

The survey showed that China's basic medical insurance program basically already provides coverage for the entire population. Within different types of the country's basic medical insurance program, the percentage of all respondents enrolled in 'urban employees' basic medical insurance' was the highest (39.8%); those enrolled in the 'new rural cooperative medical program + critical illness insurance' accounted for 33.5%; those enrolled in 'urban residents' basic medical insurance + critical illness insurance' accounted for 12.9%; those enrolled in 'urban and rural residents' basic medical insurance + critical illness insurance' and those receiving 'publicly provided medical services' both accounted for 3.2%. Among urban respondents, more than 50% were enrolled in the urban employees' basic medical insurance; among rural respondents, more than 60% were enrolled in the new rural cooperative medical program. There was little difference in the enrollment pattern across the surveyed regions. For enrollment in basic medical insurance programs, see Table 7.7.

Table 7.6 Distribution of respondents by health status and behavior (%)

Health status and behavior	Option	Percentage
Whether suffering from long-term or critical illnesses	Yes	11.4
	No	88.1
	Unclear	0.5
Frequency of physical examination	Once every half a year	9.0
	Once every year	49.0
	Once every two years or three years	19.6
	No physical examination within five years	22.3

Table 7.7 Distribution of respondents by enrollment in basic health insurance program (%)

Type		Basic health insurance program for urban employees	Basic health insurance for urban residents + Critical illness insurance	New cooperative medical scheme + Critical illness insurance	Basic health insurance for urban and rural residents + Critical illness insurance	Free medical services	None of the above	Total
Total		39.8	12.9	33.5	3.2	3.2	7.4	100.0
Regional distribution (%)	Provincial-level municipalities	56.7	15.0	14.1	2.6	5.2	6.5	100.0
	East China	41.1	11.5	32.3	3.7	3.2	8.2	100.0
	Central China	33.3	13.3	41.1	2.6	2.4	7.3	100.0
	West China	35.0	12.5	39.6	3.5	2.8	6.6	100.0
	Northeast China	37.4	14.2	32.9	2.9	3.1	9.6	100.0
Urban/rural distribution (%)	Urban areas	55.5	17.6	13.1	2.4	4.3	7.0	100.0
	Rural areas	15.5	5.5	65.0	4.4	1.5	8.1	100.0
Distribution by gender (%)	Male	38.0	11.8	35.8	3.1	3.6	7.6	100.0
	Female	42.1	14.2	30.4	3.3	2.7	7.3	100.0

7.4.1.2 Degree of satisfaction with basic medical insurance programs

Among all respondents, 68.6% believed that China's basic medical insurance programs are meeting their needs. The percentage of respondents holding this view was smaller in developed areas than it was in less developed areas. The percentage of respondents holding this view in East China (68.1%), provincial-level municipalities (66.1%) and Northeast China (62.0%) was lower than that in West China (72.7%) and Central China (69.2%). The percentage of respondents holding this view in rural areas (69.8%) was higher than that in urban areas (67.8%).

Demand for health services and health safeguards increased as age of respondents increased, while the feeling that China's basic medical insurance programs met their needs went down as age of respondents increased. Of respondents aged 18–29, 76.8% believed that China's basic medical insurance programs are meeting their needs. This figure dropped by nearly 20% in the 60–69 and 70–75 age groups. There are statistically significant differences in how satisfied different age groups are with China's basic health insurance programs. For details, see Table 7.8 and Figure 7.2.

In terms of health status, the percentage of respondents suffering from long-term or critical illnesses (55.0%) was nearly 15% lower than the percentage of healthy respondents, and there is a statistically significant difference in the degree of satisfaction of the two groups. For details, see Table 7.9.

The percentage of respondents who are satisfied with the free (publicly provided) medical services was the highest among all basic health insurance programs (over 80%). Around 70% of respondents were satisfied with other basic health insurance programs. For details, see Figure 7.3.

Table 7.8 Percentage of respondents satisfied with basic health insurance programs by region and by rural/urban status

Type		Percentage of respondents satisfied with basic health insurance programs
Total		68.6
Region	Provincial-level municipalities	66.1
	East China	68.1
	Central China	69.2
	West China	72.0
	Northeast China	62.0
Rural/urban status	Urban	67.8
	Rural	69.8

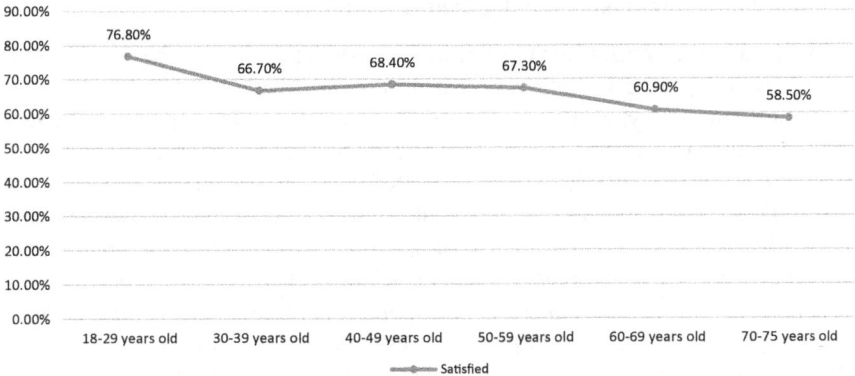

Figure 7.2 Percentage of respondents satisfied with basic health insurance programs by age group.

Table 7.9 Percentage of respondents satisfied with basic health insurance programs by health status (%)

Type		Percentage of respondents satisfied
Whether suffering from long-term or critical illnesses	Yes	55.5
	No	70.5

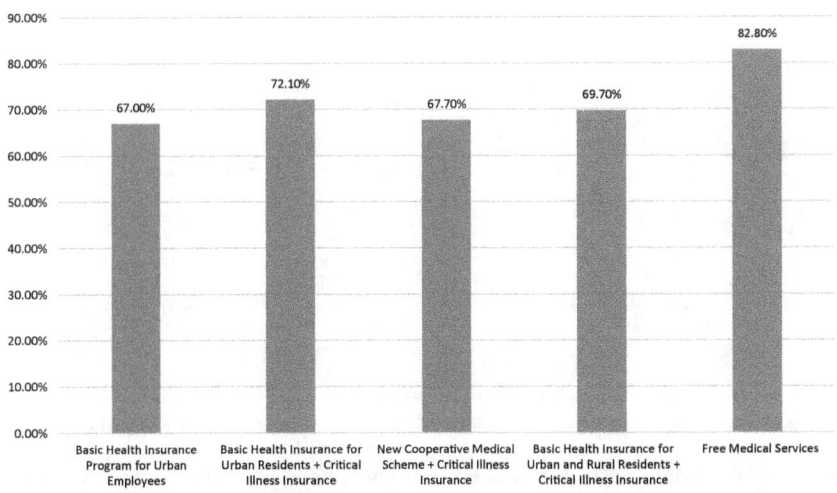

Figure 7.3 Degree of satisfaction with different basic health insurance programs.

7.4.1.3 Major reasons for the failure of (social) basic medical insurance programs to meet the needs of respondents

The most important reason for the failure of basic health insurance programs to meet the needs of respondents was that it was 'still hard to cope [financially] with critical illness.' More than one-third (36.2%) of the respondents chose this reason. Another one-third (35.8%) chose 'low percentage of reimbursements,' while 23.7% of the respondents chose 'limited scope of things that can be reimbursed.' This pattern was similar across all regions. The number of respondents who felt it was 'hard to cope with critical illness' was largest in urban areas, accounting for 39.2% of urban respondents, while the number of respondents who chose 'low percentage of reimbursements' was the largest in rural areas, accounting for 37.5% of rural respondents. For details, see Table 7.10.

With respect to income as a consideration, 'low reimbursement percentage' and 'insufficient safeguards against critical illness' (hard to cope with critical illness) were the most important reasons for the failure of basic health insurance programs to meet needs at all income levels, irrespective of which income group. More than 40% of the respondents with an annual family income of less than RMB 30,000 chose 'low percentage of reimbursements' as the most important reason. The percentage declined as income increased, however. Nearly one-half of respondents with an annual family income of RMB 150,000–500,000 chose 'insufficient safeguards against critical illness' (hard to cope with critical illness) as the most important reason. For details, see Figure 7.4.

With respect to health status, most (41.2%) of the respondents suffering from long-term or critical illness chose 'low reimbursement percentage' as the most important reason, while most healthy respondents (36.8%) chose 'insufficient safeguards against critical illness' as the most important reason. For details, see Table 7.11.

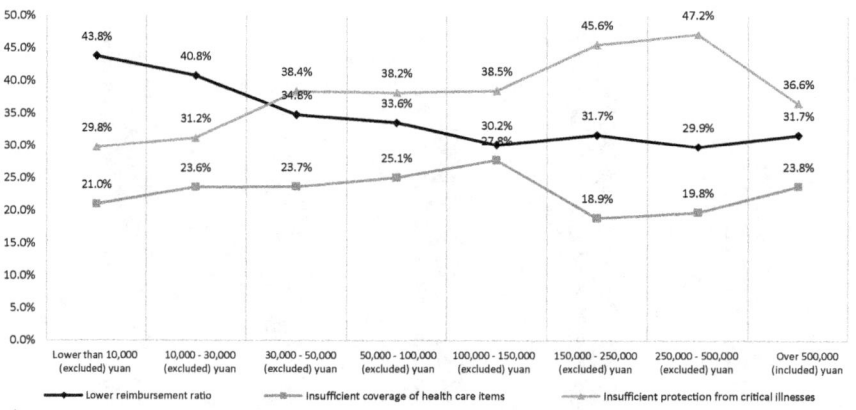

Figure 7.4 Perception of respondents about the most important reason for the failure of the basic health insurance programs to meet the needs of residents, by income level.

Table 7.10 Major reasons for the failure of basic health insurance programs to meet the needs of respondents, based on the views of respondents by region and urban/rural status (%)

Type		Low reimbursement ratio	Insufficient coverage of health care items	Insufficient protection from critical illnesses	Other reasons	Subtotal
	Total	35.8	23.7	36.2	4.2	100.0
Region	Provincial-level municipalities	38.6	17.7	37.9	5.9	100.0
	East China	35.7	23.9	37.7	2.7	100.0
	Central China	35.2	27.7	32.9	4.2	100.0
	West China	33.2	24.0	38.3	4.5	100.0
	Northeast China	39.7	23.3	31.8	5.2	100.0
Urban/rural status	Urban	34.8	22.1	39.2	3.8	100.0
	Rural	37.5	26.4	31.3	4.8	100.0

Table 7.11 Perception of respondents about the most important reason for failure of the basic health insurance programs to meet the needs of residents by health status (%)

Type		Low reimbursement ratio	Insufficient coverage of healthcare items	Insufficient protection from critical illnesses	Other reason	Sub-total
Whether suffering from long-term or critical illnesses	Yes	41.2	18.5	34.2	6.0	100.0
	No	34.6	24.8	36.8	3.8	100.0

7.4.1.4 Summary

China's basic healthcare system covers nearly 95% of China's entire population. The 'urban and rural residents' basic medical insurance,' which combines the urban residents' basic medical insurance and the new rural cooperative medical plan, is still in its infancy and covers a lower percentage of the population. About 70% of respondents believe that China's basic medical insurance programs can meet their needs. Relatively speaking, satisfaction was greater in less developed areas than it was in more developed areas. The percentage of satisfied people was lower among respondents with greater health needs, such as the elderly and those suffering from illnesses. 'Insufficient safeguards against from critical illness' and 'low percentage of reimbursements' were the two biggest reasons for the failure of the basic medical insurance programs to meet the needs of the population. One third of the respondents chose each of those as the most important reason. Respondents in vulnerable groups (such as some rural and low-income people and people suffering from illness) chose 'low percentage of reimbursements' as the most important reason China's basic medical insurance programs are not meeting their needs.

7.4.2 Evaluation of critical illness insurance

7.4.2.1 Degree of satisfaction with critical illness insurance

Among all respondents to the survey, the percentage saying that they were 'satisfied' with critical illness insurance was the highest (35.9%), followed by 'neutral' (30.1%), 'very satisfied' (25.1%), 'dissatisfied' (6.4%) and 'very dissatisfied' (2.5%). The distribution of respondents by satisfaction was similar across all regions. Relatively speaking, the percentage of respondents who were satisfied or very satisfied was highest in west China, reaching nearly 65%, and lowest in directly administered cities (55%). The percentage of respondents who were dissatisfied or very dissatisfied were highest in directly administered cities (12.9%), followed by northeast China (11.6%). Generally speaking, the degree

Table 7.12 Degree of satisfaction with critical illness insurance by region, urban/rural status, and gender (%)

Type		Very satisfied	Satisfied	Neutral	Dissatisfied	Very dissatisfied	Sub-total
	Overall	25.1	35.9	30.1	6.4	2.5	100.0
Region	Provincial-level municipalities	17.6	37.4	32.2	9.1	3.8	100.0
	East China	24.0	36.1	32.4	5.6	1.8	100.0
	Central China	27.2	33.5	30.5	6.3	2.6	100.0
	West China	27.3	37.1	27.2	6.2	2.3	100.0
	Northeast China	22.9	37.3	28.2	7.6	4.0	100.0
Urban/rural	Urban	21.7	38.9	31.0	5.8	2.7	100.0
	Rural	27.4	33.8	29.6	6.9	2.4	100.0
Gender	Male	25.9	35.6	28.0	7.1	3.3	100.0
	Female	23.8	36.2	33.0	5.5	1.4	100.0

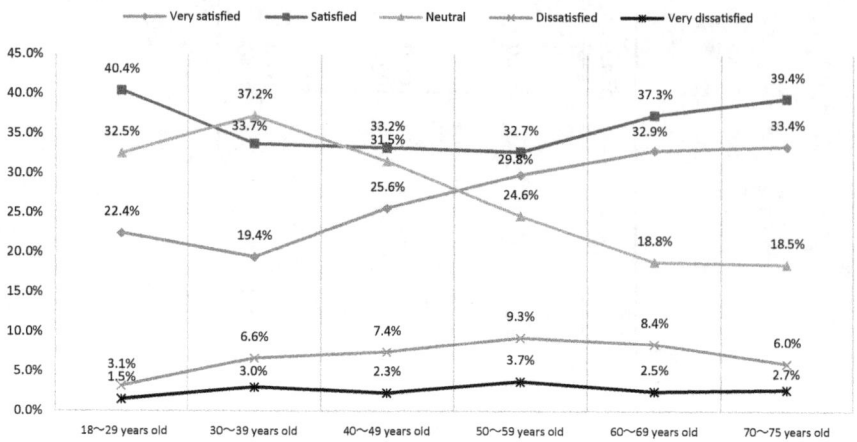

Figure 7.5 Level of satisfaction with critical illness insurance by age group.

of satisfaction in directly administered cities was the lowest. The satisfaction ratio and the dissatisfaction ratio in urban areas were lower than those in rural areas, but the percentage of respondents who were very satisfied with critical illness insurance in rural areas (27.4%) was higher than that in urban areas (21.7%). For details, see Table 7.12.

Male respondents had a higher inclination to be satisfied and also a higher inclination to be dissatisfied than women. The difference in dissatisfaction percentages was more significant (3.5%) than the difference in satisfaction percentages (1.5%). In terms of differences among age groups, the percentage of senior respondents (60–69 and 70–75 age groups) who were satisfied or very satisfied critical illness insurance was relatively higher, standing at more than 70%, while the satisfaction percentage in the 30–39 age group was the lowest, standing at about 50%. For details, see Figure 7.5.

People suffering from long-term or critical illness had relatively high rates of satisfaction as well as dissatisfaction with basic medical insurance. The difference between the two in terms of dissatisfaction was greater (around 5%, while the difference in satisfaction percentages was around 0.8%). See Table 7.13.

7.4.2.2 Analysis of the reasons for inadequacies of critical illness insurance

The survey shows that the biggest reason for feeling that critical illness insurance is inadequate is low reimbursement rate (57.4%). This is followed by cross-jurisdiction claims settlement issues (28.2%), complex claims handling process (27.8%), and too few designated healthcare facilities (25.7%). Some 62.1% of respondents in the directly administered cities chose 'low reimbursement

Table 7.13 Level of satisfaction with critical illness insurance by health status (%)

Type		Very satisfied	Satisfied	Neutral	Dissatisfied	Very dissatisfied	Sub-total
Whether suffering from long-term or critical illnesses	Yes	26.7	35.0	25.0	10.0	3.3	100.0
	No	24.8	36.1	30.8	5.9	2.4	100.0

percentage' as the most important reason, which was higher than that in east China (58.6%), central China (56.9%), west China (55.2%), and northeast China (55.0%). The top three reasons chosen by respondents in urban areas were low reimbursement ratio (57.3%), cross-jurisdiction claims settlement issues (31.9%), and complex claims handling process (28.3%), while the top three reasons chosen by respondents in rural areas were low reimbursement ratio (57.5%), complex claims handling process (27.4%), and cross-jurisdiction claims settlement issues (25.7%). See Table 7.14.

7.4.2.3 Summary

Most respondents were either satisfied or very satisfied with the coverage of critical illness insurance—less than 10% were dissatisfied or very dissatisfied, but nearly one-third of the respondents expressed a neutral attitude. People in directly administered cities have the lowest degree of satisfaction. The percentage of respondents in urban areas expressing a 'neutral' attitude was higher than that in rural areas. The percentage of respondents who were very satisfied in rural areas was higher than that in urban areas. More male respondents than female respondents gave a clear comment and were dissatisfied or very dissatisfied with critical illness insurance. The degree of satisfaction of the elderly (60–69 and 70–75 age group) was relatively high. The percentage of senior respondents who were satisfied or very satisfied was more than 70%. The degree of satisfaction in the 30–39 age group satisfaction was the lowest and the percentage was about 50%. For reasons for insufficiency of critical illness insurance, more than 50% of the respondents chose 'low reimbursement ratio.' More than 60% of respondents chose 'low reimbursement ratio' in the provincial-municipal municipalities. Respondents choosing 'cross-jurisdiction claims settlement issues,' 'complex claims handling process,' and 'too few designated healthcare facilities' accounted for more than 20%.

Table 7.14 Main reasons that respondents feel critical illness insurance is inadequate, by region and urban/rural status (%)

Type		Coverage overlapping with social insurance	Low reimbursement ratio	High out-of-pocket spending	Cross-city settlement issues	Complex claims handling process	Too few designated healthcare facilities
	Overall	14.1	57.4	24.2	28.2	27.8	25.7
Region	Provincial-level municipalities	14.4	62.1	24.2	27.9	23.7	30.0
	East China	17.7	58.6	23.7	33.0	28.6	25.8
	Central China	13.6	56.9	24.6	22.7	28.5	23.4
	West China	10.9	55.2	24.7	28.8	29.8	26.2
	Northeast China	11.5	55.0	23.0	28.4	20.9	25.5
Urban/rural	Urban	16.6	57.3	24.0	31.9	28.3	26.6
	Rural	12.3	57.5	24.3	25.7	27.4	25.1

7.5 PURCHASE OF COMMERCIAL HEALTH INSURANCE AND EVALUATION OF THAT INSURANCE

7.5.1 Purchase of commercial health insurance

7.5.1.1 *Percentage of respondents who purchased commercial health insurance*

Among the respondents, 26.2% purchased commercial health insurance. Directly administered cities had the highest percentage of respondents who had purchased commercial health insurance (32.8%), followed by east China (29.9%) and northeast China (25.5%). There were significant differences in the percentage of respondents who purchased commercial health insurance across regions. The percentage of respondents who purchased commercial health insurance was higher among urban respondents (31.5%) than rural respondents (18.1%).

The percentage of female respondent who purchased health insurance (27.3%) was higher than that of male respondents (25.4%). With respect to age distribution, the percentage of respondents aged 40–49 who purchased commercial health insurance was 31.7%, followed by people 30–39 years old (31.5%), and 18–29 years old (27.9%). The percentage of commercial health insurance buyers among elderly respondents was low—the 70–75 age group had the lowest percentage (6.2%). For details, see Tables 7.15 and 7.16.

With respect to occupation and the percentage of commercial health insurance purchased in urban areas, private business owners had the highest percentage (37.3%) of purchase of insurance, followed by employees of collective-owned units (33.5%), employees of private businesses (33.0%), and employees of state-owned units (29.9%). With respect to the percentage of purchase by occupation in rural areas, owners of township collective-owned or

Table 7.15 Percentage of respondents who purchased commercial health insurance by region and urban/rural status (%)

Type		Percentage of respondents who purchased commercial health insurance
Overall		26.2
Region	Provincial-level municipalities	32.8
	East China	29.9
	Central China	21.0
	West China	22.9
	Northeast China	25.5
Urban/rural	Urban	31.5
	Rural	18.1

Table 7.16 Percentage of respondents who purchased commercial health insurance by gender and age group (%)

Type		Percentage of respondents who purchased commercial health insurance
Gender	Male	25.4
	Female	27.3
Age (years)	18~29	27.9
	30~39	31.5
	40~49	31.7
	50~59	22.7
	60~69	11.5
	70~75	6.2

private business had the highest percentage (33.8%), followed by employees of township collective-owned or private businesses (22.7%). Farmers had the lowest percentage of purchase (11.6%). See Figures 7.6 and 7.7.

The percentage of China's population that purchases health insurance is positively correlated to education and income. The higher the education and income level, the higher the chance of purchasing health insurance. Respondents with a master's or higher degree had the highest percentage of purchase (39.0%), and respondents with primary or lower education had the lowest percentage (10.4%). With respect to income level, respondents with an annual family income of RMB 250,000–500,000 and more than RMB 500,000 had the highest percentage of purchase (49.5% and 49.0%, respectively). Respondents with an annual family income of RMB 10,000 had the lowest purchase percentage (14.2%). See Figures 7.8 and 7.9.

With respect to health status, the percentage of health insurance purchases among respondents who are suffering from long-term or critical illnesses

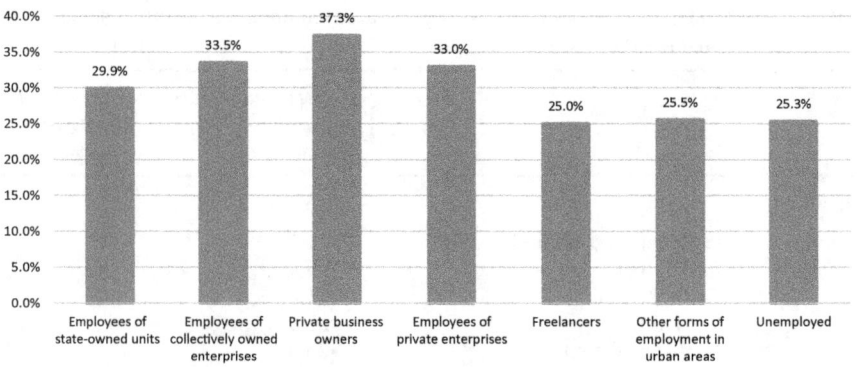

Figure 7.6 Percentage of respondents who purchased commercial health insurance in urban areas by occupation.

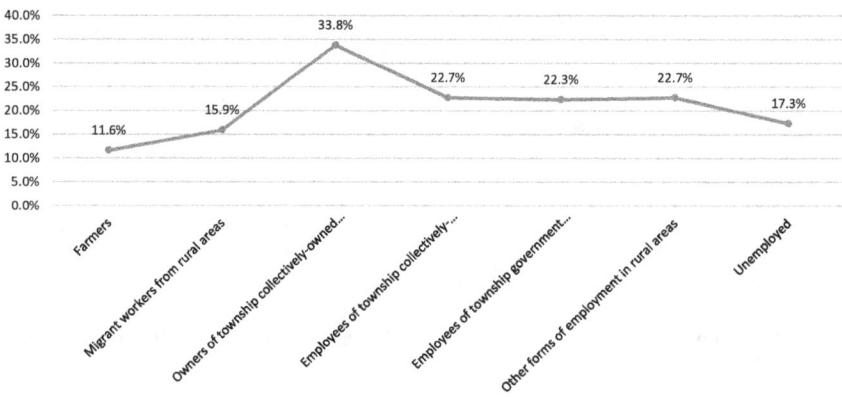

Figure 7.7 Percentage of respondents who purchased commercial health insurance in rural areas by occupation.

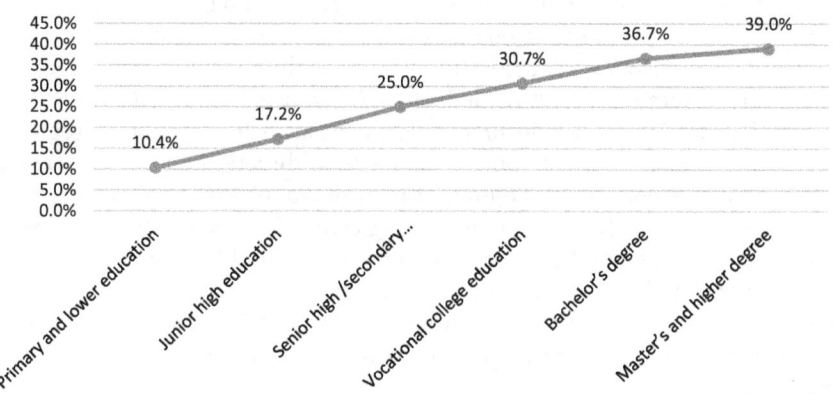

Figure 7.8 Percentage of respondents who purchased commercial health insurance by education level.

(15.4%) was lower than the percentage of purchases made by healthy respondents (27.7%). By tying that result in with income, the survey showed that the families of sick people have significantly lower income than those with people who are not sick. To a certain degree, their lack of purchasing power suppresses demand for health insurance. As to the frequency of physical examinations, respondents who had physical exams once every year and once every six months had higher percentages of purchase of health insurance (31.0% and 30.7%, respectively), while the percentage of purchase among respondents who had had no physical examination within five years was only 14.3%. There were statistically significant differences in the amount of health insurance bought by groups with different levels of health. See Table 7.17.

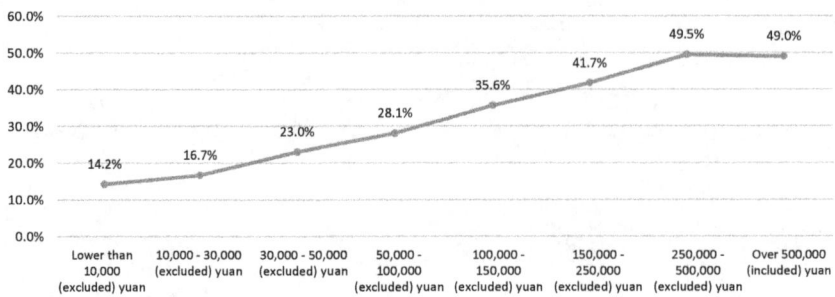

Figure 7.9 Percentage of respondents who purchased commercial health insurance by family income.

7.5.1.2 Types of commercial health insurance products purchased by respondents

Critical illness insurance dominated insurance products bought by respondents. The percentage of people who bought them reached 82.2%, followed by outpatient and hospitalization insurance (36.9%), rehabilitation insurance (13.6%), nursing care insurance (12.0%), and other insurance products (8.8%). This dominance of critical illness insurance was consistent throughout all regions. Hospitalization insurance was purchased more in directly administered cities (40.4%). The east coast held the highest percentage of people buying rehabilitation insurance (15.7%), as well as nursing care insurance (13.9%). The percentage of urban respondents who purchased critical illness insurance was higher than that of rural respondents (84% as opposed to 77.3%). The percentage of urban respondents who purchased outpatient and hospitalization insurance was higher than that of rural respondents (37.7% as opposed to 35%). See Table 7.18.

Table 7.17 Percentage of respondents who purchased commercial health insurance by health status and frequency of physical examination (%)

Type		Percentage of purchase
Whether suffering from long-term or critical illnesses	Yes	15.4
	No	27.7
	Unclear	14.3
Frequency of physical examination	Once every six months	30.7
	Once every year	31.0
	Once every two to three years	25.6
	No physical examination within five years	14.3

Table 7.18 Commercial health insurance products purchased by respondents by region and urban/rural status (%)

Type		Critical illness insurance	Outpatient and hospitalization insurance	Rehabilitation insurance	Care insurance	Others
Overall		82.2	36.9	13.6	12.0	8.8
Region	Provincial-level municipalities	78.9	40.4	11.5	9.5	9.4
	East China	85.0	38.0	15.7	13.9	5.9
	Central China	82.1	32.4	12.1	10.8	9.1
	West China	78.2	38.2	13.8	12.0	13.3
	Northeast China	89.1	31.1	12.0	12.9	7.8
Urban/rural	Urban	84.0	37.7	13.8	12.2	8.0
	Rural	77.3	35.0	12.8	11.4	11.0

With respect to age distribution, the percentage of respondents aged 30–39 years who bought critical illness insurance was higher than other age groups (87.1%), followed by the 40–49 age group (86.1%). The 70–75 age group had the highest percentage of respondents who purchased outpatient and hospitalization insurance (41.8%), followed by the 30–39 age group (40.4%). This age group also had a fairly high percentage of people buying rehabilitation and nursing care insurance (18.2% and 14.5%, respectively). See Figure 7.10.

With respect to income, the overall trend was that purchase of all kinds of commercial health insurance rose as income increased. More specifically, people with an annual income above RMB 500,000 had the highest percentage of respondents who purchased critical illness insurance (89.1%). The group with an annual income of RMB 250,000–500,000 had the highest percentage of respondents who purchased outpatient and hospitalization insurance (47.7%), followed by the group with an annual income of more than RMB 500,000 (46.9%). The group with an annual income of RMB 250,000–500,000 also had the highest percentage of respondents who purchased rehabilitation and care insurance (24.0% and 19.8%, respectively). See Figure 7.11.

7.5.1.3 *Annual premiums of commercial health insurance products purchased by respondents*

Among respondents who purchased commercial health insurance, 27.1% of all respondents who paid premiums paid in the range of RMB 1,001–3,000. Those who paid less than RMB 1,000 per year came to 24.5%. Those who paid more than RMB 10,000 per year came to just 10.2%. With respect to the geographic

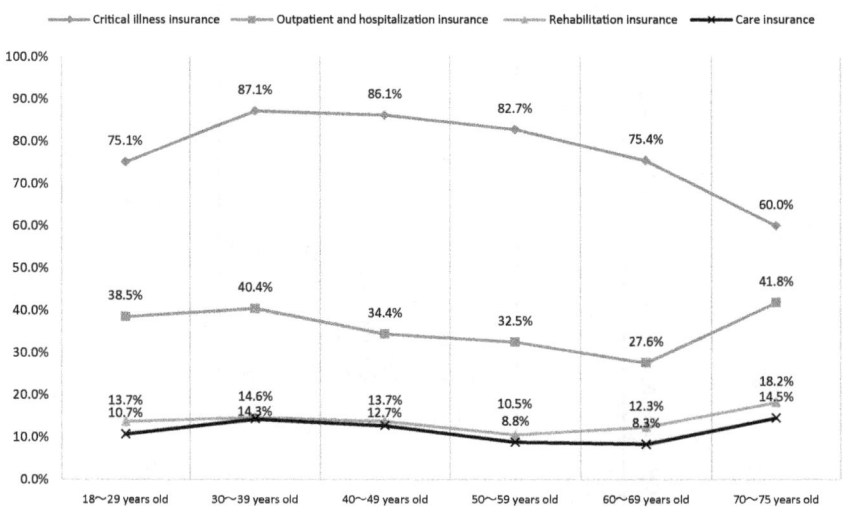

Figure 7.10 Commercial health insurance products purchased by respondents by age group.

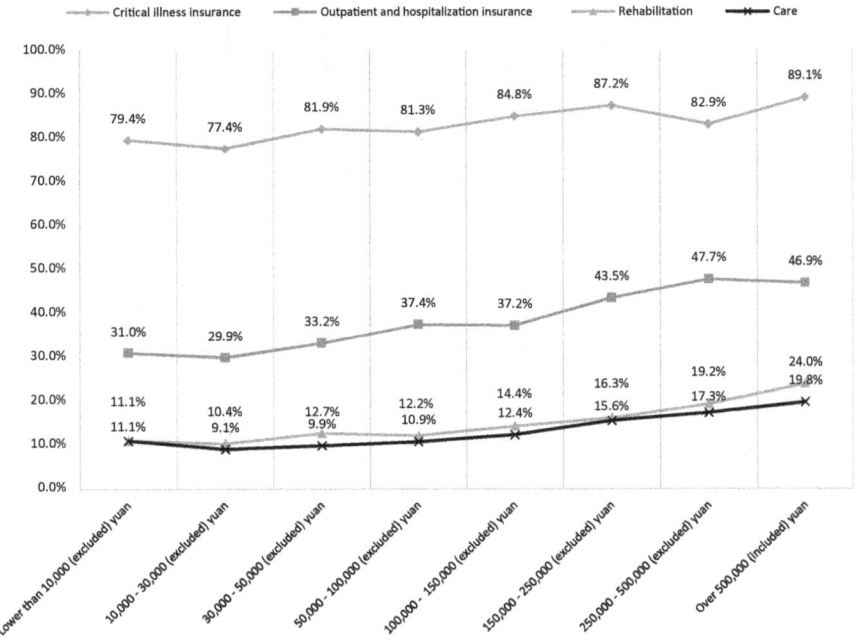

Figure 7.11 Commercial health insurance products purchased by respondents by family income.

distribution of premium payments by region, people in developed areas generally paid more than people in less developed areas. East China held the highest percentage of respondents paying RMB 3,001–5,000 per year (19.1%). Directly administered cities had the highest percentage of respondents paying more than RMB 10,000 per year (12.3%). With respect to the difference between urban and rural premium payment levels, more people in rural areas paid less than RMB 5,000 per year, and more people in urban areas paid more than that amount. See Table 7.19 for details.

With respect to how premium amounts differed among age groups, the 70–75 age group had the highest percentage of people paying less than RMB 1,000 per year in premiums (32.7%). This group also had the highest percentage paying the next level up in premiums, RMB 1,001–3,000 (34.5%). The 30–39 age group had the highest percentage of respondents who paid RMB 3,001–5,000 (21.2%) and RMB 5,001–10,000 (18.4%) for annual premiums of commercial health insurance. The 40–49 age group had the highest percentage of respondents who paid more than RMB 10,000 for annual premiums of commercial health insurance (13.1%). For details, see Table 7.20.

With respect to income levels and premiums paid by survey respondents, in general there was a positive correlation between level of income and amount of premiums that people paid for insurance. Low-income people paid less. As

Table 7.19 Distribution of annual commercial health insurance premium by region and urban/rural status (%)

Type		Below 1,000 yuan	1,001~3,000 yuan	3,001~5,000 yuan	5,001~10,000 yuan	Above 10,000 yuan	Unclear	Subtotal
	Overall	24.5	27.1	18.2	14.6	10.2	5.4	100.0
Region	Provincial-level municipalities	24.3	26.6	17.1	12.5	12.3	7.2	100.0
	East China	24.8	25.2	19.1	15.3	11.4	4.1	100.0
	Central China	25.2	26.7	18.1	15.4	8.8	5.8	100.0
	West China	24.4	29.0	18.0	15.3	7.9	5.4	100.0
	Southeast China	21.8	33.3	17.1	12.6	9.2	5.9	100.0
Urban/rural	Urban	23.8	26.6	17.8	15.1	11.1	5.6	100.0
	Rural	26.3	28.4	19.1	13.3	7.9	4.9	100.0

Table 7.20 Distribution of annual commercial health insurance premiums by age group (%)

Type		Below 1,000 yuan	1,001~3,000 yuan	3,001~5,000 yuan	5,001~10,000 yuan	Above 10,000 yuan	Unclear	Subtotal
Age (years)	18~29	29.7	28.3	18.5	9.6	6.5	7.3	100.0
	30~39	20.2	25.3	21.2	18.4	11.4	3.6	100.0
	40~49	21.4	26.2	17.5	17.8	13.1	4.0	100.0
	50~59	27.2	29.2	15.0	12.5	10.0	6.1	100.0
	60~69	29.8	28.9	9.2	9.6	9.6	12.7	100.0
	70~75	32.7	34.5	9.1	9.1	9.1	5.5	100.0

income increased, the percentage of respondents paying less than RMB 1,000 declined and the percentage paying more than RMB 10,000 rose. For example, in groups with incomes below RMB 10,000, more than one-third of the people chose to pay lower than RMB 1,000 in insurance premiums. In groups with income above RMB 500,000, the percentage of people that was willing to pay more than RMB 10,000 in premiums approached 30%. There was a statistically significant difference in the level of premiums people were willing to pay, depending on their income. See Figure 7.12.

7.5.1.4 Summary

To sum up the above, more than one-quarter of all respondents to this survey purchased commercial health insurance. The extent of purchasing power had a decisive effect on transforming potential demand into effective demand. Demand in some areas and by some groups of people was held down for economic reasons and other factors that limited purchase or made the threshold too high. Demand was lower among people in lesser developed regions, older people, low-income people, and people who are already ill. The percentage of respondents who purchased commercial health insurance was higher than the national average in developed parts of China, such as the east coast and directly administered cities. Purchase was far greater in cities than in the countryside. Purchase by young people was far greater than older age groups. A mere 6.2% of people in the 70–75 age category bought insurance. Education and income also had a similar effect. For example, the higher the degree of education and higher the income, the higher the percentage of people who bought insurance, to the extent that nearly 40% of people with higher degrees bought insurance. Nearly 50% of people whose incomes were either RMB 250,000–500,000 or above RMB 500,000 bought insurance. The percentage of people who were not yet sick that

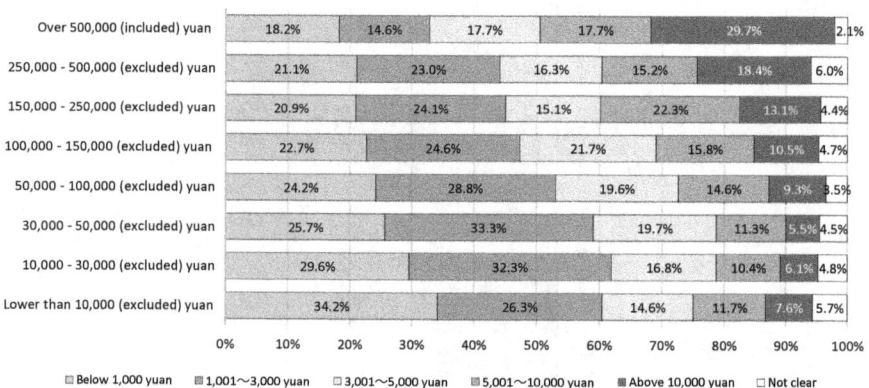

Figure 7.12 Distribution of annual commercial health insurance premiums by family income (%).

bought insurance was higher than that of people who were already sick. What's more, an awareness of health considerations had an impact on whether or not people bought insurance. Those groups with little awareness of health tended not to buy health insurance. For example, less than 15% of people who had not exercised within the past five years purchased insurance, which was vastly lower than people who exercised regularly. The difference was statistically significant.

With respect to the type of commercial health insurance products purchased by the respondents, critical illness insurance occupies an absolute dominant position (more than 80%) among purchased commercial health insurance products. The percentage of young respondents who purchased critical illness insurance was particularly high. The percentage of elderly respondents who purchased reimbursement insurance, rehabilitation insurance, and nursing care insurance in developed areas was higher than less developed areas. The percentage of high-income respondents who purchased commercial health insurance was high for each type of product.

With respect to annual premiums, the percentage of respondents who purchased commercial health insurance products with small annual premiums was higher than that of products requiring large annual premiums. More than 50% of total respondents paid less than RMB 3,000 for annual premiums of commercial health insurance; about 10% paid more than RMB 10,000. The commercial health insurance premiums paid by respondents in developed regions were relatively higher than they were in less developed areas. For example, the commercial health insurance premiums paid by respondents in east China and directly administered cities were higher than other regions, and the commercial health insurance premiums paid by the respondents in urban areas were higher than those in rural areas. Senior citizens were more inclined to purchase products requiring small annual premiums, while young people were more inclined to purchase products requiring higher premiums. Low-income people were more inclined to purchase products requiring small annual premiums, while high-income people were more inclined to purchase products requiring higher premiums.

7.5.2 Ways to purchase commercial health insurance and obtain relevant information

7.5.2.1 Ways to purchase commercial health insurance

Among the various channels through which to purchase commercial health insurance products, 74.0% of respondents purchased commercial health insurance products via physical as opposed to online channels (such physical channels included insurance agents and brokers). After that preference came collective purchase by employers (24.3%), individual purchase through WeChat and mobile apps (10.6%), and then individual purchase through Internet platforms (8.1%). With respect to distribution channels by region, namely directly administered cities, east China, central China, west China, and northeast China, the percentage of respondents choosing to purchase commercial health insurance products by themselves through physical channels was the highest in northeast China (87.1%). This was followed by west China (78.7%). The percentage of respondents who purchased health insurance products through collective purchase was the highest in directly administered cities (27.9%). The percentage of respondents who purchased health insurance products through WeChat and mobile apps (14.7%) and Internet platforms (10.5%) was the highest in east China. In rural areas, the percentage of respondents choosing to buy through physical (offline) distribution channels (76.0%) was higher than that in urban areas (73.3%). The percentage of respondents choosing collective purchase arranged by employers and WeChat and mobile apps by themselves in urban areas was higher than that in rural areas. For details, see Table 7.21.

Looking at age ranges and channels through which to purchase insurance, respondents in age groups 40–49 and 50–59 had the highest percentage of people who purchased insurance through physical channels (79.6%). The percentage of respondents choosing WeChat, mobile apps, and websites was highest in the 18–29 age group. For details, see Table 7.22.

Looking at the level of education, the higher the education, the more respondents chose to buy online, and the lower the education, the more they chose to buy through off-line channels. In addition, the higher the education, the more people bought through collective purchase by an employer. Specifically, the group with just primary school education or lower had the highest percentage of respondents choosing off-line channels (81.2%) while the group with a master's degree or higher had the lowest percentage of respondents choosing off-line channels (60.3%). The group with a master's degree or higher had the highest percentage of respondents choosing to have their unit (employer) purchase a unified insurance policy on their behalf (39.3%), while the group with junior high education had the lowest (12.9%). See Figure 7.13.

Looking at income levels and channels through which people bought insurance: families with incomes of less than RMB 30,000 were quite likely to buy insurance through physical, off-line channels (close to 80%). The second group most likely to buy through off-line channels included people with incomes over RMB 500,000 (76.6%). People with family incomes in the range of RMB 250,000–500,000 had the highest percentage of respondents who chose to buy a collective insurance policy through the unit (32.0%). See Figure 7.14.

7.5.2.2 Ways to access commercial health insurance information

The most important information channel by which people accessed information was still insurance agents who recommended policies to people, that is, the staff of insurance companies. Some 45.1% of people gained information this way. Another 19.3% accessed information via their cell phones or the Internet, 18.4% had family and friends make recommendations, and 8.8% received recommendations from their unit (employer). The percentage of people who accessed information via traditional media was very low (6.2%). This included television,

Table 7.21 Ways to purchase commercial health insurance by region and urban/rural status (%)

Type		Purchase via off-line channels (including insurance agents, brokers, etc.) by individuals	Purchase via WeChat and mobile apps by individuals	Purchase via websites by individuals	Collective purchase by employers	Other channels
Overall		74.0	10.6	8.1	24.3	3.2
Region	Provincial-level municipalities	71.1	7.5	7.8	27.9	3.2
	East China	71.1	14.7	10.5	22.6	3.2
	Central China	72.4	10.7	7.7	27.8	3.5
	West China	78.7	7.9	5.7	22.1	3.6
	Northeast China	87.1	7.0	4.8	19.3	1.1
Urban/rural	Urban	73.3	11.1	8.6	26.3	2.8
	Rural	76.0	9.2	6.6	18.7	4.2

Table 7.22 Ways to purchase commercial health insurance by age group (%)

Type		Purchase via off-line channels (including insurance agents, brokers, etc.) by individuals	Purchase via WeChat and mobile apps by individuals	Purchase via websites by individuals	Collective purchase by employers	Other channels
Age (years)	18~29	65.7	14.1	10.8	28.7	4.3
	30~39	76.1	11.8	9.0	23.4	2.4
	40~49	79.6	9.5	7.7	21.6	2.3
	50~59	79.6	5.6	3.0	19.8	3.5
	60~69	70.6	2.6	1.8	25.9	3.9
	70~75	52.7	3.6	5.5	40.0	9.1

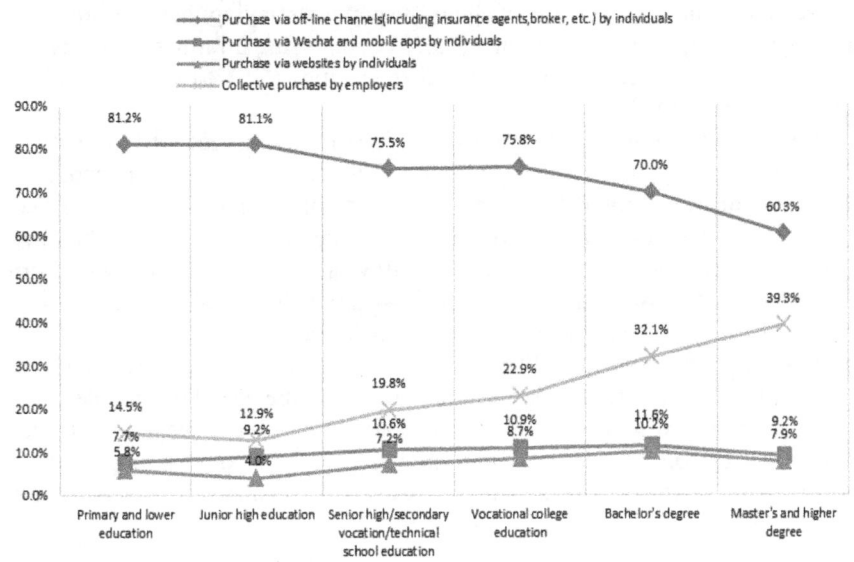

Figure 7.13 Ways to purchase commercial health insurance, by education level (%).

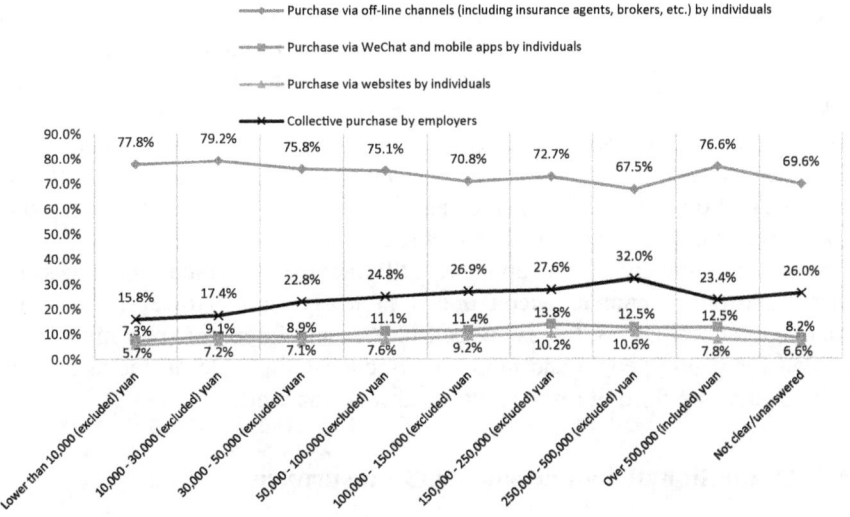

Figure 7.14 Ways to purchase commercial health insurance by family income (%).

newspapers, radio, magazines, and so on. Relative to other cities, directly administered cities had a larger percentage of respondents saying they got information through cell phone and the Internet (23.1%). Accessing information on insurance via cell phone or the Internet was higher in cities (20.1%) than in rural areas (17.2%). See Table 7.23.

Looking at the age distribution of preferred ways to access information on insurance, a fairly high percentage of people in the 70–75 age group chose to get their information from TV, newspapers, radio, and magazines (21.8%.) People in the 18–29 age range were more inclined to choose cell phones and the Internet (28.6%.) People 50–59 years old and 40–49 years old chose to get their information via the staff of insurance companies—more than half of them chose this method (57.3% and 52.8% respectively.) See Table 7.24.

Looking at the educational level in terms of preferred ways to access information on insurance, as levels of education increased, the use of cell phones and the Internet increased as the main way to learn about health insurance. In corresponding fashion, the use of television, radio, newspapers, magazines, and recommendations from insurance agents declined as a way to get information. See Figure 7.15.

7.5.2.3 Summary

Generally speaking, actual, physical, sales channels for receiving information remained dominant, and accounted for over 70% of how people learned about insurance. The use of Internet platforms, WeChat, and mobile apps was still modest, around 10% for each of these. However, in relatively well developed parts of China, where education and income levels are higher and also among young people, there is more of an inclination to use the Internet or mobile networks for purchase of insurance. Moreover, one-quarter of people enjoy insurance that is bought by their unit (employer) on a unified group basis. People with higher education and those whose families have incomes of RMB 250,000–500,000 have higher percentages of being insured in this way, also those who live in directly administered cities.

Insurance company salespeople are still the main channel for accessing information on insurance, accounting for nearly half. However, in more developed parts of China, the use of cell phones and Internet is becoming more common for young people and more highly educated people. In the age group 18–29, nearly one-third of respondents used such channels.

7.5.3 Evaluation of commercial health insurance

7.5.3.1 Degree of satisfaction with commercial health insurance

Among those who actually have commercial health insurance, 42% expressed general satisfaction in having it. Some 19% were extremely satisfied, while 33.9% indicated it was ok. The percentage of people who were dissatisfied and

Table 7.23 Ways to access commercial health insurance information by region and urban/rural status (%)

Type		TV, newspapers, radio, and magazines	Internet (including mobile Internet)	Salespersons of insurance companies	Friends and family members	Employers	Others	Subtotal
Overall		6.2	19.3	45.1	18.4	8.8	2.2	100.0
Region	Provincial-level municipalities	7.2	23.1	39.0	18.9	8.9	3.0	100.0
	East China	5.8	19.8	45.4	20.1	7.9	0.9	100.0
	Central China	5.7	20.3	43.9	17.1	9.8	3.1	100.0
	West China	6.4	17.0	50.1	15.4	9.0	2.1	100.0
	Northeast China	6.2	10.6	49.0	21.6	9.0	3.6	100.0
Urban/rural	Urban	6.5	20.1	43.5	18.7	9.0	2.2	100.0
	Rural	5.5	17.2	49.6	17.8	8.0	2.0	100.0

Table 7.24 Ways to access commercial health insurance information by age group (%)

Type		TV, newspapers, radio, and magazines	Internet (including mobile Internet)	Salespersons of insurance companies	Friends and family members	Employers	Others	Subtotal
Age (years)	18~29	4.2	28.6	32.9	22.9	9.3	2.1	100.0
	30~39	4.3	20.7	45.1	19.9	8.4	1.5	100.0
	40~49	6.6	16.2	52.8	15.7	7.0	1.8	100.0
	50~59	9.6	7.9	57.3	13.8	8.1	3.3	100.0
	60~69	16.2	4.4	49.1	11.4	14.9	3.9	100.0
	70~75	21.8	5.5	30.9	5.5	29.1	7.3	100.0

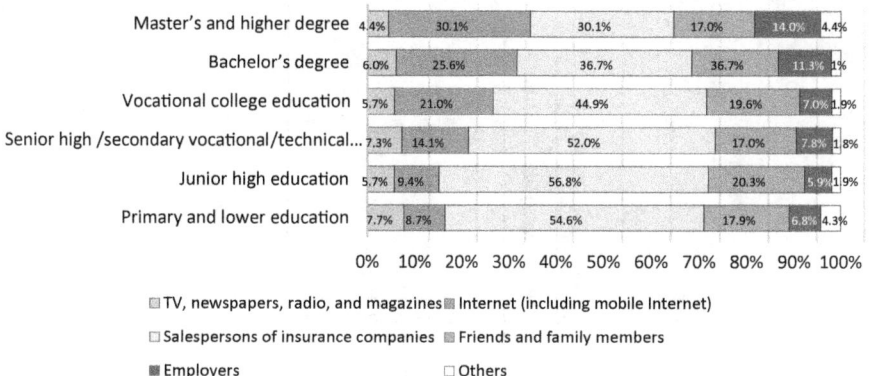

Figure 7.15 Ways to access commercial health insurance information by education level.

very dissatisfied was quite small, accounting for 4.1% and 1.0% respectively. In terms of age groups, the 18–29 age group was inclined to be most satisfied (including extremely satisfied and fairly satisfied—70% for these combined categories). The age group most inclined to be dissatisfied were older people. The age group 60–69 had 16.6% who were dissatisfied, and 70–75 had 12.7% who were dissatisfied. The age group with the highest percentage of people thinking insurance was 'just ok' was 40–49—some 36.8% of this age group felt that way. For details, see Table 7.25.

With respect to satisfaction of respondents by income level, the evaluation of health insurance in the middle and high-income groups fell mainly in the 'relatively satisfied' category. People with an annual income of RMB 250,000–500,000 were more likely to be relatively satisfied—this percentage came to 47.7%. Next were people with an income of RMB 150,000–250,000, who represented 46.1% of the relatively satisfied category. Finally, some 44.3% of people whose income surpassed RMB 500,000 felt relatively satisfied. Of all income groups, those whose income was in the range of RMB 30,000–50,000 were more likely to feel health insurance was simply ok, since 39.3% of this group felt that way. See Figure 7.16.

With respect to the types of commercial health insurance, an evaluation of 'very satisfied' was more prevalent among those who purchased critical illness insurance than other types of insurance—20.1% of respondents were pleased with that insurance. An evaluation of 'fairly satisfied' was more common for rehabilitation and nursing care insurance—these types of insurance earned only a 'fairly satisfied' evaluation among 42.4% of respondents. The satisfaction rate for the purchase of rehabilitation and nursing care insurance was slightly higher than other types, accounting for 42.4% of the total. In contrast, insurance relating to outpatient care and inpatient medical expenses was generally given an evaluation of either 'just ok' or 'not satisfied.' For details, see Table 7.26.

Table 7.25 Satisfaction with commercial health insurance by age group (%)

Type		Very satisfied	Satisfied	Neutral	Dissatisfied	Very dissatisfied	Subtotal
Overall		19.0	42.0	33.9	4.1	1.0	100.0
Age (years)	18~29	22.4	46.6	29.2	1.4	0.5	100.0
	30~39	17.6	42.7	35.6	3.1	1.1	100.0
	40~49	18.5	39.5	36.8	4.7	0.5	100.0
	50~59	17.2	36.6	36.2	7.8	2.3	100.0
	60~69	14.5	39.9	28.9	14.0	2.6	100.0
	70~75	27.3	30.9	29.1	9.1	3.6	100.0

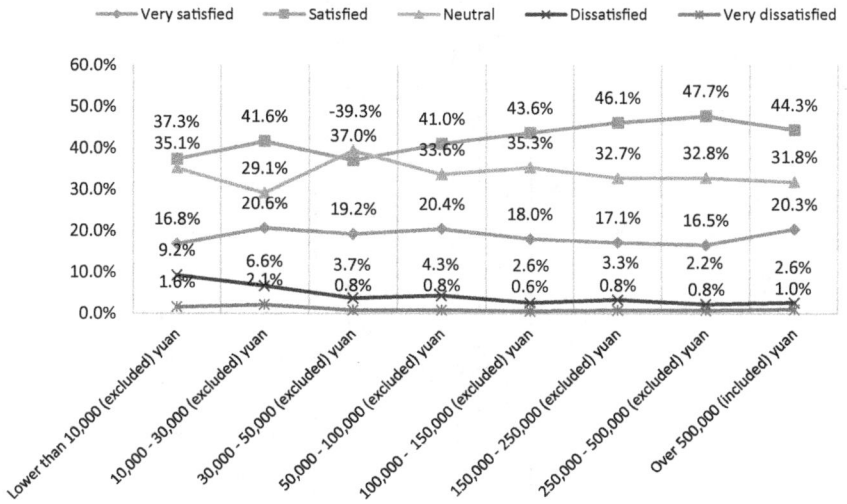

Figure 7.16 Satisfaction with commercial health insurance by family income (%).

7.5.3.2 *Analysis of the inadequacies of commercial health insurance*

Within the entire sampled population, there were three main reasons for feeling that commercial health insurance is inadequate. First, claims procedures are complex and the reimbursement is not made in a timely manner (30.2%); second, policies are too expensive (27.9%); third, insurance lacks corresponding 'health management' and 'health services' components (23.9%). With respect to these categories of sentiments, urban respondents had uniformly higher percentages of all three reasons than rural respondents. The different age groups presented many similarities overall, but in relative terms, lower age groups felt the inade-quacies more than other age groups. For example, people in the age group 18–29 had a higher percentage of feeling that claims procedures are too complex and also that types of insurance are too uniform. People in the age group 30–39 had higher percentages of all categories, that is, they felt claims procedures were too complex, policies were too expensive, there were too many restrictions on being insured, and there was too much overlap between commercial insurance and social insurance. See Table 7.27.

7.5.3.3 *Summary*

In overall terms, the degree to which people in the survey were satisfied with commercial health insurance was fairly high—that is, over 60% were in the two categories 'very satisfied' and 'fairly satisfied.' In contrast, only around 5% were either not satisfied or extremely dissatisfied. Relatively speaking, younger people were more satisfied, while older people had a less satisfied attitude. Close to half

Table 7.26 Satisfaction with commercial health insurance by type of product (%)

Type		Very satisfied	Satisfied	Neutral	Dissatisfied	Very dissatisfied	Subtotal
Type of health insurance products	Critical illness insurance	20.1	41.2	33.6	4.1	1.0	100.0
	Outpatient and hospitalization insurance	16.3	40.8	36.7	5.1	1.2	100.0
	Rehabilitation insurance	17.1	42.4	35.2	4.4	1.0	100.0
	Care insurance	17.5	42.4	34.8	4.3	1.0	100.0

Table 7.27 Perceived weaknesses of commercial health insurance by urban/rural status and age (%)

Type		Coverage overlapping with social insurance	Complex purchase procedure	Slow, complex claims handling process	Too expensive	Low product variety	Too many participation restrictions	Lacking health management and healthcare services	Other reasons
Overall		13.1	12.1	30.2	27.9	12.3	18.1	23.9	34.5
Urban/rural	Urban	14.7	12.8	32.9	29.6	13.7	20.5	25.6	30.8
	Rural	11.0	11.3	26.8	25.9	10.6	15.1	21.9	40.2
Age (years)	18~29	15.9	16.4	34.5	29.3	14.3	19.3	25.1	28.3
	30~39	16.3	12.9	35.4	33.5	14.2	21.5	26.6	27.1
	40~49	14.2	11.9	31.0	28.7	13.0	20.2	23.6	32.8
	50~59	8.9	8.5	26.2	23.2	10.4	16.2	22.7	42.6
	60~69	7.2	8.9	20.3	22.2	8.0	12.0	19.6	49.6
	70~75	6.1	7.7	16.9	20.4	7.3	9.4	21.5	54.6

of middle- and high-income groups were relatively satisfied. Of all types of insurance, satisfaction with critical illness insurance was highest—over 20%. With respect to the top three reasons given for the inadequacies of health insurance—complex claims procedures and tardy reimbursement, expensive policies, and lack of health management and health services—between 20% and 30% of the total sampled population felt this way.

7.6 FUTURE DEMAND FOR COMMERCIAL HEALTH INSURANCE

7.6.1 Long-term forecast of demand for commercial health insurance

7.6.1.1 Total size of demand for commercial health insurance

Among the respondents, 55.9% thought it was necessary to purchase health insurance in the future. In terms of regional distribution, the intent to buy was strongest in east China (60%), after which came directly administered cities (56.2%), west China (55.7%), central China (52%), and northeast China (50.9%). A higher percentage of people in urban areas felt that buying insurance would be necessary (60%) than people in rural areas (49.5%). The intent to buy was higher among women than men (59.6% as opposed to 53%). People in the age groups 18–29 and 30–39 had the strongest intent to buy insurance in the future of all groups (66.4% and 65.2% respectively.) Next came the age group 40–49 (58.4%). The intent to buy was weakest among people in the 70–75 age group (22.5%). See Tables 7.28 and 7.29.

The degree of acceptance about buying insurance increased as income increases. The peak percentage of 73.3% came from people whose family income was RMB 250,000–500,000. The percentage of people whose income was over RMB 500,000 was basically similar. See Figure 7.17.

Table 7.28 Potential demand for commercial health insurance by region and urban/rural status (%)

Type		Percentage
Overall		55.9
Region	Provincial-level municipalities	56.2
	East China	60.0
	Central China	52.0
	Western China	55.7
	Northeast China	50.9
Urban/rural	Urban	60.0
	Rural	49.5

Table 7.29 Potential demand for commercial health insurance by gender and age group (%)

Type		Percentage
Gender	Male	53.0
	Female	59.6
Age (years)	18~29	66.4
	30~39	65.2
	40~49	58.4
	50~59	44.9
	60~69	30.2
	70~75	22.5

People who already were insured had a powerful intent to continue to purchase insurance in the future (83.4%). Their intent was clearly higher than those people who were uninsured (46.1%).

7.6.1.2 Design of commercial health insurance policies

In terms of the design of health insurance products (policies), respondents to the survey were most concerned about scope of coverage and percentage of reimbursements (49.3%). Next came ease of making a claim and speed of getting reimbursed (21.5%), and after that came special healthcare services (13.7%). In terms of the difference between urban and rural areas, urban people felt a greater need for policies to have good scope of coverage and a higher reimbursement percentage than rural people (52.4% as opposed to 43.4%). In contrast, rural people focused on speed of getting reimbursed (23% as opposed to 20.7% in urban areas), and on special healthcare services (16.2% as opposed to 12.3% in urban areas.) Looking at age considerations, people above the age of 60 were quite concerned that insurance policies include coverage for special healthcare services. See Table 7.30.

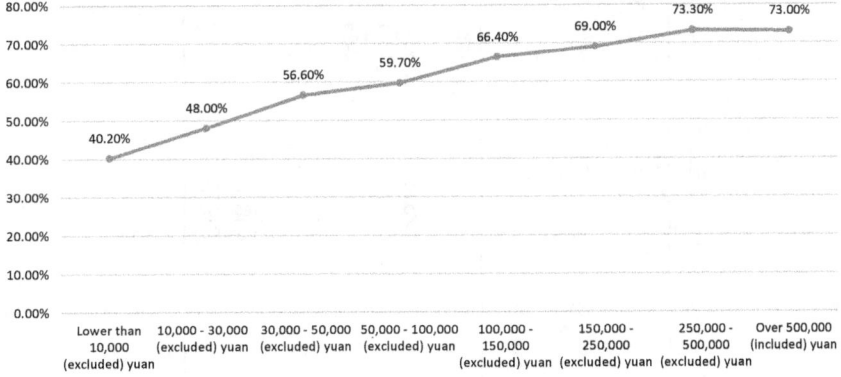

Figure 7.17 Potential demand for commercial health insurance by family income.

Table 7.30 Demand for features of commercial health insurance products by urban/rural status and age group (%)

Type		Coverage and reimbursement ratio	Price	Visibility of insurance companies	Convenience of claims handling	Special health services (appointment registration, VIP medical services)	Sub-total
Overall		49.3	6.3	9.2	21.5	13.7	100.0
Urban/rural	Urban	52.4	5.6	9.0	20.7	12.3	100.0
	Rural	43.4	7.6	9.7	23.0	16.2	100.0
Age (years)	18–29	55.2	5.3	7.9	19.6	11.9	100.0
	30–39	53.0	5.9	8.3	21.0	11.7	100.0
	40–49	43.9	7.2	10.5	23.6	14.8	100.0
	50–59	40.6	7.4	12.4	23.8	15.8	100.0
	60–69	37.6	8.0	9.2	21.7	23.4	100.0
	70–75	39.2	7.5	11.6	21.1	20.6	100.0

Looking at income levels, the higher the income the more concerned respondents were in general about scope of coverage and percentage of reimbursement. The most concern about this came from people whose incomes were RMB 250,000–500,000. In contrast, the more income increased the less likely people were to be concerned about coverage for special healthcare services—people with income of over RMB 500,000 had the lowest percentage of concern about this (8.7%), while people with income lower than RMB 10,000 had the highest percentage of concern (17.8%). People with incomes of less than RMB 50,000 were more concerned about price than people with incomes of more than RMB 50,000. See Figure 7.18.

7.6.1.3 Value-added services that affect the purchase of commercial health insurance

Among the entire population that was sampled, the top three value-added services that influenced people to buy health insurance were physical examinations (41.6%), appointment-making services at public hospitals (35.3%), and health management (31.8%). In terms of regional differences, people in directly administered cities had a higher preference for appointment-making services (42.6%), while people in the east had a higher preference for physical examinations (43.5%), but also health consultations and education (30.2%) and appoint-making services (39.7%). People in central China focused the most on appointment-making services (34.9%). In terms of urban versus rural preferences, urban people had higher percentages for all value-added services than did rural people. See Table 7.31.

Women showed higher demand for all value-added services than men. In terms of age, as age went up, the desire for health consulting and health education gradually decreased—people in the age ranges of 18–29 and 30–39 had a higher preference for all value-added services than other age ranges. See Table 7.32.

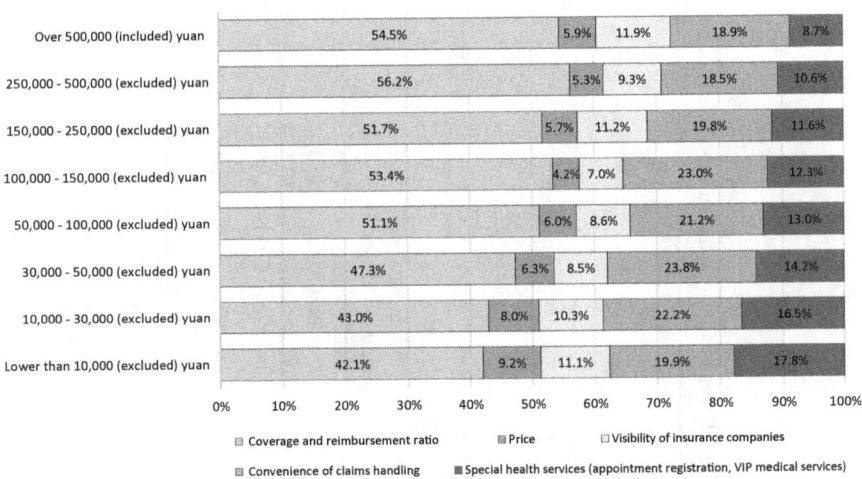

Figure 7.18 Demand for features of commercial health insurance products by family income (%).

Table 7.31 Demand for value-added services of commercial health insurance products by region and urban/rural status (%)

Type		Physical examination	Health advice and education (such as lectures, information push, etc.)	Health management (such as chronic disease management)	Public hospital appointment registration service	Special health services (such as physical examination, scaling, TCM, women's health, etc.)	Green channel for overseas medical services
Overall		41.6	26.3	31.8	35.3	18.8	9.5
Region	Provincial-level municipalities	41.2	24.0	29.2	42.6	19.9	11.0
	East China	43.5	30.2	32.2	39.7	17.9	9.8
	Central China	40.3	25.3	34.9	32.0	17.4	7.8
	West China	40.1	24.3	29.8	29.7	20.0	9.0
	Northeast China	43.4	22.6	32.6	28.9	20.2	12.5
Urban/rural	Urban	42.8	26.6	33.0	38.2	19.3	10.2
	Rural	39.3	25.7	29.6	30.0	17.8	8.3

Table 7.32 Demand for value-added services of commercial health insurance products by gender and age group (%)

Type		Physical examination	Health advice and education (such as lectures, information push, etc.)	Health management (such as chronic disease management)	Public hospital appointment registration service	Special health services (such as physical examination, scaling, TCM, women's health, etc.)	Green channel for overseas medical services
Gender	Male	40.9	25.5	30.7	34.7	16.0	9.4
	Female	42.4	27.2	33.1	36.1	21.9	9.7
Age (years)	18–29	43.5	30.2	32.8	37.2	19.6	11.1
	30–39	42.2	26.5	32.4	38.9	20.9	10.4
	40–49	41.6	25.2	30.4	32.6	17.9	9.2
	50–59	36.3	21.3	31.2	29.8	15.1	6.1
	60–69	40.8	20.1	29.6	27.9	13.7	6.2
	70–75	37.2	17.6	30.2	34.2	16.6	6.5

As income increased, the general trend was to want more appointment-making services at public hospitals as well as services that allowed for direct medical treatment overseas. The highest preference for appointment-making services was among people making more than RMB 500,000 (43.7%), and the desire for overseas medical treatment was also highest (16.8%). People making RMB 150,000–250,000 per year were most interested in physical examinations, healthy lifestyle services, and health management services. There were significant differences in the preferences for value-added services among people at different levels of income. See Figure 7.19.

In addition, people who had previously bought commercial health insurance were more interested in value-added services than people who had not bought insurance. Their percentages for all the value-added services were higher. See Table 7.33.

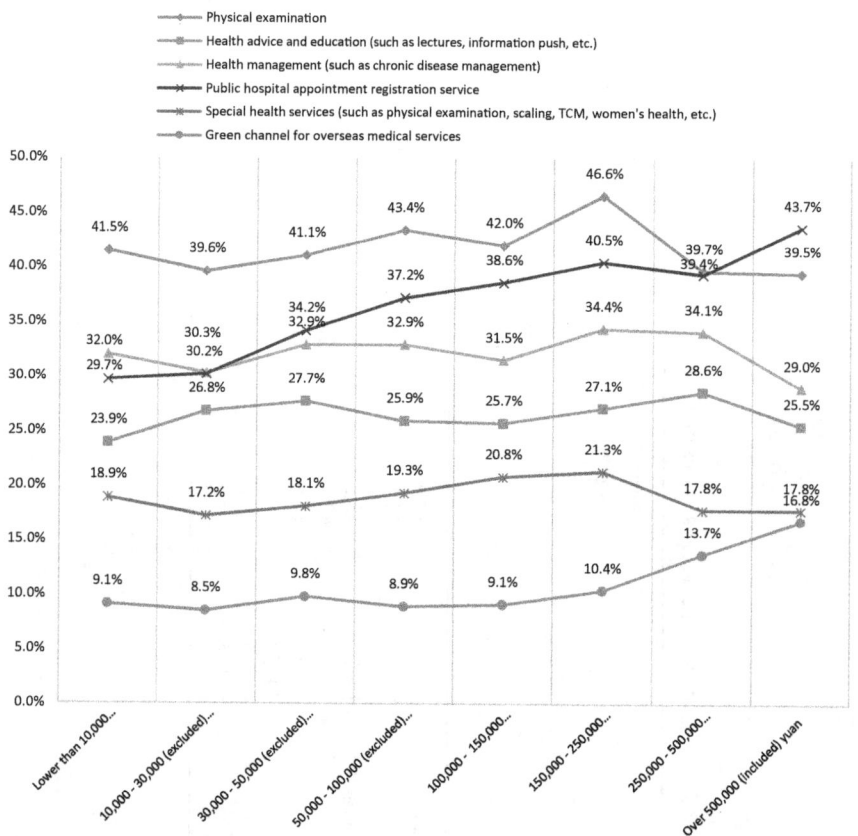

Figure 7.19 Changes in demand for value-added services by family income.

Table 7.33 Demand for value-added services depending on whether or not people already had health insurance (%)

Type		Physical examination	Health advice and education (such as lectures, information push, etc.)	Health management (such as chronic disease management)	Public hospital appointment registration service	Special health services (such as physical examination, scaling, TCM, women's health, etc.)	Green channel for overseas medical services
Whether the respondent had health insurance	Yes	36.2	22.8	26.0	30.4	15.6	8.5
	No	18.6	11.8	14.9	16.0	8.9	4.2

7.6.1.4 Desired ways to purchase commercial health insurance products

The highest percentage of respondents hoped to purchase health insurance via physical sales channels (71%). Next came purchasing via cell phone (13.9%), and then via Internet platforms (12.8%). People in rural areas were slightly more inclined to buy health insurance via physical sales channels than people in urban areas (72.2% versus 70.4%). Women were more inclined to buy via physical sales channels than men (74.7% versus 67.8%), while men were slightly more inclined to buy via online channels than women. See Table 7.34.

As income increased, the preference for buying health insurance via physical sales channels decreased. Instead, the preference for buying via WeChat, mobile client services, and Internet platforms went up. See Figure 7.20.

7.6.1.5 Summary

To summarize the above section, more than half of the people surveyed feel that they will need to buy health insurance in the future, which is substantially different from the actual situation at the present time. This feeling was stronger in economically developed areas, urban areas, and among women and younger people—the corresponding percentage was roughly 60%. Only around 20% of people in the age range 70–75 intended to buy insurance. Higher-income people were more inclined to buy—among people with family incomes of RMB 250,000–500,000, the figure came to over 70%. People who already were insured showed the strongest intent to buy health insurance (over 80%). This was significantly higher than the intent of people who currently are not insured (less than 50%).

In terms of the design of insurance products, people remain primarily interested in scope of coverage and the percentage of costs that are reimbursed. Close to 50% chose 'percentage,' while claims procedures and health services are gradually becoming of greater interest. The older population is relatively more concerned about special healthcare services. As income goes up, interest in scope of items covered under insurance and percentage of reimbursements gradually increases, while interest in healthcare services decreases.

The three value-added services of most concern to people are physical examinations, appointment-making services at public hospitals, and healthcare management. More than 30% of people selected all of these. People in economically developed regions were relatively more interested in appointment-making services, which may be related to the way access to medicine is harder in places where the highest-quality medical resources are concentrated. People in urban areas were more interested in all value-added services than people in rural areas, as were people who had already purchased health insurance. As incomes increased, the structure of people's expected consumption gradually changed—it showed an increase in appointment-making services at public hospitals and overseas medical services. People with incomes of over RMB 500,000 showed the

Table 7.34 Desired ways to purchase commercial health insurance products by urban/rural status, gender, and age group (%)

Type		Off-line channels (including insurance agents, brokers, etc.) by individuals	WeChat and mobile apps by individuals	Websites	Others	Subtotal
Overall		71.0	13.9	12.8	2.3	100.0
Urban/rural	Urban	70.4	13.9	13.7	2.1	100.0
	Rural	72.2	13.8	11.3	2.7	100.0
Gender	Male	67.8	15.4	14.4	2.4	100.0
	Female	74.7	12.1	11.0	2.2	100.0
Age (years)	18~29	67.1	16.9	15.2	0.8	100.0
	30~39	71.2	15.3	12.1	1.3	100.0
	40~49	74.4	11.7	11.9	2.0	100.0
	50~59	74.6	9.7	10.5	5.1	100.0
	60~69	71.7	8.0	12.4	7.9	100.0
	70~75	69.3	7.5	11.6	11.6	100.0

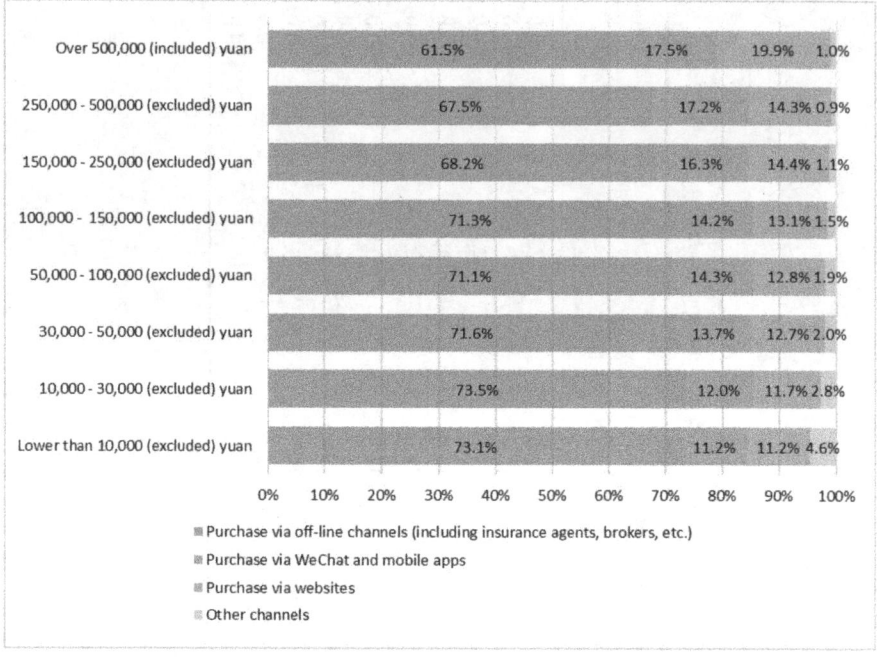

Figure 7.20 Desired ways to purchase commercial health insurance products by family income (%).

highest percentage of respondents choosing these services—over 40% and close to 20% respectively.

Physical sales channels are still the primary means by which people expect to buy commercial health insurance—over 70% of people selected this option. The percentage hoping to buy through WeChat, mobile phone client services, and Internet platforms goes up as income increases.

7.6.2 Demand for commercial health insurance in the coming year

7.6.2.1 Size of market demand for commercial health insurance

7.6.2.1.1 Intentions of the demand side

Generally speaking, 41.3% of respondents expressed willingness to buy commercial health insurance in the coming year. This willingness was strongest in east China (44.9%), after which came west China (43.3%). The weakest 'intent to purchase' was in the northeast (30.9%). Men had a stronger intent to buy than women (44.2% as opposed to 37.9%). As the age of the respondent went up, the intent to purchase commercial health insurance declined. See Table 7.35.

As income increased, the intent to purchase commercial health insurance also increased. People with incomes of less than RMB 10,000 showed the lowest intent to buy (34.6%), while those with incomes of more than RMB 500,000 showed the highest intent to buy (55.9%). See Figure 7. 21.

Looking at the categories of people with different kinds of basic medical insurance, people with publicly funded medical care showed the lowest intent to purchase commercial health insurance (36.5%), while those with urban employees' basic medical insurance were next (37.2%). People with other forms of insurance showed relatively higher intent to buy. See Table 7.36.

People who already had health insurance showed a significantly higher intent to buy in the coming year than those without health insurance (51.9% versus 34.4%). See Table 7.37.

Table 7.35 Intent to purchase health insurance in the coming year by region, gender, and age group (%)

Type		Percentage
Overall		41.3
Region	Provincial-level municipalities	36.8
	East China	44.9
	Central China	39.9
	West China	43.3
	Northeast China	30.9
Gender	Male	44.2
	Female	37.9
Age (years)	18~29	46.7
	30~39	43.0
	40~49	39.0
	50~59	32.0
	60~69	33.1
	70~75	32.7

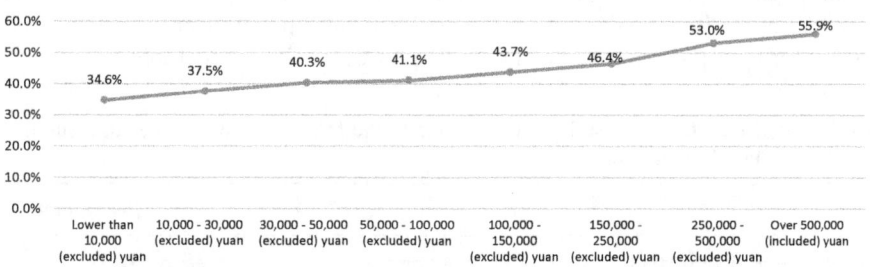

Figure 7.21 Intent to purchase health insurance in coming year by family income (%).

Table 7.36 Intent to purchase health insurance in the coming year by basic health insurance enrollment (%)

	Program	Percentage
Basic health insurance program enrolled in	Basic health insurance program for urban employees	37.2
	Basic health insurance for urban residents + Critical illness insurance	47.0
	New cooperative medical scheme + Critical illness insurance	43.7
	Basic health insurance for urban and rural residents + Critical illness insurance	45.0
	Free medical services	36.5
	None	44.1

7.6.2.1.2 Expected premiums

In overall terms, the highest percentage of respondents was willing to spend between RMB 1,001 and RMB 3,000 in the coming year on premiums (37.4%). The next highest percentage was willing to spend 'below RMB 1,000' (27.4%). The percentage of respondents in directly administered cities willing to buy was higher than all other places when premiums were at a level of RMB 3,001–5,000, RMB 5,001–10,000, and above RMB 10,000. Urban people were willing to spend more to purchase health insurance than people in rural areas. From the perspective of age of respondents, people aged 60–69 showed the intent to spend less money on health insurance (under RMB 1,000) and this intent was quite pronounced (58.6%). See Table 7.38 and Figure 7.22.

7.6.2.2 People for whom commercial health insurance is being purchased

The majority of people who were surveyed were buying health insurance for themselves (77.4%). Next came those who bought insurance for their parents (59.9%), then for spouses (57.1%), and finally for children (56.9%). All five survey regions showed the highest percentage of people buying insurance for themselves, but after that the ranking of purchases for spouses, children, and parents was different. In terms of the difference between urban and rural areas, urban people were more inclined to buy for their parents (60.6%) and children (58.3%) in addition to themselves. In contrast, rural people were more inclined to buy for their parents (58.7%) and then spouses (56.1%). See Table 7.39.

Table 7.37 Intent to purchase health insurance in the following year by health insurance enrollment (%)

Type		Percentage
Whether enrolled in health insurance program or not	Yes	51.9
	No	34.4

Table 7.38 Expected premiums in the next year by region, urban/rural status, and age group (%)

Type		Below 1,000 yuan	1,001~3,000 yuan	3,001~5,000 yuan	5,001~10,000 yuan	Above 10,000 yuan	Sub-total
	Overall	27.4	37.4	21.6	9.2	4.4	100.0
Region	Provincial-level municipalities	22.1	34.2	23.5	12.4	7.7	100.0
	East China	26.1	36.2	22.3	10.3	5.1	100.0
	Central China	31.1	37.3	20.2	7.9	3.4	100.0
	West China	28.4	41.1	20.7	7.4	2.4	100.0
	Northeast China	30.0	36.4	21.8	7.7	4.1	100.0
Urban/rural	Urban	23.2	38.2	22.8	10.5	5.3	100.0
	Rural	35.2	36.0	19.3	6.8	2.8	100.0
Age (years)	18~29	26.9	42.5	20.1	7.1	3.4	100.0
	30~39	21.7	35.1	26.0	12.2	4.9	100.0
	40~49	23.5	37.6	22.4	10.7	5.8	100.0
	50~59	39.1	31.7	18.5	7.2	3.6	100.0
	60~69	58.6	25.3	8.1	3.5	4.5	100.0
	70~75	49.2	36.9	10.8	3.1	0.0	100.0

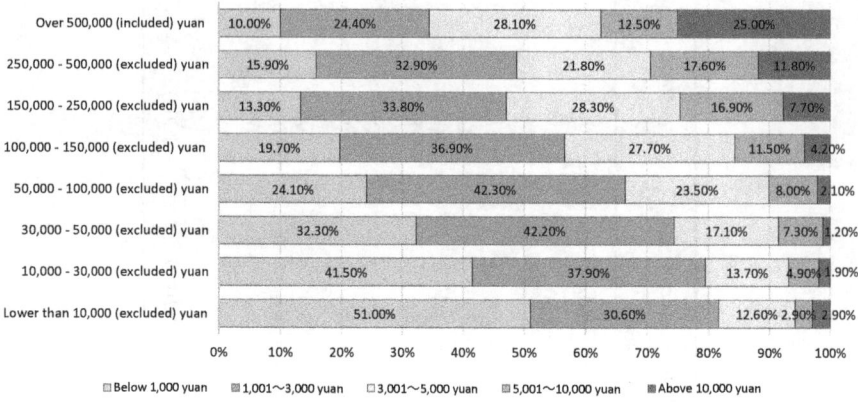

Figure 7.22 Expected premiums in coming year by family income.

As age goes up, the intent to buy commercial health insurance for oneself gradually strengthens while the intent to buy for one's parents gradually weakens. At the same time, the percentage of respondents in the age group 40–49 who chose to buy for their spouse (69.3%) was greater than all other age groups. People in the age group 30–39 were, in contrast, more inclined to buy for their children (73.7%). See Table 7.40.

7.6.2.3 Types of commercial health insurance products that respondents were most willing to buy

Of all types of health insurance, respondents indicated the strongest intent to buy critical illness insurance (82.7%). Next came insurance for outpatient and inpatient medical costs (49.5%), and after that was rehabilitation insurance (26%)

Table 7.39 People for whom health insurance is being bought in the following year, by region and urban/rural status (%)

Type		Themselves	Spouse	Children	Parents	Others
	Overall (%)	77.4	57.1	56.9	59.9	1.0
Region	Provincial-level municipalities	82.1	57.7	50.8	55.0	0.5
	East China	78.0	59.3	60.5	62.4	0.8
	Central China	73.8	51.7	53.6	57.2	0.6
	West China	76.9	57.5	58.1	63.0	1.9
	Northeast China	80.0	62.3	55.9	51.4	0.5
Urban/ rural	Urban	78.3	57.7	58.3	60.6	1.0
	Rural	75.9	56.1	54.2	58.7	1.0

Table 7.40 People for whom respondents intended to purchase health insurance in the following year, by age group (%)

Type		*Themselves*	*Spouse*	*Children*	*Parents*	*Others*
Age (years)	18~29	76.5	40.5	40.2	73.9	1.6
	30~39	76.3	67.2	73.7	63.5	0.3
	40~49	77.5	69.3	70.0	51.6	0.7
	50~59	81.1	62.4	51.1	36.2	1.2
	60~69	83.8	56.6	32.8	22.2	2.0
	70~75	83.1	44.6	24.6	16.9	0.0

and nursing care insurance (21.4%). The percentage of respondents in east China who were willing to buy insurance for outpatient and inpatient medical costs was fairly high, 51.4%. In northeast China, the percentage willing to buy rehabilitation and nursing care insurance was higher than other regions. Demand for all types of insurance was higher in urban areas than it was in rural areas. The age groups 30–39 and 40–49 were more willing to buy critical illness insurance than other age groups, while people age 60–69 were more willing to buy rehabilitation insurance (29.3%). The highest percentage of people willing to buy nursing care insurance was in the age group 70–75 (24.6%). See Table 7.41.

7.6.2.4 Summary

To sum up this section, more than 40% of respondents were willing to buy commercial health insurance in the following year. The intent to buy declined as age increased, and it went up as income went up. People with publicly funded medical care and the urban employees' medical insurance were relatively less inclined to buy. People who had already bought insurance were relatively more inclined to buy.

In the year following the survey, the amount that people expected to pay for insurance was still mainly under RMB 3,000. The amount was relatively more in directly administered cities as well as in urban versus rural areas. More than 50% of people in the age group 60–69 were inclined to pay under RMB 1,000 for insurance. As incomes increased, the amount that people expected to pay for insurance increased as well.

Other than insurance that people intended to buy for themselves (nearly 80%), the main people for whom respondents intended to buy insurance were parents, spouses, and children, in each case a choice that exceeded 50%. The intent to buy for oneself increased with age, while the intent to buy for one's parents decreased with age. People in the age group 40–49 were more inclined to buy insurance for their spouse, while people in the age group 30–39 were more inclined to buy for their children.

Critical illness insurance dominated the type of insurance people intended to buy in the coming year (more than 80%). Cost-subsidizing insurance came

Table 7.41 Types of health insurance products respondents are willing to purchase next year by region, urban/rural status, gender and age group (%)

Type		Critical illness insurance	Outpatient and hospitalization insurance	Rehabilitation insurance	Care insurance	Others
Overall		82.7	49.5	26.0	21.4	2.3
Region	Provincial-level municipalities	84.7	49.8	25.5	21.8	2.4
	East China	83.8	51.4	28.0	23.6	1.2
	Central China	80.0	44.8	22.2	17.9	2.2
	West China	81.5	50.5	25.6	19.9	3.4
	Northeast China	87.7	50.0	30.9	27.3	3.6
Urban/rural	Urban	84.5	50.3	26.7	22.5	2.0
	Rural	79.4	48.0	24.6	19.3	2.8
Gender	Male	83.1	46.7	25.7	19.6	2.4
	Female	82.2	53.2	26.3	23.7	2.1
Age (years)	18~29	79.2	55.5	28.2	21.7	2.4
	30~39	87.8	50.5	25.6	22.5	1.8
	40~49	87.2	43.3	23.6	21.2	2.0
	50~59	78.4	42.7	21.8	17.3	2.2
	60~69	66.2	40.4	29.3	18.2	5.1
	70~75	73.8	36.9	27.7	24.6	4.6

next, at nearly 50%. Rehabilitation insurance and nursing care insurance both were over 20%. The intent to buy the last three of these was higher than the percentage of actual purchase. Young people's intent to purchase critical illness insurance, and cost-subsidizing insurance for outpatient and inpatient costs was relatively high. A fairly high percentage of people in the age group 60–69 intended to buy rehabilitation insurance (nearly 30%), while around 25% of people in the age group 70–75 intended to buy nursing care insurance.

7.7 AWARENESS OF TAX INCENTIVES FOR THE PURCHASE OF COMMERCIAL HEALTH INSURANCE PRODUCTS

In overall terms, 16% of respondents were aware of the existence of tax-incentive policies. The highest awareness was in east China (18.3%), with next being directly administered cities (18%). The lowest awareness was in the northeast (10.6%). Awareness of people in cities was higher than it was in rural areas (19% as opposed to 11.5%). Awareness among people in the age group 40–49 was highest (20%), with next highest being people in the age group 30–39 (18.3%). The lowest level of awareness was among people in the age categories 60–69 and 70–75. See Table 7.42.

The awareness of tax incentives rose with level of education. People with a primary school education or less had the lowest awareness (7.2%), while people with a graduate degree and above had the highest awareness (26.9%). See Figure 7.23.

Table 7.42 Awareness of tax incentives for health insurance by region, urban/rural status and age group (%)

Type		Percentage of respondents who were aware
Overall		16.0
Region	Provincial-level municipalities	18.0
	East China	18.3
	Central China	14.3
	West China	15.4
	Northeast China	10.6
Urban/rural	Urban	19.0
	Rural	11.5
Age (years)	18~29	14.2
	30~39	18.3
	40~49	20.0
	50~59	15.5
	60~69	10.9
	70~75	9.0

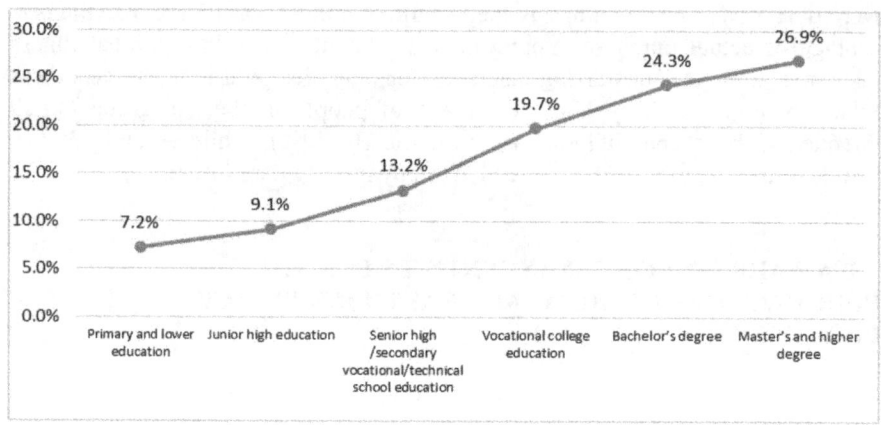

Figure 7.23 Awareness of tax incentives for health insurance by education level (%).

As income of respondents rose, awareness of tax-incentive policies showed an upward trend. People with incomes of less than RMB 10,000 had the lowest awareness (9%). In contrast, people with incomes from RMB 250,000–500,000 had the highest awareness (29%). Next to that came people whose income exceeded RMB 500,000 (26.8%). See Figure 7.24.

People who already had insurance were distinctly more aware of the related tax incentives for that insurance than people who were not insured (29.1% as opposed to 11.4%). In another regard, people with publicly funded medical services and participants in the urban employees' basic medical insurance program were the most aware of all (21.2% for the former and 21.1% for the latter). In contrast, respondents who had never participated in any basic medical insurance had the lowest awareness (9.3%). See Table 7.43.

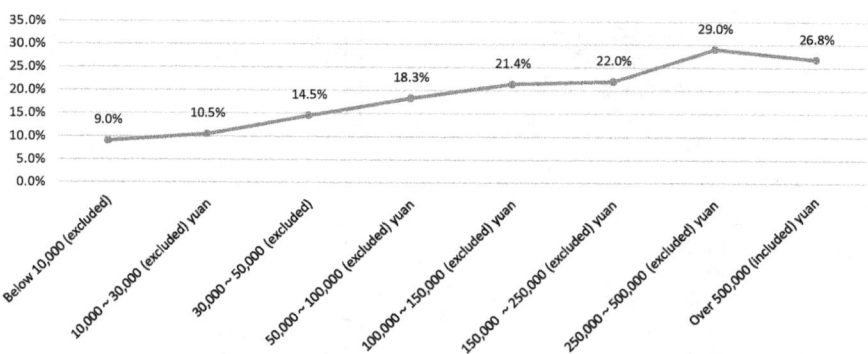

Figure 7.24 Awareness of tax incentives for health insurance by family income (%).

Table 7.43 Awareness of tax incentives for health insurance depending on whether respondents had participated in health insurance or not, and what kind of insurance (%)

Type		Ratio of awareness
Whether enrolled in any health insurance	Yes	29.1
	No	11.4
Basic health insurance programs enrolled in	Basic health insurance program for urban employees	21.1
	Basic health insurance for urban residents + Critical illness insurance	17.0
	New cooperative medical scheme + Critical illness insurance	10.8
	Basic health insurance for urban and rural residents + Critical illness insurance	14.6
	Free medical services	21.2
	None of the above	9.3

Index

Page numbers in **bold** denote tables, those in *italics* denote figures.

ACA see *Affordable Care Act 2010*
accuracy test of model (5.10) **166**
Acts and Regulations: *Affordable Care
Act 2010* 77–78, 346–348; *American
Health Care Act 2017* 78; *Beveridge
Report 1942* 80; *Commercial Health
Insurance Incentive Act 1998* 31;
Family Allowances Act in 1945 80;
Health and Social Care Act 2012 82;
Health Care Reform Bill 327; *Health
Insurance Act 1973* 39; *Health
Maintenance Organization Act 1973*
35; *Medical Insurance Bill 1883* 83;
National Assistance Act 1948 80;
National Health Act 1953 39; *National
Health Services Act 1948* 79–80;
National Insurance Act 1946 80;
Private Health Insurance Act 2007 39;
*Private Health Insurance Incentives
Bill 1996* 349; *Stabilization Act 1942*
345; *Tax Equity and Fiscal
Responsibility Act 1982* 35
adjusted gross income 346–347
administration 7–8, 68, 75, 83, 232, 240,
266–267, 275, 284, 305–306, 375, 381,
395, 398, 400; central healthcare funds
256; of health insurance business 40,
112, 133, 312–313, 363; public 43;
separating government from business
262; streamlining of 367
Affordable Care Act 2010 (Obamacare)
77–79, 250, 346–348
age groups 418, 424–425, 430–431,
433–434, 438–439, 441–442, 444, 446,
448, 450–453, 456–458, 461, 465, 467,
469–473
AGI *see* adjusted gross income

Alibaba Group (previously Alibaba Health
Insurance Co.) 323
Allianz Health Insurance Co. Ltd. 49, 131,
321
American Health Care Act 2017 78
annual family income 421, 426, 434
annual growth rate of government
spending on healthcare by country *4*
annual growth rate of national public hospital
revenues and personnel expenditures
between 2010 and 2015 (%) *406, 408*
annual income 17, 80, 349–350, 357, 438
Arrow, Kenneth 115, 223–224
Australia 31–32, 39, 63, 87, 124, 349–351;
eligibility for the universal healthcare
system 350; government 31, 349–350;
legal system 39; and participation in
commercial health insurance 31;
structured health insurance rebates 31
automatic insurance underwriting 29
average wage and index of urban
employees (unit: yuan) **178**
Aviva Claim Connect (mobile application)
26
Aviva Group, Singapore 26
awareness of tax incentives for health
insurance by education level (%) *474*
awareness of tax incentives for health
insurance by family income (%) *474*
awareness of tax incentives for health
insurance by region, urban/rural status
and age group (%) **473**
awareness of tax incentives for health
insurance depending on whether
respondents had participated in health
insurance or not, and what kind of
insurance (%) **475**

Bancassurance (channel for selling health insurance) 225

banks 149, 207, 305–306, 308–309, 342; central 305; financial regulation functions of the 305

Barmer GEK (German health insurance fund) 25

basic medical insurance 19–20, 32–34, 47–48, 51–54, 59–60, 68–69, 94–96, 99–100, 231–233, 261–262, 290–294, 334–337, 373–374, 381–388, 398; card 33; funds 32, 34, 92, 104, 174, 293, 338, 344, 358, 370, 383, 385, 399–400, 405–406; individuals' accounts 33; information system 36, 342; programs 16, 19–20, 23, 33–34, 135, 137, 198, 200–202, 208, 338, 382–384, 422, 424, 426, 428; system 26–27, 44, 51–52, 63, 65–66, 225, 227–228, 271, 273, 276–278, 369, 371, 373, 384–385, 387

BCG *see* Boston Consulting Group

behavior 37, 40, 45, 64, 92, 105, 108, 151, 224, 226, 311, 314–315, 318, 390, 396; characteristics 151; constraining 21; forbidden 310; fraudulent 105, 139, 157, 224, 262, 275, 336; improper 68, 104, 202, 269, 414; interfering 133; patterns 384; rent-seeking 235

Beijing 12, 205, 213, 219, 232, 265–266, 268, 354–355, 359, 370, 395, 397, 400–401, 417, 419

Beijing Pinggu Model 53

beneficiaries 106, 110, 176, 303

benefits 18, 79–81, 112, 139, 177, 235–238, 246, 326–328, 330, 348–349, 352–353, 404–405, 407–408, 412, 414; actual 354, 408; of commercial health insurance products involving tax preferences (RMB) **353**; consumption of 235–236; core 81; equalized 338; payment of 15, 35, 170; preferential personal tax policies 356; security plan 345; special 237, 271; theory of 235

Beveridge Report 1942 80

bianzhi system (public hospitals) 412

bidding 68, 320, 334, 336–341, 388, 399, 402; competitive 288; conducting 334; process 22, 35, 100, 174, 339–341, 399; public 341–342

bills 41, 101, 189, 327, 337, 349–350, 397, 408; as certificates of evidence 267; hospital and drug 159; self-pay portion 266; unpaid 326

Blue Book of China's Society 2

Blue Cross 40, 75, 345

Blue Shield (also known as Blue Plans) 40, 75, 345

bonds 54, 96, 308; convertible 96; financial 308; government 308

bonuses 232, 253–255, 268, 295

Boston Consulting Group 26

boundaries 34, 44, 62, 64, 88–89, 131–132, 228, 231, 395; defining 64; funding 414; jurisdictional 205

brands 57, 70, 96, 128, 188

brokers 82, 443, 445–446, 465; general insurance 82

Brown, Mark J. 115

budget planning 333; *see also* budgets

Budget Reconciliation Bill 2010 327

budgetary constraints 127, 333

budgets 79, 333, 396, 400

buildings 10, 12, 21–22, 36, 39, 54, 56–59, 97, 187–188, 190, 235, 237, 310, 390, 393; apartment 393; information technology 71; institution 94, 333; process of 70, 232, 295, 392; redundant 71

Bupa Health Insurance Co. 28

bureaucracies 235–236

business 51–54, 59, 64–71, 186–188, 264–265, 272, 307, 310–311, 319–320, 322, 324, 340–342, 355–357, 391, 394–395; activities 38, 306; actual 51, 232; arenas 80, 127, 131; capacities 60–61, 69; commercial 117; complex 158; conditions 112, 133; core 67, 86; data-intensive 205; domestic 305; expanding 57; financial services 29; foreign-related insurance 305; income 348, 372; insurance industry launch 234; new rural cooperative 101; offline 394; outsourcing 95; preferential tax-type 361; private 421, 433–434; risks 66, 93, 363; scope 73, 307, 310; specialized 86, 321; standards 22, 29, 90; tax 184, 322; technical 61, 67

business models 53–54, 67–68, 117, 324; innovative 90; insurance 323; new 127, 131; replicating 57; specialized 16

cancer 2, 144, 170, 201, 216

cantons 252

capacity 60, 130, 140–141, 181, 189–190, 294, 308, 316, 319, 340–341, 344, 395; building 333–336, 340; company's 341; financial 148, 191; independent underwriting 81; individual paying 141, 181;

capacity *continued*
   insurance service 375; productive 61;
   professional 70
capital 35, 54–55, 66, 90, 96, 277,
   279–280, 308, 316, 323, 382, 391;
   adequacy ratios 240, 308; commercial
   79; financial 323; formation 211;
   income 359; indebted 54; operations
   308; private 55; registered 336;
   requirements 54, 308
cardiovascular diseases 2, 216, 409
care 1–10, 12–19, 24–29, 32–38, 54–59,
   72–90, 110–116, 198–204, 206–217,
   247–252, 289–292, 323–335, 366–368,
   393–400, 408–413; childbirth 75;
   insurance 438, 454; managed 27, 241,
   248, 250, 289–290, 295–296, 334;
   neonatal 330; nursing home 75;
   ophthalmic 75, 81; policies 144; post-
   treatment 207; private 248; terminal 292
career development 70
cases 52, 56, 63–64, 103, 107–108, 151,
   159, 264, 272, 324, 329–330, 333, 335,
   341, 347–349; audited 269; chronic 290;
   extreme 159; representative 233, 264;
   suspicious 342
CASS *see* Chinese Academy of Social
   Sciences
CCB Life Insurance Co. 352
CCDC *see* Chinese Center for Disease
   Control and Prevention
CCGs *see* Clinical Commissioning Groups
CDRF *see* China Development Research
   Foundation
cell phones 444, 448, 464
centers 105, 107, 330, 384, 389; diagnostic
   service 389; health-examination 413;
   medical 199, 394; municipal
   administrative 264; rural cooperative
   medical insurance 264; surgical 389,
   413
central China 205, 417–418, 424, 427,
   431, 433, 443, 456, 459, 467, 470, 473
Central Government 9, 25, 48, 51, 279,
   354, 367, 374, 381, 417; documents
   366, 370, 372, 374–375, 383; issues a
   document that explicitly called for
   managing hospitals in different
   categories 370; issues a policy document
   setting up a system called the Medical
   insurance system for urban employees
   369; issues *Opinions on deepening
   reform of the institutional structures
   that govern medicine, pharmaceuticals,*

and healthcare 373; issues policies
   allowing doctors to practice medicine in
   more than one place 397; lays down a
   path for 'having China become a
   country with a social security system'
   369; and municipalities directly under
   the administration of the 306; policies
   398; upgrades the position of
   commercial insurance to being a 'key
   pillar' of the 382
chain 279–280, 384, 388; health-industry
   97; industrial 231, 277, 279, 379; long
   service 321; medical 295
changes in demand for value-added
   services by family income *462*
changes of commercial health insurance to
   health expenditures ratio between 2003
   and 2013 *374*
channels 30, 97, 190, 225, 268, 282, 308,
   379, 410, 443–446, 448; 'green'
   (expediting visits with doctors, and
   management of health-related funds) 27,
   402; important information 444;
   informal 363; off-line 444, 465; official
   propaganda 387; physical 443–444;
   purchasing 26; shared business 94
cheating 94, 224; insurance company 224;
   reimbursement system 94
Chengdu 33, 58, 392, 395
CHI compensation and compensation rate
   218
CHI in China does not cover whole life
   span *222*
CHI markets at the provincial/municipal
   level in 2014 *220*
CHI premium income and its proportion in
   life insurance premium income
   2005–2014 *218*
CHI products and market shares 2015 *219*
CHI purchasers *220*
Children's Health Insurance Program 75
China Development Research Foundation
   13–14, 16–18, 23, 25, 30
China Development Research Foundation
   Research Group 1–2, 4, 6, 8, 10, 12, 14,
   16, 18, 20, 22, 24, 26, 28, 30
China Health Insurance *see* CHI
China Insurance Regulatory Commission
   5–9, 55–56, 62–63, 112, 119, 127–128,
   133–134, 306, 309–311, 316–321, 333,
   339–340, 352–355, 361–362, 371; on
   critical illness insurance 333; and the
   development of health insurance
   products that enjoy preferential

individual income tax treatment 18; and the *Health Insurance Administrative Measures* 21–22; website of 119, 153, 165

China Pacific Insurance Company 95, 101, 104, 369, 371, 384, 399, 403

China Pacific Life Insurance Co. 262–264, 352

Chinese Academy of Social Sciences 2

Chinese Center for Disease Control and Prevention 123

Chinese commercial health insurance businesses 47, 49, 91, 127, 131, 133, 217, 243, 370

Chinese multi-tiered health care system **102, 103**

Chinese public revenue and changes in its growth rate between 2001 and 2015 *405*

CHIP *see* Children's Health Insurance Program

chronic diseases 2, 28, 201, 205–206, 211, 216, 221, 223, 231, 233, 239, 279, 282, 390, 409–410; distribution 205; lower respiratory tract 205–206; monitoring 207; non-communicable 2; non-infectious 147, 216; outpatient treatment expenses for 353

CIRC *see* China Insurance Regulatory Commission

cities 9–10, 32–33, 52, 101, 104–105, 144, 147, 265–266, 274, 278, 354–356, 397, 399–402, 417–418, 448; administered provincial-level 417; core 354; directly administered 10, 417, 428, 430–431, 433, 436, 439, 442–444, 448, 456, 459, 468, 471, 473; first-line 400; major 3, 355; pilot 381; prefecture-level 417

claims 26–27, 29, 39, 41, 50, 52, 90–91, 136–137, 139, 189, 224–227, 253–255, 265–266, 382–383, 455; false 275; handling 25–26, 29, 458; management systems 29, 91; managing 189; medical 105; rate of 189–190; reimbursement of 91, 112, 183, 189, 279; review of 15, 35; settling 234

claims settlement 86, 105, 188, 199, 264, 280–281, 335, 340, 393; costs 225; managing 91; processes 225; systems 240

Clinical Commissioning Groups 247

clinics 34, 58, 199, 275, 392, 394

co-insurance 53, 267

commercial health insurance in China 9, 14, 17, 21, 24, 43, 110–116, 121, 124, 157, 183–184, 217, 287, 319, 416; claims 372; companies 10, 19–23, 26–28, 31, 33–36, 51–52, 54, 56, 59–60, 68–70, 84–85, 92–97, 114, 173–174, 391–393; coverage 6, 371; demand for 16–17, 61, 63, 111, 113–117, 119, 125–127, 129–131, 149–155, 157–161, 167–169, 181, 189, 191, 456; development of 10, 113, 117; entities 35, 53, 61, 89, 310, 374; growth of 401; industry 10, 12, 14, 16, 18–19, 21–23, 53–55, 62, 65, 112–114, 118–119, 121, 130–131, 226–227, 320; market 45, 63, 65, 74–75, 111, 118, 121, 165, 168, 184, 189, 223, 351, 355, 358; operations 87, 132; policies 5, 457; policy holders 87; premiums 10, 13, 32, 84, 116–118, 121, 162, 217, 322, 351, 440–443; products 8–9, 11, 13–16, 32–34, 46–47, 49, 67, 93, 136–140, 352–353, 360–361, 436–439, 443–444, 458–461, 464–466; regulations 309, 332, 362; supplements 231; supply of 7, 9, 11, 43–47, 49, 51, 53, 55, 57, 59–67, 73–77, 81–85, 87–89, 91–93, 97; systems 57, 63, 187; tax incentives 32

Commercial Health Insurance Incentive Act 1998 31

commercial health insurance products purchased by respondents by age group *438*

commercial health insurance products purchased by respondents by family income *439*

commercial health insurance products purchased by respondents by region and urban/rural status (%) **437**

commercial health insurance to total health expenditures ratio between 1999 and 2009 *372*

commercial insurance 5–6, 19–20, 124–125, 261–267, 270–273, 276–277, 366–367, 374–380, 382–384, 390, 395, 398–399, 401–402, 404, 410; development of 370, 372, 411–412; insertion into the system improves efficiencies 234, 266, 276–277; participation of 208, 380; role of 369, 383

commercial insurance companies 6–8, 19–20, 22, 37–39, 232–234, 262, 264, 275–276, 292–293, 295–296, 344–345, 382–392, 394–395, 397–400, 402–404; ability to negotiate 399; external

commercial insurance companies *continued*
constraints on 395; faces losses year
after year 386; and local governments
387
common stock (financial instrument) 96
Communist Party of China 173; Central
Committee 55–56, 99, 110, 112, 128,
131; National Congress 1, 16
communities 73, 102, 350, 390;
international 72; local 417
companies 5–6, 68–70, 92–93, 107–108,
127–128, 183–184, 186–190, 267–268,
295–296, 307–308, 321, 339–342,
354–358, 398–399, 402–404; domestic
370; financial 136; headquarters 336;
low-cost 289; pharmaceutical 85,
283–284, 295–296; shareholding 402;
small 76, 250
comparison of health insurance business of
different companies in 2016 **49**
comparison of investment patterns of
commercial health insurance in hospitals
57
comparison of loss ratios of life insurance,
health insurance and accident insurance
137
compensation 53, 103–104, 169, 212–213,
217–218, 227–228, 245–246, 269–274,
308, 318–319, 337–338, 341, 353,
386–387, 397–398; amounts of 139,
270, 315, 338; disability income 177;
levels of 73, 214; maximum 386;
medical 241; payment of 232, 262,
266–267, 391; percentage of 9, 408;
post-event 221, 252, 280, 285, 289;
regressive 271; secondary 270–271,
276; settlements 94; standards 272, 338;
systems 315, 373
competition 64, 86, 114, 139, 143, 186,
190, 229–230, 255–256, 261, 336, 341,
343, 345, 403; cross-jurisdiction 205;
differentiated 398; disorderly 186, 226;
fair 330, 345; international 85; long-
term 403; normal 304; orderly 36, 64;
promoting 186; unfair 39; vicious 65,
186, 316, 402
competitiveness in insurance markets 88,
137, 223
complaints 30, 315, 344, 373; consumer
316; handling 335; health insurance 31
complementary health insurance model
72–73, 80–81, 187, 233, 247, 333, 351,
375–376
comprehensive medical reform 366–415

compulsory health insurance financing in
Netherlands *254*
confidentiality 315, 335, 342; agreements
342; file 335
consumer 33, 169; confidence 315;
decisions 31; demands 137, 366;
education 30; preferences 29, 112;
psychology 30; rights 30, 304
consumers 30–31, 115–116, 134–135,
137–141, 148–149, 157, 159, 185–187,
190, 226, 228–230, 235, 238–239,
241–242, 312–314; defrauding 31; healthy
76; high-risk 229, 242, 248; individual
117, 281; interests of 64, 308, 316, 333,
336; low-risk 228–230; potential 140, 314;
primary 236; rights and interests of 39,
138, 250, 314, 326, 330, 363
consumption 1, 115, 127, 132, 236, 238;
expected 464; experience 188;
inadequate 236; spending 142
contracts 6, 68, 104, 133, 189, 307, 311,
314, 329–330, 334, 340, 354;
authorization 311; government 35;
medical safeguard 85; standardized 343;
tender 343; terminating for false
disclosure 329
contributions 3, 19, 32, 59, 89, 102, 105,
346, 407–408; employee's 349;
individual 102, 383; industry's 59
convertible bonds 96
cooperation 37, 40, 55–56, 59, 232–233,
261–262, 265, 276–277, 283, 309–310,
316–317, 339, 341, 378–380, 390–392;
agreements 69, 93, 268, 270, 385, 392;
close 40, 73; comprehensive 388, 391;
deepening 56, 389; equity 56;
mechanisms 389; methods of 397, 410;
model of 324, 389; mutual 139; private
34; regulatory 310
correlation 113, 150, 154, 159; analysis
118, 154–155; coefficient 152, 156;
degree of 156; strong 116–117
correlation analysis of influencing factors
155
costs 25–28, 84–85, 92, 104–106,
136–137, 143–144, 158–159, 189–190,
224–225, 268–269, 271–272, 274–275,
285–286, 338–340, 383–385; contract
225; curbing 211; estimated 285; healthcare 76, 261; high 100, 262, 401;
increased 84, 202; institutional 94;
insured 65; overrun 408; pre-tax 322;
production 65; reducing 69; reimbursing
200, 221, 383–384

CPC *see* Communist Party of China
CPIC *see* China Pacific Insurance
  Company
CPS *see* Current Population Survey
critical diseases 39, 103, 173, 176; *see also*
  diseases
critical illness 10, 47–48, 67–68, 99–104,
  107–108, 138, 169, 173, 205–206, 343,
  380–381, 384–385, 422–428, 430–431,
  436–437; cases 68; costs 99–100;
  dispersed reserve funds for 256–257;
  foundations 85, 255–256; identifying
  100; incidence of 108, 175; insurance
  for 10, 13, 59, 83, 221, 339, 385;
  occurrence of 108, 132; risk of 173–174,
  404
critical illness insurance 51–52, 94–95,
  99–100, 170, 173–176, 200, 319–320,
  333–345, 385–387, 398–399, 428–432,
  436, 468, 470–471, 475; businesses 94,
  320, 336–337, 339, 341–342, 345,
  386–387; compensation 338;
  components of 174; databases 335;
  evaluation of 428; funds 7, 22, 36, 105,
  338–339, 344; models 174; operations
  339, 344; plans 22, 266, 337; products
  9, 25–26, 33, 315; programs 48, 52, 104,
  106, 198, 387; regulations on 340;
  reimbursements 175–176, 340; services
  340; sound operations and sustainable
  development of 51, 100; system
  174–175, 319, 333–334, 336, 340,
  343–344, 399; for urban and rural
  residents 51, 173
Current Population Survey 325
customers 18–19, 22–23, 26–32, 35, 87,
  94, 143, 188–189, 191, 307, 315–316,
  322, 324, 330, 349–350; groups of 20,
  181, 352; high-end 238, 280, 282; high-
  risk 229, 240; potential 391; younger 79

DAK-Gesundheit (German health
  insurance fund) 25
data 9, 123, 207; analysis 28–29, 37, 97;
  consumer 29; empirical 67, 334, 337;
  financial 406; health-insurance 59;
  historical 71, 98, 115, 267, 341; medical
  cost 240; on medical expenses and
  health insurance 2010–2015 **212**, **245**;
  mining 94, 97, 280, 394; original 150,
  154, 162; standards 40; statistical 33,
  267, 387
deaths 177, 201, 205–206, 216, 222, 317,
  409; from chronic disease 216; due to

chronic diseases 201; due to illnesses
  that turn into chronic disease 205;
  liability for 317; total 2
Debeka Insurance Company 84
degree of satisfaction with critical illness
  insurance by region, urban/rural status,
  and gender (%) **429**
degree of satisfaction with different basic
  health insurance programs *425*, 427
demand for features of commercial health
  insurance products by family income
  (%) *459*
demand for features of commercial health
  insurance products by urban/rural status
  and age group (%) **458**
demand for health insurance 61, 93, 112,
  115–116, 127, 141–142, 146, 149, 157,
  167, 170, 181, 416–417, 435
demand for value-added services
  depending on whether or not people
  already had health insurance (%) **463**
demand for value-added services of
  commercial health insurance products
  by gender and age group (%) **461**
demand for value-added services of
  commercial health insurance products
  by region and urban/rural status (%) **460**
Department of Human Resources and
  Social Security 270
departments 9, 38–39, 89, 97–98, 241,
  270, 287, 290, 310, 318, 388, 391, 404,
  408, 414; functional 306; of medical
  insurance 396; municipal financial 104;
  public-finance 275; regulatory 36, 39,
  186, 361–363; social insurance 272
description of the egg-white model **210**
desired ways to purchase commercial
  health insurance products by family
  income (%) *466*
desired ways to purchase commercial
  health insurance products by urban/rural
  status, gender, and age group (%) **465**
developed countries 13, 27, 29, 39, 78,
  86–88, 124, 144, 150, 247, 280, 284,
  358–359, 401, 413
developed regions 34, 122, 207, 406–408,
  414, 442–443, 464
developing 20, 22–23, 25–26, 29, 31,
  48–49, 71–72, 74, 85, 149, 257, 261,
  278–279, 401, 403–404; health services
  234, 380; information systems 59; new
  products 20, 29, 149, 224;
  supplementary insurance products 399,
  403

directly administered cities 10, 417, 428,
430–431, 433, 436, 439, 442–444, 448,
456, 459, 468, 471, 473
disability 13, 44, 67, 87, 169, 176–177,
180, 219, 222, 234, 292; insurance for
residents 177; insurance products 25
diseases 25, 28–29, 99, 103, 170, 201,
205–206, 221, 223, 280–281, 317, 377,
381, 409–410, 460–461; acute 216, 409;
cardiovascular 2, 216, 409;
cerebrovascular 99, 205–206; coding
37; hereditary 159; incidence of 20, 28,
61, 91, 108, 240, 256, 280, 282, 286,
289; life-threatening 409; metabolic
system 409; parasitic 409; respiratory-
system 216; spectrum of 1, 23, 25, 99,
201, 366, 409; treatment of 124, 296,
389
disposable income 17, 127, 135, 140–142,
152, 157, 181, 282, 292; and
commercial health insurance products
127; grows at a lower rate than medical
expenses 17; per capita 157; since 1978
141
distribution 2, 146–147, 150, 154, 205,
217, 221, 224–225, 417–418, 420–423,
428, 433, 438–444, 448, 456; of annual
commercial health insurance premium
by region and urban/rural status (%)
440; of annual commercial health
insurance premiums by age group (%)
441; of annual commercial health
insurance premiums by family income
(%) *442*; channels 443–444; employee
income 354; price-based 236; regional
224, 456; of respondents by annual
family income (%) **421**; of respondents
by education (%) **420**; of respondents by
enrollment in basic health insurance
program (%) **423**; of respondents by
health status and behavior (%) **422**; of
respondents by occupation (%) **421**;
wage income 168
DKV (German health insurance company)
84, 111
doctors 36, 96, 158, 262, 294–295, 349,
368, 373, 382, 389–390, 393–394,
396–398, 400, 409–410, 412; allowing
295; allowing employment in multiple
places 295, 367, 397; better 227, 295,
409; compensating 412; contracted 394;
and the fragmentation of healthcare
systems in Mexico 259; relationship
with hospitals 36

documentary materials 367, 369
documents 5–8, 96, 312, 314, 318, 329,
334–336, 344, 370–371, 374–376, 378,
380–381, 392, 397, 399; five linked 320;
important 416; official government 127,
382; public 381; relevant 26, 304, 412;
standardizing 310, 339; tendering 341;
traceable 335
DOH *see* Department of Health
Douescher, Mark P. 115
drugs 34, 224–225, 227, 240–241, 248,
252, 261, 264, 271, 277, 282, 294–296,
382, 385, 393–396; costs 21, 97; high-
priced 296, 396; imported 34; medical
388; prescribed 296; pricier 46; pushing
373
dynamic demand measurement of long-
term care expenses in China (unit 100
million yuan) **182**

east China 417–418, 424, 427, 431, 433,
439, 443–444, 456, 466–467, 470–471,
473
economic and social development 1, 3, 23,
62, 99, 124, 198, 401
economic development 2, 25, 43, 62, 89,
185, 188, 221, 257, 276, 341, 369–370,
374, 406
economic growth 88, 121–122, 158, 186;
promoting 124; rapid 3; strong 62
economic structure 88, 122, 401
education 116, 130, 148–149, 189, 318,
325, 418, 420, 434, 442, 444, 448,
459–461, 463; degree of 148, 442;
higher levels of 17, 130–131, 148, 153,
157–158, 189, 281, 448; and income
levels 434, 442, 448; levels of 17,
115–116, 130, 148, 153, 191, 221, 435,
444, 447–448, 451, 473–474
efficiency 20, 25–26, 29, 34, 89, 92, 95,
98, 100, 228, 231–232, 234, 274, 277,
409; economic 124; higher 256;
improved 231, 249; low internal 411;
lower market 224, 231; operational 342,
344; regulatory 344; upgrading 380
egg-white model *208*
electronic medical records 207
employees 32–33, 75–76, 83–84, 102, 327,
345–346, 349, 354–356, 360–361, 370,
385–387, 407, 412, 420–421, 433–434;
corporate 358; full-time 327; of
government agencies 104, 421; health
insurance 346; of private enterprises
420–421; of state-owned units 420, 433;

taxable income of 346, 360; urban 32–33, 53, 59, 95, 99, 177–178, 338, 354, 358, 369–370, 385–386, 422, 467–468, 471, 474–475

employers: collective purchase by 443, 446; contributions 347; large 76; small business 327

employment 346, 397, 420–421

EMR *see* electronic medical records

Engel's coefficient 127, 142, 152, 157–159

enrollment in China's basic medical insurance program 2001–2014 *122*

equity cooperation 56

estimation of China's population structure *147*

examinations 30, 52, 72, 93, 169, 207, 378, 460–461, 463; health 90, 326; physical 15, 28, 33–34, 55, 90, 296, 361, 422, 435–436, 459, 462, 464; systemic-type 389

exemptions (health-insurance) 184

expected premiums in coming year by family income. *470*

expected premiums in the next year by region, urban/rural status, and age group (%) **469**

expenditures 40–41, 84, 141, 171, 185, 203–204, 210, 215, 250, 258, 346, 349, 353, 396; government health 158; total health 2, 371

expenses 19–20, 34–35, 73–74, 107, 173, 175, 182, 209, 211–212, 261, 266–267, 274–275, 335–337, 339–340, 352–354; account 210, 269; checking 101; current 84; daily 126; dental 349; extra 361; individual 233; of-pocket 212, 245; operating 346; ophthalmology 349; pre-tax 281, 346; reimbursable 239, 271, 315–316, 318; supervising 272; unreasonable 36, 342

facilities 8, 15, 19–20, 22, 26, 34, 37, 46, 69, 144, 188, 261, 290, 292, 430–432; finance 292; health-care 37; healthcare 15, 22, 26, 37; management 8; medical 19–20, 261, 290; non-designated health service 34

false certificates 314

families 73–75, 126, 142, 148–149, 159, 208–209, 330–331, 346, 349–350, 361, 435–436, 444, 447–450, 456–457, 466–467; annual income 421, 426, 434; low-income 74, 250, 259

Family Allowances Act in 1945 80

Federal Poverty Level 326–327, 348

FESC *see* framework for procuring external support for commissioners'

figures 3, 10, 111, 118, 121, 144, 206, 208–209, 217, 249, 252, 270, 351, 357, 434

financial 1–3, 26, 29, 71, 77, 85–86, 102, 148, 201–202, 232–233, 305–308, 319–321, 334–335, 344, 404–406; advisers 82; bonds 308; instruments 96; management 26, 312, 320, 334–335, 337; policy environment 62; resources 3, 16, 71, 133, 400; support 71, 88, 124, 348

financing 124, 209, 211, 214–215, 237–238, 266, 276, 399–400; channels of medical expenditure in Netherlands (millions euros) *253*; levels 399; methods 238; sustainable 263, 269, 271

financing sources 233, 259; of healthcare spending in Switzerland *254*; of Mexico's public insurance *259*

fiscal revenues 2, 201, 248, 404, 416

Five-Year Plan for Medical Reform 5, 7, 10, 26, 55, 57, 128, 201–202, 360

foreign companies 48, 90, 160, 324

forty-six cities from which samples were drawn *418*

Fosun United Health Insurance Co. Ltd. 49, 323

FPL *see* Federal Poverty Level

framework 35, 83, 97, 128, 187, 247, 279, 309, 352, 361, 417; design 389; of guidelines for health insurance products 319, 361; systemic 320

'framework for procuring external support for commissioners' 35

fraud 31, 36–37, 40, 68, 92, 94, 105, 139, 157, 224, 232, 262, 329–330, 336, 342; insurance 37, 330; medical 92

functions 13, 16, 19–21, 97, 133–135, 228, 230–231, 287, 291, 293, 303, 305–306, 313, 318, 320; administrative 304; comprehensive 57; direct leadership 305; financial regulation 305; government's 399; social management 133, 311; supervisory 272

funding 71–72, 202, 204, 259, 261, 263, 271–274, 276–277, 279, 338–341, 343, 392, 398, 400, 407; cooperation 85; deficiencies 78; and expenditure of new rural cooperative medical system (RMB 100 million) **204**; items 333; levels 20, 216, 407; mechanisms 73, 407; reliable 333; standards 125, 341, 398 funds 52–53, 94–95, 100–101, 103–104, 108, 174, 256, 259, 264–275, 284–286, 360–361, 370, 385–386, 400–402, 406–408; administering 101; assembling premium 132; balancing 284, 286; central health-care 85; civil welfare 388; disability protection 388; federal 79; health insurance 7, 10, 37, 157, 389; health-related 27; management 56, 105, 268–269; medical insurance 3, 19–20, 34–36, 52–56, 104, 107, 153, 174, 271–275, 338, 369–370, 383–387, 391, 399–400, 405–408; new rural cooperative 101, 104, 214, 216, 267–268; pooling of 53, 68, 173, 284, 337, 345, 385, 387, 407; public 267, 275; public finance 98, 383; risk-adjustment 338; risk-allocation 286; risk-balancing 252, 286; social security 266–267, 273, 361; sources of 101, 174, 181, 242, 286; use of 264, 293, 360

GDP *see* gross domestic product
General China Life Insurance Co. 352
General Office of the State Council 4, 7–8, 51, 57, 62, 100–101, 131, 234, 309–310, 319, 342, 380–381, 386
German Insurance Association 84
Germany 13, 25, 29, 31, 36, 73–74, 80, 83–87, 124–125, 217, 255–257, 286, 293, 398, 401; birthplace of the modern social insurance system 83; government of 85; health insurance system 255; population 83; premium income to long-term care insurance 84
government 30–35, 51–53, 72–75, 77–79, 88–89, 91–92, 184–187, 235–238, 261–263, 266–270, 274–275, 331–332, 348–350, 369–371, 398–405; administration 83, 264, 289, 370, 374; authorities 48, 59, 268; behavior 320, 354; bonds 308; budgets 227, 412; departments 95–96, 98, 104, 185–186, 190, 232–233, 241, 335, 342, 374, 383, 390, 395, 400–401, 403; district 268–269; entities 309, 334, 390, 411, 414; expenditure 141, 198; expenditure on health 2000–2014 *142*; failures 231, 235; federal 37, 74–75, 78, 259, 327, 331, 346, 348–349; functions 69, 89, 395; healthcare expenditures 3, 141; institutions 40, 199; insurance 260, 391; municipal 33, 101, 105, 267, 274, 393, 397; policies 10, 31, 62, 128, 133,

139–140, 150, 235, 322; spending 4, 132, 159, 199, 257, 260; state 30, 259, 331–332, 346; subsidies 3, 103, 238, 251, 274, 286, 292, 332, 351; tenders 398, 402
grey correlation for the factors that influence demand for commercial health insurance 154, 158–159, 185
grey relational analysis to examine the demand for commercial health insurance 150–151, 154, 157, 186, 191
'grey system theory' 150
gross domestic product 10, 13, 17, 78, 140, 201, 261
group insurance 31–32, 67, 75–76, 169, 281, 289, 310, 327, 330, 345–346, 348, 357, 360; coverage 329; market 82; plans 346; policies 329; purchasing 281; tax incentives 347
groups 16–17, 30, 32, 56, 58–59, 122–123, 125, 223, 326, 331, 338, 345, 410, 438–439, 442–444; consumer 76; corporate 87, 93; designated 348; diagnosis-related 290; disadvantaged 101, 338; high-income 48, 147, 168, 259, 282, 350, 356, 451, 456; high-risk 79, 134, 183, 223, 230; insured 356; interest 85, 236; large 330, 405; low-income 77, 260; low-risk 76, 223, 230; minority 115; small 332, 348, 356; special-needs 280; target 227, 229, 334, 364; young 351
growth 9–10, 62, 64, 111–113, 118–119, 121, 127–128, 149–150, 157, 159, 201–202, 226–227, 243, 401, 404; annual 10, 209, 243; expenditure 204; innovative 23; long-term 143, 186; negative 119; pattern 168, 321; sound 190, 371, 403; sustainable 96, 257
growth rate 2, 118–119, 165, 168, 203, 207, 243–244, 405; annual 4, 10, 30, 211, 351, 371, 393; compound 118; geometric average 243–244; year-on-year 243
Guangdong Province 175, 383, 387
Guidance Opinion on accelerating on accelerating the development of health insurance. 127
Guidance Opinion on pilot-program reform of public hospitals 395
Guidance Opinion on the provision of critical illness insurance for urban and rural residents 99
Guidance Opinion on work related to

providing critical illness insurance for urban and rural residents 51
Guiding Opinion on launching procedures for critical illness insurance for urban and rural residents 386
Guo Pei 116

handling services, provision of 383, 387
health 1, 6–8, 39–40, 43–44, 49, 96–97, 103, 108, 110–111, 126–128, 148–149, 187–189, 375–377, 379–381, 459–461; authorities 98, 363; awareness of 27, 443; condition vs. CHI purchase *224*; education 28, 94, 290, 459; examinations 90, 326; expenditures 372, 409; government expenditures on 141–142; information 38, 59, 94, 98; levels of 1, 124, 435; maintenance organizations 27, 35, 254, 290; management 12, 14, 19, 27–28, 37–38, 44, 67, 69–70, 200, 204, 216, 389, 391–392, 409–410, 456; managing 28, 73, 222, 390; people's 1, 28, 146, 158, 216; social 171, 391; understanding of 149, 190; women's 460–461, 463
Health and Social Care Act 2012 82
Health Care Reform Bill 327
health industry 39, 58, 205, 231, 294, 363; chain 47–48, 54, 56, 65–66, 69, 88, 235, 296; developed 88; mega 204
health insurance 15–18, 27–31, 61–62, 73–76, 86–88, 114–116, 127–128, 133–144, 146–149, 167–170, 240–245, 321–323, 345–347, 362–363, 463–464; advanced commercial 74; agencies 241, 265; annual premiums of commercial 439, 443; authorities 15, 34, 37–38; awareness of 30; basic 468, 475; beneficiaries 81; business 29, 40, 49–50, 56, 64–65, 67, 76, 84, 91, 132, 135–136, 312–313, 315–316, 318–319, 321–323; in China 13, 25, 61, 139, 199, 373; claims, benefits and percentage of increase *51*; companies 15, 28, 37, 49, 66–67, 85, 112, 135, 147, 205, 240, 310–311, 316, 318, 350; compensation 10, 209; compensation (RMB 100 million) as % of total medical expenses *209*; coverage of 32, 84, 116; density and penetration *52*; developing commercial 4, 113, 128, 202, 279; developing consumption-type 26; development of 13, 31, 57, 67, 127, 136, 153, 185, 289, 322, 371, 411; existing

social 184; funding 332; funds 7, 10, 37, 157, 389; growth of commercial 19, 47, 49, 65, 67, 86, 111, 118, 131, 147, 185–186, 233–234, 322, 366, 369; growth of social 185; growth trend in China during 2000–2015 *120*; growth trend in China during 2001–2015 *120*; inadequacies of 23, 456; individual income tax policies for commercial 312–313, 319, 352, 356; industry 22, 37, 39, 128, 136, 139–140, 159, 168, 170, 280, 310–312, 314, 316–317, 319–321, 324; information systems 57, 444, 449–451; mandatory supplementary 237–240, 242, 276, 284, 286–287; market for commercial 63, 121, 124, 132, 217, 219, 223, 229, 240, 247, 251, 316, 319, 321–323, 354–355; markets 84, 223; medical 387; operations 61, 310, 361; operators 39–40, 310; personal 330, 346; policies 133, 225, 351, 389; preferential tax-type 168, 353; premium income 153–154, 162, 165, 243; premium income in China (RMB 100 million) *165*; premiums 10–11, 13, 75, 118, 168, 177, 243, 347, 349, 351, 354; premiums and percentage of health insurance premiums in life insurance premiums *11*; private 39, 80, 349–351, 359; products 5, 7, 14–18, 22, 24, 26–27, 29, 66–67, 134, 187–188, 291, 314–315, 353, 360–361, 444; programs 40, 468; providers 28, 90; purchase of commercial 122, 230, 364, 417, 433–434, 459; regulation 39; reimbursements 75, 351; risk control 87; safeguards 112; services 10, 27, 112, 379; statutory 253; supplementary 9, 73, 89, 116, 139, 185, 252–253, 256, 262, 276, 282, 292–293, 385; supplying commercial 72, 74; system 22, 34, 77, 79, 116, 125, 226, 279, 288; tax-preferential commercial 360
Health Insurance Act 1973 39
Health Insurance Administrative Measures 2006 21–22
health insurance companies 9–10, 15, 19–23, 26–29, 31–37, 40, 49, 54, 59–60, 66–70, 84–85, 89–90, 92–97, 135–137, 316; Alibaba Health Insurance Co.) 323; Barmer GEK 25; Bupa 28; CPIC Allianz Health Insurance Co. Ltd. 49, 83, 131, 321; Debeka Insurance Company 84; DKV 84, 111; Hexie

health insurance companies *continued*
Health Insurance 49, 131, 136, *143*,
152–153, 321; Kunlun Health Insurance
Co. Ltd. 49, 127–128, 131, 136, 321,
371; PICC Health Insurance Company
Limited 49, 60, 65, 104, 107–108,
127–128, 130–131, 136, 168, 175,
270–271, 321, 352, 383, 387–388; Ping
An Health Insurance Co. Ltd. 49,
127–128, 131, 136, 321, 323, 371, 394,
402; Reward Health 127–128; Sunshine
Health Insurance Co. 371
health insurance products 222, 393;
consumption-type 26; current
commercial 138; differentiated 14, 19;
diversified 7, 17; major 23, 137;
mandatory 280; needs for differentiated
health insurance products 14, 19;
personalized 25, 199; pricing of 60–61,
140; private 350; providing 15, 18;
purchasing commercial 63; purchasing
complementary 73; reform of 291;
short-term 317; short-term personal 318;
voluntary 280
*Health Maintenance Organization Act
1973* 35
health risks 17, 27, 46, 50, 114, 130, 137,
149, 233; coverage spectrum *221*;
insuring 233; personal 135
Health Savings Accounts (HSA) 79, 346
health security 1–2, 10, 19–20, 43, 124;
multi-tiered 27, 31, 72; system 1, 29, 33
health services 33, 36–38, 44, 70, 72, 75,
79, 204, 248, 374, 378, 392, 394, 453,
456; community 248; industry 88, 392;
mental 75; organizations 55; providers
37, 83; providing quality 296;
psychological 248; public 199; supply
system 36
health status 76, 114–116, 329, 422,
424–426, 428, 431, 434, 436; and
health-monitoring behavior 422;
person's 353; sub-optimal 28
healthcare 1–4, 6, 8, 19, 21, 55–57, 72,
76–77, 82–83, 124, 141, 198, 208–211,
390–391, 416; costs of 2, 72, 93, 132,
208, 217, 223, 244, 260, 368, 373;
demands 35, 110; diverse 2, 5, 122;
expenses 56, 202–203, 209, 233;
government-financed 124; insurance
systems 128, 257; management services
15, 27, 187, 464; preventive 77, 291;
private 116; products 32, 146; protection
216, 226; providers 46, 75; resources

38, 113–114, 144, 158, 201, 216, 221,
389; structures 21, 26; system reform
198, 328, 332
healthcare safeguards 26, 416; managing
105; multi-tiered 89, 93; system 10
healthcare services 1–2, 12, 14, 26, 54–55,
75, 82, 93, 115, 144, 280, 295, 382, 391,
464; comprehensive lifelong 1; industry
9, 90; preventive 28; providing
comprehensive 87; special 457, 459,
464
healthcare spending 78, 159, 254, 261;
personal 13, 411; total 9, 371
healthcare systems 18–19, 35, 37–38, 40,
55–56, 65–66, 72, 88–89, 93, 95–96, 98,
128, 234–235, 332–333, 389–390; basic
428; China's medicine and 66, 198;
government-financed 124; hybrid 124;
ideal 78; national 35, 86–87, 89; public
35, 108, 206; universal 350
'Healthy China' (concept) 1, 4, 7, 9–10,
23, 198, 243, 287, 294, 296, 416
Heilongjiang 123, 205, 213
Henan Luoyang Model 53
Herfindahl-Hirschman Index 143, 152,
154–155
Herfindahl-Hirschman Index of China's
personal insurance market in recent
years *153*
Hexie Health Insurance 49, 131, 136, *143*,
152–153, 321
HHI *see* Herfindahl-Hirschman Index
HMOs *see* health maintenance
organizations
hospitalization 13, 24, 26, 115, 248, 271,
330, 353, 437, 472; costs 353; expenses
233, 271, 338; individual 383; insurance
25, 33, 345, 436, 438, 454; rate and
hospital visits per capita covered by
basic medical insurance between 2009
and 2014 **170**
hospitals 21, 47–48, 57–59, 75, 169–170,
241, 263–264, 266–270, 275, 277,
292–295, 392–398, 400, 405–408,
412–413; choice of 81; designated 55,
190, 227, 264, 267, 274–275, 396; large
state-owned 56, 66, 207; managing 370,
395; non-local 274, 294; not-for-profit
55, 96; private 57, 70, 260, 296, 349,
400, 406; quality of 92, 290
House of Representatives, United States
327, 329–332
household income 2, 326–327
HSA *see* health savings account

human resources 51, 70, 91, 99, 107, 173, 288, 292, 337, 344, 373, 383, 404, 407, 412; departments 398; governmental 393; systems 36, 295

IAGO *see* inverse accumulated generating operation
illness 23, 25, 27, 51–52, 92, 94, 103–104, 173, 175–177, 179, 186, 188, 205–206, 388, 428; chronic 181, 201–202, 216, 221–222, 282; result of 169, 271, 273, 361, 385, 387; risks of 102, 290
illness insurance 5–6, 25, 175–176, 377, 381; critical 99, 104, 199, 336, 406; major 173, 204, 275–277, 288, 311; providers of critical 10, 51, 68, 94, 99–100, 173; rural critical 6; supplementary critical 388; sustainable development of critical 51, 100
incentives 45, 61, 68, 95, 105, 241, 260–261, 267, 278, 349, 354–355, 390, 396, 403, 407; health insurance policies 345–346; insurance policies 351; tax 9, 31–32, 62, 87, 128, 139, 167–168, 238, 346, 348, 473–475
income 17–19, 118–119, 121, 126–128, 130, 139–141, 168–169, 326–328, 346–348, 396, 442, 459, 464, 466–467, 474; amount of 185, 367; balancing 20, 336–337; employee 346; higher 125, 130, 148, 158–159, 401; household 2, 326–327; individual 281; insurance 6, 103, 138, 180; lower 325, 435; of medical insurance funds 153, 185; people's 408; person's 126, 181; pre-tax 349, 354, 358; stable 125
income levels 115–116, 118, 126–127, 141, 183, 350, 354–355, 426, 434, 439, 444, 448, 451, 459, 462; low 140, 199; person's 126–127; premium 328
income tax 18, 280, 322, 348, 356; deductions in some developed countries **359**; individual 18, 319, 355; lower corporate 280; personal 322, 357, 360; preferences 357; preferential individual 7–8; total individual 168
indicator estimate 2016–2020 (RMB 100 million) **213**, 246
Industrial and Commercial Bank of China 401
industry 21–22, 30–31, 48, 58–59, 64–65, 93–96, 98, 200, 204–205, 306–307, 309–311, 319–322, 371–372, 375, 413–415; associations 413, 415;

premiums 169; reforms 323; regulations 35; service 378; tertiary 401
influence of group insurance tax incentives on insurance purchase costs **347**
information 30–31, 37, 45–47, 150, 181, 186–188, 190–191, 241, 283, 285, 293, 362–364, 391, 404, 448; accessing 444, 448; incomplete 236; indicator systems 308; insured person's 335; medical 37, 206; patient 186, 269; platform 38, 294, 343, 361; resources 383; security 342–343; technologies 37, 56, 59, 71, 97–98, 205–206, 267, 388
information systems 29, 37, 48, 56–57, 59, 71, 97–98, 187, 264, 294, 335, 340, 342, 363, 391; business 48; health insurance 57, 444, 449–451; medical 205; standardized national health insurance 97
'informatization' of medical reform 48, 54, 57, 59, 70–71, 97–98, 207
Informatization of the Medical and Pharmaceutical Industries in China 207
inpatients 81, 270, 451, 470–471; costs 473; funds 101; hospitals 370; services 81, 101, 144
institutions 37, 41, 55, 189, 281, 289, 295, 368, 372, 375, 377–380, 391, 393, 396, 412–413; mutual-insurance 292; pharmaceutical 392
insurance 43–47, 58–61, 102–105, 111–116, 133–136, 148–149, 157–159, 183–186, 190–191, 303–309, 324–327, 379–381, 442–444, 448–451, 470–472; accident 137, 389; agencies 46, 56–58, 60, 281; agents 148, 315, 330, 443–446, 448, 465; all-purpose 134, 352, 356; annuity-type 222; awareness of 23, 114, 153; casualty 13, 60, 86, 118, 222; child 329; clauses 314–315; commercial health insurance by type of 114, 160, 169; community-based 257; comprehensive 84; compulsory automobile liability 344; consumption-type 26; cost-subsidizing 471, 473; for critical illness 219; demands for 115, 141, 148, 153, 159–160, 183, 356; disability 13, 17, 176–177, 291; domestic 58; family 364; full-coverage 270; funded 83, 85, 89, 181, 183, 270; general 330; government-funded 16; government purchases 269; investment-linked 121, 222; long-term care 5, 17, 25, 48, 83–84, 103, 138, 177, 181, 389;

insurance *continued*
long-term nursing 291; management
341; medical compensation 46; medical
occupation liability 292; new 238, 246,
263, 387; non-commercial 66; nursing
care 13, 25, 83, 177, 219, 233, 317, 436,
438, 443, 451, 471, 473; penetration and
density in China during 2000–2014 *122*;
products 6, 8, 13–14, 25–27, 60–61,
158–159, 187–188, 222, 224–225,
306–307, 314–318, 323, 325, 362–363,
376–379; public-benefiting nursing-care
291; public-benefiting type nursing 291;
regulating 290, 307, 317;
reimbursements 92; resources 139, 227,
283; rural cooperative 216, 274, 400;
social security-type 47, 181, 183; special
83–84, 291; statutory 247, 251
insurance claims 46, 98, 274; basic
medical 96; excessive 190; regular
commercial health 294
insurance companies 45–48, 65–71, 94–98,
104–105, 134–140, 188–191, 223–227,
265–270, 272–274, 282–287, 306–322,
329–337, 339–346, 353–358, 360–364;
Bupa Health Insurance Co. 28; business
of 307; CCB Life Insurance Co. 352;
China Pacific Life Insurance Co.
262–264, 352; commercial 6–8, 19–20,
22, 37–39, 232–234, 262, 264, 275–276,
292–293, 295–296, 344–345, 382–392,
394–395, 397–400, 402–404; domestic
27, 56, 59, 324; eligible 339;
encouraging commercial 110, 398;
exempting 322; foreign 90, 186, 306,
324; foreign commercial 392; foreign-
funded 48; foreign-invested 48, 186,
306; lacking the ability to analyze
medical statistics 21, 68, 224, 323, 402;
large 190, 204, 331; New China Life
Insurance Co. 65, 352; online 39, 325,
363; overseas 323–324, 363;
participation of commercial health 21,
56, 393; PICC Health Insurance Co. 49,
60, 65, 104, 107–108, 127–128,
130–131, 136, 168, 175, 270–271, 321,
352, 383, 387–388; PICC Life Insurance
Company 352; private 74–75, 251–252;
qualified 125, 343; role of commercial
health 28, 289; Shanghai Life Insurance
Co. 352; solvency of 308, 319;
specialized 29, 86; specialized health
29, 40, 90, 128, 131, 135, 316, 321, 414;
specialty health 49, 64, 136; Sunshine

Life Insurance Corporation Ltd. 56, 130,
323, 352, 392–393; Swiss Re 111;
Taikang Life Insurance Co. 58, 323, 352,
388, 390; Taikang Pension & Insurance
Co. 130; Union Life Insurance Co. 352;
Xinhua Insurance Company 392; Xinhua
Life Insurance 371
insurance contracts 46, 176, 225, 314;
commercial 85; standard 274; terminate
329
insurance coverage 115, 199–200, 251,
274, 387; basic medical 233, 237;
commercial 371; low 223; private health
251, 351
Insurance Credit Cooperation Division
305
insurance data 212, 245, 283; medical 98,
336; person's 97; social medical 187;
standardizes health 57
insurance entities 61, 280, 304, 307, 340;
private 77; qualified 382; social 185,
271–272, 275, 364
insurance exchange 78, 250, 288, 291,
326–327, 331–332; mechanism
326–327, 331–332; national 331; state-
based 332; systems 331
insurance funds 6, 19–20, 34–36, 52,
54–56, 107, 132, 187, 189, 234, 265,
274, 277, 307, 335; medical 3, 32, 34,
153, 174, 202, 271–273, 275, 293, 338,
370, 383–386, 391, 399–400, 405–406;
pooled basic medical 385; social 272,
274–275, 312, 344; total critical illness
338; urban basic medical 202
insurance handling services 374, 376,
382–383, 385–386, 389, 392, 399, 403
insurance industry 48, 51–53, 55–56, 118,
128, 130, 133–134, 138, 200, 226,
303–306, 309–311, 314–316, 371, 401;
commercial 4, 402, 411; modern 6, 234;
personal 136
insurance institutions 307, 309, 317,
376–378, 380–381; commercial 322,
337–338, 342, 364, 392; establishing
public 331
*Insurance Law of the People's Republic of
China* 303, 306–309, 312–314, 319
'insurance-managed medicine' 240
insurance market 12, 118, 139, 159, 186,
229, 279, 303, 309, 323–324, 330, 402,
411; advanced commercial health 325;
commercial 139, 411; current Chinese
health 134; domestic commercial health
136; mature commercial health 13, 121;

private medical 81; small business 331; small group 332
insurance operations 306, 318, 375–376, 414; commercial 256, 294, 376; domestic 305; social 256, 334; specialized health 16
insurance plans 31, 250, 253, 326, 331, 361; critical illness 343; medical 13, 39, 77, 264; rural cooperative 264–265
insurance policies 134, 139, 174, 223, 313–314, 323, 391, 457; basic medical 175, 336–337; collective 444; comprehensive-type commercial health 351; and the document, *Various Opinions of the State Council on promoting the development of the health services industry* 392; employee-sponsored group health 349; government-subsidized 327; long-term 137, 188; mandatory supplementary health 284, 286; medical expense 329, 341, 384, 398; non-group 349; personalized supplementary 391; preferential-tax health 356; reimbursement-type health 26; short-term commercial health 137; small business health 330; social 363; tax-preferential-type 361; unified 444
insurance premiums 120, 442; basic medical 232, 286; health 167, 346; medical 360; personal health 121, 346; private health 350; statutory health 85; supplementary health 32; total personal 10
insurance programs 68, 74, 385–386; basic health 34, 423–428, 468, 475; commercial 74; failure of basic health 426–427; federal health 348; federal social 74; medical 214, 267; new medical cooperative 268; new rural cooperative 214, 263, 267, 403, 405; new rural cooperative medical 101, 311; original new rural cooperative 263; social 74, 356; statutory health 73; urban basic medical 53, 198, 214, 227
insurance regulation 240, 303, 306–308
insurance regulators 304, 308–309, 331, 343, 361, 363–364
Insurance Regulatory Bureau of Jiangsu Province 399
Insurance Regulatory Commission 121
insurance safeguards 306, 322, 356
insurance services 5, 379, 391; basic medical 48, 54, 95, 173; health 10, 27,

112, 379; illness 6; industry 374; medical 378–379, 399, 403; modern 131; social health 388
insurance system 43, 79, 173, 207, 376, 381, 383; commercial 211, 229; complete critical 174; comprehensive critical illness 320; comprehensive social 80; current critical illness 174; existing medical 242; first compulsory medical 83; large medical 227; mature basic medical 124; modern social 83; multi-tiered medical 360, 364; national health 80, 82, 124, 131; new public-benefiting health 240, 278, 282; public 102, 259; social 63, 124; statutory basic medical 63; universal health 377; universal medical 274; urban basic medical 110, 208
intent to purchase health insurance in coming year by family income (%) *467*
intent to purchase health insurance in the coming year by basic health insurance enrollment (%) **468**
intent to purchase health insurance in the coming year by region, gender, and age group (%) **467**
intent to purchase health insurance in the following year by health insurance enrollment (%) **468**
Interim Measures for administration of the health insurance business 312–313
Interim Measures for exit of insurance companies for the factors that influence demand for commercial health insurance 320
Interim Measures for financial management of insurance companies 320, 334–335
Interim Measures for market exit of insurance companies 334, 336
Interim Regulations on the administration of the insurance industry 305, 309
internal problems 402, 411
Internal Revenue Code 346, 349
inverse accumulated generating operation 161
investment information of insurance agencies in medical institutions **58**
investment via debt instruments 96
IRC *see* Internal Revenue Code

Japan Medical Association 292
Jiangsu Jiangyin Model 53, 99, *263*
JMA *see* Japan Medical Association

jurisdictions 52, 68, 287, 307, 337, 348, 385; administrative 337; direct 354; fund-pooling 386, 396; geographic 37

knowledge 30–31, 116, 191; about insurance 30; general 31; medical 188; specialized 148
Korean life insurance industry 30
Kunlun Health Insurance Co. Ltd. 49, 127–128, 131, 136, 321, 371

labor 85, 231, 266, 310, 341, 390–391, 406
level of satisfaction with critical illness insurance by age group *430*
level of satisfaction with critical illness insurance by health status (%) **431**
LHC *see* Lifetime Health Coverage
life insurance 10, 13, 15, 26, 28–29, 58, 61, 64–65, 68, 84, 86, 118, 222, 321–322, 351; commercial 22; companies 15, 22, 29, 49–50, 61, 64, 75–77, 86, 135–136, 313, 316, 318, 321–322; income 217; models 22; plans 15; policies 217, 225; premiums 11, 49, 218; products 13, 15, 61, 222; providers 46
LifeNet (Japanese insurance company) 31
Lifetime Health Coverage initiative 350–351
local governments 20, 69, 95, 262, 275, 293, 335–336, 346, 383, 385–387, 399, 403, 405–406; and commercial insurance companies 387; procure services from the insurance company 265; required to purchase critical illness insurance from commercial insurance companies 386
long-term care 62, 84, 169, 177, 181–182, 282, 292; costs 181; expenses 181–182; insurance 5, 17, 25, 48, 83–84, 103, 138, 177, 181, 389
long-term sustainability 247, 259
Longgang District Government, Shenzhen 392
loss of income 44, 222, 234; and the cost of nursing care 13; and disability insurance 17; due to disability 67, 87, 169, 176, 219; due to illness 116; insurance 13, 219, 292
losses 44–45, 68, 71, 136, 138–139, 228–229, 268–269, 272, 275, 322–323, 334–338, 340–342, 361, 364, 399; catastrophic 133, 275; economic 132, 191; policy-type 336–337

low-income people 251–252, 428, 439, 442–443
lung cancer 2
Luoyang model 12, 95, 262, 264, *265*, 266

main reasons that respondents feel critical illness insurance is inadequate, by region and urban/rural status (%) **432**
major reasons for the failure of basic health insurance programs to meet the needs of respondents, based on the views of respondents by region and urban/rural status (%) **427**
management 5–7, 27, 34–36, 65–66, 94, 185, 187, 206, 221, 309, 314–316, 375–376, 379–380, 460–461, 463; entrusted 311, 335; fees 35, 69, 266–267, 293, 391; product 134, 310; regulatory 204, 225, 307, 309, 334, 362, 364; systems 37, 40, 48, 55, 59
Management Measures for Commercial Health Insurance 38
management services 10, 35–36, 56, 93, 334, 375, 380; convenient basic medical insurance 59; incorporated health 27, 108; providing comprehensive health risk 28
managerial medical service model *239*
market 15–18, 33–34, 45–48, 63–64, 66–67, 81–82, 88–89, 134–139, 207, 217, 220–221, 223–226, 228–231, 235–237, 278–282; access 96, 186, 313, 362, 414; based insurance rate system 317; competition 29, 64, 73, 86, 131, 143, 157–158, 160, 186, 231, 318, 333, 341, 391; demands 111, 114, 466; economy 45, 303–304, 332; exit 313, 334, 336; failure 231, 303–304; mechanisms 20, 51, 73, 82, 100, 107, 133, 185, 231, 234, 248, 277, 366, 373–374, 377; personal financial services 29, 86; prices 45, 66, 410, 412; share 26, 48, 65, 68, 81–82, 84, 124, 129, 137, 219, 331, 371, 383
market equilibrium of supplementary CHI *228*
market equilibrium of undertaking and cooperative CHI *230*
mechanisms 55, 87, 89, 94, 225, 228, 267, 273, 280, 337, 339, 341, 376, 378, 380; balancing 240, 256–257, 284, 286, 289; post-event compensation 286; risk-adjusting 278, 336

Medicaid 35, 74, 79, 348
medical: bills 41, 67–68, 99, 104, 209,
    330, 364; care 55, 58, 105, 107,
    206–207, 290, 292, 295–296, 366, 368,
    383–385, 393–394, 396, 399–400,
    408–409; costs 37–38, 93, 126,
    201–202, 208–209, 211, 227–228, 272,
    286–287, 325–326, 342, 386–387,
    391–392, 407, 470–471; devices 8, 394;
    emergency assistance 124, 208, 265;
    equipment 19, 93; fraud 92; resources
    19–21, 36, 77, 95, 112, 224, 227, 240,
    271, 274, 372–373, 382, 391, 398,
    410–412
medical assistance 131, 133, 227; large-
    sum 173; program 200; rural 95
medical behaviors 56, 87, 94–95, 107, 335,
    404; abnormal 107; dishonest 94;
    unreasonable 60
medical care 367, 410, 413; basic 100;
    emerging Internet-based 382; free 260;
    funded 248, 467, 471; inadequate 317;
    rural 260; surtax 350; system 199
medical costs 126, 189, 289; excessive
    262; high-priced 77, 110, 170, 341;
    improper 108; reducing 59, 389
medical expenditures 252–253, 287;
    catastrophic 174; current 211
medical expenses 17, 19–20, 26–28,
    54–55, 86–87, 99–100, 105, 126,
    174–176, 212, 233, 245, 326–327, 342,
    346–348; actual 46; compensating 233;
    controlled 54; expected 285; high 100,
    103, 329, 353; of individuals and
    medical service institutions 79; inflated
    78; major 101; payment of 55, 290; total
    209–211
medical financing around the world in
    2013 (%) **258**
medical institutions 40, 44–48, 54–59,
    69–70, 91–96, 105, 189–190, 264–267,
    295–296, 367–368, 370, 372–373,
    378–379, 389–392, 413–414; designated
    101, 105, 335, 389, 391, 396;
    developing non-public 54; establishing
    382; managing designated 389;
    nationwide 372; non-public 96, 404;
    private 70, 80, 296, 397; public 392,
    409, 413; reform of 47, 96
medical insurance 102–103, 169–170,
    202–204, 210–211, 214–216, 274,
    287–288, 291, 316–318, 360, 363–364,
    385–386, 390–391, 405–408, 413–414;
    administering 293, 398; corporate 322;

development of 51, 53, 185; evaluating
    288; funded 315; funds 3, 32, 34, 153,
    174, 202, 271–273, 275, 293, 338, 370,
    383–386, 391, 399–400, 405–406;
    handling of basic 68, 95, 264, 311, 383,
    386; management systems 48, 59, 107;
    managing 399, 403, 414; new rural
    cooperative 22, 99–101, 174, 265, 269,
    386, 400; private 80, 82, 125; public 86,
    226; publicly-funded 276; social 89,
    269, 315, 422; supplement to basic 34,
    88, 100, 125, 356; universal social 414;
    urban 204, 216, 271
Medical Insurance Bill 1883 83
medical insurance products 315; basic 5,
    67; commercial 33; comprehensive 370;
    designing 315; developing high-end 48,
    324; private 81
medical insurance system 85, 227, 230,
    232–234, 237, 248, 250, 260, 262,
    279, 287, 332, 389, 405, 416; basic
    26–27, 44, 51–52, 63, 65–66, 225,
    227–228, 271, 273, 276–278, 369, 371,
    373, 384–385, 387; faces severe
    challenges 260; of Germany *257*; social
    187, 199
medical reform 12, 18–19, 48, 54, 59, 70,
    97–98, 247–248, 278, 294, 373–374,
    382–383, 394–395, 404, 412; deepening
    55–56; work 199, 294
medical safeguards 48, 65, 69, 72–74, 81,
    85, 99, 105, 110–113, 131–132, 187,
    227, 234, 369, 371; funded 74; market
    230; system 33, 38, 63, 73–74, 82–84,
    88–90, 99, 101, 110, 112, 114, 124–125,
    233–235, 363, 371
medical security 44, 47–49, 52, 228, 375,
    377; services 375–376; systems 44, 47,
    49, 53, 64, 67, 261, 375–376
medical services 33–38, 44–46, 66–67,
    76–77, 82–83, 92–94, 124–126, 227,
    232–235, 289–290, 294–296, 367–368,
    389, 409–410, 412–413; basic 16, 251,
    255, 312; cooperative 376–377;
    expensive 81; high-quality 110;
    institutions 79, 317, 324; markets 87,
    393; networks 312; providers 27, 29, 35,
    38, 60
medical system 47, 82, 144, 207, 211, 264,
    296, 320, 366, 394–395, 406, 410; basic
    371, 406; new cooperative 198,
    203–204, 208, 227, 234, 371; rural
    cooperative 210, 381
Medicare 35, 74, 76, 332, 348, 398

medicine 54–57, 59, 61–62, 64, 66, 93, 225–226, 278, 283–284, 290, 293, 325–326, 373, 394–395, 411–412; costs 353; funded 369; nationalized 247; systems 377
medicine contract 410
Medigap program (United States) 291
micro policies 305
migrant workers 116, 420–421
military health benefits 75
military personnel 74, 250
Ministry of Civil Affairs 6, 51, 99, 173
Ministry of Finance 9, 51, 62–63, 99, 139, 173, 305, 319, 352, 354, 367, 370
Ministry of Health 40, 51, 99, 173, 288, 367
Ministry of Human Resources 51, 99, 173, 288, 292, 344, 407
Ministry of Public Health 395
Minutes of the meeting of branch presidents of the People's Bank of China 305
mobile phones 30
money 41, 61, 136, 149, 157, 159, 183, 225, 275, 291, 308, 346, 399, 401, 405–407; assembled to set up an insurance fund 132; disbursing 399; pretax 349; safeguarding 308
monitoring 21, 92–93, 95, 97, 101, 105, 107, 240, 264, 270, 280; active 107; continuous 241; external 92; ineffective disease 326; real-time health information 105, 264, 281, 312; real-time treatment 105; systemic 94; teams 105
monopoly 66, 295, 395–396, 407; administrative 382; of Grade Three hospitals 400; pattern 400
moral hazard 16, 45–46, 66, 87, 94, 188–189, 225, 228–229, 231, 240, 250, 289, 312, 333, 407; behavior 139, 224; of the group of consumers 139; incurred by policy holders 86; leading to aberrations in the supply and demand curve 45; and the low efficiencies in the market caused by 224; risk of 46
mortality rate 2, 159, 201
'municipal health and wellness index' 108

NAIC *see* National Association of Insurance Commission
Nantong 33, 355, 419
National Assistance Act 1948 80

National Association of Insurance Commission 329
National Development and Reform Commission 6, 51, 99, 173, 386, 396, 413
National Health Act 1953 39
National Health and Family Planning Commission 2–3, 37, 292
national health expenditure and changes in physician resources between 1985 and 1997 *368*
national health insurance revenue to personal health expenditure and total health expenditure ratio between 2001 and 2014 (%) *409*
National Health Service 19, 35, 79–80, 83, 125, 247–248, *249*, 292
National Health Services Act 1948 79–80
National Insurance Act 1946 80
national insurance exchange mechanism 331
national per capita health insurance revenue between 2001 and 2014 *411*
NDRC *see* National Development and Reform Commission
Netherlands 63, 80, 124, 211, 247, 251–254, 286; complementary health insurance 251; dental care provided by the public system 80; mandatory health insurance 251
New China Life Insurance Co. 65, 352
newspapers 30, 448–450
NHFPC *see* National Health and Family Planning Commission
NHS *see* National Health Service
northeast China 205, 417–418, 424, 427–428, 431, 433, 443–444, 456, 467, 470–471, 473
number of effective samples by province/city and urban or rural area **419**
number of hospital beds in China 2001–2014 **145**
number of medical technicians per 1, 000 people in China 2003–2013 **146**
nursing care insurance 13, 25, 177, 219, 317, 436, 438, 443, 451, 471, 473

Obamacare see *Affordable Care Act 2010*
OECD *see* Organization for Economic Co-operation and Development
online insurance companies 39, 325, 363
online insurance consumers 325
operations 37–40, 59, 61, 64, 70–71, 131, 186, 188, 264, 266–267, 303–304,

306–307, 309–310, 315–316, 398–399; actual 100, 267; industry's 186; market-oriented 107, 242, 250, 374; professional 104, 107, 127

Opinions of the CPC Central Committee and the State Council on deepening reform of the institutional structures that govern the medical, pharmaceutical, and healthcare syst 51, 55–57, 62, 64, 100, 110, 112, 128, 131, 234, 310, 371, 374–375, 392, 395

OptumRX (pharmacy benefit management company) 283

Organization for Economic Co-operation and Development 2, 4, 62, 72, 74, 208–209, 211

out-of-pocket costs and expenses 27, 32, 122–123, 132, 174–176, 212, 239, 243, 245–246, 258, 262, 372, 384

Outline of the Plan for Healthy China 2030 243

outpatients 101, 104–105, 169, 221, 233, 353, 370, 436–438, 454, 470–473; care of 451; expenditures 353; expenses 271; fees 87; services 24–25, 80; treatments 353

participation 5, 37, 39, 44, 47, 70, 292–293, 351, 358, 360, 364, 375–376, 383, 415, 417; of commercial health insurance companies in China's medical reform 56; commercial insurer's 273; equity 57; mandatory 385; promoted stable 351; voluntary 133, 259, 292

patients 19–21, 45–46, 51–52, 70, 103, 266, 269, 271, 295–296, 372–373, 386–387, 390–391, 393, 400, 408; data 25; hospitalized 384; insured 105; monopolizing 227; out-of-pocket 104; prevented 103; registered 249; self-paying 349; smoking 390

payments 60, 71, 74, 92, 101, 104, 107, 140, 232, 264–265, 280–281, 287, 290–291, 334–335, 396; adjusting 267; calculation 92; effective 55; fixed-amount 67; indemnity 60; mechanisms 92, 389, 414; post-event 266; process 277, 280, 340; ratios 68, 334; reform 94; services 207, 389; systems 104, 262–263, 275, 287

payments methods 92, 259, 290, 373, 386, 396, 414; diversified 240; health insurance 393; new 279; package of 396

payouts of health insurance schemes during 2010–2015 (expressed as percentage of personal health spending) *15*

Pearl River delta 219

penetration rate of mandatory health insurance in Netherlands *252*

pensions 404–405

people for whom health insurance is being bought in the following year, by region and urban/rural status (%) **470**

people for whom respondents intended to purchase health insurance in the following year, by age group (%) **471**

People's Bank of China 305–306, 309

People's Insurance Company of China 104, 128, 199, 268–269, 274–275, 305, 333, 369, 383, 399, 402–403

per capita 13, 17, 99, 157, 159, 170, 172, 214–216, 263, 271–272, 340–341, 356, 358–359, 407, 411; health insurance income 358, 411; healthcare expenses 121, 214; premiums 272, 321, 356

per capita medical expenses and expenditure covered by medical insurance *215*

perceived weaknesses of commercial health insurance by urban/rural status and age (%) **455**

percentage of insurance buyers in population groups with different education backgrounds *148*

percentage of out-of-pocket costs in China's total medical spending *123*

percentage of respondents 17, 23–25, 424–425, 428, 430–431, 433–436, 438–439, 442–444, 448, 464, 466, 468, 470–471, 473; about the most important reason for failure of the basic health insurance programs to meet the needs of residents by health status (%) **428**; degree of satisfaction with different basic health insurance programs *426*; satisfied with basic health insurance programs by age group *425*; satisfied with basic health insurance programs by health status (%) **425**; satisfied with basic health insurance programs by region and by rural/urban status **424**; who purchased commercial health insurance by education level *435*; who purchased commercial health insurance by family income *436*; who purchased commercial health insurance by gender and age group (%) **434**; who purchased

percentage of respondents *continued*
  commercial health insurance by health
  status and frequency of physical
  examination (%) **436**; who purchased
  commercial health insurance by region
  and urban/rural status (%) **433**; who
  purchased commercial health insurance
  in rural areas by occupation *435*; who
  purchased commercial health insurance
  in urban areas by occupation. *434*; who
  purchased health insurance by level of
  family income **24**
performance evaluation standards 22
performance evaluation system 36, 343
performance management 35
personal income 17, 381
personal insurance 13, 118, 120–121, 136,
  143, 169, 189, 327, 331, 369
personnel 29, 36, 227, 275, 335, 405–406;
  expenditures 406; headcount 306; health
  insurance management 30; marketing
  315; professional 364; qualified 343;
  rolls (registered) 412; status 397; system
  393–394, 397; technical 153
pharmaceutical suppliers 240
pharmaceuticals 19–20, 38, 47, 56–57,
  92–93, 105, 264, 283–284, 289, 296,
  363, 373
physical examinations 15, 28, 33–34, 55, 90,
  296, 361, 422, 435–436, 459, 462, 464
physicians 19, 36–37, 66, 85, 267, 292,
  295, 368, 394
PICC *see* People's Insurance Company of
  China
PICC Health Insurance Company Limited
  49, 60, 65, 104, 107–108, 127–128,
  130–131, 136, 168, 175, 270–271, 321,
  352, 383, 387–388
PICC Life Insurance Company 352
pilot programs 32–33, 95, 174, 199–200,
  281, 289, 293, 340, 344–345, 354–356,
  358; of individual income tax policies
  313, 319, 352, 356; initiatives 354;
  reform 395
Ping An Endowment Insurance Co. 388
'Ping An Health Cloud' 394
Ping An Health Insurance Co. Ltd. 49,
  127–128, 131, 136, 321, 323, 371, 394,
  402
Ping An Life Insurance Company of China
  65, 69–70, 127, 352, 369, 371, 402
Ping An Trust Co. Ltd. 392
Pinggu 48, 267–269; government 270;
  model 12, 267, *268*, 269, 311

plans 5, 7, 9, 26, 31, 35, 55, 57, 76, 78,
  105, 250, 339, 345, 347; consumer-
  directed health 251; diversified risk-
  balancing 250; group health 32;
  health-care reform 332; health insurance
  132, 330; individualized health
  management 296; lifelong critical illness
  insurance 25; new rural cooperative
  medical 262, 428; security development
  376; urban employee 266
platform 2, 19, 26, 31, 57, 59, 93, 96, 104,
  186, 238, 293–294, 296, 389–391, 394;
  consultation 188; data-sharing 186, 363;
  direct compensation 266; direct-
  payment 265; health-management 296;
  independent operating 342; information-
  sharing 414; main supply 54;
  organization 234; smart health insurance
  37, 391; third-party exchange 281, 289
policies 5–8, 18, 62, 130–131, 133,
  139–140, 167–168, 287–289, 319–320,
  322–324, 351–358, 360–364, 380–382,
  388–389, 410–411; adopted special 322;
  changing 93; commercial 358;
  comprehensive 80; employee's 84;
  expensive 456; family-based health
  insurance tax incentive 32; financial
  411; government 139, 235; group health
  75; individual 75, 360; long-term 62; for
  loss of income 219; recommendations
  88, 115, 277, 287, 411–412; reform 367,
  382; and regulations 303, 305, 307, 309,
  311, 313, 315, 317, 319, 321, 323, 325,
  327, 329, 331; relevant 70, 128, 366,
  416; social security 140; supportive 30,
  133, 322; tax 31, 63, 86–87, 140, 356,
  379, 381; tax-incentive 473–474; tax
  preference 347; underground 323–324
policy documents 366, 369, 392, 412; for
  critical illness insurance 387; five
  administrative 333; *Guiding Opinion on
  launching procedures for critical illness
  insurance for urban and rural residents*
  386; important 4
policy holders 86, 94, 97, 104, 139,
  174–177, 187, 189, 250–251, 271,
  273–275, 351, 353–354, 356, 390–391;
  of basic medical insurance 104, 168,
  293; high-risk 223; individual 353;
  inducing 316; interests of 85, 318; low-
  risk 223
population 1–2, 26, 30–32, 83–85, 99–100,
  114, 124–128, 146–147, 149–150, 159,
  181, 247–248, 259–260, 417, 428;

affluent 31; elderly 25, 62, 72–73, 201, 216; large 53, 229, 354; migrant 216; permanent 263; younger 159

portion of Central Government documents relating to commercial health insurance between 2009–2015 **375**

potential demand for commercial health insurance by family income *457*

potential demand for commercial health insurance by gender and age group (%) **457**

potential demand for commercial health insurance by region and urban/rural status (%) **456**

poverty 48, 68, 80, 94, 99, 103, 170, 173, 271, 273–274, 361, 364, 377, 385, 387

pre-tax deductions 139, 352

pre-tax purchases 133

prediction of model (5.9) **164**

prediction of model (5.10) **167**

prediction of model (5.11) **167**

predictions of demand for medical insurance by residents (2) **180**

predictions of the demand for medical insurance by residents (1) **172**

predictive values 161, 163–164, 166–167

preferences 143, 357, 443, 462, 464; higher 459; individual 235; people's 235; personal 236

preferential policies 5, 62, 65, 312, 320, 354–355

preferential tax policies 18, 63, 125, 128, 130, 135, 139, 167–168, 184–185, 236, 345, 348–349, 351–355, 357–358, 364

preferential tax treatment 5, 62, 185, 200, 202, 208, 288, 345, 348, 352, 354–358, 360–362; to buyers of health insurance 281; expanding 291; health insurance products 18; involving commercial health insurance 357, 361; and social security 139; a transfer payment to the insurance industry from the government 134

preferred stock (financial instrument) 96

premium income 48–50, 52–53, 75–76, 84, 111, 114, 117–119, 121, 127–128, 135–136, 157, 168, 218–219, 243–244, 351; achieved 128; of China's insurance industry *119*; estimate (as per growth rate) *244*; estimate (percentage of out-of-pocket expenses drops to 28% in 2020) *246*; forecast 113; and growth rate over the years *243*; of health insurance business and its proportion to that of life

insurance *50*; of health insurances (millions euros) *255*; insurance companies sharing 267; level of 219, 387; and market share of health insurers in China during 2006–2012 (unit: million yuan) **129**; percentage of 120, 411; reported 128; scale of 170, 217; total 49, 118, 136

premium payments 31, 356, 439

premium rate adjustments 317

premium subsidies 326, 349–350; capping of 328; federal government's 330; raising of 350; and security levels in three U.S. healthcare reform proposals **328**

premiums 7–10, 12–13, 75–78, 132–134, 138–139, 168–170, 176–177, 251–252, 255–256, 326–327, 329, 346–351, 355–356, 384–388, 438–439; cost of 351–352, 355, 439; employer 327; fixed-amount 228; highest 223, 230, 256; levels of 329; lowest 229–230, 276; negotiated 331; net risk 317; paying 250, 281; subsidizing 229, 331; total 48, 50, 118, 138, 219, 338

prescription drugs 75, 115, 295, 330

pressures 67, 87, 107, 186, 201, 295, 316, 322, 357–358, 369, 373, 385, 403, 405–408, 416; excessive spending 370; financial 2, 85, 404–405; moderate 358

price competition 35, 68, 253–254, 340

price-control measures 327

price wars 186, 322, 340–341, 343

prices 35–36, 45–46, 60, 115–116, 140, 225, 227, 252, 254, 256, 332, 334, 340–341, 394, 396; base 341; changing 368; drug 227, 393, 396; market-set 410; negotiated 224, 227, 240; preferential 188; product's 61; reasonable 295, 317–318; setting of 282, 294

pricing 60, 66, 78, 85, 98, 238, 250, 253, 290, 295, 316, 329, 342, 413; differential 329; inaccurate 336; market-determined 397; models 238

primary health insurance 72

private health insurance 39, 80, 349–351, 359; and the *Health Insurance Act 1973* (Australia) 39; and the *National Health Act 1953* (Australia) 39; and the *Private Health Insurance Act 2007* (Australia) 39; rebate to customers 31

Private Health Insurance Act 2007 39

Private Health Insurance Incentives Bill 1996 349

Private Health Insurance Incentives Bill 1998 349–350
private insurance 85, 115, 255, 291; compulsory 250; subsidized 332
private insurers 35, 77–78, 124, 132–134, 250
Problem of Social Costs, The 225
problems, internal 402, 411
process 45, 59, 70, 91–93, 97–100, 107, 173, 186–187, 240–241, 280–281, 290, 333–334, 339–340, 389, 391–392; competitive 190; front-end 277; management 29; post-insurance 339; risk-control 189; sampling 417
procurement 34–35, 95
products 5–8, 17–18, 23–24, 31–32, 67–68, 93, 137–139, 221–223, 229, 306–307, 312–315, 317–319, 324, 356–357, 361–362; affordable insurance 79; commercial 147; consumption-type insurance 26–27; customized 229; design 15, 19, 27, 68, 86, 312–313, 343, 352; developing insurance 25, 91, 136–137; individualized 188, 280; innovation 23, 93, 188; new 37, 49, 128; offerings 12, 93, 137, 200, 221; pricing 280, 317, 326, 329, 363; selling insurance 31, 314, 317–318, 324; short-term insurance 50, 317; special 34, 144; spectrum of 231, 282; standardized 250, 378
profitability 54, 134, 136–137, 188, 321, 342, 357
profits 68, 70, 76, 252, 256, 272, 275–276, 278, 321–322, 336–337, 340–341, 361, 364, 399, 402; fund's 311; lowering monopoly-generated 160; margins 134, 339, 361; maximizing 159; monopoly 186; operating 94; pre-tax 346; reasonable 278, 318; small 174, 273
programs 52–53, 57–58, 74, 78, 84–85, 95, 101, 268, 272, 284–285, 348, 352, 356, 417, 422–423; basic healthcare 73, 78; basic medical 78; comprehensive public security 63; employer-sponsored 76; government reimbursement 289; health promotion 329; insurance education 30; new rural cooperative medical 95, 101, 214, 216, 269, 384, 422; public healthcare 80; risk allocation 284–285; television 108; traditional medical care 77; transitional 285
projects 107, 123, 333–334, 337, 390, 400; cooperative 389; government healthcare

35; medical safeguards 107; medical service 29; supporting pilot 63
property insurance 13, 28, 40, 118, 168, 321, 351, 363
property insurance companies 15, 29, 49–50, 64, 86, 127, 322
proportional co-insuring model 269–270
protections 13, 16, 25, 28, 32, 35, 77, 80, 122, 125–126, 135, 138, 310, 312–314, 363; basic 34; better health 27; comprehensive 25, 63, 353; effective 51; higher-level 126; labor 199, 345; long-term 25, 50
providers 7, 66, 75, 79, 83, 88, 90, 92, 248, 382, 403; health insurance-plus-health management service 28; private service 83; professional service 54
provincial risk balance mechanism *286*
provisions 19, 21, 31, 36, 54, 112, 133–134, 157, 307, 315, 317, 321, 334–335, 381, 388; information disclosure 239; insufficient health security 12; mandatory insurance 78; market-entry 312; medical service 40; standardizing entry 362
public benefits 237, 253, 257, 261, 278, 282
public finance 66, 101, 255, 259–261, 263, 265–267, 273–274, 276, 285, 288, 370, 393, 400, 404–405, 413; allocations 345; authorities 275; departments 267; inputs into the funds 94
public health 100, 265, 395; agencies 132; authorities 96, 101; centers 393; insurance 124, 131–132
public hospitals 15, 33, 36–37, 55, 57, 96–97, 226–227, 295–296, 349, 370, 372–373, 394–396, 405–406, 410, 459–464; doctors 36–37; government-backed 397; institutional structure of 396–397; lacking incentives to control costs 261; managing 395; monopoly position of 36, 227, 296; municipal 400; reform of 48, 54, 96, 395
public medical institutions 12, 70, 370, 373, 378, 395, 400, 405, 407, 410, 413–414
public medical system of India *260*
purchasing power 17, 61, 79, 127, 135–136, 140, 157, 185, 190, 369, 401, 435, 442

Qingdao City 37, 388
Qingdao model 58, 388–392

qualifications 22, 96, 239, 275, 316, 321, 339, 364; legitimate 413; required 311, 336; review 101, 275; uniform 69

quality 36–37, 61, 64, 69–70, 77, 81–82, 84–85, 88–89, 91–92, 96–97, 157–158, 185–188, 277–278, 364, 379–380; care services 177; high 185, 312, 389, 402; low 326; medical 288, 290; resources 342; services 49, 233, 253

ratio 329, 353, 357, 427, 432, 458; low reimbursement 428, 431; old-age dependency 153

R&D systems 143, 342

reform 18–19, 66, 78–79, 82, 92, 97, 198–199, 262–263, 290, 364, 367, 371–376, 388–389, 393–394, 412–414; health-care 33, 330, 332; of hospitals 395; individual-account 360; of medical programs 9; policies 367, 382

regional insurance exchange mechanism 331

registration 315, 317, 458, 460–461, 463

regulations 20–22, 38–40, 63–64, 266, 293, 303–305, 307, 309–313, 319–325, 333–337, 339–341, 343, 345, 353, 361–365; administrative 21, 314, 320; departmental 98; domestic regulatory laws and 305; explicit 68, 320; independent 362; national 393; and policies 303, 305, 307, 309, 311, 313, 315, 317, 319, 321, 323, 325, 327, 329, 331; on reinsurance 310; relevant 38, 311, 324; specialized 309, 320; standardized 288, 314; strengthening 339, 363; supervisory 64; violating 310

Regulations on the Operation and Management of Health Insurance 38

regulatory authorities 39–40, 90, 319, 350

regulatory bodies 304, 307, 335, 362

regulatory policies 64, 304, 314, 319, 331, 333, 361

regulatory system 12, 21–23, 39, 88, 97, 186, 290, 305–306, 309–311, 320, 331, 339, 362, 415; effective 38, 322; forward 280; insurance 303; outdated 21

rehabilitation insurance 436, 443, 454, 470–471, 473

reimbursements 26–27, 101–102, 104, 106, 108, 173–175, 280, 282, 308, 311–312, 350, 352, 384, 426–427, 457–459; actual 10, 13, 354; compensation 244, 364; low percentage of 426, 428; payments made by the

health insurance business of life insurance companies in the U.S. from 2009 to 2015 77; procedures 291, 312; ratio of critical illness insurance in Zhanjiang **175**; second 173–174

reinsurance 240, 273–274, 310; companies 133, 240, 287; mechanisms 242, 278, 287; policies 307; products 384; purchasing 270; regulations on 310; system 274, 284

Renminbi currency 10, 47–50, 52–53, 175–176, 202–204, 207, 209–213, 215–217, 243–246, 337–339, 355–359, 384–388, 399–402, 438–439, 442–444, 19 billion estimated for disability income insurance 177; annual income of 17, 438, 451; average of 18, 216, 351; figure of 2, 128.5 billion for estimated demand for critical illness insurance 176; first tier costs in premiums per year 384

research 11, 14, 43–44, 98, 110–112, 114–116, 124, 126, 152–153, 223, 225, 354–355, 387, 389, 402–403; background 1, 110; groups 381; product 279

reserve funds 291, 308, 310

residents 10, 12, 16, 32, 102–104, 170, 172, 179–180, 189, 323–324, 349–350, 379–381, 387, 399, 423; Chinese 14, 16, 32, 123, 140, 199; critical illness insurance for urban and rural 100, 320, 334–337, 345; demands for illness insurance 175–176; employed 271; encouraged to use their basic medical insurance card to pay for fitness products and services 33; rural 9–10, 47–48, 51–52, 99–100, 103, 173–175, 319–320, 334–338, 344–345, 375, 377, 381, 384–387, 457, 468; urban 53, 95, 99–100, 102–103, 171, 173–174, 177, 189, 200, 203–204, 369, 371, 457, 459, 468; urban-rural 274–275

respondents 13–16, 18, 23, 25, 123–124, 417–418, 420–424, 426–428, 430–439, 442–444, 451, 456–457, 466, 470–471, 473–475; adult 115, 123; age distribution of 417, 420; elderly 433, 443; female 431, 433; health insurance products 472; healthy 424, 426, 435; high-income 443; male 430–431, 433; percentage of 17, 23–25, 424–425, 428, 430–431, 433–436, 438–439, 442–444, 448, 464, 466, 468, 470, 473; rural 422,

respondents *continued*
 426, 433, 436, 453; senior 430–431;
 urban 422, 426, 433, 436, 453; in
 vulnerable groups 428
revenue and expenditure of urban basic
 medical insurance (RMB 100 million)
 204
revenues, public-finance 404
Review of Economic Studies 115
reviews 39, 189, 264, 269, 272, 315, 317;
 literature 114–115, 117; social insurance
 authorities 266; systemic 107
Reward Health (Ruifude Health) 127–128
risk 21, 46, 130, 132–134, 136, 138–139,
 148–149, 189–191, 221–223, 240,
 250–252, 256–257, 269–270, 284–287,
 289–290; analysis 282; aversion 135,
 138; countering of 149, 240; degrees of
 259, 278, 315; dispersals of 158, 223,
 240, 287, 343; evaluating 284; high 40,
 229, 240, 360; insurance company
 controlling 276; levels of 278, 280; low
 223, 228, 284; medical 66, 69, 105, 107,
 335, 342; mitigating 57, 86, 91, 107,
 132, 159, 185, 188, 267, 274; operating
 46, 93, 357; preferences 135, 138;
 pricing 223, 238; rebalancing of 278;
 score of each insurance company 284,
 289; sharing 66, 267–268, 270, 272,
 401; systemic 278
risk adjustment 289, 320, 334–337; funds
 338; of insurance companies 320, 334,
 336; mechanisms 335; plans 284; pre-
 event 252, 286
risk allocation system *241*
risk balance mechanism of Germany *256*
risk balance of new public-benefiting
 insurance *285*
risk-balancing mechanisms 242, 252, 256,
 261, 277, 284, 289
risk control systems 19, 22, 37, 40, 91,
 205, 312, 363
risk-control systems, pre-event 189
risk control systems, professional 91
risk management 7, 22, 28, 46, 48, 53, 57,
 67, 135, 138, 270, 279, 309, 311–312,
 321; awareness of 189; improving 98;
 systems 315, 321; technologies 311
RMB *see* Renminbi currency
role of commercial health insurance in
 China's medical reform *296*
rural areas 10, 198, 200, 265, 338, 417,
 419–421, 423–424, 426, 430–431,
 443–444, 456–457, 464, 468, 471

rural residents 9–10, 47–48, 51–52,
 99–100, 103, 173–175, 319–320,
 334–338, 344–345, 375, 377, 381,
 384–387, 457, 468

safeguards 73–75, 77, 184–185, 221–223,
 228–230, 233–234, 236–237, 256–257,
 259, 261–262, 274, 276–279, 356,
 385–386, 388–389; complementary 248;
 insufficient 426, 428; low-level
 111–112; producing 306; real 17, 68,
 225–226; strong 237, 240, 261, 276
safeguards system 83, 126, 394; multi-
 tiered health 125; multi-tiered medical
 55–56, 69, 97, 110–111, 184, 187, 310,
 416; public medical 72; rural medical
 262; social 226–227, 372, 374
satisfaction with commercial health
 insurance by age group (%) **452**
satisfaction with commercial health
 insurance by family income (%) *453*
satisfaction with commercial health
 insurance by type of product (%) **454**
Save, Barry G. 115
security 50, 53–55, 102–103, 122, 126,
 184, 187, 229–230, 277, 282, 303,
 306–307, 369, 375–377, 379; basic 184,
 229; economic 176; financial 130; health
 insurance 13; healthcare 4, 34; high-
 level 57, 228; insured 306; management
 375; public 63; sustainable 237
security system 228–229, 328, 375; current
 social medical 62; multi-tiered health 2,
 4–5, 9, 19, 23, 34; multi-tiered medical
 43, 47, 53, 322; urban social 358
service system 107, 375, 380; excellent
 188; medical 39, 47, 54, 69, 83, 88, 90,
 95, 224, 390; traditional 394
services 19–20, 25–27, 33–34, 65–67,
 72–73, 75, 79–80, 143–144, 185–188,
 324–326, 334–337, 378–383, 391–394,
 402–403, 460–463; appointment-making
 459, 462, 464; comprehensive health
 safeguard 87, 259, 393; customer 86, 91,
 94, 316, 335, 340; diagnostic support
 391; diversified 93, 391; health-care 59,
 349; health security 27, 37; high-quality
 90, 188, 205, 247; long-term 217, 251;
 preventive 93, 330; professional 40, 48,
 311; public 108, 379
Shanghai Life Insurance Co. 352
shareholders 364, 392–393
social health insurance 27, 29, 89, 132,
 183–185, 208–209, 226, 228–232,

261–262, 265–267, 271, 276–277, 283, 287, 358; authorities 272, 275; basic-level 208, 231; departments 93, 186, 232, 270, 286, 340–342, 392; medical 16, 66, 186–187, 199, 228, 230, 233, 271, 274, 281, 311, 318, 333, 390–391, 398; programs 73; services 388

social security 38–39, 59, 63, 65, 80, 83, 93, 97–99, 211, 229–230, 232, 258–259, 288, 388, 390; accounts 360–361, 364; agencies 59–60, 345, 363; bureau 71, 386–387; departments 38, 322, 342, 344, 361, 364, 389, 393, 398, 400; funds 266–267, 273, 361; services 72

social security authorities 60, 71, 86, 96, 174, 360; and connectivity with medical institutions 57; purchasing risk coverage 232; sharing risk with commercial insurance companies 174

SOEs *see* State-Owned Enterprises

solvency 291, 308, 316, 319

sources of financing of medical care in OECD countries in 2013 *211*

spending 158–159, 181, 202, 211, 214, 259, 266–268, 270, 272–274, 283, 286, 396, 400, 405–407, 411; of China's medical insurance 202; fiscal 107, 274, 348–349; individual 202, 209; per capita of the urban fund 216, 407; personal health 15

Spring Rain Doctor (online product) 393–394, 410

Stabilization Act 1942 345

State Council 4–9, 55–57, 62, 99–100, 130–131, 234, 305–306, 308–310, 319, 351–352, 369, 371, 374–376, 378–379, 381

State-Owned Enterprises 136, 199, 307, 370, 401–402, 412

statistical chart of average wage of urban employees in China (2005–2014) *177*

statistical chart of incidence of 25 major critical diseases *176*

statistics on health expenditure of urban residents between 2001 and 2014 (yuan) **171**

statutory health insurance 83, 85, 247, 251–252, 255–256

stress management 28

subsidiaries 312, 333, 339–340; bureau-level 305; China Continent Insurance Co. 333; China Ping An Insurance Company 394; of insurance companies 340, 342; PICC 333; violating rules and regulations 336

subsidies 31, 79, 236, 238, 252, 255, 260, 263, 282, 286, 288, 326–327, 332, 348–350, 357; cost-sharing 250; direct 393; economic 141; financial 62, 99, 102; largest tax-type 349; limited 242, 282; public-finance 261, 282, 400; tax 116, 346, 349

summary of commercial health insurance policies introduced in recent years **5**

Sunshine Health Insurance Co. 371

Sunshine Life Insurance Corporation Ltd. 56, 130, 323, 352, 392–393

Sunshine Union Hospital 56, 393

supplementary insurance 18, 73, 80, 84, 115, 199, 210, 270, 282, 356, 370, 385–386, 398–399; commercial 267, 370; large-sum 358, 384; mandatory 238, 242, 385; medical 291–292, 370; new 263; products 385, 389; schemes 5

suppliers 20, 47, 49, 51, 81, 83–84, 226, 398; main 66; pharmaceutical 240

supply 45–47, 49, 60–62, 65, 67, 82, 88–89, 94, 114, 138, 170, 230, 235–236, 238, 367–368; and demand (law of) 9, 44–46, 61, 76, 135, 140, 221, 235, 395; and financing of new public-benefiting insurance *238*; of health insurance 43–44, 62, 64, 67, 380; of insurance 60–61, 176, 181, 183; of medical services 46, 201, 216, 367; normal 45–46; quality of 47, 62, 65, 69–70

sustainability 237, 242, 247–248, 250, 252–253, 255–257, 259, 261, 272–273, 276–277, 401, 414

Suzhou 33, 306, 355

Suzhou Municipal Hospital 271

Swiss Re (Swiss reinsurance company) 111

systems 19–20, 59–60, 70–72, 82–86, 97, 99–103, 110–112, 173–175, 233–234, 252–257, 259–264, 276–278, 287–289, 310–312, 402–407; advance-warning 240; current 126, 295; demand-side 373, 383; economic 226; essential-drugs 373; financial 208; funded 111, 349; grey 154; hospital 281; hybrid 124; institutional 96, 290; monopoly 372; multi-tiered 356; new 71, 199, 237, 262; protective 222; public 80–81, 86, 271, 368; reimbursement 94, 189, 227; supply-side 370, 372–373

Taicang critical illness insurance program between 2011 and 2015 (unit 10,000 yuan) **106**

Taicang Model 99, 105, 107–108, 128, 173–174, 233, 270, *271*, 272–273, 288, 337, 399
Taikang Life Insurance Co. 58, 323, 352, 388, 390
Taikang Pension & Insurance Co. 130
Taiwan 32, 185
tax benefits 18, 250, 346, 348, 354, 358, 381
tax credits 327, 348
tax deductions 32, 79, 358, 364
Tax Equity and Fiscal Responsibility Act 1982 35
tax incentives 9, 31–32, 62, 87, 128, 139, 167–168, 238, 346, 348, 473–475
tax policies 31, 63, 86–87, 140, 356, 379, 381; commercial health insurance 351, 364; implementing individual income 354; insurance-related preferential 184; pilot program of individual income 312–313, 319, 352, 356; preferential 18, 63, 125, 128, 130, 135, 139, 167–168, 184–185, 236, 345, 348–349, 351–355, 357–358, 364
taxes 18, 280, 318, 346–347, 351–353, 355, 357, 362
taxpayers 169, 313, 348, 352, 358, 360
tenders 22, 288, 311, 320, 337, 339–340, 343, 399
test of predictive model (5.9) **163**
three-layer progressive structure of China's public-benefiting commercial health insurance *283*
Tianjin 60, 205–206, 266, 352, 354, 417, 419
tobacco dependency 390
top ten average death rates nationwide from critical illness and chronic disease *206*
total and individuals' healthcare expenses in 2010–2014 (RMB 100 million) **203**
total healthcare expenditures in China *3*
total medical expenses and individual medical expenses 2010–2014 *213*
total medical expenses and sources of financing in 2009–2014 *214*
total medical expenses and sources of financing in 2013 (RMB 100 million) *215*
total revenue of life insurance companies and premium income of health insurance business in the U.S. from 2009 to 2015 *76*
transfer payments 132, 134, 284–285
treatment 7–8, 72, 75, 92, 94, 103–105, 211, 216, 274, 277, 281, 290, 292, 295,

390–391; inequitable 227; preferential personal tax 112, 133–134, 312–313, 319; procedures 207, 264; services 282; systems 295, 390–391
Trump, Pres. Donald 78–79
two-week prevalence of illness among residents in the survey area in 1998 2003; and 2008 **179**
types and percentages of health insurance purchased by respondents *14*
types of health insurance products respondents are willing to purchase next year by region, urban/rural status, gender and age group (%) **472**

UK *see* United Kingdom
Uncertain Lifetimes, Life Insurance, and the Theory of the Consumer 115
Uncertainty and the Welfare Economics of Medical Care 115
underwriting 29, 40, 78, 86, 90–91, 188, 225–226, 234, 250, 288, 311, 315, 329, 331, 341; automatic insurance 29; costs 225, 329; services 81
Union Life Insurance Co. 352
United Kingdom 19, 35–36, 63, 73–74, 79–82, 85, 124–125, 247–248, 401; commercial health insurance applicants as percentage of total population *81*; Department of Health and Human Services 35, 264, 327, 330–331, 348; government 80; health insurance company Bupa 28; medical insurance system *248*; National Health System 292; population 79, 81; supply of commercial health insurance 82
United States 35–37, 40, 72, 74–75, 79–80, 85, 87, 121, 123–125, 247, 250, 288–289, 325, 345–346, 349; focus on health management and disease prevention 27; focus on insurance education 30; health insurance market *251*; and the *Health Maintenance Organization Act 1973* 35; healthcare reform bill 326; healthcare system 325; medical insurance system *250*; and the *Tax Equity and Fiscal Responsibility Act 1982* 35; tax incentives for investors and operators of commercial health insurance companies 31
universal coverage 121, 208, 250, 255, 257, 276, 293; achieved 259, 263, 265; mandatory for all eligible people in China 326, 371; medical security

system that has 261; in place in China 277

'urban and rural residents insurance program' 22, 99, 422, 428

urban areas 338, 417, 419–421, 423–424, 426, 430–431, 433–434, 439, 443–444, 456–457, 464, 471

urban employees 32–33, 53, 59, 95, 99, 177–178, 338, 354, 358, 369–370, 385–386, 422, 467–468, 471, 474–475

urban residents 53, 95, 99–100, 102–103, 171, 173–174, 177, 189, 200, 203–204, 369, 371, 457, 459, 468

urban/rural, regional, gender and age distribution of respondents **420**

urban workers 183, 203–204, 210, 291, 358

US *see* United States

vaccinations 330

vaccines 33

value-added services 14–15, 52, 137, 237, 276, 342, 356, 361, 459–464

variables 60, 114, 116, 152, 154, 157; allied 117; exogenous 60, 62; explanatory 117; relevant 336; representative 153

variation coefficient of indicators related to urban staff medical insurance of 30 provinces and cities between 2001 and 2013 *408*

verification 97, 107; post-illness 107; post-settlement 97; procedures 52

vertical coverage 242

VHI *see* voluntary health insurance

voluntary health insurance 80, 236, 280

vulnerable groups 260, 265, 267, 291–292, 428

wages 177, 180, 322, 327, 345–346, 356, 358, 360, 370, 386, 393

ways to access commercial health

insurance information by age group (%) **450**

ways to access commercial health insurance information by education level *451*

ways to access commercial health insurance information by region and urban/rural status (%) **449**

ways to purchase commercial health insurance, by education level (%) *447*

ways to purchase commercial health insurance by age group (%) **446**

ways to purchase commercial health insurance by family income (%) *447*

ways to purchase commercial health insurance by region and urban/rural status (%) **445**

wearable devices 207, 393

WeChat and mobile apps 26, 443–446, 448, 464, 466

welfare loss caused by inadequate consumption of merit goods in private provision *236*

west China 417–418, 424, 427–428, 431, 433, 443–444, 456, 466–467, 470, 473

WHO *see* World Health Organization

workers 210, 345–347; migrant 116, 420–421; urban 183, 203–204, 210, 291, 358

World Health Organization 257, 390

World War II 345

Xinhua Insurance Company 392

Xinhua Life Insurance 371

Yaari, M.E. 115

Yan Ping 126

year-on-year growth in premium income of China's insurance industry *119*

Zhanjiang Model 173, 233, 270, 273–274, 276, 383–384

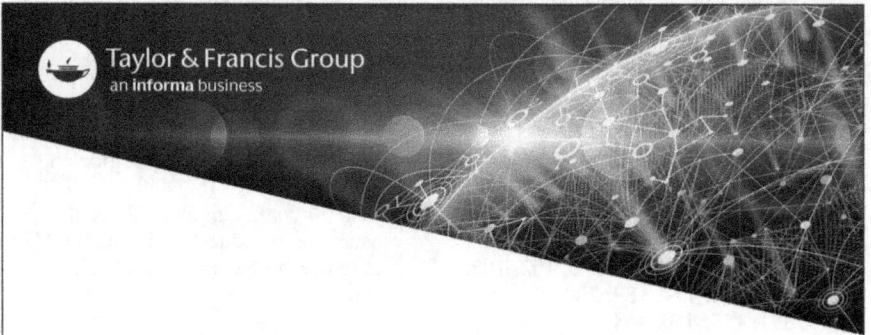
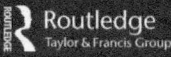
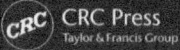